The Complete Q&A for the
NCLEX-*PN* Exam

THIRD EDITION

AUTHOR
PATRICIA A. HOEFLER, M.S.N., R.N.

CONTRIBUTING AUTHORS
Lois Walker, Ph.D., R.N.
Carol Kozik, M.S.N., R.N.
Sandra Bailey, M.S.N., R.N.
Susan W. Dockers, Ph.D., R.N.
Barbara J. Galvin, M.S.N., R.N.
Marianne Markowitz, M.S.N., R.N.
Marian L. Kovatchitch, M.S.N., R.N.

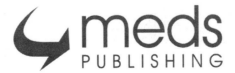

meds PUBLISHING

MEDICAL EDUCATION DEVELOPMENT SERVICES

7901 SANDY SPRING ROAD, SUITE 203

LAUREL, MARYLAND 20707

www.medspub.com

Editor: Mark Williams-Abrams

Editorial Assistant: Jen McCabe Gorman

THIRD EDITION 2006

Copies of this book may be obtained from:
MEDICAL EDUCATION DEVELOPMENT SERVICES
7901 Sandy Spring Road, Suite 203
Laurel, Maryland 20707
www.medspub.com

ISBN: 1-56533-508-2
Printed in the United States of America.

TABLE OF CONTENTS

NCLEX-PN

INTRODUCTION

SECTION I

PREPARING FOR THE EXAM

A. What You Should Know About the NCLEX-PN Exam

1. General information
   a. The first integrated exam was given in July 1982.
   b. The purpose of the exam is to determine that a candidate is prepared to practice nursing safely.
   c. The exam is designed to test essential knowledge of nursing and a candidate's ability to apply that knowledge to clinical situations.
   d. The purpose of the new test plan is to bring the exam in line with current nursing behaviors (the nursing process and decision making).
   e. Exam is "pass/fail," and no other score is given.

2. Computerized Adaptive Testing
   a. Computer program continuously scores answers and selects questions suitable for each candidate's competency level for a more precise measurement of competency.
   b. A higher weight is assigned to difficult questions so a passing score can be obtained by answering a lot of easier questions-or a smaller number of more difficult questions.
   c. Special screen design is used (see SCREEN DESIGN below).
   d. Use the mouse to move the cursor on the screen to the desired location. Double-click your mouse to select an option as your answer.
   e. A drop-down calculator also is featured. Double-click your mouse on the calculator icon, and the drop-down calculator will appear.

3. Exam schedule
   a. Given year-round.
   b. May only take a single exam in one day.
   c. Retake policy: not more than once in a three month period, with a maximum of four times in one year.

4. Number of questions and time allowed
   a. No minimum amount of time, however, a candidate must answer a minimum of 85 test questions.
   b. Maximum time is five hours, with a maximum of 205 test questions.
   c. About one out of three candidates completes the exam in less than two hours; one in three will use the complete five hours.
   d. The computer will automatically stop as soon as one of the following occurs:
      1) Candidate's measure of competency is determined to be above or below the passing standard
      2) Candidate has answered all 205 test questions

SCREEN DESIGN

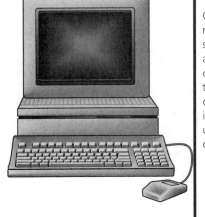

On the psychiatric unit, a nurse observes a client standing near a window and touching the glass. The client also mutters from time to time. Which comment by the nurse indicates the best understanding of the client's behavior?

1. "Why are you standing by the window and touching the glass?"

2. "There you are. I came to see if you wanted to see the video we are showing on the unit?"

3. "What are you looking at through the window?"

4. "Are you hearing voices or seeing things?"

Case Scenario and Stem   *Choices 1, 2, 3, and 4*

3) Maximum amount of time (five hours) has expired.

5. A candidate will pass by either:
   a. Answering 85 to 205 questions above the passing standard (the required weighted score) for all questions answered, within the time allowed; or
   b. Answering at least 75 questions within the time allowed and achieving the passing standard for the last 60 questions answered.

6. Types of questions
   a. All questions are multiple choice.
      1) Each question has four options
      2) The best option is the only correct answer
   b. Exam includes 25 unmarked experimental or "try-out" questions.

7. Exam procedure
   a. Look for the BEST answer to each question.
   b. It is not possible to skip questions or return to previous questions.
   c. There is a mandatory 10-minute break after first two hours and after another one-and-one-half hours.
   d. Scratch paper provided for calculations must be returned at end of exam.

8. Structure of the test plan *
   a. Safe, Effective Care Environment
      1) Coordinated Care   6 - 12%
      2) Safety and Infection Control 7 - 13%
   b. Health Promotion and Maintenance
      1) Growth and Development
         Through the Lifespan   4 - 10%
      2) Prevention and Early
         Detection of Disease   4 - 10%
   c. Psychosocial Integrity
      1) Coping and Adaptation   6 - 12%
      2) Psychosocial Adaptation   4 - 10%
   d. Physiological Integrity
      1) Basic Care and Comfort   10 - 16%
      2) Pharmacological Therapies 5 - 11%
      3) Reduction of Risk Potential 11 - 17%
      4) Physiological Adaptation   13 - 19%
   Information courtesy of the National Council of State Boards of Nursing, Inc., Test Plan 2006.

B. Schedule Your Study Time

1. The minimum time for preparation is two hours a day for six to eight weeks.
   a. Spend 1/3 of your time reviewing content.
   b. Spend 2/3 of your time answering test questions.

2. For content review, use an NCLEX-PN exam review book such as this one, which outlines content.

3. Begin with areas that are most difficult for you, or the areas that are least familiar.

4. For more detailed information on your difficult or less familiar areas, use a good nursing reference manual.

5. Review medical-surgical, pediatric, women's health, and psychiatric nursing, as well as co-ordinated care and alternate test item formats.

6. Use a body systems approach for medical-surgical and pediatric nursing areas.

7. When studying body systems and the associated diseases, remember to:
   a. Define the disease in terms of the patho-physiological process that is occurring.
   b. Identify the client's early and late manifestations.
   c. Identify the most important or life-threatening complications.
   d. Define the medical treatment.
   e. Identify and prioritize the nursing interventions associated with early and late manifestations.
   f. Identify what the nurse teaches the client/family to prevent or adapt to disease.

8. To schedule your study time:
   a. List the areas you need to review.
   b. Count the number of days you have available to study.
   c. Estimate the amount of time needed for each area.
   d. On your calendar, write the area to review, the number of questions to answer, and the amount of time needed for each study day.

C. Answer Many Questions

1. Answering questions will develop your test-taking skills.

2. Use questions similar to those on the NCLEX exam.

3. Answer a minimum of 3,000 test questions.

4. Include answering test questions in your study plan. For example, answer 100 questions each day for a month.

5. If you are at high risk, answer 5,000 test questions.

6. Use at least three different question-and-answer books, including MEDS *Complete Q&A for the NCLEX-PN* with CD-ROM.

7. Using a variety of books provides a more comprehensive preparation program.

D. Assess Your Progress

1. Each time you answer questions, check the number of questions you answered correctly.
   a. If you answer less than 65% correctly, this is a warning signal! Spend lots of time reviewing content and answering more questions in this area of nursing.
   b. If you answer 65 to 75% correctly, your performance is average. Success in this area is uncertain. Continue working with this content until your score is above 75%. Work on building your confidence by answering more questions in this area.
   c. If you answer 75 to 85% correctly, your performance is very good. Only return to this area after you have at least 75% in all other areas. Feel confident.
   d. If you answer 85 to 95% correctly, your performance is superior. Don't waste time on this. Feel very confident.

2. For each wrong answer, identify why you answered incorrectly.
   a. You may have answered a question wrong because you did not know the facts or got confused about the information.
      1) Identify this as a content weakness.
      2) Review the content again.
   b. You may have answered a question wrong because you misread the question, did not understand what it was asking, or did not know how to select the best answer.
      1) Identify this as a test-taking deficiency.
      2) For further assistance with test-taking deficiencies, we recommend MEDS test-taking book, *Successful Problem Solving & Test Taking for Nursing and NCLEX-PN Exams*.

3. Check the number of questions that you identified as difficult and went back to answer later. See how many of them you answered correctly.

SECTION II

ANSWERING QUESTIONS

A. Identify the Critical Elements in the Question

1. Identify the issue in the question
   a. The issue is the problem about which the question is asking.
   b. The issue may be a:
      1) Drug: for example, digoxin (*Lanoxin*),

furosemide (*Lasix*)
      2) Nursing problem: for example, alteration in comfort, potential for infection
      3) Behavior: for example, restlessness, agitation
      4) Disorder: for example, diabetes mellitus, ulcerative colitis
      5) Procedure: for example, glucose tolerance test, cardiac catheterization

2. Identify the client in the question.
   a. The client in the question is usually the person with the health problem.
   b. The client in a test question may also be a relative or significant other or another member of the health care team with whom the nurse is interacting.
   c. The correct answer to the question must relate to the client in the question.

3. Look for the key words.
   a. Key words focus attention on what is important.
   b. Key words may appear in bold print.
   c. Examples:
      1) During the early period, which of the following nursing procedures would be **best**?
      2) The nurse would expect to find which of the following characteristics in an **adult** diabetic?
      3) Which of the following nursing actions is **vital**?
      4) Which of the following nursing actions would be best **initially**?

4. Identify what the stem is asking and determine whether the question has a true response stem or false response stem.
   a. Be clear about what the stem is asking before you look at the options.
   b. If the question is not clear to you, rephrase it using your own words.
   c. Determine whether the question has a true response stem or a false response stem.
      1) True response stem
         a) Definition: A true response stem requires an answer that is a true statement.
         b) Examples:
            (1) Which of these interpretations is most justifiable?
            (2) The nurse would demonstrate best judgment by taking which of the following actions?

(3) The chief purpose of the drug is to:

(4) The nurse should give immediate consideration to which of the following findings?

2) False response stem

a) Definition: A false response stem requires an answer that is a false statement.

b) Examples:

(1) Which of the following nursing actions would be inappropriate?

(2) Which of the following statements by the client would indicate a need for further instruction?

(3) Which of the following describes incorrect placement of the hands during CPR?

(4) Which of the following actions would place the client at risk?

B. Use a Selection Procedure to Eliminate Incorrect Options

1. Most NCLEX questions have four options. The correct answer is the BEST answer. The other three options are "distractors."

2. Distractors are options made to look like correct answers. They are intended to distract you from answering correctly.

3. As you read each of the four options, make a decision about it:

a. This option is true (+).

b. This option is false (–).

c. I am not sure about this option (?).

4. If the stem is a true response stem:

a. An option that is true (+) might be the correct answer.

b. An option that is false (–) is a distractor. Eliminate this option.

c. An option that you are not sure about (?) is possibly the correct answer.

5. If the stem is a false response stem:

a. An option that is true (+) is a distractor. Eliminate this option.

b. An option that is false (–) may be the correct answer.

c. An option that you are not sure about (?) is possibly the correct answer.

6. Do not return to options you have eliminated.

7. If you are left with one option, that is your answer.

8. If you are left with one (+) option and one (?) option, select the (+) option as your answer.

9. If you are left with two (+) options, use strategies to select the best answer.

C. Use Test-Taking Strategies When You Are Unable to Select the Best Option

1. The Global Response Strategy

a. A global response is a general statement that may include ideas of other options within it.

b. Look for a global response when more than one option appears to be correct.

c. The global response option will probably be the correct answer.

2. The Similar Distractors Strategy

a. Similar distractors say basically the same thing using different words.

b. Since there is only one correct answer in a question, similar distractors must be wrong.

c. Eliminate similar distractors. Select for your answer an option that is different.

3. The Similar Word or Phrase Strategy

a. When more than one option appears to be correct, look for a similar word or phrase in the stem of the question and in one of the four options.

b. The option that contains the similar word or phrase may be the correct answer.

c. Use this strategy after you have tried to identify a global response option and eliminated similar distractors.

D. Answering Communication Questions

1. The NCLEX exam includes many communication questions because the ability to communicate therapeutically is essential for safe practice.

2. Identify the critical elements as in all questions. Pay particular attention to identification of the client in the question. Remember that the answer must relate to the client.

3. Learn to identify communication tools that enhance communication.

a. Being silent: Nonverbal communication.

b. Offering self: "Let me sit with you."

c. Showing empathy: "You are upset."

d. Focusing: "You say that . . ."

e. Restatement: "You feel anxious?"

f. Validation/clarification: "What you are saying is . . .?"

g. Giving information: "Your room is 423."

h. Dealing with the here and now: "At this time, the problem is . . ."

4. Learn to identify non-therapeutic communication blocks.
   a. Giving advice: "If I were you, I would . . ."
   b. Showing approval/disapproval: "You did the right thing."
   c. Using clichés and false reassurances: "Don't worry. It will be all right."
   d. Requesting an explanation: "Why did you do that?"
   e. Devaluing client feelings: "Don't be concerned. It's not a problem."
   f. Being defensive: "Every nurse on this unit is exceptional."
   g. Focusing on inappropriate issues or persons: "Have I said something wrong?"
   h. Placing the client's issues "on hold:" "Talk to your doctor about that."

5. When answering communication questions, select an option that illustrates a therapeutic communication tool. Eliminate options that illustrate non-therapeutic communication blocks.

E. Answering Questions that Focus on Setting Priorities

1. Priority-setting questions ask the test taker to identify either what comes first, is most important, or gets the highest priority.
2. Examples:
   a. What is the nurse's initial response?
   b. The nurse should give immediate consideration to which of the following?
   c. Which nursing action receives the highest priority?
   d. What should the nurse do first?
3. Use guidelines to help you to answer priority setting questions.
   a. Maslow's Hierarchy of Needs indicates that physiological needs come first.
   b. Maslow's Hierarchy of Needs indicates that when no physiological need is identified, safety needs come first.
   c. Nursing Process indicates that assessment comes first.
   d. Communication Theory indicates focusing on feelings first.
   e. Teaching/Learning Theory indicates focusing on motivation first.

SECTION III

SECTION III

PREPARING FOR EXAM TIME

A. Plan for Everything

1. Assemble everything you will need for the exam the night before:
   a. Identification: two IDs with signatures, including one with recent photograph
   b. Watch
   c. Several sharpened pencils (with erasers) for calculations
2. Plan to arrive at the test site early:
   a. Know the route to the exam site.
   b. Know how long it will take to get there.
   c. Know where you will park and if you will need coins for a parking meter.
3. Pay close attention to your own physiological needs:
   a. Dress in layers.
   b. Get a good night's sleep the night before the exam.
   c. Eat a good breakfast.
   d. Avoid stimulants and depressants.
   e. Use the bathroom just before the exam.
4. During the exam:
   a. Listen to the instructions.
   b. Pace yourself; don't spend too long on any one question.
   c. Don't let yourself become distracted. Focus your attention on answering the questions.
   d. Go with your first choice. Use test-taking strategies only when you cannot decide between close options.
   e. Keep your thoughts positive!

B. Manage Your Anxiety Level

1. Moderate levels of anxiety increase your effectiveness.
2. Don't cram the night before the exam.
3. Do something enjoyable and relaxing the night before the exam.
4. Learn and practice measures to manage your anxiety level during the exam as needed:
   a. Take a few deep breaths.
   b. Tense and relax muscles.
   c. Tell yourself positive affirmations.
   d. Visualize a peaceful scene.
   e. Visualize your success.

C. Test-Taking Tips

1. Prepare comprehensively and be sure to be well rested for the exam.

2. Read each question carefully, identifying the critical elements. Each question must be answered in sequence, and you may not skip or go back to change your answers to any questions.
3. Don't panic if the computer stops after a short time! It does not mean that you failed. The computer stops when the exam is able to determine with at least 95% certainty that you have demonstrated the ability, or inability, to practice safely at the minimal level of nursing competency.
4. It is helpful to know that most students pass by answering a maximum of 119 questions. However, you can still pass the exam even if you answered all 205 questions.
5. If you are having difficulty choosing between the best two options, use the three test-taking strategies you learned in this review:
    a. Look for the global response option.
    b. Eliminate similar distractors.
    c. Look for similar words in the question and one of the options.

6. You should anticipate that the test questions will increase in difficulty.
7. Use your scratch paper wisely. Since you cannot review earlier questions to help recall previous facts, use the scratch paper provided for calculations to remember facts from previous questions. Sometimes, information from one question is helpful in answering another question.
8. Don't panic if someone finishes before you! The test adapts to each candidate's level of ability, and it means that you may take longer to prove that you are capable of practicing competently at the beginning level of nursing.
9. Keep a positive attitude! Remember that you have learned a great amount of nursing knowledge, and the exam is only designed to determine whether you are able to practice safely at the entry level.

NCLEX-PN

Test 1

NCLEX-PN TEST 1

1. In preparation for a sigmoid colon resection, a client is receiving instructions about the colostomy that will be performed. Which statement by the client indicates to the nurse that further clarification is required?

   1. "My colostomy will begin to function seven to 10 days after surgery."
   2. "The stoma of my colostomy will appear large at first, but it will shrink over the next few weeks."
   3. "I will have to wear a colostomy bag at all times to prevent accidental leakage of stool."
   4. "My diet will not have to change dramatically. I can use a trial-and-error approach to see if any foods no longer agree with me."

2. A client with a new colostomy has been given instructions about the irrigation of his ostomy. Which action by the client would indicate to the nurse that the teaching plan has to be reviewed?

   1. 500 ml of irrigating solution is used.
   2. Warm tap water is used to irrigate the ostomy.
   3. A lubricated cone tip is inserted into the ostomy stoma to begin the irrigation.
   4. The irrigating solution bag is positioned 30 inches above the stoma.

3. A female client returns to the postoperative unit following a partial colectomy for cancer. She has a nasogastric tube set to low continuous suction and complains of a sore throat. She asks the nurse when the nasogastric tube will be taken out. Which response by the nurse is most appropriate at this time?

   1. "The doctor will discontinue the tube when your bowel sounds return."
   2. "The tube probably will be removed tomorrow, but you'll remain NPO for three to five more days."
   3. "The tube will be removed when peristalsis returns through the entire GI tract, usually in three to five days."
   4. "You'll have to ask that question of your doctor. He's the one who has to give the order to discontinue the tube."

4. A client, age 83, is admitted to the hospital with complaints of abdominal pain and distention. He has a history of no bowel movement for the past 10 days. After a diagnostic evaluation, it's determined that the client has a fecal impaction. Which treatment can the nurse anticipate will be ordered initially?

   1. Soap suds enemas until clear.
   2. Bisacodyl (Dulcolax) suppository.
   3. Oil retention enema.
   4. Tap water enema.

5. The physician orders a stool specimen to be collected for ova and parasites. What is the proper procedure for collection of this specimen by the nurse?

   1. Send the entire stool immediately to the lab.
   2. Use a sterile container.
   3. Take feces from several areas of the bowel movement.
   4. Refrigerate the specimen until it can be delivered to the lab.

6. The nurse explains to a client that preparation for a cholecystography includes:

   1. NPO after midnight.
   2. Clear liquid diet the evening before the test.
   3. Assessing for allergies to iodine or seafood.
   4. Special consent form due to the invasive nature of the procedure.

7. Following a CVA that affected the left side of the brain, an elderly client had the tube feeding removed and is ready to begin oral feedings. Which of the following nursing measures ensures the client's tolerance to liquids?

   1. Feed from right side of mouth; upright position; mouth care before feeding.
   2. Verbal encouragement; check gag reflex; feed thinned foods and liquids.
   3. Check gag reflex; feed on left side of mouth; upright position.
   4. Sensory stimulation; verbal encouragement; favorite foods.

8. A client who is 62-years-old is scheduled for coronary artery bypass. Preoperatively, the physician has ordered aspirin, 325 mg daily. Which nursing action would be most appropriate?

   1. Explain to the client that aspirin is given because of its anti-inflammatory effects.
   2. Tell the client that after surgery he will continue to take aspirin prophylactically.
   3. Question the doctor's order, since aspirin could cause postoperative bleeding.
   4. Monitor the client's temperature and report elevations to the doctor immediately.

9. In caring for a client immediately following a cardiac catheterization procedure, which of the following nurs-

ing actions is appropriate?

1. Apply warm compresses to the puncture site.
2. Assist with passive range of motion exercises.
3. Monitor the client for cardiac arrhythmias.
4. Assist the client into high Fowler's position.

10. **A client receives haloperidol (Haldol) 5 mg t.i.d. Several days later, the nurse notices that she is walking stiffly with a shuffling gait. What is the priority nursing action at this time?**

1. Take her blood pressure before her next dose.
2. Withhold the Haldol until the symptom disappears.
3. Chart her observations on the client's record.
4. Obtain an order for an antiparkinsonian drug.

11. **A client uses tamoxifen (Nolvadex) for her cancer. The nurse knows that tamoxifen has which of the following actions?**

1. Antimicrobial.
2. Anti-estrogenic.
3. Androgenic.
4. Anti-inflammatory.

12. **A client is to receive his first injection of interferon (Roferon-a) for his hairy cell leukemia. What side effects would the nurse advise the client to expect?**

1. Reduced urine output.
2. Severe vomiting and nausea.
3. Flu-like manifestations.
4. Weight gain.

13. **A client, placed on ferrous sulfate tablets twice daily as an iron supplement for anemia, asks the nurse why the doctor told her to take the medication with orange juice. The nurse most accurately informs the client that:**

1. The medication has an unpleasant taste, and the orange juice will help disguise the taste.
2. The orange juice will help avoid constipation, which is a side effect of the medication.
3. The orange juice will help the gastrointestinal tract absorb the medication more efficiently.
4. The medication can cause nausea, and the orange juice will help alleviate this problem.

14. **A client has been taking isoniazid (INH) and rifampin (Rifadin) for three weeks after being diagnosed with TB. He tells the nurse that he has noted a reddish-orange color to his urine. Which statement by the nurse is most appropriate?**

1. "I'll make an appointment for you to see the doctor this afternoon. You may have developed a bleeding problem, which is not uncommon with these

drugs."
2. "The reddish color is a side effect of the INH. Stop taking it for two to three days and the discoloration should go away. The doctor may want to change your drug therapy."
3. "The discoloration is due to rifampin. It may turn all body fluids orange-red. This is a harmless side effect."
4. "You should increase your fluid intake while on these medications. They are known to cause bladder irritation when taken together."

15. **A 43-year-old female client has had a total abdominal hysterectomy and bilateral salpingo-oophorectomy for stage III uterine cancer. Which instructions would the nurse anticipate providing?**

1. Estrogen therapy will alleviate the discomfort of surgical menopause.
2. A Papanicolaou (Pap) smear should be performed every six months.
3. Lubrication can be used to treat vaginal itching and burning.
4. Vaginal intercourse will no longer be possible.

16. **A client is being sent home on isoxsuprine (Vasodilan) for treatment of premature labor. Which of the following actions should receive priority in the nurse's discharge teaching plan?**

1. Technique for taking oral temperature.
2. How to assess her radial pulse.
3. Procedure to assess her blood sugar.
4. How to assess fetal heart rate.

17. **A 12-year-old child is being discharged from the hospital with a diagnosis of asthma. She is to be maintained on metered dose inhalers at home. The nurse is preparing a care plan on the use of cromolyn (Intal). Which of the following instructions to the parents would the nurse avoid including in the client's care plan?**

1. Intal will decrease the inflammation in your child's bronchioles.
2. Do not rely on Intal for relief of an acute attack.
3. Have your child rinse her mouth after using the puffer.
4. Your child should breathe more easily after a dose of Intal.

18. **A six-month-old male infant with AIDS has a nursing diagnosis of "altered growth and development" on the care plan. Which of the following nursing interventions will most enhance the growth and development of the child?**

1. Encourage the child to eat whatever he wants.
2. Provide therapy to help the child meet develop-

mental milestones.

3. Provide nutritional supplements in addition to an adequate diet.
4. Weigh and measure the infant on a frequent basis.

19. A nurse working with a client with agoraphobia recognizes that the most effective technique for treatment of agoraphobia is:

    1. Repeated exposure to situations that she fears.
    2. Distraction each time she brings up her problem.
    3. Teaching relaxation techniques.
    4. Gradual desensitization by controlled exposure to the situation she fears.

20. A 48-year-old man hospitalized for an obsessive-compulsive disorder has recurring thoughts that he has mouth odors that are offensive to others. He has mouth care rituals that occupy a good deal of his waking hours and caused him to be fired from his last job. The nurse knows that these manifestations most likely represent:

    1. A method of reducing anxiety.
    2. A form of manipulation to avoid work.
    3. An attention-getting strategy.
    4. A rationalization for avoiding social contact.

21. A client is scheduled for a cardiac catheterization. When he arrives for the procedure, he reports he awoke that morning with "butterflies in his stomach," a sense of restlessness, urinary frequency, and some difficulty concentrating as he drove to the hospital. The admitting nurse assesses his anxiety level as:

    1. Mild.
    2. Moderate.
    3. Severe.
    4. Panic.

22. The nurse understands in caring for a client with coronary artery disease that psychological factors such as anxiety:

    1. Contribute to both the development and progress of coronary artery disease.
    2. Cause coronary artery disease.
    3. Cannot cause coronary artery disease, but they do affect the client's prognosis.
    4. Affect the client's ability to adjust to a diagnosis of coronary artery disease but have little direct effect on treatment outcomes.

23. A 45-year-old man is admitted to the emergency room complaining of chest pain and dyspnea. He is flushed and perspiring profusely. He says, "I feel like I am going to die. Am I having a heart attack?" The medical

exam and lab work are negative. He is diagnosed with anxiety. The nurse assesses his level of anxiety as:

1. Mild.
2. Moderate.
3. Severe.
4. Panic.

24. A client explains that, for the past 10 years, she has been unable to leave her house without her husband or daughter. If she tries to go out alone, she becomes very anxious and must quickly return inside. The nurse interviewing her identifies the probable cause as:

    1. Conversion disorder.
    2. Agoraphobia.
    3. Panic disorder.
    4. Obsessive-compulsive disorder.

25. The nurse, in caring for psychiatric clients, knows that tardive dyskinesia:

    1. Is a movement disorder caused by antipsychotic drugs.
    2. Occurs within the first few days of treatment in most clients.
    3. Improves rapidly if the offending drug is discontinued.
    4. Is treated with antiparkinsonian drugs.

26. A client attends group therapy daily. The nurse understands that the most important benefit of group therapy is to:

    1. Provide the opportunity to develop social skills.
    2. Improve the client's orientation to reality.
    3. Gain support and encouragement from other persons.
    4. Develop greater insight into herself and her problems through the feedback provided by the other members.

27. In providing care to a client who is receiving ECT, the nurse knows that this treatment:

    1. Usually requires 10 days to three weeks before depression is noticeably improved.
    2. Results in a high incidence of chronic memory problems.
    3. Is effective for 60% of persons who receive it.
    4. Is used for persons who have not responded to antidepressants.

28. A client, 34, is admitted for the third time to a psychiatric hospital with a diagnosis of schizophrenia. The police found her wandering along the highway. When questioned, she was unable to give coherent answers. During the admission procedure, the nurse notices that

her appearance is unkempt and she appears to be actively hallucinating. The initial nursing assessment is:

1. Her mental status.
2. Her ability to follow directions.
3. Her perception of reality.
4. Her physical health needs.

29. In caring for a client with schizophrenic disorder who is receiving an antipsychotic medication, the nurse knows that which of the following statements about the "dopamine hypothesis" is inaccurate?

    1. Most antipsychotic drugs block the effects of dopamine and receptor sites in the brain.
    2. Amphetamine enhances dopamine activity in the brain and can cause a psychotic response that is indistinguishable from paranoid schizophrenia.
    3. The potency of antipsychotic drugs seems to be related to their antidopamine action.
    4. Schizophrenic clients excrete excessive amounts of dopamine in their urine.

30. A client is sitting by his food tray, pushing the food around on his plate. He says to the nurse, "I hate hospital food. Is this the only thing that I can get to eat?" The nurse's best response is:

    1. "What is it about the food that you dislike?"
    2. "Well, the other clients haven't complained about the food. Is something else bothering you?"
    3. "I'll call the kitchen and order something else for you."
    4. "Is there something special that you would like to eat?"

31. An 88-year-old client is admitted to the hospital with chest pain. His daughter tells the nurse that he has certain routines for his personal hygiene and for taking his medicine. The most appropriate nursing response is to:

    1. Assure the daughter that everything possible will be done to accommodate her father's needs.
    2. Ask the daughter what routines and medicines her father uses at home.
    3. Inform the daughter that the hospital has policies that have to be followed, and that you will provide the best care for her father.
    4. Tell the daughter that she should inform the doctor about her father's routines so that orders can be written to meet the client's needs.

32. When the nurse is making morning rounds, a client says, "I almost died last night." The most therapeutic nursing response is:

    1. "You made it through the night."
    2. "Patients do have dreams that they die when they are hospitalized."
    3. "Are you feeling okay now?"
    4. "That must have been frightening for you. Tell me more about it."

33. A client is told by her doctor that he has found a lump in her breast and that a biopsy would have to be done. The client states to the nurse, "Do you think it is cancer?" The best initial response by the nurse is:

    1. "You seem to be worried about what the doctor may find."
    2. "Do you have a family history of breast cancer?"
    3. "We won't know anything until the biopsy is done."
    4. "Most lumps are not cancerous, so you really shouldn't worry."

34. The nursing assistant says to the nurse, "This client is incontinent of stool three or four times a day. I get angry when I think that he is doing it just to get attention. I think adult diapers should be used for him." How should the nurse initially respond to the nursing assistant?

    1. "You probably are right. Soiling the bed is one way of getting attention from the nursing staff."
    2. "Changing his bed and cleaning him must be tiresome for you. Next time it happens, I'll help you."
    3. "It's upsetting to see an adult regress."
    4. "Why don't you spend more time with him if you think that he is behaving this way to get more attention?"

35. A hospitalized client has just found out that her mother has died of a heart attack. She is crying and has her face buried in the pillow. The most appropriate nursing response is to:

    1. Return in 15 minutes to see how the client is doing.
    2. Sit with the client for a little while.
    3. Tell the client that she will feel better in the morning.
    4. Share with the client that you lost your mother within the last year and that you know how she feels.

36. A client is seen at the clinic and is to receive an injection. When preparing to administer a medication for injection from an ampule, which action would be unsafe?

    1. Score the neck of the ampule with a file.
    2. Protect the thumb and fingers with a gauze square or alcohol wipe.

3. Snap the neck of the ampule toward the body when breaking the top free from the ampule.
4. Insert the needle into the ampule without touching the needle to the edges of the ampule.

37. **An elderly hospitalized client is to receive an x-ray. When the nurse enters the client's room and asks if the client is ready to go to x-ray, the client nods "yes." Next, the priority nursing action is:**

1. Explain the x-ray procedure to the client.
2. Help the client into a wheel chair, so that she will be ready when the transporter arrives to take her to x-ray.
3. Ask the client if she has any questions.
4. Look at the client's identification bracelet.

38. **The nurse is to apply topical ointment to the client's skin for a dermatological condition. Which action should the nurse avoid?**

1. Massaging the ointment into the skin.
2. Removing excess ointment.
3. Applying ointment with ungloved fingertips.
4. Documenting a description of the skin prior to application of the ointment.

39. **An HIV positive client is admitted to the hospital with a lung infection. Which of the following isolation categories should be implemented in order to prevent transmission of the HIV virus?**

1. Strict isolation.
2. Respiratory isolation.
3. Universal precautions.
4. Enteric precautions.

40. **A client is admitted to the hospital and a urine specimen is ordered. When obtaining a urine specimen from the client, which of the following is an inappropriate nursing action?**

1. Place the urine cup in the client's bathroom.
2. Take the full specimen cup to the lab pick up area and then place it in a clean plastic bag.
3. Attach the client's name to the specimen cup.
4. Explain to the client the procedure for obtaining a urine specimen.

41. **A client is to have a perineal examination, which requires the dorsal recumbent position. Which of the following nursing actions provides the client with the most privacy?**

1. Place a bath blanket on the client with one corner at the chest, two corners wrapped around the feet and legs, and the fourth corner draped between the client's legs.
2. Drape a draw sheet over the client's knees covering the abdomen and legs.
3. Place a bath blanket on the client, with the top at the chest and the bottom draped over the knees to cover the legs and feet.
4. Close the examination room door.

42. **A client has right-sided paralysis following a stroke. He is not able to talk, but can make gestures to make himself understood. To effectively communicate with the client, the nurse should:**

1. Speak very loudly to the client.
2. Speak quickly to the client, since his attention span may be short.
3. Use gestures while speaking slowly.
4. Wait until the family comes in, so they can interpret his behavior.

43. **An unconscious client is to have an electroencephalogram (EEG). The first nursing action is to:**

1. Notify the EEG Department that the client is ready for the scan.
2. Check to see that the client is wearing an identification bracelet.
3. Shampoo the client's hair.
4. Prepare a sedative in case the client becomes conscious prior to the procedure.

44. **During the administration of a medication, a 19-year-old client tells the nurse that he has never had that particular pill before. The best nursing action is to:**

1. Check the client's identification bracelet again.
2. Check the physician's orders to see if this is a new medication.
3. Assure the client that the medication package has his name on it.
4. Ask the client to take the medication, since the identification bracelet and medication administration record indicate the client is to receive the medication.

45. **To protect against the spread of AIDS, health care workers are encouraged to wear gloves when coming into contact with any body fluids, and to take certain other precautions. The type of precautions used in a health care facility to prevent the spread of AIDS is:**

1. Secretion precautions.
2. Enteric precautions.
3. Universal precautions.
4. Protective isolation.

46. **Before administering an injection, the nurse performs aseptic handwashing. This technique includes:**

1. Not using soap, since it causes drying of the skin.
2. Using paper towels to turn the faucet on and off.

3. The use of lotion to prevent drying.
4. Holding arms and hands upright so that all organisms will stay away from hands while washing.

47. **While administering a bed bath it is important for the nurse to maintain privacy. Which is the best method for maintaining the client's privacy?**

    1. Allow the client to wear a gown, and reach under the gown with the washcloth and towel to bathe the client.
    2. Use towels to protect the bed linen.
    3. Cover the client with a bath blanket and expose only the portion of the body that is being bathed.
    4. Use the bed sheet to cover the client during the bath.

48. **An elderly client is constantly putting her call light on. When the nurse answers the light, the client does not appear to need anything. Which action by the nurse is the least appropriate?**

    1. Ask the members of the family if they can spend more time with the client.
    2. Remove the call light from easy reach of the client.
    3. Make frequent visits to the client's room.
    4. Spend more time in the client's room while charting.

49. **A client is confused and disoriented when admitted to the hospital. The doctor has ordered bed rest. Before leaving the client's room, the most important nursing action to provide for the client's safety is:**

    1. Placing all of the client's belongings in a safe place.
    2. Placing the bed in the highest position with the side rails up.
    3. Placing the bed in the lowest position with the side rails up.
    4. Explaining where everything is in the room.

50. **A client is admitted to the hospital and the physician orders stat blood work. The laboratory technician says to the nurse, "I can't do the stat blood work because the client doesn't have an identification bracelet on." The best nursing action is:**

    1. Draw the blood for the laboratory technician, since the nurse can identify the client.
    2. Assure the laboratory technician that you will verify that he has the correct client.
    3. Obtain an identification bracelet for the client as quickly as possible.
    4. Ask the client to identify himself to the laboratory technician.

51. **A client is recovering from surgery. The nurse is pre-**
paring to irrigate his urinary catheter. To prevent injury to the mucosa of the bladder when irrigating the catheter, the nurse should:

    1. Gently compress the ball of the syringe to instill the irrigating solution.
    2. Quickly instill the irrigating solution, using some pressure to loosen any clots or mucous.
    3. After instilling the solution, apply gentle pressure to remove the irrigating solution from the bladder.
    4. Place a sterile cap on the end of the drainage tubing to protect it from contamination.

52. **In protecting the privacy of a client, the nurse should avoid reporting which of the following to a government agency?**

    1. Child abuse.
    2. Deaths.
    3. Client's change of employment.
    4. Elder abuse.

53. **Identifying the client at risk for a postpartum hemorrhage is an important part of obstetrical nursing. Which of the following clients is at the least risk for a postpartum hemorrhage?**

    1. Gravida 1, vaginal delivery after two hours of labor.
    2. Gravida 1, cesarean section for pregnancy induced hypertension (PIH).
    3. Gravida 2, Pitocin induction, vaginal delivery after seven hours of labor.
    4. Gravida 1, vaginal delivery at 29 weeks gestation after 10 hours of labor.

54. **Which finding will the nurse expect to see in a 30-week-gestation premature infant?**

    1. Good flexion.
    2. Abundant lanugo.
    3. Heel creases.
    4. Dry, flaky skin.

55. **Based upon a diagnosis of endometriosis, the nurse should expect the client to complain of:**

    1. Heavy menses.
    2. Infertility.
    3. Frequent temperature elevations.
    4. Breast tenderness.

56. **The nurse caring for a client with a diagnosis of breast cancer knows that the client's prognosis is most influenced by:**

    1. The client's age.
    2. Family history.
    3. The stage of the disease.
    4. The treatment plan.

57. The nurse understands that the primary purpose of a Pap smear is to:

    1. Screen for uterine cancer.
    2. Diagnose uterine cancer.
    3. Screen for cervical cancer.
    4. Diagnose cervical cancer.

58. A 24-year-old client who is hospitalized with toxic shock syndrome (TSS) asks the nurse to explain the cause of TSS. The nurse's best response to the client is guided by the knowledge that TSS is most commonly associated with:

    1. Multiple sexual partners.
    2. Intrauterine devices (IUD).
    3. Sexually transmitted diseases (STD).
    4. High-absorbency tampons.

59. A 45-year-old female client seen in the clinic asks the nurse whether she is entering menopause because her menstrual periods have become irregular and she has hot flashes. In assessing this client, the nurse would anticipate which symptom associated with early menopause?

    1. Elevations in body temperature above 100° F.
    2. Increases in blood pressure.
    3. Palpitations of the heart.
    4. Atrophy of the vagina.

60. A client in a women's clinic tells the nurse that her sister has just been diagnosed with cervical cancer. She tells the nurse that she wishes to be tested to rule out the possibility that she also has the disease, and asks the nurse what tests are used to diagnose this cancer. The nurse's reply is guided by the knowledge that the diagnosis of cancer of the cervix is established by:

    1. Pap smear.
    2. Endometrial biopsy.
    3. Endocervical biopsy.
    4. Dilation and curettage (D&C).

61. A client with a diagnosis of breast cancer is scheduled to have radiation therapy prior to her mastectomy. The nurse understands that the purpose of the radiation therapy at this time is:

    1. Reduction of pain.
    2. Decreasing the tumor size.
    3. Destruction of the tumor.
    4. Prevention of infection.

62. A client is given clomiphene citrate (Clomid) to treat her infertility problems. She asks the nurse, "How does this medication work? What kind of drug is it?" In re-

sponding, the nurse knows that Clomid:

    1. Stimulates ovulation.
    2. Improves cervical mucous.
    3. Treats infections.
    4. Is a hormone supplement.

63. Which of the following would indicate to the nurse that the injection of Vitamin K (AquaMEPHYTON) given to a newborn has been effective?

    1. Absence of jaundice.
    2. Minimal bleeding after circumcision.
    3. No evidence of infection.
    4. Ecchymotic area at injection site.

64. A four-year-old who had hydrocephalus is admitted to the hospital for a ventriculoperitoneal shunt. Following the shunt placement, which finding needs an immediate response from the nurse?

    1. Sleepy, very difficult to rouse.
    2. Pupils equal and reactive to light.
    3. BP 100/60, Apical pulse of 90.
    4. Urine output 33 cc in two hours.

65. An eight-year-old child complains of a stomach ache while visiting the school nurse. Which statement by the child would concern the nurse most?

    1. "My stomach ache goes away if I rest for a few minutes."
    2. "My friends are picking on me and calling me fatso."
    3. "My brother just had his appendix out."
    4. "My friends won't let me play kickball with them the way I want to."

66. When assessing a child with a cast, which observation by the nurse would cause the greatest concern?

    1. Itching at the cast site.
    2. Indentations in the cast.
    3. Swelling distal to the cast.
    4. "Hot spots" on the cast.

67. A child with a rectal temperature of 39° C has an order for acetaminophen (Tylenol) 280 mg by mouth. The label on the bottle reads 160 mg/5 cc. How many cc's should the nurse give to the child?

    1. 8.8 cc.
    2. 1.8 cc.
    3. 7.0 cc.
    4. 12.7 cc.

68. A concerned mother calls the physician's office. Her child has a respiratory infection and a temperature of

39° C orally. She needs to give her son 240 mg of acetaminophen (Tylenol). The label on her bottle at home reads 160 mg/5 cc. The nurse's most helpful response is:

1. Give 1/2 teaspoon.
2. Give 1 1/2 teaspoons.
3. Give 1 1/2 cc.
4. Give 15 cc.

69. **A child weighing 1800 gm is admitted. The nurse knows that the infant's weight in pounds is:**

1. 3.9 lbs.
2. 8.1 lbs.
3. 18 lbs.
4. 36 lbs.

70. **The nurse is working in a pediatric clinic. Which client would least likely test HIV positive?**

1. A two-month-old whose mother has been an IV drug addict for two years.
2. A 15-year-old who has been on treatment for hemophilia since infancy.
3. An eight-year-old whose best friend is HIV positive.
4. A 16-year-old who is sexually active.

71. **A 20-month-old female child is admitted for treatment of burns and investigation into the possibility of abuse. Her parents state that she climbed into the bathtub alone. Which information is most important to include in the documentation by the nurse?**

1. Treatment for the burns, parental visiting patterns and observations of the mother-child relationship.
2. Parental visiting patterns, parents' comments to nurses, and a description of the burns.
3. Observation of the mother-child relationship, the types of toys the child has, and whether the child is clean.
4. Observation of relationship between parents and the client's siblings, treatment of the burns, and the types of toys the child has.

72. **In which of the following cases would the nurse suspect physical abuse?**

1. A three-year-old female with 15% burns in a splash pattern over the face and chest, reportedly sustained when she pulled on the tablecloth and a teapot fell, spilling over her.
2. A 14-month-old male with many bruises on bony prominences, in various stages of healing. The child is reportedly clumsy.
3. A six-year-old with a spiral fracture of the tibia and fibula that reportedly occurred while riding his bicycle.

4. A nine-month-old near drowning, who reportedly climbed into the tub and turned on the water.

73. **Upon the client's return from the recovery room, the nurse observes that the fluid in the chest tube bottle has stopped fluctuating. The most appropriate interpretation of this by the nurse is:**

1. All the fluid and air has been removed.
2. The tubing may be kinked.
3. The lungs have re-expanded.
4. The suction is set too low.

74. **The nurse is preparing a seven-year-old female for hospitalization. The child had a previous hospital experience. To best prepare this child, the nurse would:**

1. Suggest role playing and provide materials.
2. Remind the child of the experience of her past hospitalization.
3. Read her a story about another child having a similar operation.
4. Tell her she is only going in to have her throat checked.

75. **A nephrectomy is scheduled tomorrow on a three-year-old client. The best preparation for this child by the nurse would be to:**

1. Demonstrate by pointing on the child's body where the incision will be made the evening before the procedure.
2. Give the preoperative sedation as ordered with a small needle so that a Band-Aid will not be needed.
3. Ask the child's parents to leave the room while the preoperative medication is administered.
4. Explain the procedure to the child in simple sentences just before giving the preoperative sedation.

76. **A general anesthesia has been given for multiple tooth extractions on a three-year-old child. He returns crying, but awake, from the recovery room. What approach by the nurse is most likely to be successful?**

1. Examine the mouth first.
2. Leave the mouth until last.
3. It really makes no difference what is done first.
4. Medicate the child for pain first.

77. **An elderly client with COPD was admitted to the pulmonary unit of the hospital. He complained of shortness of breath, lack of appetite, and difficulty sleeping. The doctor prescribed theophylline (Theo-Dur), 250 mg IV every six hours. The nurse knows that theophylline was prescribed primarily because the drug acts as a:**

1. Vasoconstrictor.

2. Analgesic.
3. Diuretic.
4. Bronchodilator.

78. **Which nursing action will be helpful in treating a client with COPD who has tenacious bronchial secretions?**

1. Maintain semi-Fowler's position as much as possible.
2. Maintain oxygen via nasal prongs at five liters per minute.
3. Encourage a low salt diet.
4. Encourage drinking six to eight glasses of water daily.

79. **The nurse caring for a client with Raynaud's disease knows that which statement about this disease is least accurate?**

1. Smoking tobacco worsens the condition.
2. Exposure to cold temperatures aggravates the condition.
3. Radial and ulnar pulses are not palpable or normal.
4. Repeated attacks of vasospasm may progress to ulceration and gangrene.

80. **In comparing skeletal traction to skin traction, the nurse knows that:**

1. Skeletal traction can be utilized longer than skin traction.
2. Clients in skin traction have more pain than those in skeletal traction.
3. Skin traction is more likely to be complicated by osteomyelitis.
4. The risk of skin breakdown is greater with skeletal traction.

81. **The client with a fracture of the right femur is placed in skeletal traction with a Thomas splint and Pearson attachment. The nurse knows that the best position for this client:**

1. Has the client's right foot on the bed in direct line with the femur.
2. Uses trochanter rolls to prevent abduction of the right leg.
3. Allows the client to turn slightly from side to side above the waist.
4. Maintains the client flat with only brief periods with her head elevated.

82. **An elderly client is admitted to the emergency department with unequal grips and aphasia. The initial nursing action for this client is to:**

1. Prepare to begin an IV infusion.
2. Raise the HOB to 30 degrees.

3. Monitor BP.
4. Explain the MRI to the client and family.

83. **A client is an insulin dependent diabetic. He is scheduled for a gallbladder x-ray in the outpatient department. He was given medication to take as a prep for this test. Which nursing action is most important when preparing the client for this test?**

1. Explain the procedure to the client, and ask if he has any questions.
2. Give the client directions to the outpatient department and the parking lot.
3. Explain to the client that he should not take his insulin before the x-ray.
4. Tell the client to take his insulin and eat breakfast before leaving home.

84. **A client sustained a spontaneous pneumothorax on the left side, and the physician inserted a chest tube to water sealed drainage connected to wall suction. While the nurse was at the bedside, the client sat up quickly and her chest tube caught on the bed rail and was pulled out. The nurse immediately sealed the opening and applied sterile Vaseline gauze, which was available at the bedside. Which nursing actions is most important initially?**

1. Call a code, since respiratory arrest is imminent.
2. Notify the charge nurse to call the physician to insert another chest tube, stat!
3. Observe the rate, depth and character of the client's respirations.
4. Document the incident immediately in the client's medical record.

85. **A client is recuperating from gallbladder surgery preformed under general anesthesia. The nurse should encourage the client to use the incentive spirometry a minimum of how many times per hour?**

1. Two.
2. Five to 10.
3. 10-15.
4. 20-25.

86. **Compared to the pain of myocardial infarction (MI), the nurse knows that the client with angina pectoris demonstrates pain that:**

1. Is relieved by rest.
2. Is substernal or retrosternal.
3. Does not radiate.
4. Is described as tightness or heaviness in the chest.

87. **The nurse would expect a client with hyper-thyroidism to report:**

1. Weight gain of 10 pounds in three weeks.
2. Constipation.
3. Sensitivity to cold.
4. Flushed, moist skin.

88. **The nurse would expect a client admitted with Cushing's syndrome to report:**

   1. Weight loss.
   2. Diarrhea.
   3. Double vision.
   4. Increased bruising.

89. **A client is admitted to the critical care unit (CCU) following a myocardial infarction. The nurse understands that digoxin (Lanoxin) has been ordered for him because the drug helps to:**

   1. Dilate the coronary arteries.
   2. Strengthen the heartbeat.
   3. Increase the electrical conductivity of the heart.
   4. Decrease calcium uptake by the cells.

90. **Which of the following statements demonstrate to the nurse that the client understands the purpose of his cardiac pacemaker?**

   1. "I won't have to worry about ever having a heart attack now that I have a pacemaker."
   2. "Now I can eat whatever I want and it won't affect my heart, since the pacemaker will take care of my heart."
   3. "Having a pacemaker means that my heart can never stop beating."
   4. "The pacemaker will help stimulate my heart to beat when my heart rate is very slow."

91. **Patient education of the client with active tuberculosis is important in helping to prevent the spread of the disease. The most effective method for the nurse to teach the client in order to help prevent the spread of infection is to:**

   1. Maintain strict isolation during the active phases of the disease.
   2. Cover nose and mouth with several layers of tissues when coughing or sneezing.
   3. Wear a protective mask while in public.
   4. Encourage the family to wear a protective mask while with the client.

92. **A client is admitted with bleeding esophageal varices. The physician has opted to use esophageal tamponade with a Sengstaken-Blakemore tube to control the bleeding. Which of the following nursing interventions is appropriate when caring for the client while the Blakemore tube is in place?**

   1. Ambulate the client four times a day.

2. Encourage clear liquids.
3. Provide mouth and nares care every two hours.
4. Maintain the manometer pressure of the esophageal balloon at all times to control bleeding.

93. **Postural drainage with percussion is ordered for a client with pneumonia. What would the nurse include in the plan for this procedure?**

   1. Perform this procedure before meals.
   2. Cup and clap lightly, to avoid causing redness to the client's skin.
   3. Administer bronchodilators after percussion and before postural drainage.
   4. Provide analgesia prior to each treatment.

94. **Which is the best action by the nurse to monitor skin integrity for a client in Buck's traction?**

   1. Instruct the client to describe any pain from under the boot.
   2. Remove the traction and boot to examine the skin every shift.
   3. Paint the skin with Betadine, which will toughen the skin to prevent breakdown.
   4. Observe for any drainage through the boot, and report to the physician immediately.

95. **While the nurse is taking a client's vital signs, an irregularity in the heart rate is noticed. Which nursing action would be most appropriate?**

   1. Request the assistance of another staff member and take an apical/radial pulse.
   2. Count the apical pulse rate for one full minute and describe the irregularity in the chart.
   3. Call the doctor and request an order for a Holter monitor recording for the next day.
   4. Take the pulse at each peripheral site and count the rate for 30 seconds.

96. **Which approach by the nurse is best when taking the blood pressure of a client with hypertension?**

   1. Measure the blood pressure under the same conditions each time.
   2. Take the blood pressure with the client sitting on the side of the bed.
   3. Place the blood pressure cuff on the right arm above the elbow.
   4. Measure the blood pressure with the client in supine position.

97. **A client has undergone a transurethral resection of the prostate to correct benign prostatic hypertrophy. He has returned from the recovery room with an indwelling urinary catheter. For several hours the urinary output has been adequate. The nurse notes, however, that the catheter has drained no urine during the last hour. What should the nurse do first?**

1. Offer the client 100 cc of oral fluids each hour.
2. Irrigate the catheter according to the postoperative orders.
3. Call the physician and request an increase in IV fluid rate.
4. Monitor the vital signs every 15 minutes for one hour.

98. A client who has been diagnosed with CHF (congestive heart failure) two days earlier begins to exhibit manifestations of left-sided heart failure. Which of the following would the nurse observe?

    1. Peripheral edema.
    2. Dyspnea.
    3. Abdominal distention.
    4. Fatigue.

99. A client is admitted with acute leukemia. The nurse can anticipate that the client will report:

    1. Nausea/vomiting, diarrhea.
    2. Fatigue, weakness.
    3. Fever, chills.
    4. Nosebleed, headache.

100. A client diagnosed with AIDS is placed on zidovudine (Retrovir) (formerly AZT). The nurse monitors the client for which life-threatening side effect of this drug?

    1. Fever.
    2. Aplastic anemia.
    3. Renal failure.
    4. Cardiac dysrhythmia.

NOTES

NCLEX-PN

Test 1

Questions with
Rationales

NCLEX-PN TEST 1 WITH RATIONALES

1. In preparation for a sigmoid colon resection, a client is receiving instructions about the colostomy that will be performed. Which statement by the client indicates to the nurse that further clarification is required?

   1. "My colostomy will begin to function seven to 10 days after surgery."
   2. "The stoma of my colostomy will appear large at first, but it will shrink over the next few weeks."
   3. "I will have to wear a colostomy bag at all times to prevent accidental leakage of stool."
   4. "My diet will not have to change dramatically. I can use a trial-and-error approach to see if any foods no longer agree with me."

   1. *No, this is a true statement that does not require further clarification. Because of the lack of bowel peristalsis after surgery and the client's NPO status, it is not unusual to see only mucous drain from the ostomy until approximately one week after surgery.*
   2. *No, this is a true statement that does not require further clarification. The stoma will be edematous at first because of the trauma of surgery and manipulation of the colon, but the stoma will shrink to a "rosebud" size within a few weeks after surgery.*
   3. ***Good work. This statement is not true and does require further clarification. Most clients with a sigmoid colostomy gain control of elimination and will only need to wear a small dressing over the site, once they know their pattern of elimination. The lower the colostomy can be placed on the colon, the more control the client may have, with less need for constant wearing of an ostomy bag.***
   4. *No, this true statement by the client does not need further clarification. Most clients have no change in their diet patterns. What bothered them before surgery (gas-producing foods) probably will bother them after surgery. For the sake of caution, clients are instructed to "try" foods and evaluate their effect upon the GI tract.*

2. A client with a new colostomy has been given instructions about the irrigation of his ostomy. Which action by the client would indicate to the nurse that the teaching plan has to be reviewed?

   1. 500 ml of irrigating solution is used.
   2. Warm tap water is used to irrigate the ostomy.
   3. A lubricated cone tip is inserted into the ostomy stoma to begin the irrigation.
   4. The irrigating solution bag is positioned 30 inches above the stoma.

   1. *Incorrect choice. The client has learned that the correct amount to be used for an irrigation is 500-1,000 ml of solution.*
   2. *Wrong choice. Tap water can be used and it should feel warm to the client's wrist. Water that is too cool can cause cramping; water that is too hot may burn the mucosal lining of the colon.*
   3. *Wrong selection. This is proper procedure for beginning the irrigation. The lubricated cone tip is inserted approximately one inch, and the solution is allowed to flow in slowly.*
   4. ***Good! You have identified the action that means the client needs further teaching. The irrigating bag should be positioned 18 to 20 inches above the height of the stoma, not 30 inches. Too much height can cause excessive pressure and force the irrigating solution in too rapidly, causing abdominal cramping.***

3. A female client returns to the postoperative unit following a partial colectomy for cancer. She has a nasogastric tube to low continuous suction and complains of a sore throat. She asks the nurse when the nasogastric tube will be taken out. Which response by the nurse is most appropriate at this time?

   1. "The doctor will discontinue the tube when your bowel sounds return."
   2. "The tube probably will be removed tomorrow, but you'll remain NPO for three to five more days."
   3. "The tube will be removed when peristalsis returns through the entire GI tract, usually in three to five days."
   4. "You'll have to ask that question of your doctor. He's the one who has to give the order to discontinue the tube."

   1. *No, this is only part of the conditions that must be present. Think about the return of total peristalsis and how that might be evidenced.*
   2. *Incorrect. The client will need the nasogastric tube for a longer period of time, because gastric and intestinal juices are still being produced, even with the NPO status. Without the tube, the accumulation of these secretions would lead to nausea/vomiting and increased discomfort for the client.*
   3. ***Yes! This will be evidenced not only by the return of bowel sounds, but also by the passing of flatus through the rectum. It is then deemed safe to pull the nasogastric tube and begin the client on a progressive diet from***

sips of clear liquids to a regular diet.

4. *Wrong choice. This statement gives no information to the client. Based on your knowledge of postoperative management of clients with a nasogastric tube, there is some information that you can share with her. This statement also uses the communication block of referring to an inappropriate person (the doctor).*

4. **A client, age 83, is admitted to the hospital with complaints of abdominal pain and distention. He has a history of no bowel movement for the past 10 days. After a diagnostic evaluation, it's determined that the client has a fecal impaction. Which treatment can the nurse anticipate will be ordered initially?**

   1. Soap suds enemas until clear.
   2. Bisacodyl (Dulcolax) suppository.
   3. Oil retention enema.
   4. Tap water enema.

   1. *No, this treatment would not be ordered initially, due to the impaction of the stool. The soap suds solution would not be able to bypass the stool to facilitate elimination. Select again.*
   2. *Incorrect. The suppository would stimulate peristalsis, but initially would be ineffective in moving the impacted stool. Try another option.*
   3. ***You are right! The initial administration of an oil retention enema will help to lubricate the impaction so that it can pass more readily through the intestine. After the mineral oil enema is given, the client is asked to retain it for 30-60 minutes. This enema then is followed with saline or soap suds enemas until the bowel is clear. At times, a digital extraction of the stool is necessary. Unless adequate lubrication is used, bowel perforation can occur with manual extraction.***
   4. *Incorrect choice. Tap water enemas are rarely used because of their hypotonic nature, which could upset the client's fluid and electrolyte status. Make another selection.*

5. **The physician orders a stool specimen to be examined for ova and parasites. What is the proper procedure for collection of this specimen by the nurse?**

   1. Send the entire stool immediately to the lab.
   2. Use a sterile container.
   3. Take feces from several areas of the bowel movement.
   4. Refrigerate the specimen until it can be delivered to the lab.

   1. ***Correct! A stool specimen for ova and parasites should be collected in its entirety, placed in a dry container free of urine, labeled correctly, and sent immediately to the labora-***

tory.

   2. *No, a sterile container is not necessary. The feces should be collected in a dry container free of urine. Select again.*
   3. *Incorrect procedure. Taking samples from various areas of the stool is done when a stool for occult blood is ordered. Choose another option.*
   4. *No! Refrigeration will kill the parasites and definitely alter the test results. Make another selection.*

6. **The nurse explains to a client that preparation for a cholecystography includes:**

   1. NPO after midnight.
   2. Clear liquid diet the evening before the test.
   3. Assessing for allergies to iodine or seafood.
   4. Special consent form due to the invasive nature of the procedure.

   1. *Incorrect. The client will be NPO from the time the contrast is given, the evening prior to the test, until the examination is completed.*
   2. *No. The client typically is given a low fat meal the evening before the x-ray examination to decrease the stimulation of the gallbladder. Make another selection.*
   3. ***Correct! An oral iodine contrast substance such as Telepaque or Oragrafin is given, because gallstones are not usually radiopaque. After administration of the iodinated substance, it takes about 13 hours for it to reach the liver and be excreted into the bile, where it's stored in the gallbladder. It's important to assess for allergies to iodine or seafood.***
   4. *Incorrect choice. Cholecystography is an x-ray examination of the gallbladder, and is not an invasive procedure. A special consent form is not needed.*

7. **Following a CVA that affected the left side of the brain, an elderly client had the tube feeding removed and is ready to begin oral feedings. Which of the following nursing measures ensures the client's tolerance to liquids?**

   1. Feed from right side of mouth; upright position; mouth care before feeding.
   2. Verbal encouragement; check gag reflex; feed thinned foods and liquids.
   3. Check gag reflex; feed on left side of mouth; upright position.
   4. Sensory stimulation; verbal encouragement; favorite foods.

   1. *No, go back and check which side would be affected with this client. This answer suggests feeding on his affected side.*
   2. *Incorrect. Thinned foods and liquids are poorly*

handled by the client with any dysphagia. Thick-ened liquids and soft foods are best. Try again.

3. ***Awesome reasoning! This includes the impor-tant points of checking to make sure the client will be able to sense the food and approaching from the unaffected side (with left-brain in-jury, right-sided involvement would be ex-pected). Feeding in the upright position best prevents choking.***

4. *No, sounded good though. Sensory stimulation may actually be counterproductive and, although the other measures may be generally helpful, they do not answer the question. Select again.*

8. **A client who is 62 years old is scheduled for coronary artery bypass. Preoperatively, the physician has ordered aspirin, 325 mg daily. Which nursing action would be most appropriate?**

   1. Explain to the client that aspirin is given because of its anti-inflammatory effects.
   2. Tell the client that after surgery he will continue to take aspirin prophylactically.
   3. Question the doctor's order, since aspirin could cause postoperative bleeding.
   4. Monitor the client's temperature and report eleva-tions to the doctor immediately.

   1. *This statement is not appropriate for the situation described in the question. Although aspirin does have an anti-inflammatory effect, cardiac clients who take 325 mg daily are taking it for its antico-agulation effect. This option is a distractor. Try another option.*

   2. *Incorrect choice. Although the client might take aspirin prophylactically following surgery to pre-vent blood clots, he should not take it preopera-tively because it may cause postoperative bleed-ing. The question is about the use of aspirin preop-eratively. This option is a distractor.*

   3. ***Excellent choice! Since aspirin interferes with the action of platelets, it may cause bleeding after the surgery. Questioning the doctor's or-der would be the best action in this case.***

   4. *This action is not the most appropriate. Although aspirin does have an antipyretic effect, this ques-tion is about the preoperative use of aspirin. The question contains no data to suggest that the client has a temperature elevation, or that he is at risk for developing a temperature elevation. Further-more, the nurse knows that cardiac clients who take 325 mg aspirin daily are taking it for its anti-coagulation effect. This option is a distractor.*

9. **In caring for a client immediately following a cardiac catheterization procedure, which of the following nurs-ing actions is appropriate?**

   1. Apply warm compresses to the puncture site.
   2. Assist with passive range of motion exercises.
   3. Monitor the client for cardiac arrhythmias.
   4. Assist the client into high Fowler's position.

   1. *This is inappropriate. Since bleeding is a major complication following a cardiac catheterization, heat is never applied. Try again!*

   2. *This is inappropriate. Since bleeding is a major complication following a cardiac catheterization, movement is limited in the involved extremity. Try again!*

   3. ***Good choice! This is appropriate. The heart muscle may be irritable following this proce-dure, and serious arrhythmias may occur.***

   > **TEST-TAKING TIP:** This is the only correct action in this question. Note also that the word "cardiac" in the stem of the question is repeated in this option — and that the issue is cardiac catheterization. Although this test-taking strategy isn't foolproof, in this question similar words present in both the question and one answer option are a good clue!

   4. *This is inappropriate. This position could obstruct arterial blood flow and lead to formation of a throm-bus. The involved extremity must be properly aligned and immobilized immediately after the procedure. Try again!*

10. **A client receives haloperidol (Haldol) 5 mg t.i.d. Sev-eral days later, the nurse notices that she is walking stiffly with a shuffling gait. What is the priority nursing action at this time?**

    1. Take her blood pressure before her next dose.
    2. Withhold the Haldol until the manifestation disappears.
    3. Chart observations on the client's record.
    4. Obtain an order for an antiparkinsonian drug.

    1. *No, this is not a necessary intervention. This would be correct if the client were experiencing postural hypotension. It is not the correct option for the manifestation of a shuffling gait. Select another option.*

    2. *No, this is not necessary. This option only would be appropriate for unusually severe extrapyrami-dal side effects. There is a better option.*

    3. Wrong choice. The nurse should chart observa-tions, but this is *not the priority action. Try again.*

    4. ***Correct. The client is experiencing parkinso-nian side effects to the Haldol. The nurse should obtain an order from the psychiatrist for an antiparkinsonian drug to counter these side effects.***

11. A client uses tamoxifen (Nolvadex) for her cancer. The nurse knows that tamoxifen has which of the following actions?

1. Antimicrobial.
2. Anti-estrogenic.
3. Androgenic.
4. Anti-inflammatory.

1. *Wrong. Tamoxifen does not have an antimicrobial effect. Try again.*
2. ***Right! Tamoxifen is used to treat cancer of the breast in both pre- and post-menopausal women. It has been shown to delay recurrences.***
3. *Wrong choice! Androgens are male hormones and can be used to treat breast cancer. Tamoxifen does not increase male hormone production. Try again.*
4. *Incorrect! Tamoxifen does not have an anti-inflammatory effect. Try again.*

12. A client is to receive his first injection of interferon (Roferon-a) for his hairy cell leukemia. What side effects would the nurse advise the client to expect?

1. Reduced urine output.
2. Severe vomiting and nausea.
3. Flu-like manifestations.
4. Weight gain.

1. *Wrong answer. Interferon is a natural body protein and does not affect the kidneys.*
2. *No, severe vomiting and nausea is not an expected side effect of interferon.*
3. ***Correct. The manifestations from interferon are usually mild and include fever, malaise, headache and chills.***
4. *Wrong choice! Weight gain is not a problem with interferon.*

13. A client, placed on ferrous sulfate tablets twice daily as an iron supplement for anemia, asks the nurse why the doctor told her to take the medication with orange juice. The nurse most accurately informs the client that:

1. The medication has an unpleasant taste, and the orange juice will help disguise the taste.
2. The orange juice will help avoid constipation, which is a side effect of the medication.
3. The orange juice will help the gastrointestinal tract absorb the medication more efficiently.
4. The medication can cause nausea, and the orange juice will help alleviate this problem.

1. *This is not correct. The medication is a tablet. Nothing is needed to disguise the taste.*
2. *No. Although constipation can be a side effect of ferrous sulfate, drinking orange juice with the tablets is not adequate to prevent constipation. This cannot be the most important reason for drinking orange juice with the medication.*
3. ***Excellent! The Vitamin C in the orange juice will help with the absorption of the iron. This is the most important reason.***
4. *Wrong choice. Some clients experience nausea when taking ferrous sulfate. Orange juice, however, will not alleviate this manifestation.*

14. A client has been taking isoniazid (INH) and rifampin (Rifadin) for three weeks after being diagnosed with TB. He tells the nurse that he has noted a reddish-orange color to his urine. Which statement by the nurse is most appropriate?

1. "I'll make an appointment for you to see the doctor this afternoon. You may have developed a bleeding problem, which is not uncommon with these drugs."
2. "The reddish color is a side effect of the INH. Stop taking it for two to three days and the discoloration should go away. The doctor may want to change your drug therapy."
3. "The discoloration is due to rifampin. It may turn all body fluids orange-red. This is a harmless side effect."
4. "You should increase your fluid intake while on these medications. They are known to cause bladder irritation when taken together."

1. *Not true! Although thrombocytopenia may occur when taking these medications, it is not a common adverse reaction. This is not the cause of the client's reddish-orange urine.*
2. *No, the reddish discoloration is not due to INH. Clients should never be instructed to periodically stop taking their medications. Try again.*
3. ***Correct. Rifampin will turn body fluids such as tears, sweat, saliva and urine an orange-red color. Advise the client of possible permanent stains on clothes and soft contact lenses.***
4. *No, these drugs are not considered to be bladder irritants. They are, however, potentially hepatotoxic agents. This response does not address the issue in the question, which is the red-orange urine reported by the client.*

15. A 43-year-old female client has had a total abdominal hysterectomy and bilateral salpingo-oophorectomy for stage III uterine cancer. Which instructions would the nurse anticipate providing?

1. Estrogen therapy will alleviate the discomfort of surgical menopause.
2. A Papanicolaou (Pap) smear should be performed every six months.
3. Lubrication can be used to treat vaginal dryness, itching and burning.
4. Vaginal intercourse will no longer be possible.

1. Incorrect. Estrogen therapy is contraindicated in clients with known uterine cancers. Select another option.
2. No. This test is used to detect cancers of the cervix or uterus. In a total abdominal hysterectomy, the uterus and cervix have been removed. Try again.
3. **Correct! Atrophic vaginal changes occur due to the loss of estrogen post operatively and may also cause pain during coitus. Lubricants may reduce the manifestations associated with the diminished mucous production.**
4. No. The client and partner may resume sexual relations after healing of the incision has occurred. The vagina remains following total hysterectomy. Try again.

16. A client is being sent home on isoxsuprine (Vasodilan) for treatment of premature labor. Which of the following actions should receive priority in the nurse's discharge teaching plan?

1. Technique for taking oral temperature.
2. How to assess her radial pulse.
3. Procedure to assess her blood sugar.
4. How to assess fetal heart rate.

1. Sorry, this is not correct! Vasodilan has no effect on body temperature, and the client therefore does not need to be taught this technique.
2. **Yes, great choice! Vasodilan frequently causes tachycardia, so the client needs to monitor her radial pulse. She is instructed to call her physician if it is 120 bpm or greater.**
3. Incorrect. Vasodilan does not affect maternal blood sugar like many of the other tocolytic agents, so the client does not need to be taught this procedure.
4. Incorrect. Vasodilan can cause maternal tachycardia, so the fetus also is at risk for an elevated heart rate. Antepartum clients, however, are instructed to count fetal movements to indicate fetal well being. Teaching them to monitor their fetus's heart rate would not be a priority.

17. A 12-year-old child is being discharged from the hospital with a diagnosis of asthma. She is to be maintained on metered dose inhalers at home. The nurse is preparing a care plan on the use of cromolyn (Intal). Which of the following instructions to the parents would the nurse avoid including in the client's care plan?

1. Intal will decrease the inflammation in your child's bronchioles.
2. Do not rely on Intal for relief of an acute attack.
3. Have your child rinse her mouth after using the puffer.
4. Your child should breathe more easily after a dose of Intal.

1. Wrong choice! Intal is a mast cell inhibitor and decreases inflammation in the bronchioles. This information is correct and should be included in the care plan. You are looking for the option that would NOT be included.
2. No, this information is correct and should be given to the client. Intal has a slow onset and will not relieve an acute asthma attack. A fast-acting bronchodilator should be given. You are looking for the option that would NOT be included.
3. Wrong choice. Intal may cause throat and mouth irritation. Rinsing or gargling after the medication will help relieve the irritation. Remember, this question has a false response stem and is asking for an answer that is NOT true.
4. **Very good! This question has a false response stem and you correctly picked the answer that is NOT true. Intal is a prophylactic medication and the client will not "feel better" after any single dose. This can lead to noncompliance. Clients need to be aware that the Intal is necessary even though its effect is not immediately felt.**

18. A six-month-old male infant with AIDS has a nursing diagnosis of "altered growth and development" on the care plan. Which of the following nursing interventions will most enhance the growth and development of the child?

1. Encourage the child to eat whatever he wants.
2. Provide therapy to help the child meet developmental milestones.
3. Provide nutritional supplements in addition to an adequate diet.
4. Weigh and measure the infant on a frequent basis.

1. No, this is not the best answer because it will not ensure that his nutritional needs are met. Try this again.
2. No. Think about Maslow's Hierarchy of Needs. Which need has priority here?
3. **Yes, that's right. If this child is behind in measurable ways on growth and development, his nutritional needs cannot be met by food alone. He needs extra supplements to help him fight infection and grow.**
4. No, this doesn't answer the question. These are assessments or means of evaluating responses, but they do not imply action toward improving or correcting the alteration in growth and development. Choose again.

19. A nurse working with a client with agoraphobia recognizes that the most effective technique for treatment of agoraphobia is:

1. Repeated exposure to situations that she fears.
2. Distraction each time she brings up her problem.

3. Teaching relaxation techniques.
4. Gradual desensitization by controlled exposure to the situation she fears.

1. *Wrong. Repeated exposure to situations she fears will create even greater anxiety. This is not the correct option.*
2. *Wrong choice! Distraction will not assist her to overcome her fear and anxiety.*
3. *Teaching relaxation techniques is helpful, but there is a better technique to treat agoraphobia.*
4. **Correct. Desensitization is a type of behavioral therapy. The client is gradually exposed to the feared situation under controlled conditions and learns to overcome the anxious response.**

20. A 48-year-old man hospitalized for an obsessive-compulsive disorder has recurring thoughts that he has mouth odors that are offensive to others. He has mouth care rituals that occupy a good deal of his waking hours and caused him to be fired from his last job. The nurse knows that these manifestations most likely represent:

1. A method of reducing anxiety.
2. A form of manipulation to avoid work.
3. An attention-getting strategy.
4. A rationalization for avoiding social contact.

1. **Correct. The ritualized behaviors of a person with an obsessive-compulsive disorder are an attempt to control anxiety.**
2. *This is not correct. The behavioral rituals performed by a person with an obsessive-compulsive disorder cannot be controlled, so they cannot be considered attempts to manipulate the environment.*
3. *This is not correct. Obsessive-compulsive behaviors may draw attention to the individual, but the individual is most often embarrassed about them and will go to great lengths to conceal the rituals from others.*
4. *No, persons with obsessive-compulsive behaviors are compelled to perform their rituals and usually derive no pleasure from carrying them out. Try again.*

21. A client is scheduled for a cardiac catheterization. When he arrives for the procedure, he reports he awoke that morning with "butterflies in his stomach," a sense of restlessness, urinary frequency, and some difficulty concentrating as he drove to the hospital. The admitting nurse assesses his anxiety level as:

1. Mild.
2. Moderate.
3. Severe.
4. Panic.

1. *Sorry. In mild anxiety, the client is alert and able to concentrate closely on the task at hand. This client is having some difficulty with concentration. He also has several physical manifestations that indicate his anxiety level is more than mild.*
2. **Good work! The combination of physical manifestations and some difficulty concentrating indicates that his level of anxiety is moderate. This is not unusual considering the intrusive medical procedure he is about to undergo.**
3. *Wrong! In severe anxiety the person is only able to focus on small details or scattered details and has a great deal of discomfort. The client was able to drive himself to the office and reported only some difficulty concentrating, so his anxiety is not severe.*
4. *Wrong! At the panic level the client is disorganized and may appear either paralyzed (unable to act) or hyperactive and agitated. The client's anxiety is not this high.*

22. The nurse understands in caring for a client with coronary artery disease that psychological factors such as anxiety:

1. Contribute to both the development and progress of coronary artery disease.
2. Cause coronary artery disease.
3. Cannot cause coronary artery disease, but they do affect the client's prognosis.
4. Affect the client's ability to adjust to a diagnosis of coronary artery disease but have little direct effect on treatment outcomes.

1. **Correct. Although theories that certain personality types (such as "Type A" persons) are prone to develop cardiac disease have been disputed, anxiety and other psychological factors are still believed to play a significant role in the development and progress of cardiac disorders.**
2. *Psychological factors are only one of the risk factors involved in the development of coronary artery disease. Psychological factors alone do not cause cardiac problems. Try again.*
3. *This statement is only partially true, so it cannot be the correct option. Anxiety and other psychological factors are believed to play a significant role in the development and progress of cardiac disorders. Try again.*
4. *Not correct. This statement is not true because psychological factors have a profound effect on treatment outcomes.*

23. A 45-year-old man is admitted to the emergency room complaining of chest pain and dyspnea. He is flushed and perspiring profusely. He says, "I feel like I am going to die. Am I having a heart attack?" The medical exam and lab work are negative. He is diagnosed with anxiety. The nurse assesses his level of anxiety as:

1. Mild.
2. Moderate.
3. Severe.
4. Panic.

1. *The severity of this client's manifestations indicate that he has more than a mild level of anxiety. This is not the correct option.*
2. *In moderate anxiety, the person's perceptual field narrows but he is able to cope with some assistance. This client's manifestations indicate a higher level of anxiety. Try again.*
3. *In severe anxiety, the person's perceptual field is scattered and he is not able to focus on anything except relieving his anxiety. This does not describe this client because he is currently immobilized. Choose another option.*
4. ***Correct. This client's manifestations indicate he is experiencing the panic level of anxiety. His manifestations are classic manifestations of a panic disorder.***

24. **A client explains that, for the past 10 years, she has been unable to leave her house without her husband or daughter. If she tries to go out alone, she becomes very anxious and must quickly return inside. The nurse interviewing her identifies the probable cause as:**

1. Conversion disorder.
2. Agoraphobia.
3. Panic disorder.
4. Obsessive-compulsive disorder.

1. *This is not the correct choice. Conversion disorder is an anxiety disorder in which the client has the physical manifestations suggesting a medical problem (such as blindness or paralysis) but for which no organic pathology can be diagnosed.*
2. ***Correct. Agoraphobia is the fear and subsequent avoidance of places or situations from which escape might be difficult. The most common form of this disorder is avoiding open public places, such as shopping malls, and fear of leaving one's home.***
3. *This is not the correct answer. Panic disorder is characterized by recurrent panic attacks that are not associated with any specific stimulus or situation, but seem to occur spontaneously.*
4. *No. Obsessive-compulsive disorders are characterized by recurrent obsessional thoughts and/or ritualized behaviors.*

25. **The nurse, in caring for psychiatric clients, knows that tardive dyskinesia:**

1. Is a movement disorder caused by antipsychotic drugs.
2. Occurs within the first few days of treatment in most clients.
3. Improves rapidly if the offending drug is discontin-

ued.
4. Is treated with antiparkinsonian drugs.

1. ***Correct! Tardive dyskinesia is a serious movement disorder caused by treatment with certain antipsychotic drugs.***
2. *Wrong. Most clients with tardive dyskinesia develop the condition after taking antipsychotics for many years. It rarely occurs shortly after beginning antipsychotic drug therapy.*
3. *Tardive dyskinesia occurs because antipsychotics block the transmission of dopamine in the basal ganglia. When the dosage of antipsychotic medication is reduced, or the drug is discontinued, dopamine is again released and floods the neurons, which demonstrate a supersensitivity to its presence. Try again.*
4. *Not correct. There currently is no treatment for tardive dyskinesia.*

26. **A client attends group therapy daily. The nurse understands that the most important benefit of group therapy is to:**

1. Provide the opportunity to develop social skills.
2. Improve the client's orientation to reality.
3. Gain support and encouragement from other persons.
4. Develop greater insight into herself and her problems through the feedback provided by the other members.

1. *Although clients in group therapy do develop better social skills, this is not the primary focus of the treatment. This is not the correct option.*
2. *Depressed persons have a negative view of themselves and their situations, and some depressed persons have delusions. Group therapy, however, is not a technique for reality orientation. This is not the correct option.*
3. *This is incorrect because this is not the most important benefit of group therapy. Be sure to read all the options before selecting the one that is the best!*
4. ***Correct. Group therapy provides benefits that occur through the feedback and validation of the other members.***

27. **In providing care to a client who is receiving ECT, the nurse knows that this treatment:**

1. Usually requires 10 days to three weeks before depression is noticeably improved.
2. Results in a high incidence of chronic memory problems.
3. Is effective for 60% of persons who receive it.
4. Is used for persons who have not responded to antidepressants.

1. *This is incorrect. ECT has a significantly more rapid*

onset of action than antidepressants and may be used for very severely depressed persons who are also highly suicidal.

2. *This is incorrect. The side effects of ECT are transient and may include short-term memory loss. It rarely causes chronic memory problems.*

3. *Incorrect statement. ECT is effective treatment for more than 80% of depressed persons who receive it. It does, however, tend to be associated with a high relapse rate.*

4. **Correct. ECT is not the first choice of treatment for most depressed persons. It is used for individuals who have not responded to antidepressants or who have had adverse reactions to these drugs.**

28. A client, 34, is admitted for the third time to a psychiatric hospital with a diagnosis of schizophrenia. The police found her wandering along the highway. When questioned, she was unable to give coherent answers. During the admission procedure, the nurse notices that her appearance is unkempt and she appears to be actively hallucinating. The initial nursing assessment is:

1. Her mental status.
2. Her ability to follow directions.
3. Her perception of reality.
4. Her physical health needs.

1. *Wrong! This is important, but it is not the highest initial priority.*

2. *No. Although this is an important part of the assessment of her mental status, it is not the highest initial priority.*

3. *Wrong choice. Her perception of reality is important for setting realistic goals and determining safety needs, but it is not the initial priority.*

4. **Correct. The client's problems may be due to a physical illness or injury, or to fluid and electrolyte imbalance. Assessing her physical health needs should be the initial priority for the nurse.**

29. In caring for a client with schizophrenic disorder who is receiving an antipsychotic medication, the nurse knows that which of the following statements about the "dopamine hypothesis" is inaccurate?

1. Most antipsychotic drugs block the effects of dopamine and receptor sites in the brain.
2. Amphetamine enhances dopamine activity in the brain and can cause a psychotic response that is indistinguishable from paranoid schizophrenia.
3. The potency of antipsychotic drugs seems to be related to their antidopamine action.
4. Schizophrenic clients excrete excessive amounts of dopamine in their urine.

1. *Wrong choice. This is an accurate statement. This*

negative response stem is asking for an option that is INACCURATE.

2. *Wrong choice. This is an accurate statement. This negative response stem is asking for an option that is INACCURATE.*

3. *Wrong choice. This is an accurate statement. The antidopamine action has been used to develop newer antipsychotic drugs. Remember, this question has a negative response stem and is asking for an option that is INACCURATE.*

4. **Correct. Schizophrenic clients do not excrete excessive amounts of dopamine in their urine. The dopamine hypothesis refers to the theory that an excess of brain dopamine may be the cause of schizophrenia.**

30. A client is sitting by his food tray, pushing the food around on his plate. He says to the nurse, "I hate hospital food. Is this the only thing that I can get to eat?" The nurse's best response is:

1. "What is it about the food that you dislike?"
2. "Well, the other clients haven't complained about the food. Is something else bothering you?"
3. "I'll call the kitchen and order something else for you."
4. "Is there something special that you would like to eat?"

1. **Very good! This response promotes communication by addressing the feelings that the client has about the food, and by asking for clarification of the statement made by the client. Clarification is a tool that promotes therapeutic communication.**

2. *Wrong. This response is defensive, focuses on inappropriate persons (the other clients) and tells the client that his feelings about the food are not valid. Asking the client if something else is bothering him may elicit an expression of feelings by the client, but it actually changes the subject. This approach is not therapeutic.*

3. *Try again! This response does not promote further communication by the client. Therapeutic communication is not developed when the nurse attempts to solve a problem without clarifying exactly what the problem is.*

4. *Try again! The response doesn't focus on the client's feelings. He states that he hates "hospital food," not just this particular meal. This is a possible indicator of other problems. The nurse needs to explore the client's feelings before offering to get other food for him. This not the best "initial" response.*

31. An 88-year-old client is admitted to the hospital with chest pain. His daughter tells the nurse that he has certain routines for his personal hygiene and for taking his medicine. The most appropriate nursing re-

sponse is to:

1. Assure the daughter that everything possible will be done to accommodate her father's needs.
2. Ask the daughter what routines and medicines her father uses at home.
3. Inform the daughter that the hospital has policies that have to be followed, and that you will provide the best care for her father.
4. Tell the daughter that she should inform the doctor about her father's routines so that orders can be written to meet the client's needs.

1. *Wrong! The daughter is the client in this question. She will interpret this response as a cliché and false reassurance. The nurse has not clarified exactly what the father's needs are! This option does not address the daughter's concerns or encourage further communication.*
2. ***Excellent! This option promotes communication and encourages the daughter to tell the nurse more about her concerns. This response also focuses on the nurse's responsibility to assess the client's needs.***
3. *Wrong! This response devalues the daughter's concerns about her father. This is a block to therapeutic communication and therefore not an appropriate nursing response.*
4. *Wrong! This response "passes the buck" to the doctor and puts the client's feelings and concerns on hold. This response inhibits communication.*

32. **When the nurse is making morning rounds, a client says, "I almost died last night." The most therapeutic nursing response is:**

1. "You made it through the night."
2. "Patients do have dreams that they die when they are hospitalized."
3. "Are you feeling okay now?"
4. "That must have been frightening for you. Tell me more about it."

1. *Wrong! At best, this response may appear to be reassuring, but in fact it does not place any value on the client's concerns or feelings. At worst, it appears to make light of what might have been a serious situation! Therapeutic responses focus on the client's feelings and promote further communication with the nurse. This is not therapeutic.*
2. *No. This response focuses on inappropriate persons ("patients" in general). It is a generalization that offers false assurance and actually contradicts the client, since he did not state that he had a dream. The nurse needs to validate and clarify the client's concerns.*
3. *This is not the most therapeutic response. The nurse may appear to be addressing the "here and now," but this simple "yes/no" question does not address*

the client's concern and thus does not encourage communication. The client might even infer that the nurse thinks his concern about dying is not valid if he is "okay" now! Although the client should be assessed for his present status, his comment to the nurse indicates that he is concerned most about "almost dying." The nurse's response should address that concern.
4. ***Excellent choice! This response directly addresses the concern of the client. The nurse uses the communication tool of empathy in responding to this client's concerns and encourages further communication with the client about them.***

33. **A client is told by her doctor that he has found a lump in her breast and that a biopsy will have to be done. The client asks the nurse, "Do you think it is cancer?" The best initial response by the nurse is:**

1. "You seem to be worried about what the doctor may find."
2. "Do you have a family history of breast cancer?"
3. "We won't know anything until the biopsy is done."
4. "Most lumps are not cancerous, so you really shouldn't worry."

1. ***Correct choice. Communication theory states that the nurse should first focus on the client's feelings. This therapeutic response uses the communication tools of empathy and restatement to address the "here and now."***
2. *Try again. This response focuses on the client's family history, not on the client's feelings. This information may be obtained after the client's feelings are addressed in order to provide data concerning the incidence of breast cancer in families. Always look for the key words in the question! The stem of the question asks which is the "best INITIAL response."*
3. *Wrong. This response does not answer the client's question or promote further expression of the client's feelings. This communication block puts the client's feelings of fear on hold.*
4. *Wrong choice. This response offers false assurance and does not encourage the client to express her feelings concerning the fear of cancer. Saying "Don't worry" devalues the client's feelings.*

34. **The nursing assistant says to the nurse, "This client is incontinent of stool three or four times a day. I get angry when I think that he is doing it just to get attention. I think adult diapers should be used for him." How should the nurse initially respond to the nursing assistant?**

1. "You probably are right. Soiling the bed is one way of getting attention from the nursing staff."

2. "Changing his bed and cleaning him must be tire-some for you. Next time it happens, I'll help you."
3. "It's upsetting to see an adult regress."
4. "Why don't you spend more time with him if you think that he is behaving this way to get more attention?"

1. *This response is not therapeutic because it does not address the nursing assistant's feelings and does not encourage expression of feelings. The communication block of showing approval can be identified by the phrase, "you probably are right."*
2. *This response shows empathy on the part of the nurse, but does not encourage any further expression of feelings. The nurse needs to obtain more information about the nursing assistant's statement concerning the client's soiling the bed purposely in order to provide therapeutic communication.*
3. ***Excellent! This response encourages further communication with the nursing assistant because it is empathetic and offers a possible explanation of the client's behavior. This response is therapeutic for the nursing assistant — who is the client in this question.***
4. *No, this is not therapeutic. The nursing assistant is the client in this question. This response begins with a non-therapeutic "why" question and does not address the feelings of the client. It also gives advice, which blocks communication. Finally, it fails to address the client's feelings.*

35. **A hospitalized client has just found out that her mother has died of a heart attack. She is crying and has her face buried in the pillow. The most appropriate nursing response is to:**

1. Return in 15 minutes to see how the client is doing.
2. Sit with the client for a little while.
3. Tell the client that she will feel better in the morning.
4. Share with the client that you lost your mother within the last year and that you know how she feels.

1. *No! This response does not promote therapeutic communication for the "here and now" of this question. By leaving, the nurse indicates to the client an unwillingness to stay with her during this stressful time. If the client wanted to communicate, there wouldn't be anyone to listen.*
2. ***Very good! The nurse lets the client know that she is important by providing time for her. Being silent is a communication tool that is appropriate during times of grieving. This response also addresses the "here and now" in this question.***

3. *This response devalues the client's feelings and puts them on hold. This response does not encourage therapeutic communication. It also offers false assurance, since the client may not feel better in the morning.*
4. *This response focuses on an inappropriate person (the nurse). This response inhibits communication since it implies that there is no need for the client to express her own feelings. There also is an assumption by the nurse that grieving is the same for everyone. This response is not therapeutic for the client.*

36. **A client is seen at the clinic and is to receive an injection. When preparing to administer a medication for injection from an ampule, which action would be unsafe?**

1. Score the neck of the ampule with a file.
2. Protect the thumb and fingers with a gauze square or alcohol wipe.
3. Snap the neck of the ampule toward the body when breaking the top free from the ampule.
4. Insert the needle into the ampule without touching the needle to the edges of the ampule.

1. *Wrong choice, this is safe! Scoring the neck of the ampule provides a place for the ampule to break easily without jagged edges. You are looking for an UNSAFE action. This question has a false response stem.*
2. *Wrong choice, this action is safe! Using a gauze or alcohol wipe protects the thumb and finger from being cut if contact is made with the hand and edges of the broken ampule. You are looking for an UNSAFE action. This question has a false response stem.*
3. ***Good, you spotted the action that is unsafe! The neck of the ampule should be broken away from the body, to prevent shattering of glass toward the hand or face.***
4. *No, this action is safe! The rim of the ampule is considered contaminated. Touching the edges with the needle will contaminate the needle. You are looking for an UNSAFE action. This question has a false response stem.*

37. **An elderly hospitalized client is to receive an x-ray. When the nurse enters the client's room and asks if the client is ready to go to x-ray, the client nods "yes." Next, the priority nursing action is:**

1. Explain the x-ray procedure to the client.
2. Help the client into a wheel chair, so that she will be ready when the transporter arrives to take her to x-ray.
3. Ask the client if she has any questions.
4. Look at the client's identification bracelet.

1. *No. Although the x-ray procedure should be explained to the client, this is not the priority nursing action.*

> **TEST-TAKING TIP:** When answering a priority-setting question, try to identify an action that addresses physiological needs or the safety of the client.

2. *No. Having the client ready for the transporter is very considerate, however, another option takes priority over this.*

> **TEST-TAKING TIP:** When answering a priority-setting question, try to identify an action that addresses physiological needs or the safety of the client.

3. *Answering any questions is an appropriate nursing action, however, this is not the priority action.*

> **TEST-TAKING TIP:** When answering a priority-setting question, try to identify an action that addresses physiological needs or the safety of the client.

4. **Excellent! This action is the priority action because it provides for the safety of the client. Once the client's identity is determined, the nurse can then proceed with the other options.**

38. **The nurse is to apply topical ointment to the client's skin for a dermatological condition. Which action should the nurse avoid?**

1. Massaging the ointment into the skin.
2. Removing excess ointment.
3. Applying ointment with ungloved fingertips.
4. Documenting a description of the skin prior to application of the ointment.

1. *Wrong choice. This action is appropriate. Massaging the ointment into the client's skin provides for penetration of the ointment into the skin. This is not the answer because the question has a false response stem; you are looking for an action to AVOID.*
2. *No, this action is appropriate. Excess ointment should be removed, since it may stain clothing or come into contact with other areas of the body, or with other objects or people. This is not the answer because the question has a false response stem; you are looking for an action to AVOID.*
3. **Correct, this action is to be avoided! Applying ointment with ungloved fingertips allows for absorption of the medication through skin pores on the fingertips, which may cause some undesirable effects to the person applying the ointment.**
4. *Wrong choice. This action is appropriate. The skin should be described to determine if the ointment*

is having a positive effect. However, this is not the answer because the question has a false response stem; you are looking for an action to AVOID.

39. **An HIV positive client is admitted to the hospital with a lung infection. Which of the following isolation categories should be implemented in order to prevent transmission of the HIV virus?**

1. Strict isolation.
2. Respiratory isolation.
3. Universal precautions.
4. Enteric precautions.

1. *Wrong. Strict isolation prevents transmission of highly contagious infections that are spread by air and contact. It may or may not be appropriate, depending upon the type of lung infection. The question, however, asks about prevention of transmission of the HIV virus, not about the lung infection.*
2. *Wrong. Respiratory isolation prevents transmission of infectious diseases over short distances via air droplets. It may or may not be appropriate, depending upon the type of lung infection. The question, however, asks about prevention of transmission of the HIV virus, not about the lung infection. HIV is not spread by air droplets, therefore, respiratory isolation is not necessary to prevent the spread of HIV.*
3. **You are correct! Universal precautions prevent the spread of infections that are transmitted by direct or indirect contact with infectious blood or other body fluids. Since this is the mode of transmission of HIV, this is the appropriate isolation precaution.**
4. *Not quite. Enteric precautions prevent the spread of infections that are transmitted by direct or indirect contact with feces. Prevention of HIV transmission involves more than protection from feces, so enteric precautions are not adequate protection.*

40. **A client is admitted to the hospital and a urine specimen is ordered. When obtaining a urine specimen from the client, which of the following is an inappropriate nursing action?**

1. Place the urine cup in the client's bathroom.
2. Take the full specimen cup to the lab pick up area and then place it in a clean plastic bag.
3. Attach the client's name to the specimen cup.
4. Explain to the client the procedure for obtaining a urine specimen.

1. *No, this is an appropriate action. The specimen cup should be placed in the client's bathroom so that it is readily available when the client has the*

urge to void. You are looking for an action that is INAPPROPRIATE.

2. **Good choice! It is inappropriate for the nurse to carry the specimen cup out of the client's room without first placing it in a clean bag to prevent possible spread of organisms. The ideal method of transporting the specimen cup is for the nurse to place it into a clean bag for transportation to the lab pick up area.**

3. *Wrong choice! This is an appropriate action. The specimen cup should be labeled with the client's identification in order to prevent erroneous reporting or mix-up of specimens in the lab. You are looking for an action that is INAPPROPRIATE.*

4. *Sorry, this is an appropriate action. Teaching the client how to obtain the specimen is part of the nurse's responsibility in order to provide the best specimen for the test. The question has a false response stem, you are looking for an action that is INAPPROPRIATE.*

41. **A client is to have a perineal examination, which requires the dorsal recumbent position. Which of the following nursing actions provides the client with the most privacy?**

    1. Place a bath blanket on the client with one corner at the chest, two corners wrapped around the feet and legs, and the fourth corner draped between the client's legs.
    2. Drape a draw sheet over the client's knees covering the abdomen and legs.
    3. Place a bath blanket on the client, with the top at the chest and the bottom draped over the knees to cover the legs and feet.
    4. Close the examination room door.

    1. **Correct! This option provides the most privacy for the client by keeping the client completely covered until the examination is performed. The examiner can lift the corner of the blanket that is between the client's legs and expose only the perineal area.**

    2. *This option does not provide much privacy since the legs are not wrapped and the sheet must be pushed up to expose the perineum, which exposes the legs and thighs. Try again.*

    3. *This is not correct. Since the blanket must be pushed up to examine the perineum, the client's legs and thighs are completely exposed.*

    4. *Wrong choice. Closing the door is appropriate but draping the client properly provides more privacy, since anyone can open the examination room door.*

42. **A client has right-sided paralysis following a stroke. He is not able to talk, but can make gestures to make himself understood. To effectively communicate with the client, the nurse should:**

    1. Speak very loudly to the client.
    2. Speak quickly to the client, since his attention span may be short.
    3. Use gestures while speaking slowly.
    4. Wait until the family comes in, so they can interpret his behavior.

    1. *No! The client is not hard of hearing.*
    2. *Wrong choice. Fast speech is difficult to understand. Also, there is no information that the client has a short attention span.*
    3. **Good work! This client is at a high safety risk, due to both impaired mobility and impaired ability to communicate. The nurse must use all appropriate means to be sure that the client understands what the nurse is saying, and to enable the client to express his needs.**
    4. *No. The client may have needs that cannot wait for the family. This option does not respect the client's needs, nor assure his comfort and safety.*

43. **An unconscious client is to have an electroencephalogram (EEG). The first nursing action is to:**

    1. Notify the EEG Department that the client is ready for the scan.
    2. Check to see that the client is wearing an identification bracelet.
    3. Shampoo the client's hair.
    4. Prepare a sedative in case the client becomes conscious prior to the procedure.

    1. *Wrong. Although the department performing the procedure should be notified, this is not the first nursing action.*
    2. **Right! Since the client is unconscious and cannot provide information, it is of utmost importance that an identification bracelet be in place.**
    3. *Wrong. Although the client's hair will need a shampoo prior to the test, one of the other actions should be performed prior to this intervention.*
    4. *No! Sedatives may be ordered by the physician prior to giving EEGs, to help the client relax. This client, however, is unconscious and does not need a sedative.*

44. **During the administration of a medication, a 19-year-old client tells the nurse that he has never had that particular pill before. The best nursing action is to:**

    1. Check the client's identification bracelet again.
    2. Check the physician's orders to see if this is a new medication.
    3. Assure the client that the medication package has his name on it.
    4. Ask the client to take the medication, since the identification bracelet and medication administration record indicate the client is to receive the medication.

1. No. Rechecking the client's identification bracelet does not resolve the question of a "new pill" for the client.
2. **Right! Checking the physician's orders will confirm if this is a new medication ordered for the client. This action addresses the client's concern and provides for the client's safety, by addressing the possibility of a medication error.**
3. No! The client's name on the medication label does not address the client's concern about a "new pill." Mistakes can be made with medications. The situation needs to be clarified further in order to provide for the client's safety and to reassure him that he is supposed to receive this pill.
4. No! The person responsible for transcribing the physician's orders onto the medication administration record could have made an error. The situation needs further clarification.

45. To protect against the spread of AIDS, health care workers are encouraged to wear gloves when coming into contact with any body fluids, and to take certain other precautions. The type of precautions used in a health care facility to prevent the spread of AIDS is:

   1. Secretion precautions.
   2. Enteric precautions.
   3. Universal precautions.
   4. Protective isolation.

   1. Wrong! Wearing gloves when coming into contact with bodily fluids is a part of secretion precautions, but the precautions used to prevent the spread of AIDS are broader than this. Try again.
   2. Wrong. Wearing gloves when coming into contact with bodily fluids is part of enteric precautions. The precautions used to prevent the spread of AIDS, however, are broader than this. Try again.
   3. **This is correct! The spread of AIDS is addressed in health care institutions by universal precautions, which include wearing gloves as well as both secretion and enteric precautions.**
   4. Wearing gloves helps protect the nurse from infection. Protective isolation, however, is designed to protect the client from infection from the nurse or others in the health care facility. Choose again.

46. Before administering an injection, the nurse performs aseptic hand washing. This technique includes:

   1. Not using soap, since it causes drying of the skin.
   2. Using paper towels to turn the faucet on and off.
   3. The use of lotion to prevent drying.
   4. Holding arms and hands upright so that all organisms will stay away from hands while washing.

1. This is not aseptic! Soap is necessary in hand washing to remove organisms from the skin. After hand washing, lotion should often be used to prevent drying and chapping, which may cause cracks in the skin that provide portals of entry for infectious organisms.
2. **Yes! Faucets have many bacteria on the handles. To prevent transmission of the bacteria, paper towels are used to turn faucets on and off.**
3. Using lotion does not clean the hands, so this option does not address the issue in the question and this cannot be the correct answer. After hand washing, however, lotion should be used as necessary to prevent drying and chapping, which may cause cracks in the skin that provide portals of entry for infectious organisms.
4. This action is incorrect because the water and organisms will run to the elbow instead of off the hand into the sink.

47. While administering a bed bath it is important for the nurse to maintain privacy. Which is the best method for maintaining the client's privacy?

   1. Allow the client to wear a gown, and reach under the gown with the washcloth and towel to bathe the client.
   2. Use towels to protect the bed linen.
   3. Cover the client with a bath blanket and expose only the portion of the body that is being bathed.
   4. Use the bed sheet to cover the client during the bath.

   1. This is not correct. The gown should be removed when performing a bed bath. It does not absorb water well and may cause the client to become chilled. Note also that the gown is not clean and may be soiled, which defeats one of the purposes of the bath, which is to cleanse the skin.
   2. Wrong choice. Using towels to protect the bed linen is appropriate during a bed bath; however, the stem of the question asks about maintaining the client's privacy. This option does not address the issue in the question.
   3. **Correct! The nurse should provide privacy by exposing only the portion of the body that is being bathed. A bath blanket should be used because it provides a covering for the client that absorbs water and avoids chilling of the client.**
   4. Wrong choice. While the bed sheet may provide privacy for the client, it does not absorb water well and will result in the client's being chilled.

48. An elderly client is constantly putting her call light on. When the nurse answers the light, the client does not

appear to need anything. Which action by the nurse is least appropriate?

1. Ask the members of the family if they can spend more time with the client.
2. Remove the call light from easy reach of the client.
3. Make frequent visits to the client's room.
4. Spend more time in the client's room while charting.

1. *Wrong choice! This action is appropriate. Family members are often willing to help in caring for a client if they are asked or given some direction. You are looking for an INAPPROPRIATE action.*
2. **Correct answer! The call light should NEVER be taken from a client! The client could fall trying to reach for the call light or attempting to get out of bed in order to get someone's attention. This action does not provide for the client's safety.**
3. *Wrong choice! This action is most appropriate. Frequently stopping by the client's room provides the client with some reassurance that someone is available to assist if needed. Many times clients feel alone and isolated, and use the call bell to get attention. You are looking for an INAPPROPRIATE action.*
4. *Wrong choice! This action would be quite appropriate. To help alleviate the client's feelings of isolation, the caregiver can perform tasks such as charting while sitting in a chair in the client's room, rather than at the nurses' station. You are looking for an INAPPROPRIATE action.*

49. A client is confused and disoriented when admitted to the hospital. The doctor has ordered bed rest. Before leaving the client's room, the most important nursing action to provide for the client's safety is:

1. Placing all of the client's belongings in a safe place.
2. Placing the bed in the highest position with the side rails up.
3. Placing the bed in the lowest position with the side rails up.
4. Explaining where everything is in the room.

1. *This action is appropriate, but it is not the most important action in providing for the client's safety. Be sure to read all the options before selecting the best one!*
2. *No! Placing the bed in the highest position puts the client at risk for falling.*
3. **Good work! This option provides for the client's safety by reducing the risk of falling.**
4. *No, the client is confused and disoriented, and may not understand explanations. Try again.*

50. A client is admitted to the hospital and the physician orders stat blood work. The laboratory technician says to the nurse, "I can't do the stat blood work because the client doesn't have an identification bracelet on." The best nursing action is:

1. Draw the blood for the laboratory technician, since the nurse can identify the client.
2. Assure the laboratory technician that you will verify that he has the correct client.
3. Obtain an identification bracelet for the client as quickly as possible.
4. Ask the client to identify himself to the laboratory technician.

1. *This is incorrect. Even though the nurse knows the client, the client must have an identification band to ensure that the name and hospital numbers match the laboratory requisitions. This is necessary to prevent errors in reporting results.*
2. *This will not adequately provide for the client's safety. In order to prevent erroneous reporting of lab results, the laboratory technician needs to match the client's name and number from the identification bracelet with those on the laboratory requisition. Try again.*
3. **Correct! The client needs an identification bracelet to provide for his safety in all aspects of hospitalization.**
4. *The client's name alone is not sufficient identification to ensure the safety of the client. Clients with the same name can be hospitalized in the same health care facility. Try again.*

51. A client is recovering from surgery. The nurse is preparing to irrigate his urinary catheter. To prevent injury to the mucosa of the bladder when irrigating the catheter, the nurse should:

1. Gently compress the ball of the syringe to instill the irrigating solution.
2. Quickly instill the irrigating solution, using some pressure to loosen any clots or mucous.
3. After instilling the solution, apply gentle pressure to remove the irrigating solution from the bladder.
4. Place a sterile cap on the end of the drainage tubing to protect it from contamination.

1. **Good technique! Gentle instillation creates a flow that helps to dilute and free sediment or debris within the lumen of the catheter, while avoiding any force or suction, which could injure the mucosa of the bladder.**
2. *Incorrect! Using force can injure tissue or cause the solution to leak from the connection. Any suction should be avoided because the mucosa of the bladder is easily injured. Removing the syringe from the catheter will break any suction created*

by vacuum.

3. *This is not correct! Using force can injure the mucosa of the bladder.*

4. *A sterile cap can help prevent a potential infection but does not protect the mucosa of the bladder from injury during irrigation. This option does not address the issue in the question.*

52. **In protecting the privacy of a client, the nurse should avoid reporting which of the following to a government agency?**

1. Child abuse.
2. Deaths.
3. Client's change of employment.
4. Elder abuse.

1. *Wrong! Child abuse must be reported. The nurse should follow the institution's procedures.*

2. *Deaths must always be reported. The nurse should follow the institution's procedures.*

3. **Very good! Changing employment is a private concern of the client. The client has the right to withhold this information.**

4. *Elder abuse is client data that must be reported. The nurse should follow the institution's procedures.*

53. **Identifying the client at risk for a postpartum hemorrhage is an important part of obstetrical nursing. Which of the following clients is at the least risk for a postpartum hemorrhage?**

1. Gravida 1, vaginal delivery after two hours of labor.
2. Gravida 1, cesarean section for pregnancy induced hypertension (PIH).
3. Gravida 2, Pitocin induction, vaginal delivery after seven hours of labor.
4. Gravida 1, vaginal delivery at 29 weeks gestation after 10 hours of labor.

1. *Wrong, this client is at high risk. A rapid labor predisposes a client to uterine atony following delivery. Any labor pattern less than three hours in length needs to be watched closely for a postpartum hemorrhage.*

2. *Wrong choice. This client is at high risk. Any operative intervention as well as PIH put this client at risk for a postpartum hemorrhage.*

3. *No, this client is at high risk. When Pitocin is used during labor, there is an increased risk for postpartum hemorrhage due to uterine atony.*

4. **Correct. This client has delivered prematurely, but the small uterus usually contracts very well after delivery. A 10-hour labor is within normal limits for a primigravida. This is the client at the least risk.**

54. **Which finding will the nurse expect to see in a 30-week-gestation premature infant?**

1. Good flexion.
2. Abundant lanugo.
3. Heel creases.
4. Dry, flaky skin.

1. *No, preterm infants are usually in an extended position rather than the state of flexion seen in the term infant.*

2. **Correct. Lanugo, a fine hair covering, is greatest between 28 and 30 weeks gestation and then begins to disappear.**

3. *No, heel creases begin to develop at the top of the foot and proceed to the heels, covering the entire foot at term. Creases are rarely seen at 30 weeks gestation.*

4. *No. In fact, the preterm infant's skin is quite transparent with veins evident. There is usually abundant vernix, the white cheese-like substance that keeps the skin soft.*

55. **Based upon a diagnosis of endometriosis, the nurse should expect the client to complain of:**

1. Heavy menses.
2. Infertility.
3. Frequent temperature elevations.
4. Breast tenderness.

1. *Wrong. The client with endometriosis often complains of painful menses but not heavy bleeding.*

2. **Good choice. The client with endometriosis most commonly has difficulty becoming pregnant and also complains of dysmenorrhea (painful menses) and dyspareunia (painful intercourse).**

3. *No, endometriosis is not related to temperature fluctuations.*

4. *No, endometriosis is not associated with breast tenderness.*

56. **The nurse caring for a client with a diagnosis of breast cancer knows that the client's prognosis is most influenced by:**

1. The client's age.
2. Family history.
3. The stage of the disease.
4. The treatment plan.

1. *Wrong. The client's age is a factor in risk assessment but it does not influence the prognosis once the diagnosis is made.*

2. *Incorrect. Family history is a risk factor for breast cancer but does not affect the prognosis.*

3. **Correct. A client's chances of survival are directly linked to the stage of the disease at**

diagnosis.

4. *Wrong. The type or combination of treatment used does not influence prognosis as greatly as early detection.*

57. **The nurse understands that the primary purpose of a Pap smear is to:**

    1. Screen for uterine cancer.
    2. Diagnose uterine cancer.
    3. Screen for cervical cancer.
    4. Diagnose cervical cancer.

    1. *Wrong. A Pap smear does not screen for uterine cancer.*
    2. *Wrong. A Pap smear is not the way to diagnose uterine cancer. Endometrial biopsy is indicated.*
    3. **Correct. When a client's Pap smear is abnormal, further testing is indicated to screen for cervical cancer. Colposcopy and endocervical biopsy are needed for diagnosis.**
    4. *No, an abnormal Pap smear indicates further testing is needed but does not confirm the diagnosis of cervical cancer.*

58. **A 24-year-old client who is hospitalized with toxic shock syndrome (TSS) asks the nurse to explain the cause of TSS. The nurse's best response to the client is guided by the knowledge that TSS is most commonly associated with:**

    1. Multiple sexual partners.
    2. Intrauterine devices (IUD).
    3. Sexually transmitted diseases (STD).
    4. High absorbency tampons.

    1. *Wrong. TSS is not associated with multiple sexual partners.*
    2. *No, IUDs are not related to the presence of TSS.*
    3. *No, the client with STDs is not at increased risk of TSS.*
    4. **Very good! The use of high-absorbency tampons has been demonstrated to be related to increased risk of TSS.**

59. **A 45-year-old female client seen in the clinic asks the nurse whether she is entering menopause because her menstrual periods have become irregular and she has hot flashes. In assessing this client, the nurse would anticipate which manifestation associated with early menopause?**

    1. Elevations in body temperature above 100° F.
    2. Increases in blood pressure.
    3. Palpitations of the heart.
    4. Atrophy of the vagina.

    1. *Wrong. The client experiencing menopause complains of hot flashes, but they are related to hor-*

monal changes, not body temperature changes.

2. *No, blood pressure changes are not related to early menopause.*
3. **Correct. The menopausal woman often complains of palpitations.**
4. *No, atrophy of the vagina rarely occurs until menopause is nearing its completion.*

60. **A client in a women's clinic tells the nurse that her sister has just been diagnosed with cervical cancer. She tells the nurse that she wishes to be tested to rule out the possibility that she also has the disease, and asks the nurse what tests are used to diagnose this cancer. The nurse's reply is guided by the knowledge that the diagnosis of cancer of the cervix is established by:**

    1. Pap smear.
    2. Endometrial biopsy.
    3. Endocervical biopsy.
    4. Dilation and curettage (D&C).

    1. *Wrong. A Pap smear is a screening tool for cervical cancer but it cannot be used to diagnose it.*
    2. *Wrong. Endometrial biopsy is used to diagnose uterine cancer, not cervical cancer.*
    3. **Correct. A biopsy of the endocervical tissue will confirm cervical cancer.**
    4. *Wrong. A D&C is useful in obtaining endometrial tissue needed to diagnose uterine cancer, not cervical cancer.*

61. **A client with a diagnosis of breast cancer is scheduled to have radiation therapy prior to her mastectomy. The nurse understands that the purpose of the radiation therapy at this time is:**

    1. Reduction of pain.
    2. Decreasing the tumor size.
    3. Destruction of the tumor.
    4. Prevention of infection.

    1. *Wrong. The preoperative use of radiation is primarily to reduce the size of the tumor.*
    2. **Correct. Reduction of the tumor size may decrease the amount of tissue surrounding the breast that will need to be removed.**
    3. *No, radiation may reduce the size of the tumor but it will not accomplish its total destruction.*
    4. *No, this is not correct. Preoperative radiation may actually increase the risk of infection rather than act as a preventive measure.*

62. **A client is given clomiphene citrate (Clomid) to treat her infertility problems. She asks the nurse, "How does this medication work? What kind of drug is it?" In responding, the nurse knows that Clomid:**

    1. Stimulates ovulation.

2. Improves cervical mucous.
3. Treats infections.
4. Is a hormone supplement.

1. ***Excellent! Clomid promotes production of FSH and LH, which in turn stimulates ovulation.***
2. No, Clomid has no effect on cervical mucous.
3. No, Clomid serves no function related to infection.
4. No, Clomid promotes hormone production but does not actually provide hormone supplements.

63. **Which of the following would indicate to the nurse that the injection of Vitamin K (AquaMEPHYTON) given to a newborn has been effective?**

1. Absence of jaundice.
2. Minimal bleeding after circumcision.
3. No evidence of infection.
4. Ecchymotic area at injection site.

1. Wrong. If Vitamin K has any effect on bilirubin that results in jaundice, it would be to elevate it.
2. ***Good work! Vitamin K is given to provide a temporary coagulation until the infant can process his/her own Vitamin K from the bowel.***
3. No, Vitamin K has no effect on treatment and prevention of infections.
4. No, areas of ecchymosis would indicate failure of Vitamin K to prevent bleeding.

64. **A four-year-old who had hydrocephalus is admitted to the hospital for a ventriculoperitoneal shunt. Following the shunt placement, which finding needs an immediate response from the nurse?**

1. Sleepy, very difficult to rouse.
2. Pupils equal and reactive to light.
3. BP 100/60, Apical pulse of 90.
4. Urine output 33 cc in two hours.

1. ***You are correct! The child may be sleepy following surgery, but should be easily roused. Lethargy could indicate increased intracranial pressure.***
2. Sorry, try again. The nurse should expect to find pupils equal and reactive to light. This indicates normal neurological function.
3. Wrong choice. These vital signs are well within normal range for a four-year-old. They do not indicate any need for action.
4. Wrong choice. A urine output of 30 cc in two hours is adequate for renal function. It does not necessitate immediate action.

65. **An eight-year-old child complains of a stomach ache while visiting the school nurse. Which statement by the child would concern the nurse most?**

1. "My stomach ache goes away if I rest for a few minutes."
2. "My friends are picking on me and calling me fatso."
3. "My brother just had his appendix out."
4. "My friends won't let me play kickball with them the way I want to."

1. Wrong choice. This would not be of highest concern. The nurse would want to make sure the child is afebrile and not in acute pain. Otherwise, this could be part of a viral illness. The nurse would want to monitor this, but it is not the most pressing issue of the choices.
2. ***Right! Children rely heavily on what other children say to them and take things said literally. Being ridiculed can lead to problems with self esteem. It's critical for the nurse to look into this statement further and try to intervene.***
3. No. Appendicitis is not contagious. The child may need reassurance or to talk about what has recently happened with the sibling. This is a somewhat normal response and would not be of major concern.
4. Wrong! Children of this age are learning and making up rules all the time. Each one wants to be the leader, and it's hard for them to not be the boss sometimes. This commonly occurs, and children need to work it out for themselves as much as possible.

66. **When assessing a child with a cast, which observation by the nurse would cause the greatest concern?**

1. Itching at the cast site.
2. Indentations in the cast.
3. Swelling distal to the cast.
4. "Hot spots" on the cast.

1. Wrong. Itching may become a concern if the child scratches under the cast, particularly with a sharp object. Client education may avoid this problem. However, itching in itself is relatively common and not of immediate concern.
2. Wrong. A wet cast should be handled by the palms rather than the fingertips in order to avoid indentations that can create pressure areas. Indentations in the cast of a child who is asymptomatic, however, are not of immediate concern.
3. ***Correct! When there is edema and swelling in the casted extremity, the cast may act as a tourniquet, cutting off circulation. Neurovascular damage can occur very quickly. In order to avoid this damage, the nurse elevates the casted extremity, monitors for edema, and reports swelling promptly.***
4. Wrong. "Hot spots" on a cast can indicate infection, and a window will often be cut so that the area can drain. While this is an important assess-

ment to make and report, it is not the highest priority listed. Read the options again, and identify a higher priority concern.

67. A child with a rectal temperature of 39° C has an order for acetaminophen (Tylenol) 280 mg by mouth. The label on the bottle reads 160 mg/5 cc. How many cc's should the nurse give to the child?

   1. 8.8 cc.
   2. 1.8 cc.
   3. 7.0 cc.
   4. 12.7 cc.

   1. *Good work! Use the formula: desired amount (280 mg) divided by amount on hand (160 mg) multiplied by the volume (5 cc).*
   2. *Wrong. This number is too low. Use the formula: desired amount divided by amount on hand, multiplied by volume.*
   3. *Wrong. This amount is too low. Use the formula: desired amount divided by amount on hand, multiplied by volume.*
   4. *Wrong. This amount is too high. Use the formula: desired amount divided by the amount on hand, multiplied by volume.*

68. A concerned mother calls the physician's office. Her child has a respiratory infection and a temperature of 39° C orally. She needs to give her son 240 mg of acetaminophen (Tylenol). The label on her bottle at home reads 160 mg/5 cc. The nurse's most helpful response is:

   1. Give 1/2 teaspoon.
   2. Give 1 1/2 teaspoons.
   3. Give 1 1/2 cc.
   4. Give 15 cc.

   1. *Wrong, too little. 240 mg/160 mg x 5 cc = 7.5 cc. There are 5 cc in a teaspoon. 7.5 cc/5 cc x 1 tsp = 1 1/2 tsp.*
   2. *Great work! 240 mg/160 mg x 5 cc = 7.5 cc. There are 5 cc in a teaspoon. 7.5 cc/5 cc x 1 tsp = 1 1/2 tsp.*
   3. *Sorry, try this again! 240 mg/160 mg x 5 cc = 7.5 cc. There are 5 cc in a teaspoon. 7.5 cc/5 cc x 1 tsp = 1 1/2 tsp.*
   4. *Try this again! 240 mg/160 mg x 5 cc = 7.5 cc. There are 5 cc in a teaspoon. 7.5 cc/5 cc x 1 tsp = 1 1/2 tsp.*

69. A child weighing 1800 gm is admitted. The nurse knows that the infant's weight in pounds is:

   1. 3.9 lbs.
   2. 8.1 lbs.
   3. 18 lbs.
   4. 36 lbs.

   1. *Good! One kilogram is equal to 2.2 pounds. The correct weight in pounds is calculated by multiplying the weight in kilograms by 2.2. There are 1000 grams in a kilogram. 1.8 kg x 2.2 = 3.96 lbs.*
   2. *No. Remember that one kilogram is equal to 2.2 pounds. Therefore, the correct weight is calculated by multiplying the weight in kilograms by 2.2. There are 1000 grams in a kilogram. 1.8 kg x 2.2 = 3.96 pounds.*
   3. *Wrong. One kilogram is equal to 2.2 pounds. The correct weight in pounds is calculated by multiplying the weight in kilograms by 2.2. There are 1000 grams in a kilogram. 1.8 kg x 2.2 = 3.96 lbs.*
   4. *Wrong! One kilogram is equal to 2.2 pounds. The correct weight in pounds is calculated by multiplying the weight in kilograms by 2.2. There are 1000 grams in a kilogram. 1.8 kg x 2.2 = 3.96 lbs.*

70. The nurse is working in a pediatric clinic. Which client would least likely test HIV positive?

   1. A two-month-old whose mother has been an IV drug addict for two years.
   2. A 15-year-old who has been on treatment for hemophilia since infancy.
   3. An eight-year-old whose best friend is HIV positive.
   4. A 16-year-old who is sexually active.

   1. *Incorrect option. This history would place the infant at high risk for HIV, since infection in utero through the placenta is a means of acquiring the virus. Many IV drug abusers are HIV positive. Select again.*
   2. *Wrong choice. This child is at risk, since the blood supply was not consistently tested until the late 1980s. Try another response.*
   3. *Correct. You recognized this is a "casual social contact" and would be considered a low risk for transmission.*
   4. *No, this adolescent is at risk. Hopefully, a condom is being used, but only abstinence offers complete protection from this form of transmission.*

71. A 20-month-old female child is admitted for treatment of burns and investigation into the possibility of abuse. Her parents state that she climbed into the bathtub alone. Which information is most important to include in the documentation by the nurse?

   1. Treatment for the burns, parental visiting patterns and observations of the mother-child relationship.
   2. Parental visiting patterns, parents' comments to nurses, and a description of the burns.
   3. Observation of the mother-child relationship, the types of toys the child has, and whether the child is clean.
   4. Observation of relationship between parents and the client's siblings, treatment of the burns, and the types of toys the child has.

1. *No, this is only partially correct. The child has two parents, as stated in the stem. Try another option.*

2. **Correct! This documentation provides information on the nurturing given by the parents to the child, care of the injury, and response.**

3. *Not the best answer. The types of toys and the cleanliness of the child are more likely to be reflections of the family's socioeconomic status than their potential for further abusive patterns. Make another choice.*

4. *No, this is not the focus. Dysfunctional families frequently treat the abused child differently than the other children in the family, but this is not frequently observable during hospitalization. Try again.*

72. **In which of the following cases would the nurse suspect physical abuse?**

   1. A three-year-old female with 15% burns in a splash pattern over the face and chest, reportedly sustained when she pulled on the tablecloth and a teapot fell, spilling over her.
   2. A 14-month-old male with many bruises on bony prominences, in various stages of healing. The child is reportedly clumsy.
   3. A six-year-old with a spiral fracture of the tibia and fibula that reportedly occurred while riding his bicycle.
   4. A nine-month-old near drowning, who reportedly climbed into the tub and turned on the water.

   1. *This is not a likely abuse case, because the history is consistent with the injury. Toddlers frequently help themselves up by pulling on objects that may be unstable. The splash of burns would occur from head downward.*
   2. *This is not a likely abuse case. Toddlers have recently mastered walking and do have many falls and collisions. Since the bruises are in various stages of healing and over bony prominences, this indicates falling on several occasions.*
   3. *This is not a likely abuse case. Spiral fractures can be caused by physical abuse, but this six-year-old child is just mastering the riding of a bicycle. This injury is consistent with having a foot caught in the spokes of the bike, which would cause the twisting and fracture.*
   4. **Good work! Maybe a nine-month-old could climb into the tub, but turn the water on? This should definitely be followed up. There seems to be a real discrepancy between the story and the expected developmental capability of the infant.**

73. **Upon the client's return from the recovery room, the nurse observes that the fluid in the chest tube bottle has stopped fluctuating. The most appropriate interpretation of this by the nurse is:**

   1. All the fluid and air has been removed.
   2. The tubing may be kinked.
   3. The lungs have re-expanded.
   4. The suction is set too low.

   1. *Highly unlikely. This would be expected to take several days. Choose again.*
   2. **Yes! The nurse should first investigate the entire length of tubing, from the collection bottle to the client, for patency. It is expected in this early postoperative period that a fluctuation would occur with each respiration.**
   3. *No, the lungs will not fully re-expand this quickly. Try again.*
   4. *Incorrect. Fluctuation should occur within the system, even if it is only to gravity drainage. Make another selection.*

74. **The nurse is preparing a seven-year-old female for hospitalization. The child had a previous hospital experience. To best prepare this child, the nurse would:**

   1. Suggest role playing and provide materials.
   2. Remind the child of the experience of her past hospitalization.
   3. Read her a story about another child having a similar operation.
   4. Tell her she is only going in to have her throat checked.

   1. **Yes, concrete experiences are the most meaningful learning for a school-aged child. This is the rationale for pediatric orientation programs. Even if there is inadequate time for her to participate in such a program, a shortened version where she could practice with a mask and other equipment in a non-threatening environment would be helpful.**
   2. *Not the best choice! Be careful! Past experiences may not have been positive, and may even have been traumatic.*
   3. *No, this isn't the best response. This is somewhat abstract, and abstract thinking is not highly developed in the seven-year-old child. Think about how you learned what an operation was really like for a client.*
   4. *Wrong! Never lie to a child. This is inappropriate under any circumstances.*

75. **A nephrectomy is scheduled tomorrow on a three-year-old client. The best preparation for this child by the nurse would be to:**

   1. Demonstrate by pointing on the child's body where

the incision will be made the evening before the procedure.
2. Give the preoperative sedation as ordered with a small needle so that a Band-Aid will not be needed.
3. Ask the child's parents to leave the room while the preoperative medication is administered.
4. Explain the procedure to the child in simple sentences just before giving the preoperative sedation.

1. This action will increase anxiety. The evening before surgery is too long before the procedure to explain to a three-year-old. Make another selection.
2. No, try again. The child does need a Band-Aid because at the age of three the child has fears of mutilation.
3. This is an incorrect action. The child needs the parents for support during the pain of the injection and for immediate comfort following it. Parents should only leave the room if that is their preference.
4. Excellent nursing judgment! The child should have an explanation at an age appropriate level just before the nurse is going to follow through. This approach promotes trust and avoids unnecessary anxiety.

76. **A general anesthesia has been given for multiple tooth extractions on a three-year-old child. He returns crying, but awake, from the recovery room. What approach by the nurse is most likely to be successful?**

1. Examine the mouth first.
2. Leave the mouth until last.
3. It really makes no difference what is done first.
4. Medicate the child for pain first.

1. Wrong. Since this is the area of discomfort, this is likely to cause more crying and uncooperative behavior.
2. Excellent! Leave the most distressing part of an exam on a toddler until the end. You must assess the child before pain medication can be administered.
3. Not true. Rethink this and try again.
4. No, this is inappropriate. An assessment is always performed immediately upon transfer from recovery. Make another choice.

77. **An elderly client with COPD was admitted to the pulmonary unit of the hospital. He complained of shortness of breath, lack of appetite, and difficulty sleeping. The doctor prescribed theophylline (Theo-Dur), 250 mg IV every six hours. The nurse knows that theophylline was prescribed primarily because the drug acts as a:**

1. Vasoconstrictor.
2. Analgesic.
3. Diuretic.
4. Bronchodilator.

1. Incorrect. This is not an action of theophylline. Also, a vasoconstrictor is contraindicated in COPD, as it would decrease blood flow to the pulmonary vasculature.
2. Incorrect. This is not an action of theophylline. An analgesic, such as acetaminophen, is used for pain control.
3. Incorrect. Although theophylline has a mild diuretic effect, this is not its primary action.
4. Correct. Theophylline acts as a bronchodilator, which helps provide maximum passageways for the exchange of air.

78. **Which nursing action will be helpful in treating a client with COPD who has tenacious bronchial secretions?**

1. Maintain semi-Fowler's position as much as possible.
2. Maintain oxygen via nasal prongs at five liters per minute.
3. Encourage a low salt diet.
4. Encourage drinking six to eight glasses of water daily.

1. Incorrect. This position will help the client to breathe more easily but does not affect the consistency of the secretions.
2. Incorrect. COPD clients are maintained on low oxygen flows of one to two liters per minute because higher levels of oxygen would impair the drive to breathe.
3. Incorrect. Although a low salt diet is indicated to limit peripheral edema, it does not affect the client's bronchial secretions.
4. Correct. Fluids will help to liquefy secretions. It is advised that the client drink six to eight glasses of fluid (preferably water) daily.

79. **The nurse caring for a client with Raynaud's disease knows that which statement about this disease is least accurate?**

1. Smoking tobacco worsens the condition.
2. Exposure to cold temperatures aggravates the condition.
3. Radial and ulnar pulses are not palpable or normal.
4. Repeated attacks of vasospasm may progress to ulceration and gangrene.

1. No, this is accurate. Vasoconstriction from the nicotine worsens the condition. Raynaud's disease is a peripheral vascular disorder of the hands in which vasospasms in the arterial wall can result in occlusion, atrophy, and possibly gangrene. You are looking for an INACCURATE statement.
2. No, this is accurate. Exposure to cold results in

vasoconstriction of the hands. Clients are advised to wear gloves in cold weather. Raynaud's disease is a peripheral vascular disorder of the hands in which vasospasms in the arterial wall can result in occlusion, atrophy, and possibly gangrene. You are looking for an INACCURATE statement.

3. **Good choice. This is inaccurate. Raynaud's disease is a peripheral vascular disorder of the hands in which vasospasms in the arterial wall can result in occlusion, atrophy, and possibly gangrene. Radial and ulnar pulses, however, are normal and palpable.**

4. *No, this is accurate. Gangrene can result from chronic vasospasms of the hands. You are looking for an INACCURATE statement.*

80. **In comparing skeletal traction to skin traction, the nurse knows that:**

    1. Skeletal traction can be utilized longer than skin traction.
    2. Clients in skin traction have more pain than those in skeletal traction.
    3. Skin traction is more likely to be complicated by osteomyelitis.
    4. The risk of skin breakdown is greater with skeletal traction.

    1. *Yes! The rationale for the use of skeletal traction is that a greater weight can be applied and the traction can be utilized longer.*
    2. *No. This is too general to be true. The client's injury and pain tolerance are two variables that would have to be assessed.*
    3. *Incorrect. The opposite is true; skeletal traction puts the client at greater risk since the wire or pin is placed through the skin into the bone, where osteomyelitis would occur.*
    4. *Too general. The client's nutritional level, hydration, and type of fracture all need to be evaluated to assess the potential for skin breakdown. All persons in traction are at high risk for skin breakdown due to limited positioning and mobility.*

81. **The client with a fracture of the right femur is placed in skeletal traction with a Thomas splint and Pearson attachment. The nurse knows that the best position for this client:**

    1. Has the client's right foot on the bed in direct line with the femur.
    2. Uses trochanter rolls to prevent abduction of the right leg.
    3. Allows the client to turn slightly from side to side above the waist.
    4. Maintains the client flat with only brief periods with her head elevated.

    1. *No, incorrect. The foot should be off the bed at all times to prevent decubitus ulcers from forming. Try again.*
    2. *No, not correct. The right leg is already stabilized by virtue of the traction and weights. Choose again.*
    3. **Terrific choice! The client may change position without disturbing the line of traction, because the counterforce is provided with counterweights, rather than by using the client's weight.**
    4. *Wrong choice. With the Thomas splint and Pearson attachment, the hips should be in a 20-degree flexed position to maintain the correct pull. Make another selection.*

82. **An elderly client is admitted to the emergency department with unequal grips and aphasia. The initial nursing action for this client is to:**

    1. Prepare to begin an IV infusion.
    2. Raise the HOB to 30 degrees.
    3. Monitor BP.
    4. Explain the MRI to the client and family.

    1. *No, this is not the first measure. Select again.*
    2. **Right! This limits the area of damage by reducing the intracranial pressure. This is a secondary prevention intervention.**
    3. *No, the key word in the question is "initial." Although monitoring blood pressure is an important assessment, this is not the initial action in this case scenario. Try this question again.*
    4. *Incorrect. Diagnosis is not the first measure; you've skipped an important intervention. Make another choice.*

83. **A client is an insulin dependent diabetic. He is scheduled for a gall bladder x-ray in the outpatient department. He was given medication to take as a prep for this test. Which nursing action is most important when preparing the client for this test?**

    1. Explain the procedure to the client, and ask if he has any questions.
    2. Give the client directions to the outpatient department and the parking lot.
    3. Explain to the client that he should not take his insulin before the x-ray.
    4. Tell the client to take his insulin and eat breakfast before leaving home.

    1. *Wrong! Any client scheduled for a test should be given an explanation and an opportunity to ask questions. However, this is not the most important nursing action in preparing the client for the test.*
    2. *No. The client should be given directions to the outpatient department and information about where to park. However, this is not the most important nurs-*

ing action in preparing him for the test.

3. *You selected the correct answer! If the client takes his insulin before the test but remains NPO as required for the procedure, hypoglycemia may result and is potentially life-threatening. Maintaining the glucose level is a physiological need, which should receive highest priority based on Maslow's Hierarchy of Needs.*

4. *No, the client should not eat breakfast. The test for which he is scheduled requires that he remain NPO. It is also very important that the client not take his insulin, because taking his insulin without eating breakfast may cause a potentially life-threatening hypoglycemia.*

84. A client sustained a spontaneous pneumothorax on the left side, and the physician inserted a chest tube to water sealed drainage connected to wall suction. While the nurse was at the bedside, the client sat up quickly and her chest tube caught on the bed rail and was pulled out. The nurse immediately sealed the opening and applied sterile Vaseline gauze, which was available at the bedside. Which nursing actions is most important initially?

1. Call a code, since respiratory arrest is imminent.
2. Notify the charge nurse to call the physician to insert another chest tube, stat!
3. Observe the rate, depth and character of the client's respirations.
4. Document the incident immediately in the client's medical record.

1. *Wrong! A chest tube being pulled out does not mean that respiratory arrest is imminent. While the left lung may collapse again, the right lung should continue to function. This is an implementation activity. The nursing process specifies that assessment should be done prior to implementation.*

2. *The charge nurse needs to notify the physician quickly. However, assessment should be done prior to notifying the physician so that the nurse can accurately report the client's condition.*

3. *Very good! Observing the rate, depth and character of the client's respirations is an assessment activity that provides additional information about her condition. The nursing process indicates that assessment should always be done first, before implementation activities.*

4. *Wrong! The incident should be documented completely in the medical record, and documentation should be done soon after the incident. However, prior to documentation, the nurse must assure that the client's condition is stable. Assessment is required to determine the client's condition.*

85. A client is recuperating from gallbladder surgery preformed under general anesthesia. The nurse should

encourage the client to use the incentive spirometry a minimum of how many times per hour?

1. Two.
2. Five to 10.
3. 10-15.
4. 20-25.

1. *Incorrect. Twice an hour would not be an efficient use of incentive spirometry to decrease the risk of atelectasis and/or pneumonia.*

2. *Good choice. Clients should use incentive spirometry five to 10 times every hour. This device is designed to motivate the client to take deep breaths, and should be included in the postoperative plan of care.*

3. *No, this number of times may tire the client and lead to decreased compliance.*

4. *No, this is beyond the reasonable expectation for a postoperative client. Postoperative breathing exercises must be balanced with turning, coughing, and the client's need for rest.*

86. Compared to the pain of myocardial infarction (MI), the nurse knows that the client with angina pectoris demonstrates pain that:

1. Is relieved by rest.
2. Is substernal or retrosternal.
3. Does not radiate.
4. Is described as tightness or heaviness in the chest.

1. *Correct! Angina pain is usually relieved by rest and/or nitroglycerin, which is not the case with MI pain.*

2. *No, both types of pain may be substernal or retrosternal. Try again.*

3. *Incorrect! Anginal pain can also radiate to the neck, jaw or arms. Choose another option.*

4. *No. Both anginal and MI pain can be described in this way! MI pain is often described as crushing or viselike and is often more severe than angina. Select again.*

87. The nurse would expect a client with hyper-thyroidism to report:

1. Weight gain of 10 pounds in three weeks.
2. Constipation.
3. Sensitivity to cold.
4. Flushed, moist skin.

1. *No. Hyperthyroidism causes an increased rate of body metabolism, so the nurse would expect the client to experience a weight loss. Make another selection.*

2. *Incorrect. Hyperthyroidism is a hypermetabolic state. The client will have increased peristalsis and diar-*

rhea, not constipation. Try another option.

3. *Not true. Clients with hyperthyroidism have an increased metabolic rate and are always "warm" due to the energy expenditure. They have heat intolerance. Choose again.*

4. ***Correct assessment! Clients with hyperthyroidism tolerate heat poorly and perspire unusually freely; the skin is flushed continuously, with a characteristic salmon color, and is likely to be warm, soft, and moist.***

88. **The nurse would expect a client admitted with Cushing's syndrome to report:**

   1. Weight loss.
   2. Diarrhea.
   3. Double vision.
   4. Increased bruising.

   1. *No, the client with Cushing's syndrome will have a weight gain due to overproduction of adrenal cortical hormone. Choose again.*
   2. *Incorrect. The gastrointestinal disturbances found in Cushing's syndrome are minimal. The major concern is for complications of peptic ulcer and pancreatitis secondary to glucocorticoid therapy. Make another selection.*
   3. *No, there is no evidence of this visual disturbance in Cushing's syndrome. The only eye complications may be glaucoma or corneal lesions. Select again.*
   4. ***Good assessment! You remembered that clients with Cushing's syndrome have thin skin, which is fragile and easily traumatized; ecchymoses and striae will often develop.***

89. **A client is admitted to the CCU following a myocardial infarction. The nurse understands that digoxin (Lanoxin) has been ordered for him because the drug helps to:**

   1. Dilate the coronary arteries.
   2. Strengthen the heartbeat.
   3. Increase the electrical conductivity of the heart.
   4. Decrease calcium uptake by the cells.

   1. *Incorrect. Digoxin is not a vasodilator. Do not confuse its action with that of nitroglycerin, which is a vasodilator used in angina pectoris. Try again.*
   2. ***Correct. Digoxin strengthens the heartbeat by increasing myocardial contractility.***
   3. *Incorrect. Digoxin does not have an effect on the electrical conductivity of the heart. Do not confuse its action with that of atropine and quinidine sulfate, which are anti-arrhythmic drugs.*
   4. *Incorrect. Digoxin is not an anti-arrhythmic drug. Try again.*

90. **Which of the following statements demonstrate to the nurse that the client understands the purpose of his cardiac pacemaker?**

   1. "I won't have to worry about ever having a heart attack now that I have a pacemaker."
   2. "Now I can eat whatever I want and it won't affect my heart, since the pacemaker will take care of my heart."
   3. "Having a pacemaker means that my heart can never stop beating."
   4. "The pacemaker will help stimulate my heart to beat when my heart rate is very slow."

   1. *Incorrect. This is a misconception about the function of a pacemaker.*
   2. *Incorrect. A low fat, low salt diet is necessary for cardiac clients to prevent further complications.*
   3. *Incorrect. The pacemaker operates on a battery pack, which needs to be monitored periodically. Also, a pacemaker cannot prevent a heart attack.*
   4. ***Correct. This is a primary purpose of a cardiac pacemaker.***

91. **Patient education of the client with active tuberculosis is important in helping to prevent the spread of the disease. The most effective method for the nurse to teach the client in order to help prevent the spread of infection is to:**

   1. Maintain strict isolation during the active phases of the disease.
   2. Cover nose and mouth with several layers of tissues when coughing or sneezing.
   3. Wear a protective mask while in public.
   4. Encourage the family to wear a protective mask while with the client.

   1. *Incorrect. Respiratory isolation, not strict isolation, is indicated for the active phases of TB.*
   2. ***Correct. Covering the nose and mouth with tissues during coughing and sneezing will prevent infectious droplets from being dispersed. Correct disposal of the tissues in a covered receptacle is also indicated.***
   3. *Incorrect. This is not necessary. The client needs to prevent the spread of infection by using tissues and good hand washing techniques.*
   4. *Incorrect. This is not necessary. Advise the family members to wash their hands after direct contact with the client.*

92. **A client is admitted with bleeding esophageal varices. The physician has opted to use esophageal tamponade with a Sengstaken-Blakemore tube to control the bleeding. Which of the following nursing interventions is**

appropriate when caring for the client while the Blakemore tube is in place?

1. Ambulate the client four times a day.
2. Encourage clear liquids.
3. Provide mouth and nares care every two hours.
4. Maintain the manometer pressure of the esophageal balloon at all times to control bleeding.

1. *No! The client must remain on bedrest while the Blakemore tube is in place to prevent accidental dislodgment, which can cause asphyxia. Choose another option.*
2. *No! The client will be NPO due to the placement of the tube. Remember that the client will be unable to swallow and may require suctioning of the oral cavity to remove secretions. Make another selection.*
3. ***Correct intervention. If the client is alert, the nurse should provide tissues, and encourage spitting of saliva into a tissue or basin. If the client is not alert, gentle suctioning may be needed.***
4. *Not correct procedure. The esophageal balloon is usually deflated in approximately 12 hours to assess if bleeding has stopped. It can be left inflated for up to 48 hours without tissue damage or severe discomfort. Choose again.*

93. **Postural drainage with percussion is ordered for a client with pneumonia. What would the nurse include in the plan for this procedure?**

1. Perform this procedure before meals.
2. Cup and clap lightly, to avoid causing redness to the client's skin.
3. Administer bronchodilators after percussion and before postural drainage.
4. Provide analgesia prior to each treatment.

1. ***Good, you selected correctly. To facilitate the client's ability to tolerate the procedure, an empty stomach is recommended.***
2. *Incorrect. Percussion, when performed correctly, causes a slight redness, even though the client's gown or a towel is placed between the percussor's hands and the client's skin. Select again.*
3. *No. Bronchodilators would be given approximately 20-30 minutes before the treatment to facilitate the drainage of secretions. Try again.*
4. *No, this would be counterproductive. This procedure is not considered painful, and the ability of the client to cough effectively following the treatment may be diminished with analgesia. Make another selection.*

94. **Which is the best action by the nurse to monitor skin integrity for a client in Buck's traction?**

1. Instruct the client to describe any pain from under the boot.
2. Remove the traction and boot to examine the skin every shift.
3. Paint the skin with Betadine, which will toughen the skin to prevent breakdown.
4. Observe for any drainage through the boot, and report to the physician immediately.

1. *Incorrect. The client can be instructed to report pain, but this is not the best method to assess skin integrity. Try again.*
2. ***Great job, this is correct. The best method of assessment is a visual inspection to pick up early signs of skin changes.***
3. *No, you're not answering the question. This is an intervention, not an assessment or monitoring function. Try again.*
4. *No, incorrect. By the time drainage has occurred, there is a serious interruption in the skin integrity. This is not the best way to determine alterations in skin integrity! Make another selection.*

95. **While the nurse is taking vital signs, an irregularity in the heart rate is noticed. Which nursing action would be most appropriate?**

1. Request the assistance of another staff member and take an apical/radial pulse.
2. Count the apical pulse rate for one full minute and describe the irregularity in the chart.
3. Call the doctor and request an order for a Holter monitor recording for the next day.
4. Take the pulse at each peripheral site and count the rate for 30 seconds.

1. *Wrong. An apical/radial pulse is used to identify a deficit between the apical and radial rates. It is not used to assess irregularity in the pulse, which is the issue in this question. This option doesn't describe the most appropriate nursing action when assessing a cardiac irregularity.*
2. ***Congratulations! When the pulse is regular, it may be counted for 15 seconds and multiplied by four, or counted for 30 seconds and multiplied by two. However, if the pulse is irregular, it must be counted for a full minute to obtain an accurate rate. The irregularity should be described in the chart.***

> **TEST-TAKING TIP:** Note that the word "irregularity" appears in the stem of the question and in this option. Although this test-taking strategy is not foolproof, in this question these similar words are a good clue!

3. *Wrong! An irregular pulse rate must be accurately counted and described and should be followed up immediately, generally by continuously monitor-*

ing the cardiac rhythm by telemetry. A Holter monitor recording the next day may be too late!

4. *Incorrect choice! Assessment of all peripheral pulses is appropriate for a client with a cardiovascular problem. That assessment, however, is related to the adequacy of circulation to each extremity rather than to regularity of the heart rate. This option does not address the issue in this question. The stem asks you to select the most appropriate nursing action when assessing a cardiac irregularity.*

96. **Which approach by the nurse is best when taking the blood pressure of a client with hypertension?**

    1. Measure the blood pressure under the same conditions each time.
    2. Take the blood pressure with the client sitting on the side of the bed.
    3. Place the blood pressure cuff on the right arm above the elbow.
    4. Measure the blood pressure with the client in supine position.

    1. ***Congratulations! This is the correct answer. The nurse should record the client's position in the chart so that the next reading may be done with the client in the same position.***

    STRATEGY ALERT! *The other three options are similar to each other in that they each describe a specific position or method. This is a broader or more global response.*

    2. *This is not the answer. The client may be sitting, lying or standing when blood pressure is measured. The nurse should record the client's position in the chart so that the reading may be done with the client in the same position each time.*
    3. *This is not the answer. The blood pressure cuff may be placed above the elbow on either the right or left arm.*
    4. *This is not the answer. The client may be sitting, lying or standing when blood pressure is measured. The nurse should record the client's position in the chart so that the reading may be done with the client in the same position each time.*

97. **A client has undergone a transurethral resection of the prostate to correct benign prostatic hypertrophy. He has returned from the recovery room with an indwelling urinary catheter. For several hours the urinary output has been adequate. The nurse notes, however, that the catheter has drained no urine during the last hour. What should the nurse do first?**

    1. Offer the client 100 cc of oral fluids each hour.
    2. Irrigate the catheter according to the postoperative orders.

    3. Call the physician and request an increase in IV fluid rate.
    4. Monitor the vital signs every 15 minutes for one hour.

    1. *Wrong. A sudden stop in urine output from the catheter following prostate surgery is probably the result of an occluded catheter. Increasing oral fluids without removing the obstruction in the catheter will just cause the client to be uncomfortable.*
    2. ***You are correct! A sudden stop in urine output from the catheter following prostate surgery is probably the result of an occluded catheter. Irrigation will remove a clot from the catheter. Note that the word "catheter" appears in the stem of the question and in the correct answer.***
    3. *Try again. A sudden stop in urine output from the catheter following prostate surgery is probably the result of an occluded catheter. Increasing IV fluids without removing the obstruction in the catheter will just cause the client to be uncomfortable.*
    4. *Wrong. Monitoring the vital signs is not relevant because there is no indication in the case situation that the vital signs are not stable.*

98. **A client who has been diagnosed with CHF (congestive heart failure) two days earlier begins to exhibit manifestations of left-sided heart failure. Which of the following would the nurse observe?**

    1. Peripheral edema.
    2. Dyspnea.
    3. Abdominal distention.
    4. Fatigue.

    1. *No, peripheral edema due to elevated venous pressure is associated with right-sided heart failure.*
    2. ***Excellent! Dyspnea is a classic manifestation of left-sided heart failure. In left-sided failure, the left atrium cannot effectively empty its contents into the ventricle so left atrial pressure rises and causes increased pulmonary hydrostatic pressure. Fluid moves from circulation into interstitial spaces and into alveoli.***
    3. *Incorrect. Abdominal distention due to elevated venous pressure is associated with right-sided failure.*
    4. *Incorrect. Fatigue due to elevated venous pressure is associated with right-sided failure.*

99. **A client is admitted with acute leukemia. The nurse can anticipate that the client will report:**

    1. Nausea/vomiting, diarrhea.
    2. Fatigue, weakness.
    3. Fever, chills.
    4. Nosebleed, headache.

1. *Incorrect. These manifestations may result from chemotherapy to treatment the leukemia, but they are not characteristic of the disease process. Select another option.*
2. ***Good choice! Fatigue and weakness secondary to anemia are the most common presenting manifestations.***
3. *No. Fever and chills may result from an infection secondary to granulocytopenia, but they are not presenting manifestations of leukemia. Try again.*
4. *No. Bleeding tendencies, such as nosebleed, may occur due to thrombocytopenia, but headache is seen when the client has meningeal leukemia. It is not a common presenting manifestation. Make another selection.*

100. **A client diagnosed with AIDS is placed on zidovudine (Retrovir) (formerly AZT). The nurse monitors the client for which life-threatening side effect of this drug?**

1. Fever.
2. Aplastic anemia.
3. Renal failure.
4. Cardiac dysrhythmia.

1. *Incorrect. Fever is not a side effect of Retrovir therapy. Choose again.*
2. ***Good! Severe bone marrow depression, resulting in anemia, is the most common life-threatening adverse reaction of Retrovir therapy.***
3. *No, Retrovir is not known as a nephrotoxic agent. It is rapidly metabolized to an inactive compound and excreted by the kidneys. Make another selection.*
4. *No, Retrovir has no known effects upon the heart. Try another option.*

NCLEX-PN

Test 2

NCLEX-PN TEST 2

1. A client is admitted to a nursing home. She has difficulty seeing and hearing. A nursing action that would place the client at risk would be:

   1. Showing the client where all of the furniture and personal items are in the room.
   2. Talking loudly to the client when entering her room.
   3. Telling the client that because of her increased risk of falling and injuring herself, she is not allowed out of her room.
   4. Assisting the client to identify the placement of food items during meals.

2. An infant is in respiratory isolation. The nurse can most effectively prevent the spread of pathogens via droplet infection by:

   1. Wearing a gown and mask when feeding the client.
   2. Using sterile gloves when changing her diapers.
   3. Having the baby wear a mask when in the playroom.
   4. Using enteric precautions when caring for the baby.

3. While changing the linen on a client's bed, how should the nurse handle the linen?

   1. Hold it close to the body to avoid dropping it.
   2. Place soiled linen on the chair until done making the bed.
   3. Hold the linen away from the body and uniform.
   4. Shake clean linen to unfold it and provide ease in making the bed.

4. A client is recovering from an appendectomy. While changing the linens on the client's bed, the nurse notes drainage from an infected wound has soiled the bed sheet. What is the best method for changing this linen?

   1. Carefully place the soiled sheet in the cloth linen bag and label it as contaminated.
   2. Spray the soiled area with a bleach solution prior to placing it in the linen bag.
   3. Carefully place the soiled sheet in a moisture-resistant plastic linen bag designated for soiled articles.
   4. Discard the sheet into a plastic trash bag.

5. During a well-child visit, the mother of a five-year-old expresses concern that her son refuses to wear his helmet while riding his bicycle. What is the appropri-

ate nursing response?

   1. "Tell him the bike doesn't leave the garage without the helmet."
   2. "It isn't that important, since he won't be riding in the road."
   3. "Gradually encourage the wearing of the helmet with small rewards."
   4. "I'll explain the potential for injury without a helmet."

6. A registered nurse, who has previously been treated for an addiction to hydromorphone (Dilaudid), is being treated on the psychiatric unit for anxiety and associated somatic manifestations. The psychiatrist orders propranolol (Inderal) for the anxiety. The client recognizes the medication and states, "There must be some mistake. I don't have any cardiac problems." Which statement offers the best nursing response?

   1. "This drug was ordered because you have a history of drug abuse and your psychiatrist doesn't want to prescribe anything that could lead to physical dependence."
   2. "This drug also has a psychiatric use. It is not only used for cardiac problems."
   3. "There is no mistake. Your psychiatrist ordered Inderal for you. Do you have a history of hypertension?"
   4. "Inderal is used to control anxiety in persons like yourself, who have a lot of physical manifestations of anxiety."

7. A confused elderly client is on strict bedrest. Which nursing intervention will provide for this client's safety?

   1. Place the client in a room away from the noise and confusion of the nurses' station.
   2. Avoid the use of nightlights, since they tend to distort images and confuse clients.
   3. Discuss with the client the need for restraints if she continues to get out of bed.
   4. Provide opportunities for regular toileting, and include this information in the client's care plan.

8. The nurse should avoid reporting which of the following events to a government agency?

   1. Births.
   2. Child abuse.

3. Marital quarrels.
4. Typhoid fever.

9. The nurse understands that which of the following is outside the scope of a client's right of privacy:

1. Not having a gunshot wound reported, upon timely request.
2. Refusing to receive visitors.
3. Wearing one's own clothing.
4. Requesting the presence of a member of the same sex during a physical examination.

10. The best nursing action to prevent the spread of infection among hospitalized clients is:

1. Using sterile technique when performing any procedure.
2. Hand washing before coming in contact with each client.
3. Wearing gloves to perform any procedure.
4. Wearing a mask and gown while performing any procedure.

11. The nurse is preparing the staffing assignment. An infant on the unit has AIDS and cytomegalovirus (CMV). Which staff person should be assigned as the primary care giver for this child?

1. An experienced practical nurse who is six months pregnant.
2. A male graduate nurse, recently oriented to pediatrics.
3. An experienced nurse's aide who is healthy.
4. A licensed practical nurse with eczema.

12. The home health nurse notes several suspicious bruises and old burns on a 10-month-old child while making an initial home visit. The priority nursing action to provide for the child's safety is:

1. Call the child protection hotline and report possible abuse.
2. Discuss the family with the physician and social worker at the next team meeting.
3. Tell the mother that child protection will be notified if injuries are noted on the next visit.
4. Carefully record the visit for follow-up.

13. At a boy scout camp the nurse encounters a child who exhibits a high-pitched inspiratory sound, and cyanosis. Describe the procedure that the nurse should institute.

1. Stand behind the child and apply an upward thrust below the xiphoid.
2. Monitor the child, and if respirations cease, use the Heimlich maneuver.

3. Bend the child forward and deliver back blows to dislodge the object.
4. Begin cardiopulmonary resuscitation.

14. The nurse is caring for a client who is paralyzed on his right side following a stroke. In preparing to give a bed bath to the client, which of the following nursing actions is best?

1. Adjust the bed to the lowest position, in case the client falls.
2. Raise the bed to the high horizontal position.
3. Put the bed in low semi-Fowler's position.
4. Unplug the bed.

15. A client is admitted with a diagnosis of premature labor. The nurse understands that which of the following drugs should be avoided when treating premature labor?

1. Magnesium sulfate.
2. Ritodrine (Yutopar).
3. Betamethasone (Celestone).
4. Terbutaline sulfate (Brethine).

16. The nurse is about to administer methylergonovine maleate (Methergine) to a postpartum client. Which assessment would have priority prior to the administration of this drug?

1. Fundus.
2. Blood pressure.
3. Apical pulse.
4. Respiratory rate.

17. You are caring for a client receiving IV magnesium sulfate to treat her severe pregnancy induced hypertension. Which assessment needs to be reported to the RN immediately?

1. Deep tendon reflexes change from +4 to +2.
2. Maternal blood pressure changes from 160/110 to 148/90.
3. Urinary output drops from 40 cc to 28 cc per hour.
4. Respiratory rate changes from 22 to 16 breaths per minute.

18. A client is admitted to the labor unit because of premature labor, with rupture of membranes. She is given betamethasone (Celestone). The nurse understands that the purpose of this drug is:

1. Uterine relaxation.
2. Fetal lung maturity.
3. Prevention of chorioamnionitis.
4. Enhancement of fetal oxygenation.

19. A client is to receive prostaglandin E2 (PGE2) vaginal suppositories to prepare the cervix for induction of labor. Which side effect should the nurse anticipate?

1. Nausea and vomiting.
2. Hypertension.
3. Vaginal bleeding.
4. Severe headaches.

20. A client with hypertension is being treated with chlorothiazide (Diuril) 500 mg. PO twice a day. In taking the client's medication history, the nurse notes that the client is a diabetic and has been taking chlorpropamide (Diabinese) 250 mg. PO daily. The nurse is aware that the potential interaction of Diabinese with Diuril may result in:

1. Hypocalcemia.
2. Hyperglycemia.
3. Aplastic anemia.
4. Hypoglycemia.

21. The nurse is to administer erythromycin (Ilotycin) to a client for preventative treatment of ophthalmia neonatorum. The nurse knows the correct technique is:

1. Inject intramuscularly in the front of the thigh.
2. Inject subcutaneously in either arm.
3. Pull down the lower eyelid and instill along the lower surface towards the nose.
4. Pull down the lower eyelid and instill along the lower surface away from the nose.

22. As you are driving home one day, a man flags you down. His car will not start and his wife is in active labor, crying that the baby is coming. Which nursing action receives the lowest priority?

1. Maintain a calm atmosphere.
2. Tie off or cut the umbilical cord.
3. Hold the baby up by the feet and rub the back after delivery.
4. Dry the newborn off.

23. The nurse checks a postpartum client's peripad and finds a large amount of rubra lochia with several clots. What is the priority nursing action?

1. Check the vital signs.
2. Check for a full bladder.
3. Check the fundus.
4. Complete a vaginal exam.

24. A client has a postpartum hemorrhage as a result of a cervical laceration. The nurse would expect to observe:

1. Continuous vaginal bleeding in the presence of a firm fundus.
2. Rapidly rising fundal height with continuous vaginal bleeding.
3. Continuous vaginal bleeding in presence of a boggy uterus.
4. Intermittent vaginal bleeding in the presence of a relaxed uterus.

25. The nurse is caring for an Rh negative obstetrical client who is to receive Rh_o (D) human immune globulin (RhoGAM). The nurse understands that which of the following is inconsistent with indications for administration of RhoGAM?

1. Birth of an Rh negative infant.
2. Amniocentesis.
3. Ectopic pregnancy.
4. Pregnancy at 28 weeks gestation.

26. A three-month-old child was admitted with a tentative diagnosis of intussusception. The parents ask the nurse how the diagnosis is made. The correct explanation by the nurse is:

1. "A small amount of tissue from the colon will be biopsied."
2. "Genotyping can identify this condition."
3. "A barium enema will be given to visualize the obstruction."
4. "An upper GI series should identify the area involved."

27. A six-month-old is in the pediatric clinic. The nurse practitioner ordered a DPT vaccine to be administered. Which finding by the nurse would cause the nurse to question the administration of the DPT vaccine?

1. Previous evidence of sensitivity to egg antigens.
2. Fever and high-pitched cry following last DPT.
3. Current rectal temperature of 100° F.
4. Currently receiving steroid therapy.

28. An eight-year-old child has a fever of 104° F upon returning from surgery. The priority nursing action is:

1. Document and continue to monitor.
2. Begin sponging with tepid water.
3. Administer acetaminophen (Tylenol) P.O. as ordered.
4. Notify the nurse in charge.

29. Nursing interventions for the child with cerebral palsy are mainly directed toward:

1. Genetic counseling.
2. Motor development.
3. Special education.
4. Seizure control.

30. A child is being admitted with otitis media. The nurse's assessment findings are most likely to include:

1. Elevated temperature and tugging on the affected ear.
2. Clear drainage from the affected ear and sore

throat.

3. Elevated temperature and rhinorrhea.
4. Anorexia and diarrhea.

31. **Which statement by a child's father indicates to the nurse that further teaching is necessary before discharging his child in a plaster cast?**

1. "After a bath, the cast must be allowed to dry completely."
2. "Petaling will prevent skin breakdown."
3. "Any odor should be reported to the doctor immediately."
4. "Elevation will reduce swelling."

32. **A two-year-old boy is brought to the emergency room with nausea and diarrhea. Which statement by the parents would most concern the nurse?**

1. "His last wet diaper smelled very strong."
2. "He is very quiet when he is playing."
3. "His lips are dry and crusty."
4. "He cries whenever I put him down."

33. **Priority nursing interventions for the child in Buck's traction are directed at:**

1. Pin site care.
2. Maintaining skin integrity.
3. Increasing calcium intake.
4. Exercising the affected extremity.

34. **The nurse caring for a nine-month-old infant knows to avoid giving the infant:**

1. Dry cold cereal.
2. Orange juice.
3. Raw carrot chunks.
4. Scrambled egg.

35. **The nurse is caring for a child who has just received a ventriculoperitoneal shunt. The nurse knows correct positioning for this client postoperatively is:**

1. Side-lying.
2. HOB elevated 30 degrees.
3. In a position of comfort for the client.
4. Supine.

36. **A two-year-old is scheduled for a cardiac catheterization. Which statement by the mother would indicate that the nurse's teaching has been successful?**

1. "I'm pleased that my child will no longer have blue spells."
2. "Although this is not a permanent repair, my baby will be some better."
3. "After this is done, we will know what has to be done for my child."

4. "My child will have a large scar following this procedure."

37. **Following hospitalization for 10 days, an 11-month-old child is quiet and sad when his mother leaves. The nurse knows this behavior indicates:**

1. An understanding of his mother's need to leave.
2. Despair at his mother's absence.
3. Protest that his source of emotional support is gone.
4. Developing autonomy.

38. **The nurse's clinical assessment of two-year-old child who is poorly nourished is most likely to include:**

1. Mother's statement that the child is a "picky eater."
2. Height and weight in the 25th percentile.
3. Observing that the child is slender and active.
4. Dry colorless hair and pale skin.

39. **A client was admitted to the hospital with an infection of his left foot. The nurse notes that he has a strong body odor and appears to be in need of a bath. The nurse notes that he is watching TV and that his left leg is cool to touch and slightly mottled. He is very abrupt in response to the nurse's questions. Which of the following data is most important for the nurse to document about the client?**

1. Appears to be comfortable, since he is watching TV.
2. Uncooperative in answering the nurse's questions.
3. Poor personal hygiene.
4. Left leg is cool to touch and slightly mottled.

40. **Which complaint by a client would lead the nurse to believe the client may be experiencing a myocardial infarction?**

1. A feeling of an intermittent strangling sensation.
2. Complaints of sudden substernal pain after an argument.
3. Feelings of numbness or weakness in arms and wrists.
4. Profuse perspiration with nausea and vomiting.

41. **After a bronchoscopy, the nurse would give immediate consideration to a client's complaint of:**

1. Blood-tinged mucous.
2. Hoarseness when speaking.
3. Irritation and discomfort when swallowing.
4. Difficulty breathing.

42. **The nurse takes precautions to prevent constipation and fecal impaction in an immobilized client. The nurse is aware that, if a client develops a fecal impaction,**

what serious complication could result?

1. Intestinal obstruction.
2. Bowel perforation.
3. Peritonitis.
4. Rectal bleeding.

43. **The nurse has just collected a liquid stool specimen for ova and parasites. The test results may be compromised if the nurse:**

1. Places the specimen into a clean container.
2. Puts the collected specimen in the refrigerator.
3. Instructs the client to defecate into a bedpan.
4. Sends only the bloody and mucoid portions of the stool.

44. **Following a gastric resection, a client is taught nutritional habits that will slow gastric emptying, helping to decrease the incidence of the "dumping syndrome." Which food selection by the client indicates to the nurse that he understands the instructions given?**

1. Ice cream.
2. Oranges.
3. Wheat bread.
4. Turkey.

45. **A client is admitted to the hospital with a diagnosis of active pulmonary tuberculosis. An immediate nursing goal is to control the spread of infection. To control the spread of active tuberculosis, the nurse would:**

1. Wear a gown and mask when caring for the client.
2. Recommend that the client wear a mask when she has visitors.
3. Teach the client how to cover her nose and mouth when she coughs or sneezes.
4. Use blood and needle precautions.

46. **A client is scheduled for a chest x-ray to rule out pneumonia. The nurse explains to the client that the preparation for the chest x-ray includes:**

1. Fasting for four hours prior to the procedure.
2. Signing a consent form for an invasive procedure.
3. Benadryl 25 mg IM prior to the procedure.
4. No special preparation.

47. **Following a total hip replacement, the nurse takes precautions to ensure that the affected hip is flexed no more than:**

1. 25 degrees.
2. 60 degrees.
3. 75 degrees.
4. 90 degrees.

48. **The client has just returned from the x-ray department after undergoing an upper GI series. Which nursing action would be appropriate at this time?**

1. Keep him NPO until the gag reflex returns.
2. Administer a cleansing enema.
3. Monitor his vital signs every 15 minutes for one hour or until stable.
4. Give milk of magnesia 30 cc P.O.

49. **A client is admitted with end stage cirrhosis of the liver. Which nursing measure would help to decrease the serum ammonia level?**

1. Administration of vitamin K (AquaMEPHY-TON).
2. Increased fluid intake.
3. Administration of diuretics.
4. Offer a low-protein, high-calorie diet.

50. **A person in a restaurant puts his hand to his throat. A nurse who sees this happen begins to administer the Heimlich maneuver. After the client falls to the floor, the nurse should:**

1. Check for the pulse.
2. Sweep the mouth.
3. Attempt to ventilate.
4. Administer five abdominal thrusts.

51. **A client received a large contusion on the head and a fracture of the femur. The nurse must be alert for possible complications. Which sign or symptom indicates a serious complication to the nurse?**

1. A change in temperature from 98.4° F to 98.2° F.
2. A blood pressure decrease from 120/90 to 112/74.
3. Increased pain at the site of the femur fracture.
4. A change in respiratory rate from 18 to 32, with increased restlessness.

52. **A client is hospitalized with chronic obstructive pulmonary disease. Oxygen per nasal cannula at two liters per minute is initiated. When the nurse made an assessment at 3:00 p.m., the client appeared to have made a good adjustment to hospitalization. At 5:00 p.m., when the nurse brought the client his dinner tray, the oxygen cannula is found on the floor. The client was angry and said, "It's about time you got here. Where am I? Where is my breakfast?" The nurse should give immediate consideration to which consideration?**

1. Has the oxygen cannula been off long enough to cause hypoxia?
2. Is the client's anger is related to being hospitalized again?
3. Does the client need a clock in the room to keep track of the time?

4. Is the client accustomed to eating meals at unusual times?

53. **A client is admitted to the hospital with a diagnosis of chest pain. The client is scheduled for a cardiac catheterization. The nurse would immediately report which assessment data about the client to the charge nurse?**

1. The client is allergic to lobster.
2. The client's father smokes heavily.
3. The client's husband died of heart disease.
4. The client is apprehensive about the procedure.

54. **A client is receiving dietary instructions after being admitted for ascites and an elevated serum ammonia level, secondary to cirrhosis. The nurse would know that the client had accurate understanding of his dietary needs if he selected a menu that was:**

1. High in protein, low in salt.
2. High in calories, moderate in protein.
3. Low in carbohydrates, high in fat.
4. Low in calcium, low in potassium.

55. **Following the completion of discharge teaching, the nurse would determine that instructions about the long-term consequences of cirrhosis were successful if the client indicates an understanding that he must refrain from:**

1. Drinking alcohol.
2. Smoking.
3. Eating spicy foods.
4. Donating blood.

56. **A client has received instructions about behaviors that put him at risk for developing hepatitis A. Which statement by the client indicates to the nurse that he has an accurate understanding of this information?**

1. "I won't donate blood anymore."
2. "I'll get a booster shot of immune serum globulin every year."
3. "I'll stop eating raw clams, even though I love them!"
4. "I won't touch another drop of alcohol."

57. **The physician has ordered a sputum specimen to be collected for culture and sensitivity. The nurse is aware that the preferable time to collect this specimen is:**

1. In the morning.
2. In the evening, after forcing fluids all day.
3. After antibiotics have been started.
4. After the client has taken an expectorant.

58. **A client had a right lobectomy yesterday and has a chest tube to suction at 20 cm of water pressure. Upon assessment of the client this morning, the nurse notes that** there is no fluctuation in the water-seal chamber. At this time, the nurse would first:

1. Increase the suction until fluctuation reappears.
2. Observe for kinks in the tubing.
3. Elevate the head of the bed to 80 degrees.
4. No action is necessary, since the lung has most likely re-expanded.

59. **A client has just returned to the unit after a right pneumonectomy. The nurse should position the client on the:**

1. Right side.
2. Left side or back.
3. Back only.
4. Right side or left side.

60. **In treating diabetic ketoacidosis (DKA), the nurse is aware that the goal of treatment is to correct which imbalance?**

1. Hypoglycemia.
2. Dehydration.
3. Hyperkalemia.
4. Respiratory acidosis.

61. **A client has been admitted to the hospital after having two seizures at work. She suddenly gives a short cry and stiffens. The initial nursing action for the client is to:**

1. Make a mental notation of the time after looking at a watch.
2. Place an oral airway in the client's mouth.
3. Loosen the clothing around the neck.
4. Turn her head to the side.

62. **To assess for correct placement of a nasogastric tube, the nurse should:**

1. Instill 30 ml of saline to assess client tolerance.
2. Instill 10 ml of air into the tube and listen for gurgling sounds with a stethoscope over the gastric area.
3. Aspirate stomach contents with a syringe.
4. Place the end of the tube in water to assess for bubbling.

63. **A 39-year-old female has had a right radical mastectomy. Which activity would the nurse anticipate will be the most difficult for this client four days postoperatively?**

1. Brushing her hair with her right hand.
2. Eating with her right hand.
3. Active-assisted range of motion of the right hand.
4. Washing her hands in a basin.

64. A colostomy has been performed on a client diagnosed with colon cancer. Postoperatively, the nurse is preparing to change the dressing. The nurse would expect the appearance of the stoma to be:

    1. Pale, with a mucoid discharge from the ostomy.
    2. Bright red, with a few drops of blood appearing from the stoma.
    3. Inclusive of a 2 cm area of eschar.
    4. Flush with the abdominal wall.

65. Physiologically, the nurse knows the difference between angina and myocardial infarction is:

    1. With angina, arterial perfusion is briefly inadequate. With myocardial infarction, arterial perfusion is cut off permanently.
    2. With angina, the enzymes SGOT, LDH, and CPK are elevated. With myocardial infarction, they are not elevated.
    3. With angina, adrenocorticosteroids are released to reduce the inflammatory reaction. With myocardial infarction, these hormones are absent.
    4. With angina, hypertension and congestive heart failure are absent. With myocardial infarction, hypertension and congestive heart failure are present.

66. A client with increasing intracranial pressure has received mannitol (Osmitrol) intravenously. The nurse would know that the mannitol has been effective if the client has which of these findings?

    1. Increased urine output.
    2. Decreased pulse rate.
    3. Elevated blood pressure.
    4. Negative Babinski reflex.

67. A male client has been given instructions about the cerebral angiogram that is scheduled for later this morning. Which statement by the client indicates to the nurse that additional teaching is needed?

    1. "The only allergy I have is to ragweed. I'm glad it won't affect this test."
    2. "I signed the special consent form last evening."
    3. "I'm glad this procedure has less risks than an MRI."
    4. "The nurse told me that I'll feel a flush as the dye is injected."

68. A physician has prescribed oral neomycin (Mycifradin Sulfate) and a neomycin enema for a client with cirrhosis who is having central nervous system changes. The nurse knows that the neomycin has been effective if which of these laboratory values are decreased?

    1. White blood cell count.
    2. Ammonia.
    3. Creatinine.
    4. Serum albumin.

69. A client is admitted for fluid replacement and a diagnosis is made of hepatitis A virus. Which nursing measure is most important to maintain in the client's plan of care?

    1. Strict bedrest.
    2. Universal precautions.
    3. Patency of the T tube.
    4. A low protein, high fat diet.

70. The nurse knows that discharge teaching is successful for a client with hepatitis A virus if the client indicates she will refrain from:

    1. Donating blood.
    2. Eating fried foods.
    3. Vacationing in a foreign country.
    4. Ordering a salad in a restaurant.

71. A client has a fractured right tibia. Immediately following cast application, the priority nursing action is to:

    1. Perform a complete neurovascular assessment.
    2. Encourage adequate nutritional intake of calcium.
    3. Air dry the cast.
    4. Monitor drainage through the cast.

72. A physician prescribes para-aminosalicylic acid (PAS) for a client who has been diagnosed with tuberculosis. To decrease the GI symptoms (nausea and vomiting) associated with PAS, the nurse should instruct the client to:

    1. Take the medication at bedtime.
    2. Ask the physician to prescribe an anti-emetic to be taken 30 minutes before the PAS.
    3. Take the medication with food or an antacid.
    4. Crush the tablets and dissolve them completely in water before swallowing.

73. A newly diagnosed diabetic with glaucoma is admitted for regulation of his blood sugar. The client receives pilocarpine (Adsorbocarpine) 2% one drop q.i.d. While instilling this drug the nurse should:

    1. Ask the client to look straight ahead.
    2. Press on the lacrimal sac for one minute after instillation.
    3. Instruct the client to squeeze his eye shut after instillation.
    4. First cleanse the eye, then wipe from the outer to the inner canthus.

74. The nurse would avoid administering terpin hydrate elixir to a client:

1. With thick respiratory secretions.
2. With an allergy to penicillin.
3. Who is pregnant.
4. With glaucoma.

75. The nurse would avoid administering an antihistamine to a client with a history of:

1. Angina.
2. Irritable bowel syndrome.
3. Sinus headaches.
4. Parkinson's disease.

76. The nurse understands that prednisone is used in treating cancers because of which effect?

1. Antimicrobial.
2. Anticoagulant.
3. Anti-inflammatory.
4. Anti-infective.

77. A two-month-old is having a well baby check-up today. The nurse will advise the parents concerning immunizations. The nurse knows that, according to current immunization guidelines, the child is due for which immunizations?

1. MMR and OPV.
2. DPT and OPV.
3. OPV, Hib and DPT.
4. DPT.

78. A five-year-old child is being seen for a well child visit in a pediatric clinic. The child's father tells the nurse that his wife recently has been diagnosed with tuberculosis. In caring for this child the nurse understands that:

1. It is likely that the child will require medication.
2. Small children do not easily contract TB, if they are otherwise healthy.
3. As long as the child has not exhibited the symptoms of night sweats and/or coughing, there is probably no infection.
4. Direct physical contact must be limited to insure the health of the child.

79. The nurse should instruct a client taking alprazolam (Xanax) that he can safely take:

1. Alcohol.
2. Meperidine (Demerol).
3. Flurazepam (Dalmane).
4. Acetaminophen (Tylenol).

80. A 36-year-old client has hypertension and is treated with chlorothiazide (Diuril). Client education should include which information?

1. Dietary sodium should be restricted to one gram daily.
2. Avoid using Diuril with other antihypertensives.
3. Orthostatic hypotension may be a side effect.
4. It is unnecessary to increase dietary potassium.

81. In caring for an elderly psychiatric client who is severely depressed, the nurse knows that elderly clients:

1. Cannot be safely treated with tricyclic antidepressants.
2. Require lower doses of antidepressants than younger clients.
3. Respond more quickly to the therapeutic effects of antidepressants than younger clients.
4. Can be treated safely and effectively with all antidepressants.

82. An unconscious 18-year-old man is brought to the emergency room for a heroine overdose. After the client regains consciousness, he is transferred to the substance abuse treatment unit. The signs and symptoms of heroin withdrawal are written in the nursing care plan. Which behavior should the nurse anticipate will occur early in the withdrawal process?

1. Vomiting and diarrhea.
2. Sneezing and rhinorrhea.
3. Restlessness and irritability.
4. Yawning and diaphoresis.

83. In caring for a client being treated for withdrawal syndrome, the nurse knows that many drugs are associated with a life-threatening abstinence syndrome. However, this is not true for all addictive drugs. Which of the following drug groups is least likely to present a medical crisis during withdrawal?

1. Narcotics.
2. Barbiturates.
3. Alcohol.
4. Benzodiazepines.

84. A high school student speaks to the school nurse about a friend who is abusing cocaine. He wants to know the best way to influence his friend to stop. The nurse's response is based on what knowledge about cocaine?

1. Cocaine use rarely interferes with academic or career activities.
2. Cocaine abuse is difficult to treat because of its abstinence syndrome.
3. Cocaine does more psychological harm than physical damage.
4. Cocaine use is highly reinforcing.

85. In caring for alcoholic clients, the nurse knows that the category of drugs commonly used to manage alcohol withdrawal is:

   1. Antipsychotic drugs.
   2. Barbiturates.
   3. Anti-anxiety agents.
   4. Anticonvulsants.

86. After detoxification, the client begins the rehabilitation phase of treatment. He tells the nurse that he cannot imagine living his life without alcohol. The nurse's best response is based on the knowledge that the client will:

   1. Be more successful if he focuses on goals for short periods of time, such as "today" or "this week."
   2. Likely drink again when under stress.
   3. Not be successful if he is not strongly motivated.
   4. Require treatment with Antabuse to maintain sobriety.

87. An unconscious 18-year-old man is brought to the emergency room by two friends, who report he took an overdose of heroin. A narcotic antagonist, naloxone (Narcan) is administered. After giving the medication, the nurse should monitor this client closely for signs of:

   1. Respiratory depression.
   2. Seizure activity.
   3. Nausea.
   4. Kidney failure.

88. A client's husband asks to speak to the nurse about what effects he and his wife should expect after she is treated with electroconvulsive therapy (ECT). He says, "I know it will improve her depression, but couldn't it also turn her into a vegetable?" After explaining that ECT will not cause any brain damage, what additional information can the nurse ethically give him?

   1. "The main side effects are temporary and may include mild confusion, a slight headache, and short-term memory problems."
   2. "Most clients have no adverse effects to this treatment. In rare cases it has been known to cause fractures resulting from the induced seizure."
   3. "Some clients with cardiac problems have been known to have a heart attack, but we will monitor her closely to be certain this does not happen."
   4. "There are no permanent adverse effects associated with this treatment. The only common side effect is short-term memory problems that last for a few weeks."

89. The nurse admitting a client to the psychiatric unit asks what factors, such as a recent change in his life, may

have contributed to his hospitalization. He replies, "Change . . . change is money . . . when you have money you make the change." This statement is an example of:

   1. Clanging.
   2. Echolalia.
   3. Perseveration.
   4. Flight of ideas.

90. The nurse is to instruct a client to recognize beginning signs of lithium toxicity, which include:

   1. Nystagmus, irregular tremor, decreased urine output.
   2. Tinnitus, blurred vision, slurred speech.
   3. Incoordination, muscle twitching, severe diarrhea.
   4. Mild ataxia, coarse hand tremors, difficulty concentrating.

91. A newly admitted client in the alcoholic treatment unit tells the nurse he has not had anything to drink for 24 hours prior to admission. He complains of feeling anxious and shaky. Based on the nurse's knowledge of alcohol withdrawal, what other behaviors could the nurse expect the client to display during the early phase of his alcohol withdrawal?

   1. Coarse tremors, tachycardia, insomnia.
   2. Confusion, visual hallucinations, delusions.
   3. Disorientation, confabulation, memory deficits.
   4. Incoordination, impaired thinking, irregular eye movements.

92. An elderly client is admitted to the hospital for surgery after finding a lump in his right testicle. He asks the nurse, "Do you think the doctor will find cancer?" The best response by the nurse initially is:

   1. "Most lumps found in the testicles are benign."
   2. "It must be difficult for you not to know what the doctor will find."
   3. "I think that you should discuss this with your doctor."
   4. "It might be, but the doctor won't know until the surgery is performed."

93. A client is taught to do colostomy care for herself prior to discharge. She says to the nurse, "I don't think that I will be able to take care of this colostomy myself." Which of the following is the most helpful response by the nurse?

   1. "Don't worry about it. Most clients feel like that at first."
   2. "What part of the colostomy care are you having trouble with?"
   3. "In time, you will become better at this than I am."

4. "A home health nurse will be visiting you, so if you have any problems, she can help you."

94. **A 76-year-old client was admitted to the hospital for surgery for a fractured hip. The client says to the nurse, "I guess I've lived long enough, and my number's up." How should the nurse respond initially?**

1. "You are in really good shape for your age."
2. "This is just a minor setback. You will be on your feet in no time."
3. "You feel that your life is ending?"
4. "The doctors and nurses are going to take good care of you while you are here. There's nothing to worry about."

95. **A client is in the hospital because of severe weight loss and refusal to eat. The physician ordered the insertion of a nasogastric tube for feeding. The nurse finds the client with the tube removed. The client tells that nurse that he "doesn't need that thing." The most appropriate response by the nurse is:**

1. "You shouldn't have done that! Now I have to put it down again."
2. "Why did you pull that tube out? Do you want to die?"
3. "Tell me what you don't like about the tube."
4. "Your doctor is going to be very upset with you for doing this."

96. **A client is scheduled for a cardiac bypass surgery in the morning. Before the surgery, she states to the nurse, "I don't think I'm going to have the surgery. Everybody has to die sometime." The best response by the nurse is:**

1. "If you don't have the surgery, you will most likely die sooner."
2. "There are always risks involved with surgery. Why have you changed your mind about the operation?"
3. "Cardiac bypass surgery must be very frightening for you. Tell me how you feel about the surgery."
4. "I will call your doctor to in and talk to you."

97. **A male nurse received a doctor's order to catheterize one of his female clients. The client says, "I'm not going to allow a male nurse to catheterize me." The therapeutic nursing response is:**

1. "Your doctor is a male. Would you let him catheterize you?"
2. "I've done this many times with no problems."
3. "You can explain to your doctor why the catheter wasn't inserted."
4. "You appear to be upset. Let me find a female nurse to help with the procedure."

98. **An elderly male client is to have Foley urinary catheter care daily. Which of the following is the best action to provide for the client's privacy during this treatment?**

1. Pull the curtain around the client's bed.
2. Cover the penis with a towel while performing catheter care.
3. Close the door to the client's room.
4. Ask the client's roommate to leave until the treatment is finished.

99. **A client is hospitalized for a surgical procedure. The most important nursing intervention when administering the preoperative medication is:**

1. Have the client void before going to the operating room.
2. Put the side rails up, and instruct the client to remain in bed.
3. Ask the client if she has signed all of the admission forms for the surgery.
4. Have the family leave, since the medication will decrease the client's inhibitions and she may say or do something that is out of character for her.

100. **An elderly, confused client is on bed rest. Which nursing intervention is not consistent with providing safe care for this client?**

1. Provide regular toileting.
2. Explain to the client that she should use the call light if she needs to get up.
3. Place the side rails in the up position and check on the client often.
4. Initiate the proper use of restraints.

NCLEX-PN

Test 2
Questions with Rationales

NCLEX-PN TEST 2 WITH RATIONALES

1. **A client is admitted to a nursing home. She has difficulty seeing and hearing. A nursing action that would place the client at risk would be:**

   1. Showing the client where all of the furniture and personal items are in the room.
   2. Talking loudly to the client when entering her room.
   3. Telling the client that because of her increased risk of falling and injuring herself, she is not allowed out of her room.
   4. Assisting the client to identify the placement of food items during meals.

   1. *This action is appropriate. Since the client has difficulty seeing, the nursing staff should familiarize her with the location of pertinent items in her room.*

   > **TEST-TAKING TIP**: *This question has a false response stem. The correct answer is an option that is NOT appropriate.*

   2. *This action is appropriate. A client who is sight and hearing impaired needs to be alerted to the presence of another individual when entering the room. This can be done by speaking loudly enough for the client to hear.*

   > **TEST-TAKING TIP**: *This question has a false response stem. The correct answer is an option that is NOT appropriate.*

   3. **Correct! Confining the client to her room is NOT appropriate. She has sensory deprivation and is at risk for falling, but she should not be isolated from others. She can be assisted by staff when attending other activities. This INAPPROPRIATE action is the correct answer to the question because the question has a false response stem.**

   > **SAFETY ALERT!** *A client with sensory deprivation is at risk for injury, because of impaired ability to perceive danger.*

   4. *Wrong choice! It is important that the client know where food items are located to prevent potential burns, spills, and other injuries.*

   > **TEST-TAKING TIP**: *This question has a false response stem. The correct answer is an option that is NOT appropriate.*

2. **An infant is in respiratory isolation. The nurse can most effectively prevent the spread of pathogens via droplet infection by:**

   1. Wearing a gown and mask when feeding the client.
   2. Using sterile gloves when changing her diapers.
   3. Having the baby wear a mask when in the playroom.
   4. Using enteric precautions when caring for the baby.

   1. *Yes! This question seeks to identify the main threat to the general population from this client's infection. To prevent the spread of pathogens to others, the nurse must ensure that respiratory secretions are not transmitted. During feeding and burping of the infant, the respiratory secretions will become mixed with the formula. When the baby burps, there is risk of spreading the pathogens via droplet as well as by contact with the nurse's uniform. Wearing a gown and mask will decrease the probability of transmitting the organisms.*
   2. *This will not prevent the transmission of respiratory secretions. Try another option.*
   3. *An infant in respiratory isolation should not leave the room. Taking the baby to the playroom is inappropriate. It is also inappropriate to put a mask on an infant! This option cannot be the answer.*
   4. *Wrong choice! Enteric precautions are not appropriate for a baby in respiratory isolation. They will not prevent the transmission of respiratory secretions.*

3. **While changing the linen on a client's bed, how should the nurse handle the linen?**

   1. Hold it close to the body to avoid dropping it.
   2. Place soiled linen on the chair until done making the bed.
   3. Hold the linen away from the body and uniform.
   4. Shake clean linen to unfold it and provide ease in making the bed.

   1. *Wrong! Holding clean linen next to the body can transfer organisms from the uniform to the clean linen. Holding dirty linen next to the body can transfer organisms from the soiled linen to the uniform. Either action results in contamination and transfer of organisms.*
   2. *Wrong! Soiled linen is contaminated and will further contaminate the surfaces of the chair. All soiled linen should be placed directly into the laun-*

dry hamper in order to prevent contamination of other surfaces.

3. **Right! The linen should be held away from the uniform. Since the nurse must go from client to client, any organisms present on the uniform can be transferred from one client to another.**

4. *Opening linens by shaking them causes movement of air. Air currents can carry dust and organisms about the room, resulting in potential infection. This is not the correct answer.*

4. **A client is recovering from an appendectomy. While changing the linens on the client's bed, the nurse notes drainage from an infected wound has soiled the bed sheet. What is the best method for changing this linen?**

   1. Carefully place the soiled sheet in the cloth linen bag and label it as contaminated.
   2. Spray the soiled area with a bleach solution prior to placing it in the linen bag.
   3. Carefully place the soiled sheet in a moisture-resistant plastic linen bag designated for soiled articles.
   4. Discard the sheet into a plastic trash bag.

   1. *No. A cloth linen bag does not protect the laundry employees from exposure to the soiled sheet and organisms that may be present on the sheet.*
   2. *Incorrect! Spraying the soiled area of the sheet does not destroy any organisms that may be present on other parts of the sheet but cannot be seen. Spraying the sheet is not practical, since the sheet will be effectively disinfected during laundering. Also, using a cloth linen bag does not protect the laundry employees from exposure to the soiled sheet.*
   3. **You are right! Placing the sheet in a moisture-resistant plastic bag protects the laundry employees and others that may come in contact with the bag from exposure to organisms that may be present in the soiled linen.**
   4. *Wrong choice! Discarding linen is neither appropriate nor cost-effective. Proper handling by placing the linen in a moisture-resistant bag will protect the nurse and other employees, and the sheet will be effectively disinfected during laundering.*

5. **During a well-child visit, the mother of a five-year-old expresses concern that her son refuses to wear his helmet while riding his bicycle. What is the appropriate nursing response?**

   1. "Tell him the bike doesn't leave the garage without the helmet."
   2. "It isn't that important, since he won't be riding in the road."
   3. "Gradually encourage the wearing of the helmet with small rewards."
   4. "I'll explain the potential for injury without a

helmet."

1. **Yes. Even though this may sound very tough, it is direct, and it is an appropriate method of obtaining compliance. The parent must believe that the helmet is necessary and apply the rule consistently.**

2. *This is not a true statement! Any fall, anywhere, can potentially cause a head injury.*

3. *No, this response implies inconsistency. Children respond more favorably to consistency. A reward system should not be necessary, since this is expected rather that an optional behavior. This child is at risk for head injury. Try again.*

4. *The nurse's explanation is not likely to be effective. This child is at risk for head injury. Try again.*

6. **A registered nurse, who has previously been treated for an addiction to hydromorphone (Dilaudid), is being treated on the psychiatric unit for anxiety and associated somatic manifestations. The psychiatrist orders propranolol (Inderal) for her anxiety. The client recognizes the medication and states, "There must be some mistake. I don't have any cardiac problems." Which statement offers the best nursing response?**

   1. "This drug was ordered because you have a history of drug abuse and your psychiatrist doesn't want to prescribe anything that could lead to physical dependence."
   2. "This drug also has a psychiatric use. It is not only used for cardiac problems."
   3. "There is no mistake. Your psychiatrist ordered Inderal for you. Do you have a history of hypertension?"
   4. "Inderal is used to control anxiety in persons like yourself, who have a lot of physical manifestations of anxiety."

   1. *This is not the best option. The client's history of drug abuse may be a factor, but it is not the primary reason why Inderal was ordered. Read all the options before selecting the best one!*
   2. *This is a true statement, but it is not the best response to the client's comments. The nurse can give her a better explanation. Try again — and read all the options before selecting the best one!*
   3. *This is not correct. Inderal is used to treat hypertension, but this is not the reason it was prescribed for the client. Select the option that correctly addresses the client's question.*
   4. **Correct. Somatic manifestations of anxiety, like the client's, are often treated effectively with the beta-blockers. Her history of narcotic abuse probably also was a factor in her psychiatrist's decision to prescribe Inderal because it is not associated with physical dependence. This is the best option, because it is the most accurate response to the client's question.**

7. **A confused elderly client is on strict bedrest. Which nursing intervention will provide for this client's safety?**

    1. Place the client in a room away from the noise and confusion of the nurses' station.
    2. Avoid the use of nightlights, since they tend to distort images and confuse clients.
    3. Discuss with the client the need for restraints if she continues to get out of bed.
    4. Provide opportunities for regular toileting, and include this information in the client's care plan.

    1. *This is an inappropriate nursing action. Any client who is confused should be placed in a room near the nursing station—not away from it. Try again!*
    2. *This is inappropriate. A nightlight is generally used for confused clients, because it decreases image distortion and enhances reality. Also, the use of a nightlight helps orient clients to the hospital environment.*
    3. *This option is a good distractor, because it implies that by talking to the client, the nurse may be able to lessen her confusion. Wrong! If the client is confused, then the issue of safety requires that the nurse should focus on how to adapt the client's environment to decrease the risk of accidents.*
    4. ***Excellent! This client is confused, which means there is a high safety risk due to decreased ability to perceive danger. Providing opportunities for regular toileting helps ensure that the client's basic needs for elimination will be met, and will greatly reduce the risk of the client's falling while trying to get up and go to the bathroom without the assistance of the nurse. This nursing action provides for the comfort and safety of the client, and it should be recorded in the plan of care.***

8. **The nurse should avoid reporting which of the following events to a government agency?**

    1. Births.
    2. Child abuse.
    3. Marital quarrels.
    4. Typhoid fever.

    1. *This is not correct. Births are required to be reported. The nurse should follow the institution's procedures.*
    2. *This is not correct. Child abuse must be reported, and the nurse should follow the institution's procedures.*
    3. ***Very good! Marital quarrels are not subject to reporting requirements. This client data is protected by the client's right to privacy.***
    4. *Typhoid fever, a communicable disease, must be reported.*

9. **The nurse understands that which of the following is outside the scope of a client's right of privacy:**

    1. Not having a gunshot wound reported, upon timely request.
    2. Refusing to receive visitors.
    3. Wearing one's own clothing.
    4. Requesting the presence of a member of the same sex during a physical examination.

    1. ***Good work! Gunshot wounds must be reported. The nurse should follow the institution's procedures.***

    > **TEST-TAKING TIP:** *This question has a false response stem and is asking you to identify the option that is FALSE.*

    2. *Wrong choice. Clients have the right to maintain privacy by choosing their company, and they may choose not to receive visitors. You are looking for something that is NOT a privacy right of the client.*
    3. *Wrong choice. The client has the right to wear personal clothing unless it interferes with medical procedures. An example of a situation where personal clothing would interfere is surgery. You are looking for something that is NOT a privacy right of the client.*

    > **TEST-TAKING TIP:** *Words like "generally" tend to make a statement true. However, this question has a false response stem and is asking you to identify the option that is FALSE.*

    4. *Wrong choice. The client does have this right, and such a request should be respected by the nurse. You are looking for something that is NOT a privacy right of the client.*

10. **The best nursing action to prevent the spread of infection among hospitalized clients is:**

    1. Using sterile technique when performing any procedure.
    2. Hand washing before coming in contact with each client.
    3. Wearing gloves to perform any procedure.
    4. Wearing a mask and gown while performing any procedure.

    1. *Sterile technique is not required for every procedure. Using sterile technique while administering medications or similar interventions is neither necessary nor practical. Aseptic technique is appropriate for most non-invasive procedures.*
    2. ***Great! Hand washing has been found to be the most effective action in preventing spread of infection among clients. This activity inhibits the transfer of organisms from one client to another.***

3. *Gloves should be worn if there is any chance of the nurse coming in contact with body fluids. However, gloves are not necessary for procedures such as administration of oral medications, where exposure to body fluids is not likely to occur.*

4. *It is not necessary to wear a gown and mask for all procedures. In addition, although wearing a gown and mask protects the nurse, it does not effectively protect the client. This is not the best option.*

11. **The nurse is preparing the staffing assignment. An infant on the unit has AIDS and cytomegalovirus (CMV). Which staff person should be assigned as the primary care giver for this child?**

    1. An experienced practical nurse who is six months pregnant.
    2. A male graduate nurse, recently oriented to pediatrics.
    3. An experienced nurse's aide who is healthy.
    4. A licensed practical nurse with eczema.

    1. *No. You probably selected this nurse due to her experience. This would place the nurse's fetus at undue risk, since pregnant women should avoid exposure to CMV. Select another option.*
    2. ***Good choice. A graduate nurse should be able to carry out the care, maintaining appropriate technique based on the principles of communicable disease transmission. Note the reasons why the other options are incorrect: Option 1 would place the nurse's fetus at undue risk. Option 3 is not correct because this client should have a licensed caregiver above the level of nurse's aide. And Option 4 is incorrect because the eczema puts this nurse at risk for infection.***
    3. *No, although the aide is "healthy" and experienced, this client should have a licensed caregiver. The implied level of care is above that of the aide.*
    4. *No, this nurse is at risk for injury from this assignment. She has open areas on her skin, which is the body's first line of defense from communicable disease. Make another choice.*

12. **The home health nurse notes several suspicious bruises and old burns on a 10-month-old child while making an initial home visit. The priority nursing action to provide for the child's safety is:**

    1. Call the child protection hotline and report possible abuse.
    2. Discuss the family with the physician and social worker at the next team meeting.
    3. Tell the mother that child protection will be notified if injuries are noted on the next visit.

4. Carefully record the visit for follow-up.

1. ***Absolutely correct! As a mandated reporter the nurse is obligated to report any cases of suspected abuse. The reporter does not need to prove the case, just report the facts known. This is the law. This is also the first action to take in providing for the child's safety.***
2. *No! The nurse could be considered negligent according to the laws of the state within which the nurse practices, because this is too long a delay before possible action that could protect the child.*
3. *No, this action will drive the family underground and will not help you develop a therapeutic relationship with the mother. She is likely not to be at home the next time you visit. Choose again.*
4. *No, you didn't do anything that will either stop the abuse or initiate an immediate investigation. Hint: What does "mandated reporter" mean?*

13. **At a boy scout camp the nurse encounters a child who exhibits a high-pitched inspiratory sound, and cyanosis. Describe the procedure that the nurse should institute.**

    1. Stand behind the child and apply an upward thrust below the xiphoid.
    2. Monitor the child, and if respirations cease, use the Heimlich maneuver.
    3. Bend the child forward and deliver back blows to dislodge the object.
    4. Begin cardiopulmonary resuscitation.

    1. ***Yes, you have correctly evaluated the data as a child with an inadequate gas exchange, and then selected the correct procedure for the Heimlich maneuver on a child.***
    2. *No, do not delay treatment! The cyanosis and high-pitched inspiratory sound indicate an inadequate gas exchange. This child needs assistance now!*
    3. *No, this is the treatment for an infant with an airway obstruction. Identify the treatment for a school age child.*
    4. *Why would you do this? There is no indication in the assessment that a cardiac arrest has occurred, and the child has distinct signs of an airway obstruction and inadequate gas exchange. Most children are primary respiratory arrests. This is not the correct emergency intervention for this case scenario.*

14. **The nurse is caring for a client who is paralyzed on his right side following a stroke. In preparing to give a bed bath to the client, which of the following nursing actions is best?**

    1. Adjust the bed to the lowest position, in case the client falls.
    2. Raise the bed to the high horizontal position.
    3. Put the bed in low semi-Fowler's position.

4. Unplug the bed.

1. *This is incorrect, because it does not permit the nurse to use proper body mechanics.*
2. **This is the correct answer. The high horizontal position is the most efficient and safest way for the nurse to bathe the client, since it permits the nurse to use proper body mechanics.**
3. *This is incorrect, because it does not permit the nurse to use good body mechanics.*
4. *Unplugging the bed serves no purpose. Try again.*

15. **A client is admitted with a diagnosis of premature labor. The nurse understands that which of the following drugs should be avoided when treating premature labor?**

1. Magnesium sulfate.
2. Ritodrine (Yutopar).
3. Betamethasone (Celestone).
4. Terbutaline sulfate (Brethine).

1. *Sorry. Magnesium sulfate, the drug of choice for treating pregnancy induced hypertension, also is commonly used to treat premature labor. Which drug is NOT used to treat premature labor?*
2. *Incorrect. Ritodrine inhibits contractility of the uterine smooth muscle and is an FDA approved drug to treat preterm labor. Which drug is NOT used to treat premature labor?*
3. **Correct choice in this difficult question! Although betamethasone often is given to mothers in premature labor, its purpose is to promote lung maturity in the fetus. It is not used to treat premature labor _per se_.**
4. *Wrong. Terbutaline relaxes uterine smooth muscle and often is used to treat preterm labor. Which drug is NOT used to treat premature labor?*

16. **The nurse is about to administer methylergonovine maleate (Methergine) to a postpartum client. Which assessment would have priority prior to the administration of this drug?**

1. Fundus.
2. Blood pressure.
3. Apical pulse.
4. Respiratory rate.

1. *Wrong. Evaluation of the fundus is not an important assessment in considering the administration of Methergine.*
2. **Excellent! Elevation of blood pressure is a common side effect of Methergine. Assessment prior to administration is indicated, and the medication should not be given if the BP is above 140/ 90.**

3. *No, the apical pulse has no bearing on the administration of Methergine.*
4. *No, the respiratory rate has no bearing on the administration of Methergine.*

17. **You are caring for a client receiving IV magnesium sulfate to treat her severe pregnancy induced hypertension. Which assessment needs to be reported to the RN immediately?**

1. Deep tendon reflexes change from +4 to +2.
2. Maternal blood pressure changes from 160/110 to 148/90.
3. Urinary output drops from 40 cc to 28 cc per hour.
4. Respiratory rate changes from 22 to 16 breaths per minute.

1. *Wrong. A decrease in deep tendon reflexes would be an expected response to magnesium sulfate. We do not become concerned unless the reflexes disappear altogether.*
2. *Incorrect. A drop in blood pressure is likely to be seen in the client who is receiving magnesium sulfate.*
3. **Good choice! Magnesium sulfate is excreted through the kidneys, so adequate urinary output is necessary to prevent magnesium toxicity. Any urinary output less than 30 cc per hour is a cause for concern.**
4. *Wrong. One would expect to see a reduction in respiratory rate in the client receiving magnesium sulfate. We do not become concerned unless the rate goes below 14 breaths per minute.*

18. **A client is admitted to the labor unit because of premature labor, with rupture of membranes. She is given betamethasone (Celestone). The nurse understands that the purpose of this drug is:**

1. Uterine relaxation.
2. Fetal lung maturity.
3. Prevention of chorioamnionitis.
4. Enhancement of fetal oxygenation.

1. *Wrong. Betamethasone has no effect on uterine contractions.*
2. **Correct. Betamethasone is a glucocorticoid that acts to accelerate fetal lung maturity.**
3. *Wrong. Betamethasone has no effect on prevention of uterine infections.*
4. *No, betamethasone promotes fetal lung maturity but has no effect on fetal oxygenation.*

19. **A client is to receive prostaglandin E2 (PGE2) vaginal suppositories to prepare the cervix for induction of labor. Which side effect should the nurse anticipate?**

1. Nausea and vomiting.
2. Hypertension.
3. Vaginal bleeding.
4. Severe headaches.

1. *Good job! Clients who receive prostaglandin E2 often experience nausea and vomiting. Often anti-emetic drugs are given.*
2. *No, prostaglandin E2 does not cause hypertension.*
3. *Wrong, vaginal bleeding is not an effect of prostaglandin E2.*
4. *No, severe headaches are not related to prostaglandin E2.*

20. A client with hypertension is being treated with chlorothiazide (Diuril) 500 mg. PO twice a day. In taking the client's medication history, the nurse notes that the client is a diabetic and has been taking chlorpropamide (Diabinese) 250 mg. PO daily. The nurse is aware that the potential interaction of Diabinese with Diuril may result in:

1. Hypocalcemia.
2. Hyperglycemia.
3. Aplastic anemia.
4. Hypoglycemia.

1. *Wrong choice. Hypocalcemia does not result from the combined use of Diuril and Diabinese. Choose again.*
2. *Correct! Thiazides, such as Diuril, may decrease the effectiveness of Diabinese, resulting in hyperglycemia. Diabetic clients require close monitoring and may require increased antidiabetic medication.*
3. *Not true. Aplastic anemia is a life-threatening side effect of Diabinese therapy (and all oral hypoglycemic agents). It is not a result of a drug-drug interaction between Diuril and Diabinese.*
4. *Incorrect. Hypoglycemia is the most common side effect of Diabinese therapy and does not result from an interaction between Diuril and Diabinese.*

21. The nurse is to administer erythromycin (Ilotycin) to a client for preventative treatment of ophthalmia neonatorum. The nurse knows the correct technique is:

1. Inject intramuscularly in the front of the thigh.
2. Inject subcutaneously in either arm.
3. Pull down the lower eyelid and instill along the lower surface towards the nose.
4. Pull down the lower eyelid and instill along the lower surface away from the nose.

1. *Wrong. Ilotycin is given in the eyes, not IM.*
2. *No, Ilotycin is not given subcutaneously.*
3. *Wrong. The ointment is instilled from the inner cannula of the eye outward away from the nose.*

4. *Yes. This describes the correct technique for administration of erythromycin ointment.*

22. As you are driving home one day, a man flags you down. His car will not start and his wife is in active labor, crying that the baby is coming. Which nursing action receives the lowest priority?

1. Maintain a calm atmosphere.
2. Tie off or cut the umbilical cord.
3. Hold the baby up by the feet and rub the back after delivery.
4. Dry the newborn off.

1. *Wrong choice! This is a priority action. Remaining calm is very important to both the mother and the father. If they see that the nurse is calm and confident they will relax. You are looking for an action that is NOT important at this time.*
2. *Correct — it is not necessary to cut or tie the cord. This measure can wait until transfer has been made to a hospital with no adverse effect to the mother or infant.*
3. *Wrong, this is a priority action! Holding the baby by the feet will promote drainage of fluid from the airways and rubbing the baby's back will stimulate respirations. You are looking for an action that is NOT important at this time.*
4. *No, this is a priority action! Warmth is very important for the newborn. Wiping the baby off decreases the risk of heat loss via evaporation. You are looking for an action that is NOT important at this time.*

23. The nurse checks a postpartum client's peripad and finds a large amount of rubra lochia with several clots. What is the priority nursing action?

1. Check the vital signs.
2. Check for a full bladder.
3. Check the fundus.
4. Complete a vaginal exam.

1. *This is not the priority. The vital signs are important but will not help you in identifying the reason for bleeding.*
2. *This is not the priority. A full bladder may cause uterine atony — but before you check the bladder, you should check the fundus.*
3. *Excellent! The primary cause of early postpartum bleeding is uterine atony manifested by a relaxed, boggy uterus. Checking the fundus will give you critical information that the RN will need to convey to the physician.*
4. *Wrong. Vaginal exam would allow diagnosis of vaginal hematomas, but assessing the client vaginally is usually the role of the physician. This cannot be the first nursing action.*

24. A client has a postpartum hemorrhage as a result of a cervical laceration. The nurse would expect to observe:

1. Continuous vaginal bleeding in the presence of a firm fundus.
2. Rapidly rising fundal height with continuous vaginal bleeding.
3. Continuous vaginal bleeding in presence of a boggy uterus.
4. Intermittent vaginal bleeding in the presence of a relaxed uterus.

*1. **Correct. When the postpartum hemorrhage is caused by a laceration anywhere in the birth canal, the uterus will remain contracted and the fundus will be firm.***
2. This is incorrect. When there is a laceration the bleeding will all be obvious, rather than collecting within the uterus.
3. This is incorrect. When the fundus is boggy the cause of the bleeding is uterine atony, not a laceration.
4. This is incorrect. Normally, the lochial discharge following delivery is intermittent, corresponding to the uterine contractions. When the uterus is boggy, the bleeding may become continuous.

25. The nurse is caring for an Rh negative obstetrical client who is to receive Rh_o (D) human immune globulin (RhoGAM). The nurse understands that which of the following is inconsistent with indications for administration of RhoGAM?

1. Birth of an Rh negative infant.
2. Amniocentesis.
3. Ectopic pregnancy.
4. Pregnancy at 28 weeks gestation.

*1. **Correct. When an Rh negative mother gives birth to an Rh negative baby, she does not need RhoGAM. She only needs it following the birth of an Rh positive infant.***
2. Wrong. This is an indication for the administration of RhoGAM, because of the risk that Rh positive blood cells from the fetus will enter the Rh negative mother's blood.
3. No, termination of an ectopic pregnancy is an indication for the administration of RhoGAM in an Rh negative mother.
4. Wrong. This is an indication for the use of RhoGAM. RhoGAM is given at 28 weeks to all Rh negative mothers, just in case they are carrying an Rh positive baby.

26. A three-month-old child was admitted with a tentative diagnosis of intussusception. The parents ask the nurse how the diagnosis is made. The correct explanation by the nurse is:

1. "A small amount of tissue from the colon will be biopsied."
2. "Genotyping can identify this condition."
3. "A barium enema will be given to visualize the obstruction."
4. "An upper GI series should identify the area involved."

1. Wrong. You're probably thinking about Hirschsprung's disease. The pathophysiology of intussusception is not a defect of nerve innervation and the disorder does not always occur in the colon.
2. Wrong. Genotyping would be used for hereditary disease. This is not a factor in intussusception.
*3. **Correct. A barium enema is given, which may also treat the condition by nonsurgical means. The telescoping of the bowel, which characterizes intussusception, may be reduced by the hydrostatic pressure of the barium enema.***
4. Incorrect. This procedure is too high up to see this problem. This is more likely to be used for the diagnosis of peptic ulcer.

27. A six-month-old is in the pediatric clinic. The nurse practitioner ordered a DPT vaccine to be administered. Which finding by the nurse would cause the nurse to question the administration of the DPT vaccine?

1. Previous evidence of sensitivity to egg antigens.
2. Fever and high-pitched cry following last DPT.
3. Current rectal temperature of 100° F.
4. Currently receiving steroid therapy.

1. Incorrect. Severe anaphylactic egg sensitivity would represent a contraindication to administration of measles and mumps vaccine, but not DPT.
*2. **Yes, most definitely! These are both manifestations of an untoward response to DPT, and are indicative of neurologic reaction. If a full dose of pertussis vaccine were to be given again, it might cause an encephalopathy.***
3. Incorrect. Mild fever, in the absence of other manifestations, is not a reason to withhold DPT vaccine. Try another response.
4. Incorrect. OPV, not DPT, is the vaccine that should be withheld if the child is receiving steroid therapy. It is a live vaccine and the child may respond in an unpredictable manner.

28. An eight-year-old child has a fever of 104° F upon returning from surgery. The priority nursing action is:

1. Document and continue to monitor.
2. Begin sponging with tepid water.
3. Administer acetaminophen (Tylenol) P.O. as ordered.
4. Notify the nurse in charge.

1. *No! This could be dangerous! An action is required generally in temperatures over 102° F. Select again.*
2. *Not the best answer, but you're on the right track. This option would require an order. Try again.*
3. *No, it's too early postoperatively to give P.O. medication and you are missing a problem. Reread the question and select again.*
4. **Yes, this needs to be reported immediately! This is beyond the normal postoperative finding and it may indicate an adverse reaction to the anesthetic. Tylenol will take too long to work and the P.O. route is questionable immediately postoperatively. Tepid baths may be in order but, first, the charge nurse needs this information.**

29. **Nursing interventions for the child with cerebral palsy are mainly directed toward:**

    1. Genetic counseling.
    2. Motor development.
    3. Special education.
    4. Seizure control.

    1. *Incorrect. Although there may be a genetic cause of the child's cerebral palsy, this counseling will not improve this client's functioning. Try again.*
    2. **Terrific! The pathology of cerebral palsy is located in the brain's motor centers, so the interventions most helpful in the child's development will be directed toward improving motor function. PT, OT and speech therapies are most are often employed.**
    3. *Not true! Intellectual deficits are not a consistent finding in children with cerebral palsy. Select another option.*
    4. *Incorrect. Seizures are not necessarily associated with cerebral palsy. Try again.*

30. **A child is being admitted with otitis media. The nurse's assessment findings are most likely to include:**

    1. Elevated temperature and tugging on the affected ear.
    2. Clear drainage from the affected ear and sore throat.
    3. Elevated temperature and rhinorrhea.
    4. Anorexia and diarrhea.

    1. **Yes, this is the classic picture of the child with otitis media. A middle ear infection is painful and the organism will cause an elevated temperature.**
    2. *No, the clear drainage is more likely CSF drainage, and the sore throat would probably be unrelated to that type of drainage. Otitis media drainage is purulent.*

3. *Incorrect. Elevated temperature may occur, but rhinorrhea refers to clear drainage from the nose, which is usually due to allergies, "cold" manifestations or CSF drainage.*
4. *Close, but not the most specific to otitis media. Any sick young child may experience loss of appetite and diarrhea, but these do not indicate an otitis. Select again.*

31. **Which statement by a child's father indicates to the nurse that further teaching is necessary before discharging his child in a plaster cast?**

    1. "After a bath, the cast must be allowed to dry completely."
    2. "Petaling will prevent skin breakdown."
    3. "Any odor should be reported to the doctor immediately."
    4. "Elevation will reduce swelling."

    1. **Good work, this dad does need some more instruction! A plaster cast must be kept dry or it will simply fall apart.**
    2. *Wrong choice. The father has understood correctly. Petaling does in fact help to keep the edges of the cast from crumbling and will help prevent irritation and skin breakdown. You are looking for an INCORRECT statement by the father.*
    3. *Wrong choice. The father has a correct understanding. The father should call the doctor if an odor is detected from the cast, because this may indicate skin breakdown under the cast and it should be investigated. You are looking for an INCORRECT statement by the father.*
    4. *No, the father has correctly understood that elevation will reduce swelling. This instruction should include elevating the extremity above the heart. You are looking for an INCORRECT statement by the father.*

32. **A two-year-old boy is brought to the emergency room with nausea and diarrhea. Which statement by the parents would most concern the nurse?**

    1. "His last wet diaper smelled very strong."
    2. "He is very quiet when he is playing."
    3. "His lips are dry and crusty."
    4. "He cries whenever I put him down."

    1. *Wrong option! Strong smelling urine may indicate concentrated urine, but the child is still voiding.*
    2. *Wrong choice! A lethargic child may be cause for alarm, but this child is still playing, and the parents give no indication of decreased alertness.*
    3. **Excellent choice! A dry and crusty mouth are classic signs of dehydration, which would be**

a cause for immediate concern.

4. *Sorry, wrong choice! A sick child, or a child in a new situation, may be fearful and irritable, and may cry to be held. This in itself is an expected finding.*

33. **Priority nursing interventions for the child in Buck's traction are directed at:**

1. Pin site care.
2. Maintaining skin integrity.
3. Increasing calcium intake.
4. Exercising the affected extremity.

1. *Incorrect. This would be necessary with skeletal traction only. Try again.*
2. **Yes, you got it! Buck's traction is skin traction. Frequent observations, as well as keeping the linen straight, are priority interventions.**
3. *No! This is contraindicated in all clients on bedrest, since renal calculi may develop. An adequate calcium intake is advised. Try again.*
4. *Oops, you probably didn't read this option carefully! It says the AFFECTED extremity. The unaffected extremity should be exercised, not the affected (broken) one.*

34. **The nurse caring for a nine-month-old infant knows to avoid giving the infant:**

1. Dry cold cereal.
2. Orange juice.
3. Raw carrot chunks.
4. Scrambled egg.

1. *Wrong choice, because this food is very appropriate. The child is developing her pincer grasp and eye-hand coordination. Choose again, looking for the inappropriate food.*
2. *Wrong choice, because juices are normally introduced at six months. Choose again, looking for the inappropriate food. Make another choice.*
3. **Yes, this food could present a real potential for choking and should wait until the child has more teeth. Table foods should be well cooked up until one year of age.**
4. *No, this is fine. Eggs often can be introduced safely at six months, especially in children with no history of allergies. Choose again, looking for the inappropriate food.*

35. **The nurse is caring for a child who has just received a ventriculoperitoneal shunt. The nurse knows correct positioning for this client postoperatively is:**

1. Side-lying.
2. HOB elevated 30 degrees.
3. In a position of comfort for the client.
4. Supine.

1. *Not preferred for this situation. You probably were thinking of safe positioning to prevent aspiration, but there is a more important issue to consider. Try again.*
2. **Correct. The elevation helps to decrease pressure in the brain and encourages the drainage from the shunt.**
3. *No. It sounds like a nice thing to do, but not in the immediately postoperative period.*
4. *Definitely unsafe! Remember, supine means lying on the back. Try again.*

36. **A two-year-old is scheduled for a cardiac catheterization. Which statement by the mother would indicate that the nurse's teaching has been successful?**

1. "I'm pleased that my child will no longer have blue spells."
2. "Although this is not a permanent repair, my baby will be some better."
3. "After this is done, we will know what has to be done for my child."
4. "My child will have a large scar following this procedure."

1. *Not true. This implies that the mother believes that the cardiac catheterization is corrective.*
2. *Not true. This is not palliative surgery. Try again.*
3. **Yes, this is a diagnostic procedure that is done to provide information on the exact nature and extent of the cardiac defect.**
4. *Not true. A cardiac catheterization leaves a very small opening where a fine catheter is inserted. Make another selection.*

37. **Following hospitalization for 10 days, an 11-month-old child is quiet and sad when his mother leaves. The nurse knows this behavior indicates:**

1. An understanding of his mother's need to leave.
2. Despair at his mother's absence.
3. Protest that his source of emotional support is gone.
4. Developing autonomy.

1. *Oops, did you note the age of this child? Choose again.*
2. **Yes, this is an indication that separation anxiety has progressed beyond the stage where protest is demonstrated. This may have consequences after hospitalization.**
3. *Wrong choice. This is only partly true. Look at the behaviors that are stated in the question and try again.*
4. *Wrong. This child is too young to be working on the development of autonomy. He is still in the*

stage of trust development with his primary caregiver. Try again.

38. **The nurse's clinical assessment of two-year-old child who is poorly nourished is most likely to include:**

    1. Mother's statement that the child is a "picky eater."
    2. Height and weight in the 25th percentile.
    3. Observing that the child is slender and active.
    4. Dry colorless hair and pale skin.

    1. *Not really helpful. Many toddlers are described as picky eaters by their families, because they are too busy to sit for meals. Select again.*
    2. *This is adequate amount of growth and does not describe a poorly nourished child. Try another response.*
    3. *No. Slender and active describes a healthy child. Make another choice.*
    4. **Yes, this is the classic picture of a poorly nourished child. Inadequate nutrients may cause a low hemoglobin, which will cause pale skin, and since the body is poorly nourished the hair is dry, brittle, and lacking in color.**

39. **A client was admitted to the hospital with an infection of his left foot. The nurse notes that he has a strong body odor and appears to be in need of a bath. The nurse notes that he is watching TV and that his left leg is cool to touch and slightly mottled. He is very abrupt in response to the nurse's questions. Which of the following data is most important for the nurse to document about the client?**

    1. Appears to be comfortable, since he is watching TV.
    2. Uncooperative in answering the nurse's questions.
    3. Poor personal hygiene.
    4. Left leg is cool to touch and slightly mottled.

    1. *Wrong choice. This assessment does not address the client's present health care problem. Make another choice.*
    2. *Wrong choice. Although the nurse may be concerned about this situation, the client's communication skills are not related to his present health care problem. Try again.*
    3. *Wrong choice. Poor personal hygiene may have contributed to the cause of the client's health care problem. This option is a possible answer but it is not the most important assessment. Read the other options!*
    4. **Very good! This answer gives a description of the left leg. Since an infection of the left foot is the reason for the client's hospitalization, charting this parameter is very important.**

40. **Which complaint by a client would lead the nurse to**

believe the client may be experiencing a myocardial infarction?

    1. A feeling of an intermittent strangling sensation.
    2. Complaints of sudden substernal pain after an argument.
    3. Feelings of numbness or weakness in arms and wrists.
    4. Profuse perspiration with nausea and vomiting.

    1. *Wrong, try again! A feeling of an intermittent strangling sensation is related to angina. Angina is characterized by pain or discomfort that is intermittent or acts at intervals.*
    2. *Wrong choice! Angina is caused by loss of blood flow or oxygen to the heart muscle. This discomfort or pain is temporary and is frequently caused by stress such as an argument.*
    3. *Wrong! Feelings of numbness or weakness are characteristics of angina. These feelings are associated with a decrease of oxygen to the heart muscle.*
    4. **Excellent! This is the only option that is characteristic of a myocardial infarction. This is a priority assessment. Any client demonstrating extreme sweating, nausea and vomiting may be experiencing a heart attack. Immediate medical help is needed. In a myocardial infarction, a portion of the heart muscle is destroyed because of a blocked blood supply. This is an assessment question that focuses on what the nurse needs to identify for a client who may be experiencing a myocardial infarction.**

41. **After a bronchoscopy, the nurse would give immediate consideration to a client's complaint of:**

    1. Blood-tinged mucous.
    2. Hoarseness when speaking.
    3. Irritation and discomfort when swallowing.
    4. Difficulty breathing.

    1. *No, this is not a priority assessment. Blood-tinged mucous and sputum is normal after this procedure. The bronchoscope, when inserted, may cause trauma to the tissue of the larynx, trachea or bronchi.*
    2. *No, this is not a priority assessment. The client may complain of hoarseness after the bronchoscopy because of trauma to tissue of the larynx and the trachea.*
    3. *No, this is not a priority assessment. This is a normal manifestation after a bronchoscopy. The swallowing reflex is usually blocked for about six hours after the procedure. Initially the client may have some discomfort and difficulty when the swallowing reflex is restored.*
    4. **Good choice! This is a priority assessment that**

needs immediate medical treatment. The difficulty in breathing may be caused by edema in the larynx or trachea and is a serious complication.

42. The nurse takes precautions to prevent constipation and fecal impaction in an immobilized client. The nurse is aware that, if a client develops a fecal impaction, what serious complication could result?

   1. Intestinal obstruction.
   2. Bowel perforation.
   3. Peritonitis.
   4. Rectal bleeding.

   1. Yes. A fecal impaction is the presence of either hardened or putty-like feces in the rectum and sigmoid colon. If the condition is not relieved, intestinal obstruction can occur.
   2. Wrong. Although this complication could occur during digital removal of the fecal impaction, it is not a complication of the impaction itself.
   3. Wrong. Peritonitis is an inflammation of the peritoneum caused by the introduction of bacteria into the abdominal cavity. A fecal impaction is contained within the bowel and therefore cannot cause peritonitis.
   4. Wrong. Rectal bleeding is seen in clients with hemorrhoids or certain types of bowel pathology, but a fecal impaction does not cause rectal bleeding.

43. The nurse has just collected a liquid stool specimen for ova and parasites. The test results may be compromised if the nurse:

   1. Places the specimen into a clean container.
   2. Puts the collected specimen in the refrigerator.
   3. Instructs the client to defecate into a bedpan.
   4. Sends only the bloody and mucoid portions of the stool.

   1. No, this would be proper procedure and would not negate the test results. Ova and parasites are detected by microscopic examination. A sterile container is needed for specimens that are to be cultured. You are looking for an action that will make the test results INACCURATE.
   2. You have identified the incorrect action. A liquid stool specimen for ova and parasites must be sent immediately to the lab and examined within 30 minutes, to preserve the "life" of any ova. If it cannot be examined within 30 minutes, then some of the specimen should be placed in a preservative.
   3. No, this would not affect the test results. The client could be instructed to use a bedpan or bedside commode to collect the stool specimen. The specimen, however, must remain free from urine con-

tamination.
   4. No, this would be the correct portion of the specimen to collect if the entire stool cannot be sent to the laboratory. You are looking for an action that will make the test results INACCURATE.

44. Following a gastric resection, a client is taught nutritional habits that will slow gastric emptying, helping to decrease the incidence of the "dumping syndrome." Which food selection by the client indicates to the nurse that he understands the instructions given?

   1. Ice cream.
   2. Oranges.
   3. Wheat bread.
   4. Turkey.

   1. Correct. Foods that are high in fat are recommended, because fat tends to slow down gastric emptying.
   2. Incorrect. Oranges, or any fruit, are not useful in helping to delay gastric emptying.
   3. No, wheat bread or high fiber foods are not known to slow gastric emptying. The bulk provided by these foods helps to increase peristaltic activity and thus prevent constipation, but not the "dumping syndrome."
   4. No. Turkey is a high protein food but it has not been identified as producing the desired effect of delayed or slowed gastric emptying.

45. A client is admitted to the hospital with a diagnosis of active pulmonary tuberculosis. An immediate nursing goal is to control the spread of infection. To control the spread of active tuberculosis, the nurse would:

   1. Wear a gown and mask when caring for the client.
   2. Recommend that the client wear a mask when she has visitors.
   3. Teach the client how to cover her nose and mouth when she coughs or sneezes.
   4. Use blood and needle precautions.

   1. No. The mask would be appropriate, but there is no need for a gown. Try again.
   2. Incorrect. The correct procedure would be for visitors, as well as all health care providers, to wear a mask when in the room. Choose again.
   3. Good choice! Teaching this, along with proper hand washing, will help prevent the spread of the infection, which is by droplet nuclei.
   4. No, tuberculosis is not transmitted via the blood. Make another selection.

46. A client is scheduled for a chest x-ray to rule out pneumonia. The nurse explains to the client that the preparation for the chest x-ray includes:

1. Fasting for four hours prior to the procedure.
2. Signing a consent form for an invasive procedure.
3. Benadryl 25 mg IM prior to the procedure.
4. No special preparation.

1. *No, there is no fasting requirement prior to a chest x-ray. Try again.*
2. *Incorrect. A chest x-ray is not an invasive procedure. Make another selection.*
3. *Incorrect. Benadryl, an antihistamine, would not be indicated prior to a chest x-ray, since no dye is used. Choose again.*
4. ***Excellent! You recalled that a chest x-ray is a non-invasive procedure requiring no special preparation.***

47. Following a total hip replacement, the nurse takes precautions to ensure that the affected hip is flexed no more than:

1. 25 degrees.
2. 60 degrees.
3. 75 degrees.
4. 90 degrees.

1. *No. The client will need to flex the affected hip more than 25 degrees in order to transfer from bed to chair, etc. Make another selection.*
2. ***Absolutely correct! The affected hip is not to be flexed more than 45 to 60 degrees. Limited flexion is maintained during transfers and when sitting, with encouragement to maintain the operative hip in extension.***
3. *Incorrect. This amount of flexion may jeopardize the positioning of the femoral head component in the acetabular cup. Choose a safer option.*
4. *No! Dislocation may occur with this angle flexion, as it exceeds the limits of the prosthesis. Make another selection.*

48. The client has just returned from the x-ray department after undergoing an upper GI series. Which nursing action would be appropriate at this time?

1. Keep him NPO until the gag reflex returns.
2. Administer a cleansing enema.
3. Monitor his vital signs every 15 minutes for one hour or until stable.
4. Give milk of magnesia 30 cc P.O.

1. *Incorrect. The client did not need to have his throat anesthetized for this procedure. The gag and cough reflex remain intact. Choose again.*
2. *Not necessary. This protocol would be appropriate after a barium enema. Make another selection.*
3. *Not needed. Unless the client became symptomatic during the exam, there is no need to monitor his vital signs so closely. The procedure does not*

interfere with the cardiovascular status; the vital signs would be monitored per daily routine. Try again.
4. ***Correct! The laxative would be essential to facilitate the passage of the barium through the alimentary tract. The stool should be checked for barium color and consistency to determine that all the barium has been evacuated.***

49. A client is admitted with end stage cirrhosis of the liver. Which nursing measure would help to decrease the serum ammonia level?

1. Administration of vitamin K (AquaMEPHY-TON).
2. Increased fluid intake.
3. Administration of diuretics.
4. Offer a low-protein, high-calorie diet.

1. *Incorrect choice. Vitamin K would be given to promote blood clotting and reduce the risk of hemorrhage. Try again.*
2. *No. An increased fluid intake would be indicated only to correct any fluid losses from perspiration and fever. This action would not decrease the serum ammonia level. Choose another option.*
3. *Not correct. Diuretics would be ordered to decrease edema and ascites, but would not affect the serum ammonia level. Make another selection.*
4. ***Correct choice. Ammonia is one of the end products of protein metabolism. A low-protein, high-calorie diet will reduce the source of ammonia and promote adequate carbohydrates for energy requirements while "sparing" protein from breakdown for energy.***

50. A person in a restaurant puts his hand to his throat. A nurse who sees this happen begins to administer the Heimlich maneuver. After the client falls to the floor, the nurse should:

1. Check for the pulse.
2. Sweep the mouth.
3. Attempt to ventilate.
4. Administer five abdominal thrusts.

1. *Incorrect. If there is no air moving it is not appropriate to progress to the pulse check. Try again.*
2. ***Congratulations, you are correct. The mouth sweep is performed in case the object is high enough in the oral cavity to allow for removal.***
3. *No, this is not the correct sequence as taught by the American Heart Association or the Red Cross. Make another selection.*
4. *Not yet. Several steps are missing. Rethink this and try again.*

51. A client received a large contusion on the head and a fracture of the femur. The nurse must be alert for possible complications. Which manifestation indicates a serious complication to the nurse?

    1. A change in temperature from 98.4° F to 98.2° F.
    2. A blood pressure decrease from 120/90 to 112/74.
    3. Increased pain at the site of the femur fracture.
    4. A change in respiratory rate from 18 to 32, with increased restlessness.

    1. *Incorrect choice! This change in temperature is not significant.*
    2. *Try again! This change in blood pressure is not significant.*
    3. *Wrong, try again. Pain at the fracture site is expected.*
    4. ***Good choice! Increased respiratory rate and increased restlessness are manifestations that indicate possible fat embolism. Fat embolism is a serious complication following the type of fracture sustained by the client. Fat emboli may be trapped in lung tissue, leading to respiratory manifestations and mental disturbances.***

    STRATEGY ALERT! Note that the word "fracture" appears in the stem of the question and in Option 3, which is a distractor! Knowing the ranges for normal vital signs is very important. You should always use your nursing knowledge first, and use strategies only when you do not know the answer.

52. A client is hospitalized with chronic obstructive pulmonary disease. Oxygen per nasal cannula at two liters per minute is initiated. When the nurse made an assessment at 3:00 p.m., the client appeared to have made a good adjustment to hospitalization. At 5:00 p.m., when the nurse brought the client his dinner tray, the oxygen cannula is found on the floor. The client was angry and said, "It's about time you got here. Where am I? Where is my breakfast?" The nurse should give immediate consideration to which consideration?

    1. Has the oxygen cannula been off long enough to cause hypoxia?
    2. Is the client's anger is related to being hospitalized again?
    3. Does the client need a clock in the room to keep track of the time?
    4. Is the client accustomed to eating meals at unusual times?

    1. ***Congratulations! The need for oxygen is a physiological need. The client's apparent confusion may be a result of decreased oxygen to the brain. The nurse should give immediate consideration to this physiological need.***

Maslow's Hierarchy of Needs indicates that physiological needs receive first priority.

2. *The case scenario tells us that the client is angry. What he says, however, does not support the idea that he is angry about being hospitalized. This statement also indicates a psychological consideration as the explanation for the client's behavior. It first must be determined if his behavior is due to a physiological need. Maslow's Hierarchy of Needs indicates that physiological needs receive first priority.*
3. *Wrong! The client appears to be confused about the time, because he is asking for his breakfast when it is 5:00 p.m. A clock in his room may help to keep him oriented to the time of day. This, however, is not the most immediate concern of the nurse. This option gives a psychological rationale for the client's behavior. This rationale should be explored only after the nurse makes sure that his behavior was not due to a physiological need. Maslow's Hierarchy of Needs indicates that physiological needs receive first priority.*
4. *Wrong. This option gives a psychological rationale for the client's behavior. This reason should be explored only after the nurse determines that his behavior is not due to a physiological need. Maslow's Hierarchy of Needs indicates that physiological needs receive first priority.*

53. A client is admitted to the hospital with a diagnosis of chest pain. The client is scheduled for a cardiac catheterization. The nurse would immediately report which assessment data about the client to the charge nurse?

    1. The client is allergic to lobster.
    2. The client's father smokes heavily.
    3. The client's husband died of heart disease.
    4. The client is apprehensive about the procedure.

    1. ***Good! Since lobster and the contrast dye used for a cardiac catheterization both contain iodine, the client may have an allergic reaction during the procedure. The doctor who will be doing the procedure needs to know this information immediately to ensure the client's safety. Maslow's Hierarchy of Needs indicates that when no physiological need exists, safety needs should get priority attention.***
    2. *Wrong! The fact that the client's father smokes heavily may be a risk factor for her but it is not an immediate threat to her safety.*
    3. *Wrong! The client's statement that her husband died of heart disease may be an indication of fear on the part of the client. According to Maslow's Hierarchy of Needs, the need for a sense of security is a higher level need. Priority should be placed on the need for safety.*
    4. *Wrong! Apprehension about the procedure indicates a need for security, which is a higher level need according to Maslow's Hierarchy of Needs.*

Priority should be placed on the need for safety.

54. **A client is receiving dietary instructions after being admitted for ascites and an elevated serum ammonia level, secondary to cirrhosis. The nurse would know that the client had accurate understanding of his dietary needs if he selected a menu that was:**

1. High in protein, low in salt.
2. High in calories, moderate in protein.
3. Low in carbohydrates, high in fat.
4. Low in calcium, low in potassium.

1. *No, this diet is not therapeutic for this client. A high protein diet is indicated only when the client with cirrhosis has no ascites or edema and exhibits no signs of impending coma. Low salt would be appropriate for the client with ascites to reduce fluid retention. Try again for a more correct answer.*
2. **Correct choice. The client needs calories to promote liver tissue healing, but moderate to low protein intake to decrease ammonia production (a result of protein metabolism). Excessively high levels of ammonia in the blood are a primary cause of the neurologic changes that constitute hepatic encephalopathy, a dangerous complication of cirrhosis.**
3. *Incorrect. The client needs a therapeutic diet to promote healing of the liver and to prevent further ammonia production. A high fat diet is indicated when the goal is to delay gastric emptying, as in clients with "dumping syndrome" secondary to a gastric resection.*
4. *No, this type of diet is not indicated in clients with cirrhosis. Electrolyte disturbances are not indicated in the manifestations listed above.*

55. **Following the completion of discharge teaching, the nurse would determine that instructions about the long-term consequences of cirrhosis were successful if the client indicates an understanding that he must refrain from:**

1. Drinking alcohol.
2. Smoking.
3. Eating spicy foods.
4. Donating blood.

1. *Absolutely! The intake of alcohol and the administration of hepatotoxic drugs must be restricted completely. Excessive alcohol intake is the major causative factor in fatty liver and its consequences.*
2. *No. Although smoking is a poor health habit, it is not connected to cirrhosis and long-term consequences of the disease.*
3. *Incorrect. Avoiding a spicy diet is indicated if the client has manifestations of gastric disease, not*

liver disease.
4. *Wrong choice. Clients with infectious diseases, such as hepatitis B, are taught to avoid donating blood. Cirrhosis is not an infectious disorder.*

56. **A client has received instructions about behaviors that put him at risk for developing hepatitis A. Which statement by the client indicates to the nurse that he has an accurate understanding of this information?**

1. "I won't donate blood anymore."
2. "I'll get a booster shot of immune serum globulin every year."
3. "I'll stop eating raw clams, even though I love them!"
4. "I won't touch another drop of alcohol."

1. *Incorrect. Hepatitis A is rarely, if ever, transmitted via blood, nor is there any danger of contacting hepatitis A from the equipment used in the blood collection process at blood banks.*
2. *Not necessary. Passive immunity to hepatitis A can be conferred for six to eight weeks by the administration of immune serum globulin during the incubation period, if the treatment is instituted within two weeks of exposure. A booster shot every year would not be appropriate.*
3. **Yes! Individuals who eat raw or steamed shellfish or who work with animals imported from areas where hepatitis A is endemic are at increased risk.**
4. *Wrong choice. Alcohol is associated with cirrhosis. Drinking alcohol does not put a client at risk for contacting hepatitis A. Alcohol is prohibited for four months following recovery from hepatitis, but the case scenario does not state that this is the case. Don't "read into" the question by assuming information that is not stated!*

57. **The physician has ordered a sputum specimen to be collected for culture and sensitivity. The nurse is aware that the preferable time to collect this specimen is:**

1. In the morning.
2. In the evening, after forcing fluids all day.
3. After antibiotics have been started.
4. After the client has taken an expectorant.

1. **Correct! Generally, the deepest specimens are obtained in the early morning. The client is instructed to rinse his mouth prior to expectorating into the sterile container. It's preferable to collect the specimen before breakfast.**
2. *No. Although forcing fluids (especially clear liquids) will help to thin the secretions, the evening hours are not the best time. Select another option.*
3. *Incorrect choice! Recall that any specimen ordered*

for culture and sensitivity should be obtained before antibiotic therapy is started in order to prevent interference with test results. Try again.

4.   No, this is not the best time. Expectorants can contaminate the specimen. Make another selection.

58.   A client had a right lobectomy yesterday and has a chest tube to suction at 20 cm of water pressure. Upon assessment of the client this morning, the nurse notes that there is no fluctuation in the water-seal chamber. At this time, the nurse would first:

1.   Increase the suction until fluctuation reappears.
2.   Observe for kinks in the tubing.
3.   Elevate the head of the bed to 80 degrees.
4.   No action is necessary, since the lung has most likely re-expanded.

1.   *No. This action will have no effect upon the water seal compartment. Recall that the amount of suction is controlled by the water level in the suction-control bottle (i.e., 20 cm level). Turning up the suction will only increase the bubbling! Make another selection.*

2.   ***Good choice! Fluctuation of the water level in the tube shows that there is effective communication between the pleural cavity and the drainage bottle. A decrease in fluctuation one day after surgery most likely means that the tubing is obstructed by blood clots, fibrin, or kinking.***

3.   *No, elevating the head of the bed will not affect the water-seal bottle. Absence of fluctuation indicates a problem within the system. Choose another option.*

4.   *Highly unlikely! Lung re-expansion will not occur within 24 hours after a lobectomy, which takes at least two or three days and needs to be confirmed by a chest x-ray. Try again!*

59.   A client has just returned to the unit after a right pneumonectomy. The nurse should position the client on the:

1.   Right side.
2.   Left side or back.
3.   Back only.
4.   Right side or left side.

1.   ***Excellent choice! After a pneumonectomy, the operative side should be dependent so that fluid in the pleural space remains below the level of the bronchial stump, and the inoperative side can fully expand.***

2.   *No! Positioning the client on his left side — the inoperative side — may compromise complete ventilation of the only lung that the client has.*

Choose again.

3.   *No, this answer is only partially correct. There is another position available that would not compromise the client's respirations. Make another selection.*

4.   *No, the nurse would not want to position the client in such a way as to impair his gas exchange. Think through the surgical results and make another choice.*

60.   In treating diabetic ketoacidosis (DKA), the nurse is aware that the goal of treatment is to correct which imbalance?

1.   Hypoglycemia.
2.   Dehydration.
3.   Hyperkalemia.
4.   Respiratory acidosis.

1.   *No! Diabetic ketoacidosis is caused by an absence or markedly inadequate amount of insulin. This results in hyperglycemia, with blood glucose levels varying from 300 to 800 mg/dl. Choose again.*

2.   ***Correct choice! The hyperglycemia of DKA leads to polyuria and polydipsia with volume depletion. Clients with severe DKA may lose an average of 6.5 liters of water.***

3.   *Incorrect. The hyperglycemia of DKA leads to electrolyte loss, especially potassium. Try to recall the pathophysiology of this process, and make the correct selection.*

4.   *No. In DKA, there is an excess production of ketone bodies because of the lack of insulin. Ketone bodies are acids, and their accumulation in the circulation leads to metabolic acidosis. Choose another option.*

61.   A client has been admitted to the hospital after having two seizures at work. She suddenly gives a short cry and stiffens. The initial nursing action for the client is to:

1.   Make a mental notation of the time after looking at a watch.
2.   Place an oral airway in the client's mouth.
3.   Loosen the clothing around the neck.
4.   Turn her head to the side.

1.   ***Correct! A major responsibility of the nurse is to observe and record the sequence of manifestations. Duration of each phase of the attack is part of the assessment.***

2.   *No. If an aura precedes the seizure, then a padded tongue blade can be inserted between the teeth to reduce the possibility of the tongue or cheek being bitten. The nurse should never attempt to pry open jaws that are clenched in a spasm to insert anything.*

3. *Incorrect. Although this is part of nursing management, it is not the initial intervention. Try again.*
4. *Not the initial action. This is a useful intervention after the seizure to help prevent aspiration. The other appropriate intervention is to protect the head from striking a hard surface during the seizure. Choose again.*

62. To assess for correct placement of a nasogastric tube, the nurse should:

1. Instill 30 ml of saline to assess client tolerance.
2. Instill 10 ml of air into the tube and listen for gurgling sounds with a stethoscope over the gastric area.
3. Aspirate stomach contents with a syringe.
4. Place the end of the tube in water to assess for bubbling.

1. *Incorrect and a hazardous procedure! This could be dangerous if the tube was in the lungs and not the stomach. Select a safer action.*
2. *Incorrect. This method does not provide for a sufficient amount of air to reach the stomach and make any gurgling sounds. At least 30 ml of air is needed. There is a safer and more reliable method among the options given. Try again.*
3. **Absolutely correct! Placement should be checked by aspirating gastric contents with a syringe and testing the pH of the aspirate.**
4. *Never, never! This could be dangerous to the client if the tube was incorrectly positioned in the lungs. The client could aspirate the water in the glass. Select a safer, more reliable option.*

63. A 39-year-old female has had a right radical mastectomy. Which activity would the nurse anticipate will be the most difficult for this client four days postoperatively?

1. Brushing her hair with her right hand.
2. Eating with her right hand.
3. Active-assisted range of motion of the right hand.
4. Washing her hands in a basin.

1. **Good reasoning. Moving the arm away from the body (abduction) would be the most difficult, and usually would be the last type of movement to be regained by the post-mastectomy client.**
2. *No, this isn't too difficult. The arm motion necessary for eating mainly involves the hand, wrist, and elbow. Select again.*
3. *Incorrect. This is an early postoperative activity. Active-assisted means that the client does what she is able with the nurse assisting. Try again.*
4. *No, this isn't too difficult. The affected arm can be held low, and only the fingers and wrist moved. Make another choice.*

64. A colostomy has been performed on a client diagnosed with colon cancer. Postoperatively, the nurse is preparing to change the dressing. The nurse would expect the appearance of the stoma to be:

1. Pale, with a mucoid discharge from the ostomy.
2. Bright red, with a few drops of blood appearing from the stoma.
3. Inclusive of a 2 cm area of eschar.
4. Flush with the abdominal wall.

1. *No. This would indicate a reduced blood supply. Mucous may be present but it does not indicate a functioning or healthy stoma. Select again.*
2. **Great! A small amount of blood from the stoma would be acceptable and indicates a healthy bowel with a good blood supply.**
3. *No, this indicates tissue death, either from a burn or gangrene. This stoma is not healthy. Try another selection.*
4. *Not likely. As the stoma matures it will shrink, but immediately after surgery the stoma is usually edematous. A stoma flush with the abdomen is not desirable, since it will be difficult to ensure maintenance of skin integrity.*

65. Physiologically, the nurse knows the difference between angina and myocardial infarction is:

1. With angina, arterial perfusion is briefly inadequate. With myocardial infarction, arterial perfusion is cut off permanently.
2. With angina, the enzymes SGOT, LDH, and CPK are elevated. With myocardial infarction, they are not elevated.
3. With angina, adrenocorticosteroids are released to reduce the inflammatory reaction. With myocardial infarction, these hormones are absent.
4. With angina, hypertension and congestive heart failure are absent. With myocardial infarction, hypertension and congestive heart failure are present.

1. **Correct. The arterial supply is inadequate in angina but permanently blocked in a myocardial infarction. This is the best answer!**
2. *Wrong! In fact, the opposite is true: after an infarction, the enzymes are elevated. Since there is no muscle or tissue damage in angina, the enzymes are not elevated. This is a distractor. Try again!*
3. *This is a good distractor, but it is incorrect. There is no inflammatory reaction in a myocardial infarction. Were you confused by this option? When you are deciding between two options, always choose what you know for sure!*
4. *This option looks like a possibility. The statement is false, however, because these are complications that may be associated with either angina or*

a myocardial infarction. They are not characteristic of just one of these conditions. This option is a distractor. Try again!

66. A client with increasing intracranial pressure has received mannitol (Osmitrol) intravenously. The nurse would know that the mannitol has been effective if the client has which of these findings?

1. Increased urine output.
2. Decreased pulse rate.
3. Elevated blood pressure.
4. Negative Babinski reflex.

1. ***Correct! Mannitol, an osmotic diuretic, helps to remove fluid from the body as well as from the brain, thus decreasing intracranial pressure. An increased urinary output is the desired effect.***
2. *Incorrect. Mannitol's action does not affect the pulse rate directly. The drug's primary action is related to the increased intracranial pressure and measures to relieve it.*
3. *No, mannitol will not elevate the blood pressure. In fact, the blood pressure may decrease as a result of the drug's major action.*
4. *Not true. A negative Babinski reflex is a normal response, elicited by scraping an object along the sole of the foot. A positive Babinski reflex indicates an abnormality in the motor control pathways leading from the cerebral cortex.*

67. A male client has been given instructions about the cerebral angiogram that is scheduled for later this morning. Which statement by the client indicates to the nurse that additional teaching is needed?

1. "The only allergy I have is to ragweed. I'm glad it won't affect this test."
2. "I signed the special consent form last evening."
3. "I'm glad this procedure has less risks than an MRI."
4. "The nurse told me that I'll feel a flush as the dye is injected."

1. *No, this statement indicates that the client knows the need for allergy identification. The contraindication is allergy to iodine or shellfish because of the iodine base to the contrast media used. Other allergies are not as significant.*
2. *No, this statement indicates that the client knows that a special consent form is indicated because a cerebral angiogram is an invasive procedure. The consent form should be signed after the physician gives the client information about possible risks of the procedure (cerebral bleed, allergic reaction to the dye, internal bleeding at the puncture site).*

3. ***Yes, the client needs further teaching! This procedure, because of its invasive nature, has more risks than an MRI. Risks include a cerebral bleed, allergic reaction to the dye, or internal bleeding at the puncture site.***
4. *No, this statement is true and means that the client understands a particular sensation felt during the procedure. Clients also report feelings of warmth in the face, behind the eyes, or in the jaw, teeth, tongue, and lips, and a metallic taste when the dye is injected.*

68. A physician has prescribed oral neomycin (Mycifradin Sulfate) and a neomycin enema for a client with cirrhosis who is having central nervous system changes. The nurse knows that the neomycin has been effective if which of these laboratory values are decreased?

1. White blood cell count.
2. Ammonia.
3. Creatinine.
4. Serum albumin.

1. *Incorrect. A decreased white blood cell count would be evident after antibiotic therapy for an infection. Cirrhosis is not an infectious process.*
2. ***Yes. The antibiotic neomycin sulfate is given to reduce the number of intestinal bacteria capable of converting urea to ammonia. As the serum ammonia level decreases, the central nervous system changes decrease. Keeping the serum ammonia level within normal limits will help to decrease the chances of hepatic encephalopathy.***
3. *No. Creatinine is a measure of kidney glomerular filtration, not liver function, and would not be affected by neomycin therapy.*
4. *Wrong. Serum albumin levels are not affected by neomycin sulfate, an antibiotic. In cirrhosis, the serum albumin level is already decreased due to altered protein metabolism.*

69. A client is admitted for fluid replacement and a diagnosis is made of hepatitis A virus. Which nursing measure is most important to maintain in the client's plan of care?

1. Strict bedrest.
2. Universal precautions.
3. Patency of the T tube.
4. A low protein, high fat diet.

1. *Try again! Rest is promoted to prevent undue fatigue and to decrease metabolic demands, however, strict bedrest rarely is necessary. The client usually has bathroom privileges.*
2. ***Good choice! Since the mode of transmission of this virus is the fecal oral route, universal***

precautions will prevent contamination of the nurse and others.

3. *Incorrect. A T-tube is not warranted for treatment of hepatitis A virus. A T-tube is used when the common bile duct is edematous and prevents the flow of bile.*

4. *Incorrect. Nutritional deficits can easily occur due to increased metabolic demands. With hepatitis A virus, the metabolism of fats is altered and they usually are poorly tolerated. A high protein diet is recommended to promote liver healing and improve activity tolerance.*

70. **The nurse knows that discharge teaching is successful for a client with hepatitis A virus if the client indicates she will refrain from:**

1. Donating blood.
2. Eating fried foods.
3. Vacationing in a foreign country.
4. Ordering a salad in a restaurant.

1. **Correct. Once a person has been infected with hepatitis A virus, they can never donate blood.**

2. *Incorrect. Dietary fat is not contraindicated, although it may not be well tolerated. The client should recover and be able to tolerate fats within two months.*

3. *Incorrect. It is not necessary for the client to refrain from vacationing. This in itself has no direct correlation to hepatitis A virus.*

4. *Incorrect, although the fear is real if the initial cause of hepatitis A was from eating at a restaurant. It is not necessary for the client to refrain from eating in restaurants.*

71. **A client has a fractured right tibia. Immediately following cast application, the priority nursing action is to:**

1. Perform a complete neurovascular assessment.
2. Encourage adequate nutritional intake of calcium.
3. Air dry the cast.
4. Monitor drainage through the cast.

1. **Good choice! Neurovascular compromises must be detected in the early stages to avoid irreversible and permanent damage.**

2. *Incorrect. Generally good dietary habits are encouraged rather than just calcium intake, even though calcium promotes healing and bone repair.*

3. *Incorrect. Using unnatural ways to dry the cast is contraindicated. Drying of the cast does not take priority.*

4. *Incorrect. Monitoring of drainage is important to validate the amount, yet it is not a priority.*

72. **A physician prescribes para-aminosalicylic acid (PAS) for a client who has been diagnosed with tuberculosis. To decrease the GI manifestations (nausea and vomiting) associated with PAS, the nurse should instruct the client to:**

1. Take the medication at bedtime.
2. Ask the physician to prescribe an anti-emetic to be taken 30 minutes before the PAS.
3. Take the medication with food or an antacid.
4. Crush the tablets and dissolve them completely in water before swallowing.

1. *Incorrect. The normal dosage of PAS is 10-12 grams daily in three or four doses. It could not be taken all at one time.*

2. *Wrong. There should not be a need for this intervention. If the nausea and vomiting were that severe, a change in medication therapy would be indicated. There is another option that will help decrease the side effects without the use of additional drugs.*

3. **Exactly! Nearly all clients taking PAS report GI irritation of one form or another. Taking the drug with food or an antacid prevents some but not all of the irritation produced by the large amount of drug contained in a normal dose.**

4. *No. This intervention, although perfectly acceptable, will not decrease the GI manifestations. PAS is not well tolerated by most clients, but there is an intervention that will help decrease the severity of the nausea and vomiting. Try again.*

73. **A newly diagnosed diabetic with glaucoma is admitted for regulation of his blood sugar. The client receives pilocarpine (Adsorbocarpine) 2% one drop q.i.d. While instilling this drug the nurse should:**

1. Ask the client to look straight ahead.
2. Press on the lacrimal sac for one minute after instillation.
3. Instruct the client to squeeze his eye shut after instillation.
4. First cleanse the eye, then wipe from the outer to the inner canthus.

1. *Incorrect. When instilling eye drops, the client is instructed to look upward since they are less likely to blink in this position.*

2. **Correct. This prevents the medication from running out of the eye and down the duct.**

3. *Incorrect. Squeezing can injure the eye and push out the medication. The client should be instructed to close the eyelids but not to squeeze them shut.*

4. *Incorrect. If the eye needs cleaning, the proper direction to wipe is from the inner to outer canthus. Wiping from the outer to inner canthus would*

cause contamination of the lacrimal duct and possibly the other eye.

74. The nurse would avoid administering terpin hydrate elixir to a client:

1. With thick respiratory secretions.
2. With an allergy to penicillin.
3. Who is pregnant.
4. With glaucoma.

1. *Wrong. Expectorants, such as terpin hydrate, are used to liquefy and mobilize secretions. Thick respiratory secretions would be an indication for their use, not a contraindication. The nurse could administer the drug.*
2. *No, the nurse could administer the drug. There is some cross-allergic reaction between penicillin and the cephalosporin antibiotics, but none between penicillin and terpin hydrate. This would not contraindicate use.*
3. **Yes! There is a high alcohol content in the terpin hydrate elixir. Alcohol can cross the placental barrier and is associated with fetal abnormalities. If a pregnant client requires use of an expectorant, guaifenesin is considered a safer choice.**
4. *No, the nurse could administer the drug. You may be thinking of the anticholinergics. Expectorants have no ophthalmic actions. Glaucoma would not be a concern.*

75. The nurse would avoid administering an antihistamine to a client with a history of:

1. Angina.
2. Irritable bowel syndrome.
3. Sinus headaches.
4. Parkinson's disease.

1. **Correct! The anticholinergic effects of antihistamines can cause tachycardia and extra myocardial oxygen demand.**
2. *No, this is not a contraindication. The effect of antihistamines on the bowel is minimal, and would not be considered life-threatening. Actually, some anticholinergics are given to relieve the manifestations of irritable bowel syndrome.*
3. *No, this is not a contraindication. Sinus headaches may be caused by allergies. These headaches could be relieved by the use of an antihistamine.*
4. *No, this is not a contraindication. Occasionally antihistamines are used for treatment of Parkinson's disease because of their anticholinergic effect.*

76. The nurse understands that prednisone is used in treating cancers because of which effect?

1. Antimicrobial.
2. Anticoagulant.
3. Anti-inflammatory.
4. Anti-infective.

1. *Incorrect. Prednisone does not have an antimicrobial effect. Antimicrobials are antibiotics, like penicillin.*
2. *Incorrect. Anticoagulants are drugs like heparin and warfarin (Coumadin). They interfere with blood clotting.*
3. **Correct. Prednisone has a wide variety of effects, but its anti-inflammatory properties help with the treatment of cancers by suppressing swelling.**
4. *No, anti-infectives include antibiotics or antimicrobials. Try again.*

77. A two-month-old is having a well baby check-up today. The nurse will advise the parents concerning immunizations. The nurse knows that, according to current immunization guidelines, the child is due for which immunizations?

1. MMR and OPV.
2. DPT and OPV.
3. OPV, Hib and DPT.
4. DPT.

1. *Incorrect. MMR is not given until the child is 15 months. Earlier immunization has proven ineffective.*
2. *Partially correct. DPT and OPV are given together at two months, but you are missing something. Try again.*
3. **Yes! OPV (oral polio), Hib (Haemophilus influenzae type b), and DPT (diphtheria, pertussis, tetanus) reflect the current recommendation for immunization of two-month-old children.**
4. *No, this answer is incomplete. DPT only protects the child from the diseases of diphtheria, pertussis and tetanus. This does not meet the current standards.*

78. A five-year-old child is being seen for a well child visit in a pediatric clinic. The child's father tells the nurse that his wife recently has been diagnosed with tuberculosis. In caring for this child the nurse understands that:

1. It is likely that the child will require medication.
2. Small children do not easily contract TB, if they are otherwise healthy.
3. As long as the child has not exhibited the manifestations of night sweats and/or coughing, there is probably no infection.
4. Direct physical contact must be limited to insure the health of the child.

1. *Right! The most common source of infection to a child is an adult within the immediate household. Prophylactic medication and/or treatment for active disease are a high probability for this child.*
2. *No. Children are at high risk when someone in their household has active tuberculosis. In addition, children in this age group have frequent illness, which makes them susceptible hosts.*
3. *No. Manifestations such as coughing are not reliable in small children, so this would be an empty reassurance. Screening with Tine and then PPD would be more appropriate indicators. Try again.*
4. *No. How is TB usually transmitted? That's right-- by droplet. Make another selection.*

79. **The nurse should instruct a client taking alprazolam (Xanax) that he can safely take:**

    1. Alcohol.
    2. Meperidine (Demerol).
    3. Flurazepam (Dalmane).
    4. Acetaminophen (Tylenol).

    1. *Wrong! A client taking Xanax should be instructed to avoid the use of alcohol because the central nervous system depressant effects will be potentiated and could lead to accidental overdose and death. Try again.*
    2. *Wrong! Clients on Xanax should avoid the use of other CNS depressants, such as Dalmane, because of their potentiation effects.*
    3. *Wrong! Clients on Xanax should avoid other benzodiazepine drugs, such as Dalmane, because of the potentiation effects.*
    4. *Correct! This client could safely take acetaminophen. All the other drugs should be avoided.*

80. **A 36-year-old client has hypertension and is treated with chlorothiazide (Diuril). Client education should include which information?**

    1. Dietary sodium should be restricted to one gram daily.
    2. Avoid using Diuril with other antihypertensives.
    3. Orthostatic hypotension may be a side effect.
    4. It is unnecessary to increase dietary potassium.

    1. *Wrong choice! Diuril is a thiazide diuretic that causes sodium loss in the urine. Sodium restriction is not indicated.*
    2. *Incorrect. Diuril is sometimes used with other antihypertensive medications to counteract the effect of sodium retention.*
    3. *Correct choice! Thiazide diuretics such as Diuril may cause orthostatic hypotension. This information should be included in the teaching plan.*
    4. *No, Diuril is a thiazide diuretic and causes potassium loss in the urine. Increased dietary intake or potassium supplements are indicated.*

81. **In caring for an elderly psychiatric client who is severely depressed, the nurse knows that elderly clients:**

    1. Cannot be safely treated with tricyclic antidepressants.
    2. Require lower doses of antidepressants than younger clients.
    3. Respond more quickly to the therapeutic effects of antidepressants than younger clients.
    4. Can be treated safely and effectively with all antidepressants.

    1. *Wrong choice. A careful assessment must be done to rule out clients with cardiac problems or glaucoma. An elderly client who does not have these medical problems can safely be treated with antidepressants, especially those that have a lower incidence of anticholinergic side effects.*
    2. *Correct. Elderly clients are treated with lower doses because of their increased sensitivity to the anticholinergic and cardiovascular side effects.*
    3. *Incorrect. Response rates can take up to three or four weeks for all clients, regardless of age.*
    4. *This is not the correct choice. It is best to avoid treating elderly clients with certain antidepressants that have a higher incidence of anticholinergic or orthostatic hypotensive side effects.*

82. **An unconscious 18-year-old man is brought to the emergency room with heroine overdose. After the client regains consciousness, he is transferred to the substance abuse treatment unit. The signs and manifestations of heroin withdrawal are written in the nursing care plan. Which behavior should the nurse anticipate will occur early in the withdrawal process?**

    1. Vomiting and diarrhea.
    2. Sneezing and rhinorrhea.
    3. Restlessness and irritability.
    4. Yawning and diaphoresis.

    1. *This is not correct. Vomiting and diarrhea are usually late, rather than early, signs of heroin withdrawal.*
    2. *This is not correct. Sneezing and rhinorrhea are usually late, rather than early, signs of heroin withdrawal.*
    3. *Correct. Restlessness, irritability, piloerection (gooseflesh), tremors, and loss of appetite are all early signs of heroin withdrawal.*
    4. *This is not correct. Yawning and diaphoresis are usually late, rather than early, signs of heroin withdrawal.*

83. **In caring for a client being treated for withdrawal syndrome, the nurse knows that many drugs are associ-**

ated with a life-threatening abstinence syndrome. However, this is not true for all addictive drugs. Which of the following drug groups is least likely to present a medical crisis during withdrawal?

1. Narcotics.
2. Barbiturates.
3. Alcohol.
4. Benzodiazepines.

*1. **Very good! The abstinence syndrome following narcotic abuse is uncomfortable but is not life-threatening.***
2. This is not correct. The abstinence syndrome associated with barbiturate abuse can involve seizures and lead to death.
3. This is not correct. Alcohol withdrawal can involve seizures and lead to death if not medically managed.
4. This is not correct. The abstinence syndrome associated with the prolonged use of benzodiazepine anti-anxiety agents can involve seizures and lead to death.

84. A high school student speaks to the school nurse about a friend who is abusing cocaine. He wants to know the best way to influence his friend to stop. The nurse's response is based on what knowledge about cocaine?

1. Cocaine use rarely interferes with academic or career activities.
2. Cocaine abuse is difficult to treat because of its abstinence syndrome.
3. Cocaine does more psychological harm than physical damage.
4. Cocaine use is highly reinforcing.

1. This is not correct. Cocaine use is frequently associated with family, financial, academic, and career disruptions.
2. This is not the best option. Cocaine abuse results in a powerful psychological dependence. Repeated abuse is associated with an abstinence syndrome of fatigue, depression, prolonged sleep and increased appetite with overeating. This abstinence syndrome is unpleasant but not life-threatening unless the depression becomes suicidal.
3. This is not correct. Medical complications of cocaine use include severe weight loss, hepatitis, cerebrovascular stroke, and cardiac arrest.
*4. **Correct. Because of cocaine's effects on the neurotransmitters that regulate mood and other psychological processes, it is highly reinforcing of self-administration. Cocaine abuse is very difficult to treat. Some abusers are treated successfully as outpatients, but many require inpatient treatment programs.***

85. In caring for alcoholic clients, the nurse knows that the category of drugs commonly used to manage alcohol withdrawal is:

1. Antipsychotic drugs.
2. Barbiturates.
3. Anti-anxiety agents.
4. Anticonvulsants.

1. This is not correct. Antipsychotics are used to treat psychotic manifestations. They are not used to manage alcohol withdrawal.
2. This is not correct. Barbiturates are potent central nervous system depressants. They are not used during alcohol withdrawal.
*3. **Correct. Anti-anxiety agents, such as chlordiazepoxide (Librium) and diazepam (Valium), are long acting central nervous system depressants that are used to treat alcohol withdrawal. They are substituted for alcohol during the withdrawal process to prevent the occurrence of delirium tremens and to minimize withdrawal manifestations.***
4. This is not correct. Magnesium sulfate or other anticonvulsants may be used to prevent seizures during detoxification in clients with a history of seizures. Anticonvulsants, however, are not commonly used in alcohol withdrawal for clients who do not have a history of seizures.

86. After detoxification, the client begins the rehabilitation phase of treatment. He tells the nurse that he cannot imagine living his life without alcohol. The nurse's best response is based on the knowledge that the client will:

1. Be more successful if he focuses on goals for short periods of time, such as "today" or "this week."
2. Likely drink again when under stress.
3. Not be successful if he is not strongly motivated.
4. Require treatment with Antabuse to maintain sobriety.

*1. **Correct. Clients are less overwhelmed by the thought of sobriety when they set short-term goals that focus on "today" or "this week." Dealing with shorter periods of time is more manageable. The AA maxim, "One day at a time," is a reflection of this principle.***
2. This could be true, but it is not the best option because it would not be the basis for a helpful response for this client.
3. Motivation is important but the statement by the client does not indicate a lack of motivation. Moreover, motivation alone is not sufficient to maintain sobriety. The client must also develop the skills to maintain sobriety. Can you identify the basis for a therapeutic response that addresses the client's concerns?
4. Wrong! Antabuse is used for individuals who lack

the ability to abstain from alcohol without fear of adverse consequences. There is no data to indicate that this client requires Antabuse, since he is just beginning his rehabilitation program.

87. An unconscious 18-year-old man is brought to the emergency room by two friends, who report he took an overdose of heroin. A narcotic antagonist, naloxone (Narcan) is administered. After giving the medication, the nurse should monitor this client closely for signs of:

1. Respiratory depression.
2. Seizure activity.
3. Nausea.
4. Kidney failure.

1. Congratulations! Narcan displaces the opioid from the receptor sites in neurons and dramatically reverses the effects of the drug overdose. The client must still be monitored closely, however, because Narcan has a short duration of action and its effect may wear off before the overdosed drug has been sufficiently eliminated. If the client returns to a coma, naloxone must be given again.

2. This is not correct. Seizure activity is not associated with either heroin overdose or the use of Narcan.

3. This is not correct. Nausea is not associated with either heroin overdose or the use of Narcan. Nausea, however, is one of the late developing manifestations of heroin withdrawal.

4. This is not correct. Kidney failure is not associated with either heroin overdose or the use of Narcan.

88. A client's husband asks to speak to the nurse about what effects he and his wife should expect after she is treated with electroconvulsive therapy (ECT). He says, "I know it will improve her depression, but couldn't it also turn her into a vegetable?" After explaining that ECT will not cause any brain damage, what additional information can the nurse ethically give him?

1. "The main side effects are temporary and may include mild confusion, a slight headache, and short-term memory problems."
2. "Most clients have no adverse effects to this treatment. In rare cases it has been known to cause fractures resulting from the induced seizure."
3. "Some clients with cardiac problems have been known to have a heart attack, but we will monitor her closely to be certain this does not happen."
4. "There are no permanent adverse effects associated with this treatment. The only common side effect is short-term memory problems that last for a few weeks."

1. Correct. The main side effects are mild disorientation and confusion immediately after the treatment, a slight headache, and short-term memory problems. Information about the treatment should be presented by the treating psychiatrist, but the nurse should reinforce this information and answer any questions the client and family may have.

2. Incorrect. There are several possible adverse effects to ECT, but fractures is not one of them. Before receiving the treatment, the client is medicated with a muscle relaxant to prevent any muscle contractions, and resulting fractures, during the brain seizure.

3. This option is factually incorrect correct and would be inappropriate to present to a client or family member. Clients receive a complete medical history and physical exam before being scheduled for ECT. In addition, any client with heart disease should receive a cardiology consultation and clearance before receiving ECT. ECT is not done when a client has a history of recent myocardial infarction or aneurysm.

4. This option, while technically correct, is not truthful. Whenever general anesthesia is used there is a small risk of death. Clients need to be accurately informed of both the risks and benefits so they can make an informed decision.

89. The nurse admitting a client to the psychiatric unit asks what factors, such as a recent change in his life, may have contributed to his hospitalization. He replies, "Change . . . change is money . . . when you have money you make the change." This statement an example of:

1. Clanging.
2. Echolalia.
3. Perseveration.
4. Flight of ideas.

1. Correct. Clanging is speech in which sounds, rather than conceptual relationships, govern word choice. It is most commonly associated with schizophrenia and mania.

2. Wrong choice! Echolalia is the repetition or "echoing" of the words or phrases of others. This is not the correct option.

3. Wrong. Perseveration is the persistent repetition of words or ideas so that once an individual uses a particular word it recurs. It is most commonly associated with organic mental disorders or schizophrenia.

4. Sorry. Flight of ideas refers to a nearly continuous flow of accelerated speech with abrupt changes from topic to topic before the original topic is completed. It is most frequently associated with manic episodes but is also seen in other conditions.

90. The nurse is to instruct a client to recognize beginning signs of lithium toxicity, which include:

1. Nystagmus, irregular tremor, decreased urine output.
2. Tinnitus, blurred vision, slurred speech.
3. Incoordination, muscle twitching, severe diarrhea.
4. Mild ataxia, coarse hand tremors, difficulty concentrating.

1. *These are signs of severe lithium intoxication. The key word in this question is "beginning." Read the options again, and identify the signs of beginning intoxication.*
2. *These are signs of moderate lithium intoxication. The key word in this question is "beginning." Read the options again, and identify the signs of beginning intoxication.*
3. *These are signs of moderate lithium intoxication. The key word in this question is "beginning." Read the options again, and identify the signs of beginning intoxication.*
4. ***Very good! If these manifestations occur, the client should stop the medication and call his or her psychiatrist immediately. The client should also call the psychiatrist if vomiting, diarrhea, tinnitus, blurred vision, nystagmus, decreased urine output, seizures, or irregular pulse — the manifestations of moderate or severe lithium toxicity — occur. Lithium toxicity can lead to cardiac arrest and death.***

91. A newly admitted client in the alcoholic treatment unit tells the nurse he has not had anything to drink for 24 hours prior to admission. He complains of feeling anxious and shaky. Based on the nurse's knowledge of alcohol withdrawal, what other behaviors could the nurse expect the client to display during the early phase of his alcohol withdrawal?

1. Coarse tremors, tachycardia, insomnia.
2. Confusion, visual hallucinations, delusions.
3. Disorientation, confabulation, memory deficits.
4. Incoordination, impaired thinking, irregular eye movements.

1. ***Correct. The earliest signs of alcohol withdrawal are anxiety, anorexia, insomnia, and tremor. Tachycardia of 120-140 beats per minute persists throughout withdrawal. Pulse rates are closely monitored during the withdrawal process to assess the client's condition and need for medication.***
2. *This is not correct. The onset of confusion, visual hallucinations, and delusional activity indicates delirium tremens, now called alcohol withdrawal delirium, which is a potentially fatal complication of alcohol withdrawal that occurs when the withdrawal process has not been medically managed. It begins the second or third day after the client's last drink and lasts 48 to 72 hours.*

3. *This is not correct. Disorientation, confabulation and memory deficits are manifestations of alcohol amnestic disorder or Korsakoff's syndrome. Thiamine deficiency, a physical disorder associated with chronic alcoholism, is thought to cause this syndrome.*
4. *This is not correct. Incoordination, impaired thinking, and irregular eye movements are seen in Wernicke's syndrome, a rare disorder of central nervous system metabolism associated with thiamine deficiency and seen chiefly in chronic alcoholics.*

92. An elderly client is admitted to the hospital for surgery after finding a lump in his right testicle. He asks the nurse, "Do you think the doctor will find cancer?" The best response by the nurse initially is:

1. "Most lumps found in the testicles are benign."
2. "It must be difficult for you not to know what the doctor will find."
3. "I think that you should discuss this with your doctor."
4. "It might be, but the doctor won't know until the surgery is performed."

1. *Wrong. This statement does not allow the client to express his fears concerning cancer. This response blocks communication between the client and the nurse.*
2. ***Very good! This response promotes communication by allowing the client to express his feelings.***
3. *Referring the client's concern to the doctor puts the client's concern on hold and is not a therapeutic nursing response. The client's feelings and concerns need to be addressed by the nurse. Try again.*
4. *This response does not help the client to explore his feelings and is not a therapeutic nursing response. Choose another option.*

93. A client is taught to do colostomy care for herself prior to discharge. She says to the nurse, "I don't think that I will be able to take care of this colostomy myself." Which of the following is the most helpful response by the nurse?

1. "Don't worry about it. Most clients feel like that at first."
2. "What part of the colostomy care are you having trouble with?"
3. "In time, you will become better at this than I am."
4. "A home health nurse will be visiting you, and can help you if you have any problems."

1. *This response may appear to be reassuring to the client, but it actually inhibits further communica-*

tion by devaluing the client's feelings. The client is saying "I can't," and the nurse is saying "Don't worry about it." This is not a therapeutic response.

2. *Very good! Addressing the client's concerns is a goal of therapeutic communication. The communication tool that is used in this response accepts the client's feelings and seeks clarification of the client's concerns.*

3. *This response contradicts the client and devalues the client's feelings. The client is saying "I can't," and the nurse is saying "Yes, you can." This is not a therapeutic response.*

4. This is a common practice for a client with a colostomy. However, this response does not obtain further *information about the client's feelings. Clarification of the client's concerns is necessary for further interventions that meet the client's needs.*

94. **A 76-year-old client was admitted to the hospital for surgery for a fractured hip. The client says to the nurse, "I guess I've lived long enough, and my number's up." How should the nurse respond initially?**

1. "You are in really good shape for your age."
2. "This is just a minor setback. You will be on your feet in no time."
3. "You feel that your life is ending?"
4. "The doctors and nurses are going to take good care of you while you are here. There's nothing to worry about."

1. *This response does not address the client's concerns. He has made a statement that implies he is going to die. The nurse needs to explore these feelings further to be able to promote therapeutic communication. This response devalues the client's feelings and is an inhibitor to effective communication.*

2. *This response devalues the client's feelings about dying, and it also uses trite and false assurance, which inhibit communication. The nurse needs to address this client's feelings of doom.*

3. *Excellent! This response uses restatement and clarification of the client's feelings to promote therapeutic communication. It addresses the client's immediate concerns.*

4. *This response focuses on inappropriate persons (the doctors and nurses) and not on the client. The feelings of the client concern death, but this response devalues his feelings by using superficial and false reassurance.*

95. **A client is in the hospital because of severe weight loss and refusal to eat. The physician ordered the insertion of a nasogastric tube for feeding. The nurse finds the client with the tube removed. The client tells that nurse that he "doesn't need that thing." The most appropriate response by the nurse is:**

1. "You shouldn't have done that! Now I have to put it down again."
2. "Why did you pull that tube out? Do you want to die?"
3. "Tell me what you don't like about the tube."
4. "Your doctor is going to be very upset with you for doing this."

1. *Wrong! This response indicates that the nurse is inconvenienced by the client's actions. Furthermore, "You shouldn't have done that!" is a judgmental statement, which is non-therapeutic. This is not an appropriate response.*

2. *This response is judgmental because it implies that the client did something wrong. It may also imply that he did it because he wants to die, and the nurse does not know the client's reason for his action. The nurse's response also puts the client on the defensive by requesting an explanation with a "why" question, which is a block to therapeutic communication.*

3. *Correct. This response allows the client to tell the nurse how he feels about the tube and what it means to him. It promotes therapeutic communication and doesn't judge the client's actions. This response is therapeutic for the client.*

4. *This response focuses not on the client but on the doctor. It also expresses the opinion of the nurse, which is not important. The response is judgmental in that it implies that the client did something that is wrong. Therapeutic communication promotes the expression of the client's feelings. This option doesn't promote any communication and is not therapeutic.*

96. **A client is scheduled for a cardiac bypass surgery in the morning. Before the surgery, she states to the nurse, "I don't think I'm going to have the surgery. Everybody has to die sometime." The best response by the nurse is:**

1. "If you don't have the surgery, you will most likely die sooner."
2. "There are always risks involved with surgery. Why have you changed your mind about the operation?"
3. "Cardiac bypass surgery must be very frightening for you. Tell me how you feel about the surgery."
4. "I will call your doctor to come in and talk to you."

1. *Wrong! This response devalues the client's feelings and is a block to any further communication!*

2. *The first part of this response addresses the procedure but not the client's fear. The second part is an illustration of requesting an explanation. The nurse has asked a question beginning with the word*

"why." This can be intimidating and is a communication block. To be therapeutic, the response should address the client's feelings. Select again.

3. ***Very good! The nurse's response shows empathy and focuses on the client's feelings in a non-threatening way, by using the communication tool of clarification.***

4. *This response does not address the client's feelings and puts the client's feelings on hold. Choose another option.*

97. **A male nurse received a doctor's order to catheterize one of his female clients. The client says, "I'm not going to allow a male nurse to catheterize me." The therapeutic nursing response is:**

1. "Your doctor is a male. Would you let him catheterize you?"
2. "I've done this many times with no problems."
3. "You can explain to your doctor why the catheter wasn't inserted."
4. "You appear to be upset. Let me find a female nurse to help with the procedure."

1. *This response focuses on an inappropriate person (the doctor), focuses on an inappropriate issue (whether the client would allow the doctor to catheterize her), and devalues the client's feelings. The response places the client on the defensive and is not therapeutic.*

2. *This response focuses on an inappropriate person (the nurse), focuses on an inappropriate issue (the nurse's competency), and does not address the client's feelings or concerns. This response is not therapeutic for the client.*

3. *This response refers the client to an inappropriate person (the doctor) and fails to ensure that an ordered procedure is performed, which might endanger the client. This response is not professional.*

4. ***Good choice! This response shows empathy, responds to the client's concern, and offers a possible solution to the problem. This is the best of the four options for this question. The other options are not client centered, and are defensive and unfocused.***

98. **An elderly male client is to have Foley urinary catheter care daily. Which of the following is the best action to provide for the client's privacy during this treatment?**

1. Pull the curtain around the client's bed.
2. Cover the penis with a towel while performing catheter care.
3. Close the door to the client's room.
4. Ask the client's roommate to leave until the treatment is finished.

1. ***Correct! Pulling the curtain provides the most privacy for the client. With the curtain pulled,*** *neither the roommate nor anyone entering the room will have visual access to the client or the treatment being performed.*

2. *This action is inappropriate. Performing catheter care includes cleansing and inspection of the urinary meatus. This cannot be accomplished if the penis is covered.*

3. *While closing the door provides some privacy for the client, anyone can open the door and unnecessarily expose the client to the person entering the room and others in the hallway. There is a better option.*

4. *It is not necessary for the client's roommate to leave the room while catheter care is performed. Also, anyone can open the door and unnecessarily expose the client to the person entering the room and others in the hallway. There is a better option.*

99. **A client is hospitalized for a surgical procedure. The most important nursing intervention when administering the preoperative medication is:**

1. Have the client void before going to the operating room.
2. Put the side rails up, and instruct the client to remain in bed.
3. Ask the client if she has signed all of the admission forms for the surgery.
4. Have the family leave, since the medication will decrease the client's inhibitions and she may say or do something that is out of character for her.

1. *Sorry, this is not the answer. Although it is standard preoperative care to have clients void prior to surgery, the nurse should have the client void before administering the preoperative medication.*

> **TEST-TAKING TIP:** *The stem of the question asks about administering the preoperative medication — not about preoperative preparation of the client. This option does not address the issue in the question.*

2. ***Yes! Preoperative medications may cause the client to become disoriented, drowsy, and unsteady when walking. It is very important that the side rails are up and the client remain in bed in order to protect the client from an injury caused by a fall.***

> **SAFETY ALERT!** *Preoperative medications are identified as a priority risk factor, because they impair the client's ability to perceive and respond to danger.*

3. *No, this is not an appropriate nursing action! The necessary forms should be signed prior to surgery, but the client does not know what forms are required by the hospital. It is the nursing staff's responsibility to check the forms for completion.*

4. *No, this is not an appropriate nursing action! Although preoperative medications can alter a*

person's behavior, educating the family about the possible side effects is more appropriate than separating the family at this time, when support for the client is important.

100. An elderly, confused client is on bed rest. Which nursing intervention is not consistent with providing safe care for this client?

   1. Provide regular toileting.
   2. Explain to the client that she should use the call light if she needs to get up.
   3. Place the side rails in the up position and check on the client often.
   4. Initiate the proper use of restraints.

   1. No. This is an important and necessary nursing action. When a confused, elderly client has the physiological need to void or have a bowel movement, an attempt is usually made to find a bathroom. This attempt may result in a fall for the confused client.

> **TEST-TAKING TIP:** *Since this question has a false response stem, the correct answer is something that will NOT help prevent a fall.*

   2. *Excellent! If the client is confused, as identified in the case scenario, she is not likely to remember instructions concerning the use of the call light. This action is not likely to prevent a fall, and does not provide for the client's safety. Since this question has a false response stem, the answer is something that will NOT prevent a fall.*

> **SAFETY ALERT!** *This client is confused, and thus may not be able to perceive danger.*

   3. Wrong. The side rails should be in the up position to prevent the client from falling out of bed, and to serve as a reminder to the client to remain in bed.

> **TEST-TAKING TIP:** *Since this question has a false response stem, the correct answer is something that will NOT help prevent a fall.*

   4. Wrong. If the client is assessed and it is determined that she needs to be restrained in order to avoid injury, then restraints may be applied, and the physician notified of the situation. Note that the option provided for the PROPER use of restraints.

> **TEST-TAKING TIP:** *Since this question has a false response stem, the correct answer is something that will NOT help prevent a fall.*

NCLEX-PN

Test 3

NCLEX-PN TEST 3

1. **The nurse knows which action is the most common cause of invasion of a client's privacy?**

   1. Over-exposing a client during a treatment or examination.
   2. Failing to pull the curtain while performing a treatment or examination.
   3. Talking about the client to other staff members who are not involved with the care of the client, or within hearing of the public.
   4. Helping a client with a tub bath.

2. **A 55-year-old client is hospitalized following myocardial infarction. He is to be transferred from a cart to a bed in a room on a unit. When transferring the client from a cart to his bed, the priority nursing action is to:**

   1. Have the client place his arms on his chest.
   2. Lock the wheels on the cart and the bed.
   3. Have at least four people to help with the transfer.
   4. Use a draw sheet to move the client.

3. **A client has left-sided weakness secondary to a stroke. In assisting him out of bed, which nursing action would be most appropriate?**

   1. Allow the client to do as much of the transfer as possible.
   2. Lock the wheels of the bed and wheelchair.
   3. Place the client's hands around the nurse's neck for support.
   4. Place the front of the wheelchair at a right angle to the bed.

4. **The doctor has ordered restraints for a very agitated client. When applying restraints to the client, which nursing action is inappropriate?**

   1. Using the least restrictive type of restraint that will effectively protect the client from injury.
   2. Fastening the restraints to the bed frame.
   3. Tying the restraint with a knot that cannot be undone easily, in order to prevent the client from untying it.
   4. Explaining to the client and family the type of restraint and the reason for applying the restraint.

5. **During administration of medications to a client, the priority nursing action is to:**

   1. Help the client swallow medications without aspirating by keeping the head in a neutral position.
   2. Identify the client by checking the client's identification bracelet and asking for his name.
   3. Keep all prepared medications in sight.
   4. Check the client for desired or undesired drug effects within an hour after administration of the medication.

6. **A client puts her call light on and tells the nurse that she has to urinate. The client has had a Foley catheter in place since her surgery two days ago. The appropriate nursing action is to:**

   1. Remind the client that she has a Foley catheter in place and does not need to go to the bathroom.
   2. Replace the Foley catheter with a new catheter.
   3. Explain to the client that the urge to void is a common occurrence for clients who have urinary catheters.
   4. Check the catheter and tubing for kinks and note the urine output in the drainage bag.

7. **An adolescent client had surgery on his foot and has just been returned to his room from the recovery room. The initial assessment indicates that he is stable. An hour later, his roommate turns on the call light and tells the nurse that the client has gotten up and hopped on one foot to the bathroom, using his IV pole for support. What should the nurse do first?**

   1. Open the bathroom door to assess if the client is okay.
   2. Help the client back to bed and get him a urinal.
   3. Explain to the client that it is not safe for him to be hopping around on one foot.
   4. Get a wheelchair and help the client back to bed when he is done in the bathroom.

8. **An elderly client is on strict bed rest. While making an occupied bed for this client, which action should the nurse take to maintain proper body mechanics?**

   1. Place the bed in semi-Fowler's position.
   2. Place the bed in a low horizontal position.
   3. Ask the client to move to the foot of the bed.
   4. Place the bed in a high horizontal position.

9. **The nurse is caring for a client who is visually impaired from a childhood injury. When ambulating this client, the most important nursing action is:**

   1. Not to leave the client alone in an unfamiliar area.
   2. To stand on the client's non-dominant side.
   3. To have the client use his dominant hand to reach out for barriers or landmarks.
   4. To describe the route to be taken and remove any

obstacles.

10. **The nurse in a long-term care facility is ambulating a newly admitted, frail, elderly client. The nurse provides for the client's safety by:**

    1. Allowing the client to get up and walk unsupervised.
    2. Using a transfer belt if the client is unsteady.
    3. Allowing the client to shuffle when walking.
    4. Walking two feet behind the client in case of a fall.

11. **An elderly client is confused. The charge nurse says that the client is constipated and is to have a soap suds enema. As the nurse is explaining the procedure, the client states that she doesn't think that she is supposed to have an enema. At this time, the nurse should:**

    1. Tell the client that her doctor must have ordered the procedure.
    2. Assure the client that although the procedure sounds unpleasant, she will feel better afterwards.
    3. Check the client's chart for the doctor's order to help clarify the situation.
    4. Record on the chart that the client refused the enema.

12. **While transferring a client with left-leg weakness from the bed to a wheelchair, the most important nursing action is to:**

    1. Have the seat of the wheelchair at a right angle to the bed.
    2. Lock the wheels on the bed and the wheelchair.
    3. Allow the client to do as much as possible to increase his sense of independence.
    4. Have the client lock his hands around the nurse's neck to provide the client with a sense of security.

13. **A postoperative client is ambulatory and wishes to go to the day room. While the nurse is walking down the hall with the client, the client says that she feels faint and starts to fall. The nurse would:**

    1. Grasp the client around the waist and hold her up so she doesn't fall and injure herself.
    2. Hold the client up against the wall to keep her from falling.
    3. Ease the client gently to the floor.
    4. Ask another client to get some help while supporting the client to prevent her from falling.

14. **A client is to be transferred from her bed to a stretcher, in order to be transported to surgery for a fractured hip. The priority nursing action is to:**

    1. Provide for the client's privacy with a blanket.
    2. Lock the wheels on the stretcher and the bed.
    3. Have four people available for lifting the client.
    4. Provide a lifting device to assist with moving the client.

15. **A client is to receive medication for control of tachycardia and an irregular heart rate. The nurse obtains the following vital signs prior to administering this medication: blood pressure 98/54; pulse 48; respirations 30; temperature 98° F. The client's skin is cool, with cyanosis of the fingers and lips. Based on this data, the priority nursing action is to:**

    1. Administer the medication as ordered by the physician.
    2. Omit the medication for a day or two, depending on the client's response and manifestations.
    3. Notify the charge nurse concerning the client's status before administering the medication.
    4. Give the client one half of the ordered dose.

16. **The first, most important nursing action when a nurse discovers a fire in a client's room is to:**

    1. Pull the fire alarm and notify the hospital operator.
    2. Close fire doors and client room doors.
    3. Remove the client from the room.
    4. Place moist towels or blankets at the threshold of the door of the room with the fire.

17. **A mother expresses concern about her infant's lack of eye muscle control at two days of age. Her neighbor's daughter is mentally retarded and her eyes cross the same way. What is the nurse's best reply?**

    1. "You should probably talk to the doctor about your concerns."
    2. "Newborns all lack the ability to control eye movement until they are three to four months of age."
    3. "I will take the baby back to the nursery and assess other neuromuscular activity."
    4. "It's nothing to worry about."

18. **A mother is concerned about her infant, who was born large for gestational age at 39 weeks gestation. She has heard that fat babies become fat children and she wants to limit her baby's intake during the next days. What is the nurse's best response?**

    1. "You will need to discuss this with the baby's doctor."
    2. "LGA babies are at risk for hypoglycemia. The baby needs additional calories at this time."
    3. "Don't worry, babies always lose weight anyway, no matter what they eat."
    4. "Let's try feeding the baby one ounce at each feeding and see how he tolerates it."

19. The nurse is to administer naloxone (Narcan) to an infant weighing 3.5 kg. The suggested dosage is 0.1 mg per kg, and the drug is supplied in a vial labeled 0.4 mg/ml. How much will the nurse administer to the infant?

    1. 0.35 cc.
    2. 0.62 cc.
    3. 0.87 cc.
    4. 1.1 cc.

20. Which of the following clinical manifestations would the nurse expect to see in a client with an ectopic pregnancy?

    1. Acute abdominal pain, with or without vaginal bleeding at 11 weeks gestation.
    2. Large amount of vaginal bleeding with menstrual-type discomfort at 10 weeks gestation.
    3. Severe nausea and vomiting with abdominal pain at 15 weeks gestation.
    4. Rapidly enlarging uterus with a rise in blood pressure at 10 weeks gestation.

21. Which of the following clinical findings would the nurse expect to find in a client with a hydatidiform mole?

    1. Bright red vaginal bleeding.
    2. Excessive uterine enlargement.
    3. Fetal heart rate irregularities.
    4. Rapidly dropping human chorionic gonadotropin levels (hCG).

22. The nurse is caring for a client with an abruptio placenta. The nurse would expect clinical findings to include:

    1. Large amount of bright red vaginal bleeding, with or without pain.
    2. Moderate to large amount of bright red vaginal bleeding, with decreasing fundal height.
    3. Abdominal pain with or without bright red vaginal bleeding.
    4. Intermittent abdominal pain with bright red vaginal bleeding.

23. The nurse is teaching a client who is to receive danazol (Danocrine) to treat her endometriosis. Which of the following effects should the nurse teach the client to expect as a result of this drug?

    1. No periods.
    2. Weight loss.
    3. Breast enlargement.
    4. Hair loss.

24. The nurse is to administer silver nitrate to a newborn, as protection against blindness related to exposure to gonorrhea in the process of delivery. Which of the following

is inconsistent with a normal response to silver nitrate instillation into the newborn's eyes?

    1. Edema.
    2. Inflammation.
    3. Purulent drainage.
    4. Crusty appearance.

25. The nurse has just given a rubella vaccine to a client who is two days postpartum. Which statement by the client would alert the nurse to the client's need for further instruction?

    1. "I may get a low-grade fever after this shot."
    2. "I will still need to have a rubella titer when I get pregnant next time."
    3. "As long as I don't get flu-like manifestations in the next four days I can conceive any time I want."
    4. "I may experience a stinging feeling at the site where I got the shot."

26. An obstetrical client is to receive oxytocin (Pitocin). The nurse knows that the use of Pitocin for induction of labor is contraindicated in:

    1. Post term pregnancy.
    2. Prolonged rupture of membranes at 38 weeks gestation.
    3. Positive contraction stress test at 38 weeks gestation.
    4. Mild preeclampsia at 38 weeks gestation.

27. The nurse is to administer naloxone (Narcan) to a newborn infant. The nurse understands that the use of Narcan in a newborn is warranted in the case of respiratory depression related to:

    1. Narcotics given to the mother in labor.
    2. Maternal drug use.
    3. Hyaline membrane disease.
    4. Meconium aspiration.

28. A seven-year-old with newly diagnosed asthma is admitted. He is receiving theophylline (Theo-Dur). He complains of nausea and headache, and says his "heart is pounding." The nurse should:

    1. Report these manifestations to the RN immediately.
    2. Document and reassess in 30 minutes.
    3. Sit down with him and provide reassurance.
    4. Provide distraction with a quiet game.

29. A 10-month-old is scheduled for OR. The preoperative medication is ordered IM, and the volume will amount to 1.5 cc. The nurse should give the injection in the:

    1. Deltoid muscle.

2. Gluteus maximus.
3. Rectus femoris.
4. Vastus lateralis.

30. **A 12-year-old is admitted with possible appendicitis. Which order should the nurse question with the charge nurse before implementing?**

    1. NPO.
    2. Fleets enema today.
    3. Medicate with Demerol (meperidine) 50 mg every four hours PRN.
    4. Temperature every four hours.

31. **Following several episodes of vomiting combined with increasing temperature in a two-year-old toddler, the nurse is to assess the client for dehydration. The best indicator of dehydration is:**

    1. A listless appearance.
    2. BP of 90/58.
    3. Depressed fontanel.
    4. Specific gravity of 1.010.

32. **The observation by the nurse that would assist in the diagnosis of pyloric stenosis is:**

    1. Projectile vomiting.
    2. Effortless regurgitation.
    3. Distended abdomen.
    4. Improvement with frequent burping.

33. **A child is admitted with possible streptococcal infection. Twenty-four hours later, the throat culture result is positive. The nurse interprets this information as indicating:**

    1. Antibiotic therapy has been successful.
    2. Nothing of clinical significance.
    3. The child should be placed on isolation.
    4. An organism has been identified.

34. **When planning the discharge of a child receiving warfarin (Coumadin) therapy, the nurse should teach the parents to:**

    1. Monitor for signs of bleeding.
    2. Discontinue if there are signs of viral infection.
    3. Check pulses before administration.
    4. Administer the medication subcutaneously.

35. **When planning to teach families about Reye's syndrome, it is important for the nurse to know that Reye's syndrome is:**

    1. Avoidable.
    2. Untreatable.
    3. Caused by hepatic failure.
    4. Poorly understood.

36. **A school age child with neuroblastoma becomes anorexic, with periods of nausea after beginning chemotherapy. The best nursing intervention is to:**

    1. Allow him to eat whatever he wants, at any time.
    2. Force him to eat balanced meals.
    3. Encourage high quality nutritious foods.
    4. Increase proteins and fats.

37. **Which activity would the nurse encourage in order to meet the developmental needs of a 12-month-old hospitalized client?**

    1. A cradle gym across crib.
    2. Push-pull toys.
    3. Finger paints.
    4. A stick horse.

38. **The nurse caring for a client with pediatric leukemia knows that the most important measure to prevent complications and death is:**

    1. Proper administration of iron.
    2. Prevention of infection.
    3. Monitoring intake and output.
    4. Pupil checks q2h to evaluate intracranial pressure.

39. **A three-year-old is hospitalized with nephrotic syndrome. The nurse would expect to find:**

    1. Hematuria, fever, increased output.
    2. Elevated blood pressure, puffy eyes, hematuria.
    3. Poor appetite, frothy urine, weight gain.
    4. Bulging fontanel, elevated BP, albuminuria.

40. **A 12-year-old child is admitted with possible acute appendicitis. Which sign would indicate to the nurse that the condition is becoming worse?**

    1. Sudden increase in abdominal pain.
    2. Diarrhea and vomiting.
    3. Loss of appetite.
    4. Temperature rise from 100° F to 101° F.

41. **A client is admitted to the emergency room with a sharp object in his eye. What is the most important action for the nurse to take immediately?**

    1. Remove the foreign object.
    2. Irrigate the eye with copious amounts of normal saline.
    3. Carefully place sterile gauze over the object to cover the eye.
    4. Instill a topical anesthetic to reduce his pain.

42. **An elderly client develops acute pulmonary edema secondary to congestive heart failure. The physician orders rotating tourniquets. Which action by the nurse demonstrates accurate understanding of this procedure?**

1. The nurse places the client flat in bed with a small pillow.
2. Tourniquets are applied to each extremity for 15 minutes and then released.
3. The nurse checks for the presence of an arterial pulse in the extremity after applying a tourniquet.
4. When the procedure is completed, the tourniquets are released in a clockwise manner, one every five minutes.

43. The physician has ordered an indwelling urinary catheter for a male client. Where should the nurse tape the catheter to prevent pressure on the urethra at the penoscrotal junction?

    1. Medial thigh.
    2. Upper abdomen.
    3. Mid-abdominal region.
    4. Lateral thigh.

44. A client is transferred from the recovery room to the special care unit after a radical neck dissection. At this time, which vital sign would receive the highest priority by the nurse?

    1. Temperature.
    2. Pulse.
    3. Respirations.
    4. Blood pressure.

45. During a home visit, the wife of your client collapses. There is no pulse or respirations. Which of the following accurately describes the CPR the nurse would provide?

    1. 5 to 1 ratio of compressions to ventilations, at a rate of 100 beats/min.
    2. 15 to 2 ratio of compressions to ventilations, at a rate of 80 beats/min.
    3. 15 to 2 ratio of compressions to ventilations, at a rate of 100 beats/min.
    4. 5 to 1 ratio of compressions to ventilations, at a rate of 80 beats/min.

46. An elderly female has fallen, fracturing her left hip. She is admitted in Buck's traction and scheduled for intramedullary nailing. The nurse knows that the reason for Buck's traction in this client is to:

    1. Reduce muscle spasm.
    2. Provide for total immobility.
    3. Promote healing of the fracture.
    4. Allow for a 20 pound weight to be applied.

47. A female client has a history of frequent episodes of cystitis. Which statement by the client would indicate to the nurse that she needs further teaching about measures to prevent the reoccurrence of cystitis?

1. "I drink plenty of liquids during the day, usually two to three quarts."
2. "I often like to take baths instead of showers."
3. "I try to empty my bladder every two to three hours."
4. "I use an oral contraceptive for birth control."

48. A client diagnosed with chronic renal failure is started on hemodialysis. During the procedure, heparin sodium is added to the blood. The nurse knows that the heparin has been effective if the client remains free of:

    1. Thrombi.
    2. Infection at the fistula site.
    3. Chills and fever.
    4. Hypertension.

49. A client has just been catheterized and has an indwelling Foley catheter in her bladder. If all of the following actions were taken, improper technique was used when the nurse:

    1. Cleansed the client's urinary meatus with soap and water prior to inserting the catheter.
    2. Placed the client in the lithotomy position.
    3. Inserted the catheter one to two inches further into the urinary meatus when urine was observed in the catheter tubing.
    4. Used sterile normal saline to inflate the retention balloon on the catheter.

50. When attempting to obtain information from a hearing impaired client, the nurse should:

    1. Face the client and speak slowly.
    2. Speak frequently and exaggerate lip movements.
    3. Speak loudly.
    4. Speak directly into the impaired ear.

51. An elderly client is diagnosed with benign prostatic hypertrophy. Which of the following nursing interventions is contraindicated following a prostatectomy?

    1. Administration of analgesics as ordered.
    2. Notifying the physician of excessive clots.
    3. Irrigation of the Foley catheter as ordered and PRN.
    4. Rectal temperatures taken every four hours for the first 24 hours.

52. A client is admitted with a complaint of weight loss of 12 pounds in the last two months, despite increased appetite. She also is experiencing increased perspiration, fatigue, and restlessness. A diagnosis of hyperthyroidism is made. Which measure is essential for the nurse to include in her plan of to prevent thyrotoxic crisis?

1. Provide a quiet, low stimulus environment.
2. Administer aspirin as ordered for any sign of hyperthermia.
3. Maintain the client's NPO status until her anorexia subsides.
4. Observe the client carefully for signs of hypocalcemia.

53. A client is post-craniotomy and is progressing well. While he is sitting in a chair, the nurse notices that he begins to experience a grand mal seizure. The most important nursing action is to:

1. Provide oxygen.
2. Restrain the client.
3. Insert an airway.
4. Lower the client to the floor.

54. When changing dressings for an HIV positive client, the nurse should remember to wash hands and to:

1. Wear a mask.
2. Wear gloves.
3. Maintain strict isolation.
4. Wear a gown and gloves.

55. While caring for a client 24 hours following surgery, the priority nursing action is to:

1. Monitor his comfort level.
2. Encourage the client to verbalize his fears.
3. Observe safety precautions.
4. Instruct the client in self-care skills.

56. A client has had a right total hip replacement and is three days postoperative. When the nurse and nursing assistant are transferring her to a chair, she cries out in pain. Which observation by the nurse would lead to the suspicion of a dislocated hip prosthesis?

1. Shortening of the right leg.
2. Bulging in the right hip area.
3. Adduction of the left leg.
4. Loose hip joint movement on the right side.

57. The nurse knows that a signed consent form is necessary for which procedure?

1. Magnetic resonance imagery (MRI).
2. Cerebral arteriogram.
3. Computed tomography (CT scan).
4. Echoencephalography.

58. A client is admitted with a T2-T3 spinal cord transection. Nursing care for a client with T2-T3 spinal cord transection includes care for what type of paralysis?

1. Hemiplegia.
2. Paraplegia.

3. Quadriplegia.
4. Paresthesia.

59. A client had a right total hip replacement three days ago. When transferring from the bed to the chair, the client suddenly complains of sharp, severe pain in the right hip area. The nurse interprets this to mean that the client most likely:

1. Suffered a dislocation of the hip prosthesis.
2. Put too much weight on the right leg when transferring into the chair.
3. Experienced muscle spasms in the right leg.
4. Developed a blood clot in the right hip area.

60. Which action by the nurse would indicate that the client has an understanding of measures to be taken to prevent hip dislocation following a total hip replacement?

1. Keeping the affected leg adducted at all times.
2. Using a trochanter roll when the client is supine.
3. Maintaining the affected hip in the flexed position.
4. Keeping the client in the supine position.

61. A client undergoes surgery for a hip replacement. In the postoperative period, the nurse must instruct the client to avoid which action while sitting in a chair?

1. Crossing his legs.
2. Elevating his feet.
3. Flexing his ankles.
4. Extending his knees.

62. When inserting a nasogastric tube in a comatose client for internal tube feedings, it is inappropriate for the nurse to:

1. Measure the amount of the tube to be inserted.
2. Lubricate the distal portion of the tube.
3. Tilt the client's head back when inserting the tube.
4. Check placement of the tube.

63. Prior to a paracentesis procedure for a client with ascites, the nurse should encourage the client to:

1. Drink two liters of water.
2. Empty his bladder.
3. Cleanse the abdominal area thoroughly.
4. Eat a meal high in sodium.

64. A client is admitted with esophageal varices. The most appropriate nursing action that will decrease the risk of esophageal bleeding is to:

1. Apply an ice collar.
2. Maintain semi-Fowler's position.
3. Administer stool softeners.

4. Provide a diet high in Vitamin D.

65. **A client is admitted to the emergency room for an acute asthmatic attack. At this time, the initial nursing action for this client is to:**

1. Assist the client to a high Fowler's position.
2. Offer oral fluids to loosen secretions.
3. Monitor respiratory rate for changes.
4. Reduce all unnecessary environmental stimuli.

66. **A client has sustained a gunshot wound to her left side and has a closed water seal drainage system attached to a chest tube. The nurse notices continuous bubbling in the water seal collection immediately after insertion of the chest tube. Which action should the nurse take?**

1. Notify the physician immediately.
2. Clamp the chest tube.
3. Continue to monitor for continuous bubbling.
4. Reposition the client.

67. **Which nursing intervention will help to prevent the development of postoperative thrombophlebitis?**

1. Have the client sit with her feet touching the floor.
2. Apply gentle leg massage.
3. Encourage the client to ambulate.
4. Place pillows under the client's knees.

68. **The nurse knows that which finding would contribute to rheumatic endocarditis?**

1. Congestive heart failure.
2. Tuberculosis.
3. Streptococcus throat infection.
4. Coronary artery disease.

69. **After a myocardial infarction, the nurse knows that which vital signs assessment may indicate cardiogenic shock?**

1. BP - 180/100, P - 90 and irregular.
2. BP - 130/80, P - 100 and regular.
3. BP - 90/50, P - 50 and regular.
4. BP - 80/60, P - 110 and irregular.

70. **A client is seen in the health clinic with manifestations of urinary burning and urgency. Which diagnostic test can the nurse anticipate will be ordered to diagnose the possibility of a urinary tract infection?**

1. Clean-catch midstream urine.
2. Catheterized urine.
3. Intravenous pyelogram (IVP).
4. Random urine specimen.

71. **Following cataract surgery, which comment made by the client to the nurse should be reported immediately to the charge nurse?**

1. "My eye itches, but I'm trying not to scratch it."
2. "I need something for this pain in my eye. I can hardly stand it."
3. "It's really hard to see with one eye patched. I'm afraid of falling."
4. "No one has taught me how to change this eye dressing or apply the ointment."

72. **Which statement made to the nurse by a diabetic client on insulin would indicate the need for further teaching?**

1. "It's important to measure the correct dosage of insulin at eye level."
2. "The insulin should be injected at a 90-degree angle."
3. "I'll remember to rotate sites so that each site is used only once a month."
4. "If I increase my exercise, I know that I will have to increase my insulin dosage."

73. **A client is to receive Regular Humulin insulin (Humulin R) 10 Units and NPH Humulin insulin (Humulin N) 30 Units subcutaneously at 7:30 a.m. The nurse can anticipate the onset of insulin action to occur at:**

1. 7:30 a.m.
2. 8:00 a.m.
3. 9:00 a.m.
4. 9:30 a.m.

74. **A hospitalized client is disoriented, confused, and agitated, and is receiving lorazepam (Ativan). Because the client is receiving Ativan, which nursing action is a priority?**

1. Observing the client for early signs of tardive dyskinesia.
2. Warning the client not to drive her automobile or engage in activities that require alertness.
3. Frequently checking the client's serum level of medication.
4. Monitoring the client closely when she ambulates.

75. **The physician has prescribed clindamycin (Cleocin) 300 mg P.O. every six hours for a client diagnosed with an upper respiratory tract infection. In order to facilitate maximum drug absorption, the nurse should instruct the client to take Cleocin:**

1. With meals or a snack.
2. On an empty stomach.
3. With a full glass of water at six-hour intervals around the clock.
4. With an antacid or glass of milk.

76. **A client calls the doctor's office and reports that he has developed diarrhea secondary to taking clindamycin (Cleocin). At this time, the nurse would:**

1. Report the diarrhea to the physician for appropriate treatment.
2. Advise the client to take the medicine with food to decrease GI distress.
3. Instruct the client to take kaolin/pectate (Kaopectate) over-the-counter at the same time as his oral dose of Cleocin.
4. Recommend that the client take a bulk-forming agent such as psyllium (Metamucil) while on Cleocin, but to report any bloody stools immediately.

77. A client is complaining of gastric problems while taking his demeclocycline (Declomycin) and asks if it is all right to take his antacid along with the medication. What is the best response by the nurse?

1. "Sure, if it helps, go right ahead."
2. "It would be better to take the medication with milk."
3. "Antacids will block the absorption of the medication and you will not get the full effect. Let's ask your doctor to switch you to another form of tetracycline."
4. "You should take all medications on an empty stomach."

78. The nurse is reviewing the client's history prior to administration of theophylline (Theo-Dur). Which factor, if true about this client, would indicate the need for increased Theo-Dur dosage? The client:

1. Is over 70 years of age.
2. Is also taking levothyroxine (Synthroid) for "thyroid difficulties."
3. Has difficulty swallowing.
4. Smokes cigarettes.

79. The nurse who is assigned to care for a child with cerebral palsy understands that the aim of therapy is to:

1. Assess the child's assets and potentialities and capitalize on these in the habilitative process, while ignoring limitations.
2. Reverse abnormal functioning and restore brain damage through rehabilitation.
3. Provide a therapeutic program that avoids subjecting the child to frustrating experiences that decrease his achievement.
4. Develop an individualized therapeutic program that uses the child's assets and abilities and provides experiences that permit him to achieve success as well as help to cope with frustration and failure.

80. A client, 35 years old, was admitted to the hospital for possible gall bladder surgery. Following a gall bladder x-ray, the doctor decided that a cholecystectomy was necessary. The nurse's preoperative teaching should include which information?

1. Many clients are admitted to the intensive care unit after this type of surgery.
2. Minor discomfort is expected in the operative site during the first few postoperative days.
3. Moving as little as possible will decrease the discomfort following this procedure.
4. Learning to cough and deep breathe will help prevent postoperative respiratory breathing complications.

81. A 30-month-old male is being admitted with asthma. To decrease the stress of hospitalization for the toddler, the nurse should:

1. Explain procedures and routines.
2. Encourage contact with children of the same age.
3. Provide for privacy.
4. Encourage rooming-in.

82. A client taking lithium is discharged. After five days, she tells the nurse that she is still having difficulty with hyperactivity. She asks how long it will take for her lithium to be effective. The best explanation by the nurse is:

1. "Each person is different. Lithium usually takes one to two weeks to be effective."
2. "We are monitoring your blood level to see when it is in the therapeutic range. At that point your manifestations should be controlled."
3. "You should see an immediate improvement. I will call your psychiatrist so she can increase your dose."
4. "You will begin to see some improvement when your blood level reaches the therapeutic range, but it still may be a while before your manifestations are controlled."

83. The nurse finds an elderly client standing in a puddle of water in the hallway of the unit. The nurse does not know this client. What is the nurse's initial action?

1. Ask the client for her name and room number.
2. Wipe up the water until the floor is completely dry.
3. Call the supervisor for assistance in identifying the client.
4. Have the client wait in the lounge until security arrives.

84. After a series of nine ECT treatments, a client reports that his depressive manifestations are gone. However, he does complain of short-term memory loss. The initial nursing action is to:

1. Report the problem immediately to his psychiatrist.
2. Encourage him to ventilate his feelings about the problem.
3. Explain that this memory loss is only temporary, and his memory will return to normal in four to eight weeks.
4. Tell him that this is a side effect of the treatment, and he can expect his memory to return to normal in five to ten days.

85. **When caring for elderly clients who are treated with antidepressant medication, the nurse knows that:**

1. They will probably require a higher doses of medication than a younger person.
2. Psychotherapy and medication together are usually more effective than either alone in treating elderly depressed clients.
3. Antidepressant medications are not usually tolerated well by elderly clients because of their many side effects.
4. Antidepressants are expensive medications, and the potential results may not be worth their cost.

86. **Although most depressed clients do not attempt suicide, an estimated 80% of persons with depression do have suicidal thoughts. In caring for an elderly widower with agitated depression who has trouble sleeping, the nurse considers that his risk of suicide is:**

1. No different than for any other depressed client.
2. Lower than that of an elderly man who has never married.
3. Quite low.
4. Extremely high.

87. **A 30-year-old single man who works as a computer analyst is admitted to the hospital with a diagnosis of bipolar depression, acute manic episode. When taking a nursing history, the nurse would identify which information that would support this diagnosis?**

1. He describes himself as a "loner" with a history of being withdrawn and aloof in relationships.
2. His paternal grandfather had mood swings all his life and died in a mental institution.
3. He had a similar episode when in college. He dropped out of school without finishing his degree, and his friends say he was never the same again.
4. His parents were divorced when he was a young child.

88. **Before administering lithium, the nurse checks the** client's latest lab report for her serum lithium level and notes a level of 1.2 mEq/L. What is the best action for the nurse to take next?

1. Administer the next prescribed dose of lithium.
2. Suggest the blood test be repeated.
3. Withhold the next dose of lithium and notify the psychiatrist of the lab results.
4. Ask the client how she is feeling, to identify any untoward effects.

89. **When a client's mother comes to visit, the client does not acknowledge her greeting and lies down on her bed, curling up into the fetal position. After talking with the client's mother, the nurse returns to the client's room. The client is still lying in a fetal position. What action by the nurse would be most therapeutic at this time?**

1. Ask the client to get up and put away the clothing her mother has brought in.
2. Ask the client why she responded to her mother that way.
3. Sit in a chair next to the bed and ask the client to talk about what happened when her mother visited.
4. Explain unit expectations about how visitors are to be treated.

90. **A depressed client has not bathed or changed her clothes during the two days she has been on the psychiatric unit. When the nurse suggests that she take a shower, the client states an emphatic "No!" and turns her back to the nurse. What is the best action for the nurse to take initially?**

1. Withdraw and return at a later time.
2. Question the client about her resistance to showering.
3. Get another staff member to help get the client into the shower.
4. Tell her she will be much more acceptable to other people on the unit if she cleans up and changes her clothes.

91. **The nurse is caring for a client who is mourning a recent loss. The nurse understands that it is inaccurate to state that mourning:**

1. Is a normal response to loss.
2. Functions to free the individual from an attachment to the lost object so that future relationships can be established.
3. Is accompanied by a growing realization that the loss has occurred.
4. Occurs only in humans.

92. After her first night in the hospital, a depressed client complains of feeling too tired to get out of bed in the morning. In planning how to deal with this therapeutically, the nurse is guided by the knowledge that:

    1. Helping to mobilize the client physically will also help to improve her emotional state.
    2. Most people do require more rest when they are depressed.
    3. It is best to wait until the client indicates that she is ready to participate in structured activities.
    4. Encouraging the client to get up and come out on the ward will only increase her feelings of worthlessness and guilt.

93. The nurse learns that a depressed client is an expert at crewel embroidery. The nurse asks the client if she will teach her crewel work. Which of the following is the best rationale for this nursing intervention?

    1. To assess the client's ability to communicate clearly.
    2. To distract the client from thinking about her problems.
    3. To reinforce the client's identity as a homemaker.
    4. To use the client's strengths to build self-esteem.

94. The nurse tells the client that a catheter must be inserted to collect a urine specimen. The client pulls the covers to her neck. She glances at the open door and says, "Someone might see me out there!" At this time, the best nursing action is to:

    1. Explain the procedure to the client.
    2. Obtain some assistance, since the client does not appear to be comfortable and may be resistant to the procedure.
    3. Close the door and assure the client that you will cover her as much as possible during the procedure.
    4. Gather all of the needed equipment before starting the procedure.

95. A client is admitted to the hospital with abdominal pain. She overhears her doctor and nurse discussing cancer of the liver. Later, she says to her nurse, "Having cancer of the liver must be a terrible thing." Which of the following nursing responses is most helpful?

    1. "Yes, it is a terrible disease."
    2. "What made you think about cancer of the liver?"
    3. "Any kind of cancer is terrible, but you can't live without a liver."
    4. "Yes, it is. A client on this floor has it, and it's sad for everyone."

96. The nurse is teaching a client about self breast exams when the client states that she doesn't understand why she is being taught this since she doesn't plan on doing it anyway. The best nursing response is:

    1. "The self breast exam is taught to women to detect any lumps or changes in the breast which can be an early sign of cancer, and early treatment has a higher rate of cure."
    2. "You're right. If you don't plan on doing the exam, then I don't need to show you how to do it."
    3. "If you don't plan on doing the exam yourself, then you should have your doctor do it at your annual check up."
    4. "It is your body, and you have the right to do whatever you choose."

97. A daughter has come to take her mother home from the hospital after a colostomy. The daughter tells the nurse that she doesn't know how she is going to care for her mother's colostomy. The nurse's most helpful response to the daughter is:

    1. "Your mother can take care of her colostomy without difficulty."
    2. "What part of your mother's care are you concerned about?"
    3. "A home health nurse will be stopping by tomorrow. If you have any questions, you can ask her."
    4. "It is quite simple. I'll make sure that her colostomy bag is clean before she leaves."

98. A client is scheduled for a mastectomy in the morning. Her daughter says to the nurse, "I should call my brother and sister and have them here in the morning, just in case something goes wrong." The most helpful nursing response is:

    1. To ask the mother if she would like her children there in the morning.
    2. To suggest to the daughter that she ask her mother how she feels about that.
    3. To say to the daughter, "If your brother and sister want to be here, they are welcome."
    4. To ask the daughter what she knows about her mother's surgery and diagnosis.

99. A disruptive 10-year-old child is having difficulty interacting with other children on the unit. Which nursing action would be best initially?

    1. Have a unit conference with other staff members and discuss strategies to solve the problem.
    2. Talk to the child about the behavior that is causing the problem and identify possible solutions.
    3. Tell the other children to stop teasing the client and to observe for changes in the client's behavior.

4. Tell the client's mother that she needs to talk to her son about his disruptive behavior.

100. **A client is paralyzed from the waist down. He is to be up in a chair three times a day. What is the best nursing approach when transferring the client from a bed into a wheelchair?**

1. Place the wheelchair close to the foot of the bed.
2. Utilize the principles of body mechanics while providing a safe transfer for the client.
3. Slide the client to the edge of the bed, keeping the nurse's back straight and using a rocking motion to pull the client.
4. Place the nurse's arms under the client's axillae from the back of the client.

NOTES

NCLEX-PN

Test 3
Questions with
Rationales

NCLEX-PN TEST 3 WITH RATIONALES

1. The nurse knows which action is the most common cause of invasion of a client's privacy?

   1. Over-exposing a client during a treatment or examination.
   2. Failing to pull the curtain while performing a treatment or examination.
   3. Talking about the client to other staff members who are not involved with the care of the client, or within hearing of the public.
   4. Helping a client with a tub bath.

   1. *Wrong choice! It is true that only the body part that is involved in an examination or treatment should be exposed, in order to provide as much privacy as possible for the client. This is not, however, the most common violation of privacy.*
   2. *Wrong choice! It is true that the curtain should be closed whenever a client is to have a treatment or examination that may expose body parts. This is not, however, the most common violation of privacy.*
   3. **Correct! No information about the client, including personal concerns, diagnosis, and treatment, should be discussed with anyone who is not involved in the care of the client. Talking about the client is the most common cause of invasion of privacy in the health care setting. The nurse should take special care not to compromise this right by discussing client care in such places as elevators, restaurants, or other areas that are accessible to the public and where the discussion might be overheard.**
   4. *Although there is loss of privacy for the client when assisting with a tub bath, this action is performed when necessary to provide for the safety of the client. This nursing intervention is not an invasion of privacy.*

2. A 55-year-old client is hospitalized following myocardial infarction. He is to be transferred from a cart to a bed in a room on a unit. When transferring the client from a cart to his bed, the priority nursing action is to:

   1. Have the client place his arms on his chest.
   2. Lock the wheels on the cart and the bed.
   3. Have at least four people to help with the transfer.
   4. Use a draw sheet to move the client.

   1. *Wrong choice. Although placing the arms across the chest helps protect the client's arms from injury, this option is not the priority. Be sure to read all the options before selecting the best one.*

   2. *Right! Locking the wheels stabilizes the cart and bed, preventing the client from falling between them during the transfer. This is the priority action for transferring a client.*
   3. *Four people may or may not be the number needed for a transfer. The number will depend on the size of the client and the size of the persons performing the transfer. The case situation does not provide enough information for this to be the correct option.*
   4. *Wrong choice. Although a draw sheet is often used to transfer clients between two level horizontal surfaces, this is neither a requirement nor a priority action. Try again.*

3. A client has left-sided weakness secondary to a stroke. In assisting him out of bed, which nursing action would be most appropriate?

   1. Allow the client to do as much of the transfer as possible.
   2. Lock the wheels of the bed and wheelchair.
   3. Place the client's hands around the nurse's neck for support.
   4. Place the front of the wheelchair at a right angle to the bed.

   1. *Incorrect. While it is important to encourage self care to the extent that is appropriate, this client has left-sided weakness and is at risk for falling. The nurse needs to prioritize so that the client's safety is the most important factor.*
   2. **Correct. The bed and wheelchair must both be stabilized to prevent the client from falling and being injured.**
   3. *Incorrect. Holding onto the nurse's neck places undue stress on the neck and back. If the client loses his balance and falls, the nurse, as well as the client, is at risk for injury. The client should place his hands on the nurse's shoulders.*
   4. *Incorrect. With this option, the client would have to turn almost 180 degrees to get into the chair. The wheelchair should be placed parallel to the bed.*

4. The doctor has ordered restraints for a very agitated client. When applying restraints to the client, which nursing action is inappropriate?

   1. Using the least restrictive type of restraint that will effectively protect the client from injury.
   2. Fastening the restraints to the bed frame.
   3. Tying the restraint with a knot that cannot be undone easily, in order to prevent the client from untying it.

4. Explaining to the client and family the type of restraint and the reason for applying the restraint.

1. *No, this action is appropriate. Over-restraining a client can intensify the problems caused by immobility. The question asks you to identify an action that is INAPPROPRIATE. Try again!*

2. *Wrong choice, this is a correct nursing action. The bed frame, rather than the side rails should be used to attach the restraints because the bed frame is more stable. Lowering side rails that have restraints attached can result in injury to the client. The question asks you to identify an INAPPROPRIATE action. Make another selection.*

3. **Correct choice, this is something that the nurse should not do! Restraints should be tied with knots that can be undone easily, in case the client's well being necessitates removal of the restraints. To protect the client from releasing the restraints, the knot should be placed where the client cannot reach it.**

4. *Wrong choice, this is a correct nursing action. Restraints can increase the client's confusion and cause anger and hostility in the client and family. An explanation concerning the client's safety can help to promote understanding and cooperation. The question asks you to identify an INAPPROPRIATE action. Make another choice.*

5. **During administration of medications to a client, the priority nursing action is to:**

1. Help the client swallow medications without aspirating by keeping the head in a neutral position.
2. Identify the client by checking the client's identification bracelet and asking for his name.
3. Keep all prepared medications in sight.
4. Check the client for desired or undesired drug effects within an hour after administration of the medication.

1. *Wrong choice. Maintaining the head in a neutral or slightly flexed position is an appropriate nursing action that facilitates the movement of tablets or capsules down the esophagus and into the stomach. This question, however, requires use of the nursing process. This option is an implementation action, not the priority assessment action. Make another choice.*

2. *Very good! Identification of the client helps to ensure that the medication will be given to the right client. This is one of the "five rights" to be checked before administering medications: the right client, the right drug, the right dose, the right route, and the right time.*

3. *Wrong choice. Keeping prepared medications in sight is important in assuring that the right medication will be administered in the right dose. The nurse can ensure that the medications will not be*

disturbed and will not be taken by others. However, this nursing action is part of the implementation phase of the nursing process. Can you identify the priority assessment action?

4. *Wrong choice. Evaluating the client's response to a medication is important for identifying undesired signs of toxicity or side effects. For example, after administering a narcotic pain medication, the nurse might observe signs of respiratory depression. The nurse may also evaluate whether the medications are helpful, which can be seen in relief of pain. Evaluation, however, is the last phase of the nursing process. Can you identify the priority assessment action?*

6. A client puts her call light on and tells the nurse that she has to urinate. The client has had a Foley catheter in place since her surgery two days ago. The appropriate nursing action is to:

1. Remind the client that she has a Foley catheter in place and does not need to go to the bathroom.
2. Replace the Foley catheter with a new catheter.
3. Explain to the client that the urge to void is a common occurrence for clients who have urinary catheters.
4. Check the catheter and tubing for kinks and note the urine output in the drainage bag.

1. *Incorrect! Although a Foley catheter is in place, it may not be patent, which can result in distention of the bladder and cause the client to feel the urge to void. This action does not meet the client's needs.*

2. *Incorrect, try again! A new catheter might be necessary to meet the client's needs, but the nurse must assess the situation further to determine the cause of the client's urge to void.*

3. *Try again! The urge to void usually occurs upon initial insertion of the Foley catheter, not two days afterwards. There are several possible reasons for the client having urgency, and the nurse must attempt to discover the cause in order to meet the client's needs.*

4. *Yes! Checking the equipment is the best nursing action, since data will be obtained which will assist the nurse with problem solving. This is a nursing process question, and assessment is always the first nursing action in this type of question.*

7. An adolescent client had surgery on his foot and has just been returned to his room from the recovery room. The initial assessment indicates that he is stable. An hour later, his roommate turns on the call light and tells the nurse that the client has gotten up and hopped on one foot to the bathroom, using his IV pole for support.

What should the nurse do first?

1. Open the bathroom door to assess if the client is okay.
2. Help the client back to bed and get him a urinal.
3. Explain to the client that it is not safe for him to be hopping around on one foot.
4. Get a wheelchair and help the client back to bed when he is done in the bathroom.

1. *Incorrect choice! Even though the client should not have hopped to the bathroom, the nurse should respect his privacy and knock on the door to determine if he is okay.*
2. *Wrong choice! The client will have to hop back to bed with the nurse helping him, which is not a very stable method of ambulation. This is not safe.*
3. *This intervention is appropriate, but it is not the priority action. Getting the client safely back to bed is the priority issue for the nurse.*
4. ***Good choice! Since the client is already in the bathroom, allow him to void, and then return him to his bed safely in a wheel chair. This is an implementation question, and the stem asks you to prioritize the actions. This option meets the physiological and safety needs of the client.***

8. **An elderly client is on strict bed rest. While making an occupied bed for this client, which action should the nurse take to maintain proper body mechanics?**

1. Place the bed in semi-Fowler's position.
2. Place the bed in a low horizontal position.
3. Ask the client to move to the foot of the bed.
4. Place the bed in a high horizontal position.

1. *Incorrect! The bed cannot be made correctly while in the semi-Fowler's position. Making the bed while it is in semi-Fowler's position will cause the nurse to reach while making the head of the bed, which places strain on the musculoskeletal system. It will also cause the linen to pull out when the bed is placed in the horizontal position.*
2. *This is incorrect. Bending over to reach a bed in low position causes more stress on the small muscles of the back.*
3. *This is not an appropriate nursing action. The client should be kept in good body alignment.*
4. ***Great choice! In order to use good body mechanics, the bed should be in a high horizontal position. This prevents bending and excess stretching by the nurse.***

9. **The nurse is caring for a client who is visually impaired from a childhood injury. When ambulating this client, the most important nursing action is:**

1. Not to leave the client alone in an unfamiliar area.

2. To stand on the client's non-dominant side.
3. To have the client use his dominant hand to reach out for barriers or landmarks.
4. To describe the route to be taken and remove any obstacles.

1. ***Correct! A client with a visual impairment should not be left alone in an unfamiliar environment because of the increased risk of injury.***
2. *The client can use the non-dominant hand to hold on to the nurse's arm during ambulation, since the dominant hand should be utilized for feeling objects. Although this is a correct nursing action, it is not the most important action for the nurse to take. Try again.*
3. *The dominant hand should be utilized for feeling objects or barriers since it is stronger and more developed than the non-dominant hand. This is not, however, the most important action for the nurse to take in this situation. Try again.*
4. *Describing the route helps familiarize the client with surroundings and decreases the sense of social isolation. Removing obstacles provides for the client's safety. It is not, however, the most important nursing action in this situation. Try again.*

10. **The nurse in a long-term care facility is ambulating a newly admitted, frail, elderly client. The nurse provides for the client's safety by:**

1. Allowing the client to get up and walk unsupervised.
2. Using a transfer belt if the client is unsteady.
3. Allowing the client to shuffle when walking.
4. Walking two feet behind the client in case of a fall.

1. *This is incorrect. The client's abilities should be assessed before allowing him or her to move around unsupervised. This frail elderly client may be at risk for falling. Try again.*
2. ***Great choice! The use of a transfer belt helps to hold the client steady while ambulating.***
3. *This is incorrect, since shuffling may cause the client to fall. Try again.*
4. *This is incorrect, since the client may fall forward! Try again.*

11. **An elderly client is confused. The charge nurse says that the client is constipated and is to have a soap suds enema. As the nurse is explaining the procedure, the client states that she doesn't think that she is supposed to have an enema. At this time, the nurse should:**

1. Tell the client that her doctor must have ordered the procedure.
2. Assure the client that although the procedure sounds unpleasant, she will feel better afterwards.
3. Check the client's chart for the doctor's order to help clarify the situation.

4. Record on the chart that the client refused the enema.

   1. *Wrong. This option ignores the client's concern about whether or not she is really supposed to have an enema. Make another selection.*
   2. *No, try again. The fact that the client doesn't think she is supposed to have an enema needs to be addressed. This option does not give any credibility to the client's concerns. Try again.*
   3. **Good choice! Looking at the doctor's orders will help to clarify the situation and will reassure the client that the procedure was ordered for her.**
   4. *This action is incorrect because the client didn't refuse the enema. Make another selection.*

12. **While transferring a client with left-leg weakness from the bed to a wheelchair, the most important nursing action is to:**

   1. Have the seat of the wheelchair at a right angle to the bed.
   2. Lock the wheels on the bed and the wheelchair.
   3. Allow the client to do as much as possible to increase his sense of independence.
   4. Have the client lock his hands around the nurse's neck to provide the client with a sense of security.

   1. *This is incorrect. This position would require the client to pivot 180 degrees to get into the seat of the wheel chair. The seat of the wheelchair should be parallel with and next to the bed for ease of access for the client.*
   2. **Correct! Locking the wheels of both bed and wheelchair provides for the client's safety by not allowing the equipment to move away from the client, thereby risking an injury from a fall.**
   3. *This is not correct. Although encouraging independence is important, the client's safety is the most important consideration. A client with a weakened lower extremity is at risk for falling.*
   4. *This is wrong! The client can place his hands on the shoulders of the nurse but not around the nurse's neck. If the client slips, all of client's weight will be placed on the cervical vertebrae of the nurse, which could cause a spinal cord injury.*

13. **A postoperative client is ambulatory and wishes to go to the day room. While the nurse is walking down the hall with the client, the client says that she feels faint and starts to fall. The nurse would:**

   1. Grasp the client around the waist and hold her up so she doesn't fall and injure herself.
   2. Hold the client up against the wall to keep her from falling.
   3. Ease the client gently to the floor.

4. Ask another client to get some help while supporting the client to prevent her from falling.

   1. *This is not correct. Preventing injury to the client is the most important action. This option may result in both the client and the nurse falling, putting both individuals at risk for injury.*
   2. *Holding the client against the wall will not prevent the fall and may cause injury to the client from the impact against the wall. Make another choice.*
   3. **Right! Easing the client gently to the floor is the best action, since it protects both individuals from injury.**
   4. *This is incorrect. Attempting to hold a client who is fainting upright places the nurse at risk for injury. If the client becomes too heavy, then the client may be injured if the nurse becomes fatigued and can no longer support her. Choose another option.*

14. **A client is to be transferred from her bed to a stretcher, in order to be transported to surgery for a fractured hip. The priority nursing action is to:**

   1. Provide for the client's privacy with a blanket.
   2. Lock the wheels on the stretcher and the bed.
   3. Have four people available for lifting the client.
   4. Provide a lifting device to assist with moving the client.

   1. *Covering the client with a blanket for privacy provides for the client's comfort and self-esteem. Maslow's Hierarchy of Needs, however, identifies self-esteem as a high level need. Look for an option that addresses a more basic need.*
   2. **Excellent! Locking the wheels on the bed and the stretcher stops their movement and helps prevent client falls between the bed and the stretcher. Safety is the priority in this case scenario.**
   3. *If the nurse requires help with a transfer, the number of assistants required will depend upon the situation. More or fewer people may be needed to assist the nurse. This action might be appropriate, but it cannot be the best option. Look for a nursing intervention that identifies a top priority action.*
   4. *A transfer device can assist with transferring a client from a bed to a stretcher by decreasing the amount of strength and energy required by the nurses or persons who are performing the transfer. This action might be appropriate, but it cannot be the best option. Look for an option that identifies a top priority action.*

15. **A client is to receive medication for control of tachycardia and an irregular heart rate. The nurse obtains the following vital signs prior to administering this medication: blood pressure 98/54; pulse 48; respirations 30;**

temperature 98° F. The client's skin is cool, with cyanosis of the fingers and lips. Based on this data, the priority nursing action is to:

1. Administer the medication as ordered by the physician.
2. Omit the medication for a day or two, depending on the client's response and manifestations.
3. Notify the charge nurse concerning the client's status before administering the medication.
4. Give the client one half of the ordered dose.

1. *Administering a medication that decreases the heart rate to a client with a pulse of 48 is inappropriate, since the pulse rate may decrease even further. A pulse rate of 48 does not fall within the normal range, and results in a physiological need for oxygen for this client. Make another choice.*
2. *Withholding the medication is a possible nursing action, since the result of this action may be a increase in pulse rate. However, withholding the medication alone does not address all of the physiological needs identified in the case scenario. Try again.*
3. **Very good! The assessment data gathered by the nurse indicate that the client is exhibiting manifestations that are not within the normal parameters. A pulse rate of 48 results in a physiological need for oxygen for this client. The charge nurse will need to notify the physician. Withholding the medication until the physician has been notified addresses the immediate physiological need of the client. The information needs to be communicated to the physician, who will determine which medical interventions are necessary.**
4. *Changing or altering an ordered medication is a medical intervention, not a nursing action! Make another choice.*

16. The first, most important nursing action when a nurse discovers a fire in a client's room is to:

1. Pull the fire alarm and notify the hospital operator.
2. Close fire doors and client room doors.
3. Remove the client from the room.
4. Place moist towels or blankets at the threshold of the door of the room with the fire.

1. *This is an appropriate action. Pulling the fire alarm and alerting the hospital operator notifies the appropriate individuals who are needed to fight a fire. But this is not the first nursing action! The immediate safety of the client in the room with the fire takes priority. Make another choice.*
2. *No! This action does not address the immediate safety of the client in the room with the fire! After providing*

for the safety of this client, closing fire doors and other clients' room doors will help prevent the spread of a fire to other areas of the hospital and help prevent smoke and fumes from entering their rooms. What should the nurse do first?
3. **Right! The client in the room with the fire is at highest risk for injury. The smoke from a fire can deprive a client of adequate oxygenation, and the fire poses a direct threat to the safety of this client. Moving this client to safety receives first priority.**
4. *No! Placing moist towels or blankets at the threshold of the door where the smoke is coming from helps prevent the smoke and fumes from entering other areas. This is an inappropriate action in this case scenario because the fire is in the client's room! The client is at risk for injury and oxygen deprivation. The immediate safety of the client in the room with the fire takes priority. Try again.*

17. A mother expresses concern about her infant's lack of eye muscle control at two days of age. Her neighbor's daughter is mentally retarded and her eyes cross the same way. What is the nurse's best reply?

1. "You should probably talk to the doctor about your concerns."
2. "Newborns all lack the ability to control eye movement until they are three to four months of age."
3. "I will take the baby back to the nursery and assess other neuromuscular activity."
4. "It's nothing to worry about."

1. *Wrong! This suggests there could be a problem that the physician needs to know about.*
2. **Good choice. Lack of eye muscle control is present in all newborns. This mother needs to know this so she will not think this is abnormal. This response is therapeutic because it addresses the client's concerns and provides correct information.**
3. *No, this statement suggests that the lack of eye muscle control warrants further assessment of the newborn.*
4. *Wrong. This statement is not therapeutic. It does not reassure the mother that this finding is normal, and it ignores her fears.*

18. A mother is concerned about her infant, who was born large for gestational age at 39 weeks gestation. She has heard that fat babies become fat children and she wants to limit her baby's intake during the next days. What is the nurse's best response?

1. "You will need to discuss this with the baby's doctor."
2. "LGA babies are at risk for hypoglycemia. The

baby needs additional calories at this time."

3. "Don't worry, babies always lose weight anyway, no matter what they eat."

4. "Let's try feeding the baby one ounce at each feeding and see how he tolerates it."

1. *Wrong. The LGA baby is at risk for hypoglycemia, and it is within the practical nurse's role to explain this to the mother.*

2. **Correct. This baby's caloric intake is very important to prevent hypoglycemia over the next few days.**

3. *Wrong. This answer does not address the mother's suggestion to limit the infant's caloric intake.*

4. *No. This intake is insufficient to meet the newborn's caloric needs and prevent hypoglycemia.*

19. **The nurse is to administer naloxone (Narcan) to an infant weighing 3.5 kg. The suggested dosage is 0.1 mg per kg, and the drug is supplied in a vial labeled 0.4 mg/ml. How much will the nurse administer to the infant?**

1. 0.35 cc.
2. 0.62 cc.
3. 0.87 cc.
4. 1.1 cc.

1. *Sorry, try again.*
2. *Sorry, try again.*
3. **Very good!**
4. *Sorry, try again.*

20. **Which of the following clinical manifestations would the nurse expect to see in a client with an ectopic pregnancy?**

1. Acute abdominal pain, with or without vaginal bleeding at 11 weeks gestation.
2. Large amount of vaginal bleeding with menstrual-type discomfort at 10 weeks gestation.
3. Severe nausea and vomiting with abdominal pain at 15 weeks gestation.
4. Rapidly enlarging uterus with a rise in blood pressure at 10 weeks gestation.

1. **Correct! Rarely does an ectopic pregnancy progress further than 12 weeks gestation. As the fetus grows, it causes ischemia in the fallopian tube, which results in severe pain. Once the tube ruptures, the client will display signs of shock immediately. Vaginal bleeding, if present, is usually minimal.**

2. *Wrong. An ectopic pregnancy is rarely associated with large amounts of vaginal bleeding, and the discomfort is always severe.*

3. *Incorrect. Ectopic pregnancy is not related to the*

presence of nausea and vomiting.

4. *Wrong. When a client has an ectopic pregnancy, there are no products of conception in the uterus, and therefore no enlarging uterus. Blood pressure elevation is not related to ectopic pregnancy unless it is related to the pain prior to rupture.*

21. **Which of the following clinical findings would the nurse expect to find in a client with a hydatidiform mole?**

1. Bright red vaginal bleeding.
2. Excessive uterine enlargement.
3. Fetal heart rate irregularities.
4. Rapidly dropping human chorionic gonadotropin levels.

1. *Wrong. The client with a hydatidiform mole often has vaginal discharge, but it is most often brownish in color.*

2. **Correct. A rapidly enlarging uterus is characteristic of a growing hydatidiform mole. It is often accompanied by severe nausea and vomiting and signs of pregnancy induced hypertension in the first trimester.**

3. *No, when the client has a hydatidiform mole there is no developing fetus and therefore no fetal heart rate.*

4. *When the client has a hydatidiform mole there is usually elevated levels of serum hCG.*

22. **The nurse is caring for a client with an abruptio placenta. The nurse would expect clinical findings to include:**

1. Large amount of bright red vaginal bleeding, with or without pain.
2. Moderate to large amount of bright red vaginal bleeding, with decreasing fundal height.
3. Abdominal pain with or without bright red vaginal bleeding.
4. Intermittent abdominal pain with bright red vaginal bleeding.

1. *Wrong. The client with an abruptio placenta always has abdominal pain. The bleeding may or may not be visible.*

2. *Incorrect. When the placenta separates prematurely, there is internal bleeding, which will cause a rapidly rising fundal height.*

3. **Correct choice. When the placenta separates, there is always bleeding, but it may or may not be evident. As the blood accumulates in the uterus the severity of the abdominal pain increases.**

4. *No, the pain associated with an abruptio placenta is constant, not intermittent. Whenever a client complains of intermittent pain, labor must be considered.*

23. **The nurse is teaching a client who is to receive danazol (Danocrine) to treat her endometriosis. Which of the**

following effects should the nurse teach the client to expect as a result of this drug?

1. No periods.
2. Weight loss.
3. Breast enlargement.
4. Hair loss.

1. *Right. While a client is on Danazol, ovulation is suppressed and no periods will occur.*
2. *This is incorrect. In fact, weight gain is a common side effect of Danazol.*
3. *This is incorrect. On the contrary, a reduction in breast size is commonly reported by the client on Danazol.*
4. *This is incorrect. Clients report very oily skin and hair, but not hair loss, while taking Danazol.*

24. The nurse is to administer silver nitrate to a newborn, as protection against blindness related to exposure to gonorrhea in the process of delivery. Which of the following is inconsistent with a normal response to silver nitrate instillation into the newborn's eyes?

1. Edema.
2. Inflammation.
3. Purulent drainage.
4. Crusty appearance.

1. *Wrong. Edema is often seen around the eyes after instillation of silver nitrate. You are looking for a response that is NOT normal.*
2. *Wrong. There is often mild inflammation in the eyes after administration of silver nitrate. You are looking for a response that is NOT normal.*
3. *Correct. Purulent drainage is suggestive of infection, not an expected response to silver nitrate.*
4. *No. Crusty appearance is a normal occurrence following silver nitrate in the eyes. You are looking for a response that is NOT normal.*

25. The nurse has just given a rubella vaccine to a client who is two days postpartum. Which statement by the client would alert the nurse to the client's need for further instruction?

1. "I may get a low-grade fever after this shot."
2. "I will still need to have a rubella titer when I get pregnant next time."
3. "As long as I don't get flu-like manifestations in the next four days I can conceive any time I want."
4. "I may experience a stinging feeling at the site where I got the shot."

1. *No, the client's statement is accurate. Clients often get a low-grade fever after receiving rubella vaccine.*

2. *No, the client's statement is accurate. A rubella titer is part of the routine blood work at the start of each pregnancy. There are times when a rubella positive client may be negative at a later examination.*
3. *Correct. Whenever a client receives rubella vaccine, she should not conceive for at least three months. This client needs further teaching.*
4. *No, the client's statement is accurate. Clients often report discomfort in the area of the injection.*

26. An obstetrical client is to receive oxytocin (Pitocin). The nurse knows that the use of Pitocin for induction of labor is contraindicated in:

1. Post term pregnancy.
2. Prolonged rupture of membranes at 38 weeks gestation.
3. Positive contraction stress test at 38 weeks gestation.
4. Mild preeclampsia at 38 weeks gestation.

1. *Wrong. Induction of labor with Pitocin is suggested in post term pregnancies.*
2. *Incorrect. When the client is near term with prolonged rupture of membranes, Pitocin induction is indicated.*
3. *Correct. With a positive contraction stress test, the fetus has repeated deceleration of fetal heart in response to uterine contractions. Prolonged use of Pitocin could compromise this fetus's oxygen supply.*
4. *No, this is not a contraindication. When a client has mild preeclampsia near term, delivery of the infant is recommended, and the use of Pitocin is the suggested method of induction.*

27. The nurse is to administer naloxone (Narcan) to a newborn infant. The nurse understands that the use of Narcan in a newborn is warranted in the case of respiratory depression related to:

1. Narcotics given to the mother in labor.
2. Maternal drug use.
3. Hyaline membrane disease.
4. Meconium aspiration.

1. *Correct. Narcan is used to reverse respiratory depression due to acute narcotic toxicity such as use of narcotics in labor.*
2. *No; in fact, the use of Narcan in the drug addicted infant could result in immediate withdrawal manifestations.*
3. *No, Narcan has no effect on hyaline membrane disease.*
4. *No, Narcan has no effect on meconium aspiration respiratory distress.*

28. A seven-year-old with newly diagnosed asthma is admitted. He is receiving theophylline (Theo-Dur). He complains of nausea and headache, and says his "heart is pounding." The nurse should:

    1. Report these manifestations to the RN immediately.
    2. Document and reassess in 30 minutes.
    3. Sit down with him and provide reassurance.
    4. Provide distraction with a quiet game.

    1. *Yes! It's important to recognize tachycardia as a side effect of aminophylline and its derivatives.*
    2. *No, there is not likely to be any change in this finding after giving it more time. Some action is required, so choose again.*
    3. *Incorrect. There is no information in the stem that would imply anxiety. You have "read into" the question. Try again.*
    4. *Incorrect. There is no information in the stem about pain or anxiety. Select again.*

29. A 10-month-old is scheduled for OR. The preoperative medication is ordered IM, and the volume will amount to 1.5 cc. The nurse should give the injection in the:

    1. Deltoid muscle.
    2. Gluteus maximus.
    3. Rectus femoris.
    4. Vastus lateralis.

    1. *Incorrect. This muscle in the arm is too small and undeveloped in the infant. It is sometimes used to give small doses of emergency medications that are to be absorbed quickly and in small volume. Select again.*
    2. *Incorrect. Until a child walks, the gluteus maximus (buttocks) is too undeveloped, and this child is only 10 months old. Try again.*
    3. *Wrong. This doesn't even exist! If you've never heard of an answer, it's probably not correct. In other words, "go with what you know" when answering test questions. Select again.*
    4. *Yes, this is the preferred site for this injection in the infant. This is the lateral aspect of the thigh.*

30. A 12-year-old is admitted with possible appendicitis. Which order should the nurse question with the charge nurse before implementing?

    1. NPO.
    2. Fleets enema today.
    3. Medicate with Demerol (meperidine) 50 mg every four hours PRN.
    4. Temperature every four hours.

    1. *No, this order is fine. It is appropriate to rest the bowel before surgery. This child may have to go to surgery as an emergency. Look for an action that is INAPPROPRIATE for the care of this child.*
    2. *Good work! Enemas and laxatives are contraindicated, since they increase the volume in the bowel and may cause rupture.*
    3. *No, this is an appropriate order. Pain medication is often prescribed, since appendicitis may cause acute pain. Look for an action that is INAPPROPRIATE for the care of this child.*
    4. *No, this order is fine. Since appendicitis is an inflammatory process, fever may be evident. Look for an action that is INAPPROPRIATE for the care of this child.*

31. Following several episodes of vomiting combined with increasing temperature in a two-year-old toddler, the nurse is to assess the client for dehydration. The best indicator of dehydration is:

    1. A listless appearance.
    2. BP of 90/58.
    3. Depressed fontanel.
    4. Specific gravity of 1.010.

    1. *Not the best choice. By itself, a listless appearance is not enough information to determine that the child is dehydrated. There could be other reasons for this appearance, such as exhaustion, nausea, or generalized illness appearance.*
    2. *Wrong, you've forgotten the normals for this age group. Try again.*
    3. *Very good! Before the fontanels are closed, they are a good source of information about hydration level. Depressed fontanels means the infant is dehydrated; bulging fontanels indicates increased intracranial pressure.*
    4. *Wrong. Although the specific gravity is a good source of information on hydration, this is a normal result. Try again.*

32. The observation by the nurse that would assist in the diagnosis of pyloric stenosis is:

    1. Projectile vomiting.
    2. Effortless regurgitation.
    3. Distended abdomen.
    4. Improvement with frequent burping.

    1. *Very good, you are correct. There is forceful vomiting due to the hypertrophic enlargement of the pyloric muscle, which does not allow for emptying of the stomach contents.*
    2. *Wrong. This is a manifestation of gastroesophageal reflux (GER), which is due to the lower esophageal (cardiac) sphincter's being relaxed or in-*

competent. A different muscle is involved in the pathophysiology of pyloric stenosis. Make another choice.

3. *Incorrect. This child will show muscle wasting and dehydration. The classic finding in the abdomen of a child with pyloric stenosis is the olive shaped mass, which is sometimes palpable. Select again.*

4. *Incorrect. This is not symptomatic of pyloric stenosis. The child with an incompetent lower esophageal (cardiac) sphincter who has gastroesophageal reflux will improve with positioning in high Fowler's and frequent burping during feedings. Try again.*

33. **A child is admitted with possible streptococcal infection. Twenty-four hours later, the throat culture result is positive. The nurse interprets this information as indicating:**

    1. Antibiotic therapy has been successful.
    2. Nothing of clinical significance.
    3. The child should be placed on isolation.
    4. An organism has been identified.

    1. *Wrong. This is an incorrect understanding of the result. Make another selection.*
    2. *Not true. Choose again.*
    3. *Wrong choice. Whenever a child is suspected of being infectious, isolation should be initiated immediately upon admission. Select again.*
    4. **Yes, that is right. A positive culture indicates that an organism has been grown in the culture medium.**

34. **When planning the discharge of a child receiving warfarin (Coumadin) therapy, the nurse should teach the parents to:**

    1. Monitor for signs of bleeding.
    2. Discontinue if there are signs of viral infection.
    3. Check pulses before administration.
    4. Administer the medication subcutaneously.

    1. **Yes, you obviously understand that warfarin is an anticoagulant and can increase the chance of bleeding.**
    2. *Incorrect. This drug is not associated with any side effects that would require it to be discontinued because of viral illness. Try again.*
    3. *No, warfarin does not affect the heart or blood vessels directly, so pulse checks are not indicated. Try again.*
    4. *Incorrect. You may be thinking about Heparin, which is a relative of warfarin. Select again.*

35. **When planning to teach families about Reye's syndrome, it is important for the nurse to know that Reye's syndrome is:**

    1. Avoidable.
    2. Untreatable.
    3. Caused by hepatic failure.
    4. Poorly understood.

    1. **Yes! Reye's syndrome is associated with the presence of specific diseases and the use of aspirin.**
    2. *Not true. This is a serious diagnosis, but if it is recognized early, treatment can be successful. Choose another option.*
    3. *Incorrect. This syndrome causes hepatic failure. You switched cause for effect. Try again.*
    4. *Wrong. Fortunately, this is not true. Since we do understand a lot about this syndrome, there are fewer cases every year. Select again.*

36. **A school-age child with neuroblastoma becomes anorexic, with periods of nausea after beginning chemotherapy. The best nursing intervention is to:**

    1. Allow him to eat whatever he wants, at any time.
    2. Force him to eat balanced meals.
    3. Encourage high quality nutritious foods.
    4. Increase proteins and fats.

    1. **Correct. When the nausea is absent, offering small amounts of favorite foods is the best way to improve intake.**
    2. *Never force a child to eat. This is unlikely to be successful if the child does not feel hungry. Select another option.*
    3. *Not the best answer. The child can be encouraged, but this will not ensure that a balanced, nutritious diet will appeal to a nauseated child. Try again.*
    4. *No, protein and fat are not appealing to someone who has a loss of appetite. Carbohydrates should be given to protect the fat and protein stores in the body. Choose again.*

37. **Which activity would the nurse encourage in order to meet the developmental needs of a 12-month-old hospitalized client?**

    1. A cradle gym across crib.
    2. Push-pull toys.
    3. Finger paints.
    4. A stick horse.

    1. *Incorrect. Although this encourages fine motor skills, you have not matched the age of the client with the activity that is needed to improve skills. This could also be a safety issue, since the child may be able to stand and could strangle on the cradle gym. Try again.*
    2. **Great, correct choice! Walking is the skill that**

is being perfected at this age, and push-pull toys will encourage the client to walk unaided.

3. *Incorrect. Reread the question and think about the skill level of this age child. Try again.*

4. *Incorrect. This is beyond the ability of the client and could be a safety concern. Make another selection.*

38. **The nurse caring for a client with pediatric leukemia knows that the most important measure to prevent complications and death is:**

1. Proper administration of iron.
2. Prevention of infection.
3. Monitoring intake and output.
4. Pupil checks q2h to evaluate intracranial pressure.

1. *No, the pathophysiology of the anemia in leukemia isn't a lack of iron. Select another option.*

2. **Yes! The leading cause of death from leukemia is infection, since WBCs are immature.**

3. *No, this disease does not affect fluid balance directly. Think about the pathology of the disease as well as the treatment, and make another selection.*

4. *Incorrect. Frequent pupil checks are not often a part of the care of the child with leukemia. You've missed the most common cause of death in leukemia, and how this would be detected or prevented. Try again.*

39. **A three-year-old is hospitalized with nephrotic syndrome. The nurse would expect to find:**

1. Hematuria, fever, increased output.
2. Elevated blood pressure, puffy eyes, hematuria.
3. Poor appetite, frothy urine, weight gain.
4. Bulging fontanel, elevated BP, albuminuria.

1. *Only part of this response is correct. Hematuria may occur but it is rarely gross. Fever is not a manifestation unless there is a secondary infection. Outputs are diminished, not increased. Try again.*

2. *Only part of this response is correct. Microscopic hematuria may be seen, but elevated blood pressure is a manifestation of glomerulonephritis, not nephrotic syndrome. Puffy eyes is a manifestation of nephrotic syndrome. Choose again.*

3. **Excellent! All three of these are seen in nephrotic syndrome. Anorexia is an expected manifestation. The frothy urine is due to loss of albumin into the urine, and the syndrome also results in weight gain due to edema.**

4. *Incorrect. In a three-year-old, fontanels are not assessed. There is no increase in intracranial pressure, and blood pressure is normal. Choose again.*

40. **A 12-year-old child is admitted with possible acute appendicitis. Which sign would indicate to the nurse that the condition is becoming worse?**

1. Sudden increase in abdominal pain.
2. Diarrhea and vomiting.
3. Loss of appetite.
4. Temperature rise from 100° F to 101° F.

1. **Correct! This may indicate that the appendix has ruptured. The RN should be notified and vital signs obtained.**

2. *Incorrect. While it is true that these manifestations are seen in appendicitis, they may also be seen in the child with a viral infection. This is one reason why it is difficult to diagnose appendicitis.*

3. *No, anorexia is a non-specific manifestation. It is not a sign of the condition becoming more severe. Select again.*

4. *Not correct. Temperature in itself is not usually helpful in making the diagnosis of ruptured appendicitis, especially not at 101° F, which is still within the expected findings when a virus is the cause. Try again.*

41. **A client is admitted to the emergency room with a sharp object in his eye. What is the most important action for the nurse to take immediately?**

1. Remove the foreign object.
2. Irrigate the eye with copious amounts of normal saline.
3. Carefully place sterile gauze over the object to cover the eye.
4. Instill a topical anesthetic to reduce his pain.

1. *Incorrect. Removal of a sharp object by the nurse is contraindicated since more damage can be done. An ophthalmologist should be notified immediately.*

2. *Incorrect. Copious irrigation with normal saline is the treatment of choice for chemical burns to the eye, not for a puncture wound.*

3. **Correct. Sterile gauze should be placed carefully to absorb the drainage and to protect the eye from infection.**

4. *Incorrect. Although a topical anesthetic is often instilled in the eye to reduce pain during eye examination, it is not done initially.*

42. **An elderly client develops acute pulmonary edema secondary to congestive heart failure. The physician orders rotating tourniquets. Which action by the nurse demonstrates accurate understanding of this procedure?**

1. The nurse places the client flat in bed with a small pillow.

2. Tourniquets are applied to each extremity for 15 minutes and then released.
3. The nurse checks for the presence of an arterial pulse in the extremity after applying a tourniquet.
4. When the procedure is completed, the tourniquets are released in a clockwise manner, one every five minutes.

1. *No! Remember that the client is in the ultimate stage of pulmonary congestion and feels as if she is suffocating. She should be positioned upright, with legs and feet down if possible. Choose again.*
2. *Incorrect. Tourniquets are applied to three of four extremities, and rotated every 15 minutes in a clockwise pattern. Make another selection.*
3. ***Correct! The tourniquets are applied to three of four extremities securely enough to impede venous return to the heart, but not so tightly that they interfere with arterial flow to each extremity.***
4. *No. When the procedure is finished, the tourniquets are released in a clockwise pattern, one every 15 minutes. This slow release allows for gradual return of blood from the extremities back into the general circulation.*

43. **The physician has ordered an indwelling urinary catheter for a male client. Where should the nurse tape the catheter to prevent pressure on the urethra at the penoscrotal junction?**

1. Medial thigh.
2. Upper abdomen.
3. Mid-abdominal region.
4. Lateral thigh.

1. *No, taping in this area would not eliminate the penoscrotal angle and could lead to a fistula. Choose again.*
2. *Incorrect. This section of the abdomen would not be possible to reach without putting undo pressure on the catheter and the retention balloon. Make another selection.*
3. *No. The mid-abdominal region would not be comfortable for the client nor would it allow for the downward flow of urine via gravity into the drainage bag. This is not the preferred taping site. Choose another option.*
4. ***Good choice! The lateral thigh or lower abdomen are the recommended sites to eliminate the penoscrotal angle and prevent the formation of a urethrocutaneous fistula.***

44. **A client is transferred from the recovery room to the special care unit after a radical neck dissection. At this time, which vital sign would receive the highest priority by the nurse?**

1. Temperature.
2. Pulse.
3. Respirations.
4. Blood pressure.

1. *Incorrect. Although this vital sign is important to detect the presence of infection, it is not the highest priority at this time. Choose another option.*
2. *No. The pulse will give an assessment of the client's cardiovascular status, which is necessary to detect early signs of shock, but it is not the priority after radical neck surgery. Try again.*
3. ***Excellent choice! Patency of the airway and respiratory function are always evaluated first, particularly after radical neck surgery.***
4. *Not the correct choice. Blood pressure assessment is needed to monitor cardiovascular status, but there is another assessment that always takes precedence. Make another selection.*

45. **During a home visit, the wife of your client collapses. There is no pulse or respirations. Which of the following accurately describes the CPR the nurse would provide?**

1. 5 to 1 ratio of compressions to ventilations, at a rate of 100 beats/min.
2. 15 to 2 ratio of compressions to ventilations, at a rate of 80 beats/min.
3. 15 to 2 ratio of compressions to ventilations, at a rate of 100 beats/min.
4. 5 to 1 ratio of compressions to ventilations, at a rate of 80 beats/min.

1. *No, this is incorrect. Go back and reread the question. Try again.*
2. *Incorrect. You have selected the correct ratio, but the rate is not fast enough.*
3. ***Excellent! One-person CPR is performed with 15 compressions and 2 ventilations. It is necessary to give the compressions at a rate of 100 per minute, since you are pausing after every 15 compressions to give the ventilations. This actually results in approximately 60 compressions per minute to the client.***
4. *No, this is not one-person CPR. Try again.*

46. **An elderly female has fallen, fracturing her left hip. She is admitted in Buck's traction and scheduled for intramedullary nailing. The nurse knows that the reason for Buck's traction in this client is to:**

1. Reduce muscle spasm.
2. Provide for total immobility.
3. Promote healing of the fracture.
4. Allow for a 20 pound weight to be applied.

1. ***Right! This is the correct option. Buck's traction usually is used initially to reduce the se-***

vere muscle spasm that is mainly responsible for the pain associated with a fracture of the femoral head.

2. *Incorrect. Although the client's mobility is limited by traction, the affected leg is the only part that should be immobilized. The client will be allowed to turn and exercise the unaffected limbs.*

> **TEST-TAKING TIP:** *Be wary of any response that uses absolutes, like the word "total" in this option.*

3. *No, not likely. Only persons who are inoperable would have Buck's traction used for the whole course of treatment. The usual course of treatment includes surgical reduction and pinning.*

4. *No, this is incorrect. Buck's is skin traction, and the limit for weight is usually five to 10 pounds. If greater weight is needed, skeletal traction must be used.*

47. **A female client has a history of frequent episodes of cystitis. Which statement by the client would indicate to the nurse that she needs further teaching about measures to prevent the reoccurrence of cystitis?**

    1. "I drink plenty of liquids during the day, usually two to three quarts."
    2. "I often like to take baths instead of showers."
    3. "I try to empty my bladder every two to three hours."
    4. "I use an oral contraceptive for birth control."

    1. *Wrong choice. This measure is correct and would help to decrease the incidence of bladder infections. A fluid intake of 2,000 to 3,000 ml per day is ideal to provide "natural irrigation" and prevent urinary stasis. Look for a statement by the client indicating an INCORRECT action.*
    2. **Good work. This statement indicates a knowledge deficit on the part of the client. Women who suffer frequent urinary tract infections are encouraged to shower rather than take tub baths, because a tub bath is more likely to cause irritation and contamination of the urethra.**
    3. *Incorrect choice. This measure is appropriate and would prevent urinary stasis, which is a leading cause of urinary tract infections. Look for a statement by the client indicating an INCORRECT action.*
    4. *Wrong choice. This measure would not affect the urinary tract and has no correlation to the frequent episodes of urinary tract infections experienced by the client. Look for a statement by the client indicating an INCORRECT action.*

48. **A client diagnosed with chronic renal failure is started on hemodialysis. During the procedure, heparin so-**

dium is added to the blood. The nurse knows that the heparin has been effective if the client remains free of:

1. Thrombi.
2. Infection at the fistula site.
3. Chills and fever.
4. Hypertension.

1. **Yes! Heparin is used to prevent clotting of the blood. This anticoagulant acts to block the conversion of prothrombin to thrombin and fibrinogen to fibrin. Heparin is necessary during hemodialysis to prevent clot formation as the blood is passed, via a pump, through a semipermeable membrane.**
2. *Incorrect. Heparin does not have anti-infective properties. Try again.*
3. *Incorrect. Heparin is not an antipyretic. Try again.*
4. *Wrong. Heparin is not a vasoconstrictor. The process of dialysis acts to decrease blood pressure as fluid is removed from the circulating blood volume. Try again.*

49. **A client has just been catheterized and has an indwelling Foley catheter in her bladder. If all of the following actions were taken, improper technique was used when the nurse:**

1. Cleansed the client's urinary meatus with soap and water prior to inserting the catheter.
2. Placed the client in the lithotomy position.
3. Inserted the catheter one to two inches further into the urinary meatus when urine was observed in the catheter tubing.
4. Used sterile normal saline to inflate the retention balloon on the catheter.

1. **Good choice, this action is incorrect! Even if this was done prior to beginning the procedure, the cleansing of the urinary meatus must be done with an antiseptic solution to decrease the chance of bacteria being introduced into the urinary meatus.**
2. *No, this is proper technique. The lithotomy position provides for the best visualization of the urinary meatus. Most clients are placed in the dorsal recumbent position with knees bent and legs apart, but the lithotomy position is appropriate and would not be judged improper technique.*
3. *No, this is proper technique. It allows for advancement of the catheter and the retention balloon, which is distal to the openings on the end of the catheter. Advancing the catheter further after urine is sighted in the tubing prevents the retention balloon from remaining in the urinary meatus, which can cause pain for the client if inflated in this area.*
4. *No, this is proper technique. Sterile normal saline can be used to inflate the retention balloon. The*

key word is STERILE.

50. When attempting to obtain information from a hearing impaired client, the nurse should:

1. Face the client and speak slowly.
2. Speak frequently and exaggerate lip movements.
3. Speak loudly.
4. Speak directly into the impaired ear.

1. ***Correct. You should always face the hearing impaired client and accentuate your words without exaggerating lip movements.***
2. *Incorrect. Speaking frequently will not aid the client in hearing, and exaggerated lip movements are contraindicated.*
3. *Incorrect. Shouting over employs normal speaking movements, which may cause distortion and be too loud for the client.*
4. *Incorrect. Speaking directly into the impaired ear is contraindicated. Moving closer and toward the better ear will facilitate communication.*

51. An elderly client is diagnosed with benign prostatic hypertrophy. Which of the following nursing interventions is contraindicated following a prostatectomy?

1. Administration of analgesics as ordered.
2. Notifying the physician of excessive clots.
3. Irrigation of the Foley catheter as ordered and PRN.
4. Rectal temperatures taken every four hours for the first 24 hours.

1. *Wrong choice, this action is appropriate. Postoperative pain is usually mild, but expected. A non-narcotic analgesic is usually ordered. Note that the question has a false response stem, so you are looking for an intervention that is CONTRAINDICATED.*
2. *Wrong choice. This action is appropriate and the question has a false response stem. You are looking for an intervention that is CONTRAINDICATED. Bright red bleeding or excessive clots could indicate hemorrhage, in which case the physician should be notified.*
3. *Wrong choice, this action is appropriate. Irrigation of the catheter will ensure patency by preventing clots from blocking the catheter, thereby causing bladder distension and possibly fresh bleeding. You are looking for an action that is CONTRAINDICATED.*
4. ***Correct choice, this is contraindicated. Rectal temperatures are not taken because of the close proximity of the prostate and rectum, and the potential of causing damage.***

52. A client is admitted with a complaint of weight loss of 12 pounds in the last two months, despite increased appetite. She also is experiencing increased perspiration, fatigue, and restlessness. A diagnosis of hyperthyroidism is made. Which measure is essential for the nurse to include in her plan of to prevent thyrotoxic crisis?

1. Provide a quiet, low stimulus environment.
2. Administer aspirin as ordered for any sign of hyperthermia.
3. Maintain the client's NPO status until her anorexia subsides.
4. Observe the client carefully for signs of hypocalcemia.

1. ***Good choice! Thyrotoxic crisis usually occurs in response to a stressor, and the client should not be exposed to other clients in the room who are very sick. Visitors should maintain a calm environment.***
2. *Wrong! Although fever is an additional stressor, aspirin is contraindicated since it displaces the thyroid hormone from plasma proteins, and results in active thyroid hormone in the blood, which may exacerbate a thyrotoxic crisis. Aspirin would not properly be ordered for this client.*
3. *Wrong! Anorexia, nausea, and vomiting may precede thyrotoxic crisis, but the case scenario does not include this data. The question states that the client is losing weight despite increased appetite. The client should be encouraged to eat a high protein, high caloric diet to maintain weight and prevent negative nitrogen balance.*
4. *Incorrect. Hypocalcemia is a clinical finding in hypoparathyroidism, and does not play a role in preventing thyroid storm.*

53. A client is post-craniotomy and is progressing well. While he is sitting in a chair, the nurse notices that he begins to experience a grand mal seizure. The most important nursing action is to:

1. Provide oxygen.
2. Restrain the client.
3. Insert an airway.
4. Lower the client to the floor.

1. *Not the first priority. Oxygen is provided if needed, but only if the client becomes hypoxic.*
2. *Never! Restraints are contraindicated, as they may cause the client to harm himself during the seizure. Resistance against strong muscle contractions may cause injury.*
3. *Never! Forcing the jaw apart while a client is experiencing a seizure can cause permanent damage to teeth and gums.*
4. ***Great job! When a client begins a seizure in a***

chair, the nurse should gently lower him to the floor to protect him from injury.

54. When changing dressings for an HIV positive client, the nurse should remember to wash hands and to:

    1. Wear a mask.
    2. Wear gloves.
    3. Maintain strict isolation.
    4. Wear a gown and gloves.

    1. Incorrect. Masks are not necessary. Goggles should be used if splatter is likely.
    2. Correct! Gloves are necessary and, besides hand washing, are the best protection from HIV clients.
    3. Incorrect. Universal precautions are required to care for HIV positive clients, not strict isolation.
    4. Incorrect. This is necessary only if the nurse's clothing may become contaminated.

55. While caring for a client 24 hours following surgery, the priority nursing action is to:

    1. Monitor his comfort level.
    2. Encourage the client to verbalize his fears.
    3. Observe safety precautions.
    4. Instruct the client in self-care skills.

    1. No, this is not the priority. Although comfort is important, safety is the priority.
    2. No, this is not the priority. Although fears need to be identified so they can be explored, safety is the priority.
    3. Good choice! Safe nursing care takes precedence over any other nursing interventions.
    4. No, this is not the priority. Although learning proper skills to care for IOL is important, safety is the priority.

56. A client has had a right total hip replacement and is three days postoperative. When the nurse and nursing assistant are transferring her to a chair, she cries out in pain. Which observation by the nurse would lead to the suspicion of a dislocated hip prosthesis?

    1. Shortening of the right leg.
    2. Bulging in the right hip area.
    3. Adduction of the left leg.
    4. Loose hip joint movement on the right side.

    1. Correct choice! One of the classic indicators of prosthetic dislocation is shortening of the affected leg, along with an inability to move it, abnormal rotation, and increased discomfort.
    2. Incorrect. Dislocation of the prosthesis will not result in any visible bulging in the surgical area. Make another selection.
    3. No. A prosthetic dislocation will not result in

changes to the unaffected leg. Try again.
4. Incorrect choice. Dislocation of the prosthesis will result in an inability to move the affected leg. Choose another option.

57. The nurse knows that a signed consent form is necessary for which procedure?

    1. Magnetic resonance imagery (MRI).
    2. Cerebral arteriogram.
    3. Computed tomography (CT scan).
    4. Echoencephalography.

    1. No, the MRI is a noninvasive and painless procedure that uses a powerful magnetic field to obtain images of different body areas. Choose another option.
    2. Yes! The cerebral arteriogram is considered invasive, with the injection of contrast material into a selected artery to study the cerebral circulation. A consent is required.
    3. Incorrect. The CT scan makes use of a narrow beam of x-ray to scan the body in successive layers. CT is a noninvasive and painless procedure.
    4. No. Echoencephalography is the recording of sound waves in response to ultrasound signals created by a transducer positioned over specific areas of the head. It is a noninvasive test.

58. A client is admitted with a T2-T3 spinal cord transection. Nursing care for a client with T2-T3 spinal cord transection includes care for what type of paralysis?

    1. Hemiplegia.
    2. Paraplegia.
    3. Quadriplegia.
    4. Paresthesia.

    1. Incorrect. Hemiplegia, paralysis of an arm and leg on the same side of the body, is seen after a cerebral vascular accident. Choose again.
    2. Correct! Paraplegia, paralysis of both legs, is seen after a spinal cord transection below T1.
    3. Wrong. Quadriplegia, paralysis of all four extremities, is seen with spinal cord transections in the cervical vertebrae above C4. An injury at C2-3 is usually rapidly fatal. Make another selection.
    4. Wrong. Paresthesia is burning or tingling sensations due to pressure on nerves or circulatory impairment. It is not a form of paralysis. Try another option.

59. A client had a right total hip replacement three days ago. When transferring from the bed to the chair, the client suddenly complains of sharp, severe pain in the right hip area. The nurse interprets this to mean that the client most likely:

1. Suffered a dislocation of the hip prosthesis.
2. Put too much weight on the right leg when transferring into the chair.
3. Experienced muscle spasms in the right leg.
4. Developed a blood clot in the right hip area.

1. **Correct choice. Signs of hip prosthesis dislocation include severe pain, external rotation of the hip with noticeable shortening of the leg, and a palpable bulge over the head of the femur.**
2. *Incorrect. The client would express some discomfort if this happened, but should not have sharp, severe pain.*
3. *Incorrect. Remember that the pain is in the right hip area. Muscle spasms would result in pain in the right thigh or calf area.*
4. *Incorrect. A blood clot (or hematoma) would cause a feeling of increased pressure or tightness in the hip area, but not sharp, severe pain with a sudden onset. Sudden, sharp severe pain in the operative site would indicate another serious problem.*

60. **Which action by the nurse would indicate that the client has an understanding of measures to be taken to prevent hip dislocation following a total hip replacement?**

1. Keeping the affected leg adducted at all times.
2. Using a trochanter roll when the client is supine.
3. Maintaining the affected hip in the flexed position.
4. Keeping the client in the supine position.

1. *Wrong. The leg should be ABDUCTED, that is, away from the midline — not ADDUCTED. This is usually accomplished through an abductor pillow that is placed between the client's legs and kept there at all times. Try again.*
2. **Correct. The trochanter roll will prevent external rotation of the hip. This roll can be made from a bath blanket and should extend from the crest of the ilium to the midthigh. It acts as a mechanical wedge under the projection of the greater trochanter and prevents the femur from rolling.**
3. *No, the hip should NOT be maintained in a flexed position, especially one greater than 60 degrees. Limited flexion is maintained during transfers and when sitting in a chair. Try again.*
4. *No, this is not correct. After surgery, the client can be in the supine position or can turn to the unoperated side. The client is not to sleep on the operated side until this position is cleared with the surgeon.*

61. **A client undergoes surgery for a hip replacement. In the postoperative period, the nurse must instruct the client to avoid which action while sitting in a chair?**

1. Crossing his legs.
2. Elevating his feet.
3. Flexing his ankles.
4. Extending his knees.

1. **Good work, the client should NOT cross his legs. After hip replacement, the client must maintain his legs in a state of abduction in order to prevent dislocation of the prosthesis. Crossing his legs involves adduction, which is to be avoided. Also to be avoided is 90-degree hip flexion.**
2. *Wrong choice. Elevating his feet would not put the client at risk for prosthetic displacement. Which action by this client would be harmful?*
3. *Wrong choice, this position is actually good for the client! It's part of ankle exercises that help to decrease the chance of thrombophlebitis after surgery. Which action by this client would be harmful?*
4. *Wrong choice, extending his knees would not increase hip flexion beyond a 90-degree angle. The client must keep the abductor pillow in position and is encouraged to keep the operative hip in extension. He cannot do this easily without extending his knees. Which action by this client would be harmful?*

62. **When inserting a nasogastric tube in a comatose client for internal tube feedings, it is inappropriate for the nurse to:**

1. Measure the amount of the tube to be inserted.
2. Lubricate the distal portion of the tube.
3. Tilt the client's head back when inserting the tube.
4. Check placement of the tube.

1. *No, this action is correct. Measurement from the tip of the client's nose to the ear lobe to the xiphoid process is the measurement considered to be approximately equal to the distance necessary for stomach placement. This question is asking for something that is NOT appropriate to do. Try again.*
2. *Wrong choice. Remember, this question has a negative response stem and is looking for something NOT to do when inserting a nasogastric tube. Lubricating the tube allows it to pass through the nostril easier.*
3. **Good work! This action is incorrect, since it makes it difficult to swallow, and increases the likelihood of introducing the tube into the trachea.**
4. *Wrong choice. Remember, this question has a negative response stem. This is a correct action, because placement needs to be verified to ensure that the tube is not in the trachea or lungs. This question asked for something that was NOT appropriate to do. Try again.*

63. **Prior to a paracentesis procedure for a client with ascites, the nurse should encourage the client to:**

 1. Drink two liters of water.
 2. Empty his bladder.
 3. Cleanse the abdominal area thoroughly.
 4. Eat a meal high in sodium.

 1. *Incorrect. Fluids are restricted to 1 to 1.5 liters daily for clients with ascites.*
 2. ***Good choice! Voiding will help avoid puncture of the bladder when the trocar is inserted into the abdomen.***
 3. *Incorrect, because cleansing of the skin with an antiseptic solution on the lower abdomen is done during the procedure by a physician or nurse, not by the client.*
 4. *Incorrect. Sodium is restricted to 800 mg in order to induce a negative sodium balance and permit diuresis.*

64. **A client is admitted with esophageal varices. The most appropriate nursing action that will decrease the risk of esophageal bleeding is to:**

 1. Apply an ice collar.
 2. Maintain semi-Fowler's position.
 3. Administer stool softeners.
 4. Provide a diet high in Vitamin D.

 1. *Incorrect. An ice collar cannot control portal hypertension.*
 2. *Incorrect. This plays no role in decreasing the risk of bleeding for this client.*
 3. *Good choice! Bleeding occurs as a result of straining when stooling. It is therefore appropriate to decrease any possibility of straining by administering stool softeners.*
 4. *Incorrect. Foods high in Vitamin D help to stimulate the active transport of calcium and phosphorous, but play no role in controlling bleeding.*

65. **A client is admitted to the emergency room for an acute asthmatic attack. At this time, the initial nursing action for this client is to:**

 1. Assist the client to a high Fowler's position.
 2. Offer oral fluids to loosen secretions.
 3. Monitor respiratory rate for changes.
 4. Reduce all unnecessary environmental stimuli.

 1. ***Correct. This position should be initiated first in order to lower abdominal organs to facilitate breathing.***
 2. *Wrong! A client in an acute attack is unable to take oral fluids, parenteral fluids are necessary to route medications and liquefy secretions.*
 3. *Incorrect. Tachypnea can indicate hypoxemia. Initially, however, changing her position in order to*

 promote adequate ventilation is most important.
 4. *Wrong choice! The initial goal is to promote oxygenation, then the nurse can begin to allay fears.*

66. **A client has sustained a gunshot wound to her left side and has a closed water seal drainage system attached to a chest tube. The nurse notices continuous bubbling in the water seal collection immediately after insertion of the chest tube. Which action should the nurse take?**

 1. Notify the physician immediately.
 2. Clamp the chest tube.
 3. Continue to monitor for continuous bubbling.
 4. Reposition the client.

 1. *Wrong choice. Bubbling that occurs immediately after insertion is normal.*
 2. *Wrong. This would be done only to determine a leak if the tube became dislodged or if the bubbling continued. Clamping prevents external air from entering pleural space.*
 3. ***Good job! Fluid and air initially rush out from intrapleural space under high pressure, so the nurse would watch for continuous bubbling.***
 4. *Wrong! This would not have any effect on leakage from the chest tube. Select another option.*

67. **Which nursing intervention will help to prevent the development of postoperative thrombophlebitis?**

 1. Have the client sit with her feet touching the floor.
 2. Apply gentle leg massage.
 3. Encourage the client to ambulate.
 4. Place pillows under the client's knees.

 1. *Wrong. This position will help to prevent orthostatic hypotension, not thrombophlebitis.*
 2. *No. This is contraindicated, since it may cause a thrombus to become an embolus.*
 3. ***Yes! Early ambulation promotes optimal cardiovascular function and helps to prevent thrombus formation.***
 4. *No. Pillows under knees (popliteal area) will impede circulation; pressure here should be avoided.*

68. **The nurse knows that which finding would contribute to rheumatic endocarditis?**

 1. Congestive heart failure.
 2. Tuberculosis.
 3. Streptococcus throat infection.
 4. Coronary artery disease.

 1. *Incorrect. A history of congestive heart failure has no correlation with rheumatic endocarditis. Try to recall the pathophysiology of the disease process, and choose again.*

2. *No, there is no connection between TB and rheumatic endocarditis. Select another option.*

3. ***Excellent! You recalled that a streptococcal infection (usually group A beta-hemolytic streptococcus) is a major cause of endocarditis.***

4. *No, there is no connection between coronary artery disease and rheumatic endocarditis, which affects the heart's valves. Make another selection.*

69. **After a myocardial infarction, the nurse knows that which vital signs assessment may indicate cardiogenic shock?**

1. BP - 180/100, P - 90 and irregular.
2. BP - 130/80, P - 100 and regular.
3. BP - 90/50, P - 50 and regular.
4. BP - 80/60, P - 110 and irregular.

1. *Incorrect. These vital signs are not seen in a shock-like state. Choose again.*

2. *No, these vital signs are within normal limits. Recall the pathophysiology of shock, and make a more appropriate selection.*

3. *You're partially right. The client in cardiogenic shock will be hypotensive, but will not have bradycardia. Try to find the best option.*

4. ***Good assessment! The classic signs of cardiogenic shock are low blood pressure, rapid and weak pulse, cold, clammy skin, decreased urinary output, and cerebral hypoxia.***

70. **A client is seen in the health clinic with manifestations of urinary burning and urgency. Which diagnostic test can the nurse anticipate will be ordered to diagnose the possibility of a urinary tract infection?**

1. Clean-catch midstream urine.
2. Catheterized urine.
3. Intravenous pyelogram (IVP).
4. Random urine specimen.

1. ***Correct! A clean-catch urine specimen is the routine test of choice to diagnose a urinary tract infection. It is designed to eliminate as much external contamination of the specimen as possible by cleansing the labia and midstream collection into a sterile container.***

2. *No, this technique is too invasive, uncomfortable, and expensive for the diagnosis of a urinary tract infection. Try again.*

3. *Incorrect. The IVP is a radiologic test that visualizes the urinary tract. It is ordered in suspected disease or urinary tract dysfunction. It is not used to diagnose a urinary tract infection. Make another selection.*

4. *No, this collection of urine may result in external contamination of the specimen. Choose another option.*

71. **Following cataract surgery, which comment made by the client to the nurse should be reported immediately to the charge nurse?**

1. "My eye itches, but I'm trying not to scratch it."
2. "I need something for this pain in my eye. I can hardly stand it."
3. "It's really hard to see with one eye patched. I'm afraid of falling."
4. "No one has taught me how to change this eye dressing or apply the ointment."

1. *Incorrect choice. This comment is often made by clients as the healing process begins. Clients are instructed not to rub or place pressure on the eyes. This comment would not require the attention of the charge nurse.*

2. ***Correct! Following cataract surgery, the client is advised to immediately report any pain in the eye, decrease in vision, or increased discharge. The client should normally need nothing stronger than acetaminophen for eye discomfort. The nurse should know that eye pain after surgery may indicate acute angle glaucoma, which can cause permanent damage to the optic nerve if not treated promptly.***

3. *Incorrect choice. This comment does need to be addressed by the nurse, but it does not require the attention of the charge nurse. Reassurance can be given to the client without intervention needed by the charge nurse.*

4. *Wrong. This issue does not have priority. Another statement made by the client can result in serious, permanent injury if not addressed immediately.*

72. **Which statement made to the nurse by a diabetic client on insulin would indicate the need for further teaching?**

1. "It's important to measure the correct dosage of insulin at eye level."
2. "The insulin should be injected at a 90-degree angle."
3. "I'll remember to rotate sites so that each site is used only once a month."
4. "If I increase my exercise, I know that I will have to increase my insulin dosage."

1. *Incorrect choice. The client's statement is correct and means that the client knows the proper technique for measuring an insulin dosage. Remember this fundamental principle from your first nursing course: any medications drawn up in a syringe should be checked at eye level for accuracy of dose. Look for an INCORRECT statement by the client.*

2. *Incorrect choice. This true statement means that the client needs no further teaching on the technique for injecting the insulin. Insulin needles are*

shorter than regular subcutaneous needles and can be given at a 90-degree angle into the tissue without fear of injecting into the muscle. Look for an INCORRECT statement by the client.

3. Incorrect choice, this statement suggests that the client knows how to prevent lipodystrophy. When insulin is repeatedly injected into the same place over a period of time, depressions in the fat beneath the skin (lipodystrophy) can occur. Rotation of sites can help minimize this problem. Look for an INCORRECT statement by the client.

4. **Yes! This statement indicates that the client needs further teaching. Muscular activity improves utilization of glucose by using it for energy. Exercise also makes the insulin receptors on cells more sensitive to the hormone and thus improves utilization of the available glucose. Once a client begins to follow a regular exercise program, he probably will need to take LESS insulin.**

73. A client is to receive Regular Humulin insulin (Humulin R) 10 Units and NPH Humulin insulin (Humulin N) 30 Units subcutaneously at 7:30 a.m. The nurse can anticipate the onset of insulin action to occur at:

   1. 7:30 a.m.
   2. 8:00 a.m.
   3. 9:00 a.m.
   4. 9:30 a.m.

   1. Incorrect. Humulin insulin, given subcutaneously, cannot have an immediate onset of action. It will take some time for the insulin to be absorbed by the tissue.

   2. **Yes. The onset of action for Regular Humulin insulin is one-half to one hour, with a peak effect in two to four hours.**

   3. Incorrect. Ninety minutes before onset of action is typical for the intermediate-acting insulins when they are given alone. Recall that regular Humulin insulin was also given at the same time as the NPH Humulin insulin.

   4. Wrong choice. A two-hour onset of action is seen with the long-acting insulins, such as Humulin L, or with the intermediate insulins (Humulin N) when given alone.

74. A hospitalized client is disoriented, confused, and agitated, and is receiving lorazepam (Ativan). Because the client is receiving Ativan, which nursing action is a priority?

   1. Observing the client for early signs of tardive dyskinesia.
   2. Warning the client not to drive her automobile or engage in activities that require alertness.
   3. Frequently checking the client's serum level of medication.
   4. Monitoring the client closely when she ambulates.

1. Wrong. Tardive dyskinesia is an adverse effect of antipsychotics, not Ativan. This is not the correct option.

2. This is not a priority for the client while she is hospitalized. Try again.

3. Serum levels are checked frequently when elderly clients are taking the tricyclic antidepressants and lithium, but this is not necessary for Ativan. Choose another option.

4. **Correct. Elderly clients may become dizzy or ataxic when taking benzodiazepines, like Ativan. They should be monitored closely when they are out of bed and ambulatory, to prevent falls and possible injuries.**

75. The physician has prescribed clindamycin (Cleocin) 300 mg P.O. every six hours for a client diagnosed with an upper respiratory tract infection. In order to facilitate maximum drug absorption, the nurse should instruct the client to take Cleocin:

   1. With meals or a snack.
   2. On an empty stomach.
   3. With a full glass of water at six-hour intervals around the clock.
   4. With an antacid or glass of milk.

   1. No! With oral administration, Cleocin is well absorbed (90%) if administered before meals. Food decreases the absorption of the drug. Select again.

   2. **Correct! As with most antibiotics, Cleocin is best taken one hour before or two hours after meals, with a full glass of water to facilitate its absorption.**

   3. Not the best choice. Although the instructions to take with a full glass of water and at six-hour intervals are correct, these actions will not ensure the maximal drug absorption. Make another selection.

   4. No! The Cleocin may bind with the antacid or milk and significantly delay the drug's absorption. Choose another option.

76. A client calls the doctor's office and reports that he has developed diarrhea secondary to taking clindamycin (Cleocin). At this time, the nurse would:

   1. Report the diarrhea to the physician for appropriate treatment.
   2. Advise the client to take the medicine with food to decrease GI distress.
   3. Instruct the client to take kaolin/pectate (Kaopectate) over-the-counter at the same time as his oral dose of Cleocin.
   4. Recommend that the client take a bulk-forming agent such as psyllium (Metamucil) while on Cleocin, but to report any bloody stools immediately.

1. *Excellent choice! A serious adverse reaction to Cleocin is pseudomembranous colitis, which has diarrhea as its major manifestation. Clients should not try to self-treat, but should report any diarrhea to the physician immediately. The nurse needs to stress the importance of observing stools for blood and mucous and reporting appearance and quantity of fecal material expelled.*

2. Incorrect. To minimize diarrhea, food should be avoided one to two hours before and after ingestion of Cleocin. Try again.

3. Wrong choice! Kaolin decreases the absorption of Cleocin if taken concurrently. If it is ordered, it should be taken no sooner than two hours after or at least three to four hours before taking the antibiotic again. Choose another option.

4. Wrong choice. Taking a bulk-forming agent will not resolve the problem. It is true that the client should report any bloody or tarry stools immediately, but he also needs treatment for the diarrhea. Make another selection.

77. A client is complaining of gastric problems while taking his demeclocycline (Declomycin) and asks if it is all right to take his antacid along with the medication. What is the best response by the nurse?

1. "Sure, if it helps, go right ahead."
2. "It would be better to take the medication with milk."
3. "Antacids will block the absorption of the medication and you will not get the full effect. Let's ask your doctor to switch you to another form of tetracycline."
4. "You should take all medications on an empty stomach."

1. No. This would be an inappropriate response because an antacid will inhibit absorption of the drug.
2. Wrong response! Taking any of the tetracyclines with milk or antacids will inhibit absorption.
3. *Great choice! This is the best response because it explains why the client should not take an antacid and it does not cause noncompliance by allowing the client to just suffer with side effects.*
4. No! Taking ALL medications on an empty stomach would not be correct advice.

78. The nurse is reviewing the client's history prior to administration of theophylline (Theo-Dur). Which factor, if true about this client, would indicate the need for increased Theo-Dur dosage? The client:

1. Is over 70 years of age.
2. Is also taking levothyroxine (Synthroid) for "thyroid difficulties."
3. Has difficulty swallowing.
4. Smokes cigarettes.

1. No! Generally, the elderly need a DECREASED dosage, because of decreased hepatic and renal function.
2. No! There are many medications that interact with theophylline. Synthroid, however, is not one of them. If the client is hyperthyroid, theophylline is used cautiously. The client on synthroid is most likely euthyroid if the medication is dosed correctly.
3. A client who has difficulty swallowing may use a "sprinkle" preparation in food. This preparation enables the client to receive the correct dose. A higher dosage is not indicated.
4. *Good work! Cigarette smoking decreases the serum levels and therefore the therapeutic effects. Heavy cigarette smokers require higher doses of theophylline.*

79. The nurse who is assigned to care for a child with cerebral palsy understands that the aim of therapy is to:

1. Assess the child's assets and potentialities and capitalize on these in the habilitative process, while ignoring limitations.
2. Reverse abnormal functioning and restore brain damage through rehabilitation.
3. Provide a therapeutic program that avoids subjecting the child to frustrating experiences that decrease his achievement.
4. Develop an individualized therapeutic program that uses the child's assets and abilities and provides experiences that permit him to achieve success as well as help to cope with frustration and failure.

1. Although this goal is stated in general terms, the last part of the statement is not appropriate—ignoring any aspect of the client's health problem is never an aim of therapy! Make another choice.
2. Incorrect. Brain damage cannot be reversed or restored. This is a false statement, and this option should be eliminated. Make another choice.
3. Wrong. It cannot be an aim of therapy to avoid frustrating experiences; this would be unrealistic. Although this option might appear to be a possibility and is stated in general terms, it is not correct. Make another choice.
4. *You chose the correct answer! This goal statement includes recognizing the client's assets and helping him cope with frustrations and failures due to his limitations.*

TEST-TAKING TIP: *This option is a global response. It states appropriate goals of therapy in general terms and it also includes the correct part of Option 1. When you are having difficulty identifying the correct option, look for a statement that is a global response.*

80. A client, 35 years old, was admitted to the hospital for possible gall bladder surgery. Following a gall bladder x-ray, the doctor decided that a cholecystectomy was necessary. The nurse's preoperative teaching should include which information?

    1. Many clients are admitted to the intensive care unit after this type of surgery.
    2. Minor discomfort is expected in the operative site during the first few postoperative days.
    3. Moving as little as possible will decrease the discomfort following this procedure.
    4. Learning to cough and deep breathe will help prevent postoperative respiratory breathing complications.

    1. This is not a true statement. Following cholecystectomy, clients usually return to the general nursing unit from the post anesthesia recovery room. This option is a distractor. Try again!

    2. This is not a true statement. Following cholecystectomy, clients usually experience acute pain in the operative site for several days.

    3. Moving as little as possible is contraindicated following surgery because it contributes to the complications associated with immobility. Clients are encouraged to turn, cough, deep breathe, and ambulate postoperatively to decrease the possibility of complications. Acute postoperative discomfort can be managed by giving medications as ordered.

    4. Good choice! A demonstration and return demonstration of coughing and deep breathing will facilitate the client's ability to participate in her care postoperatively. Coughing and deep breathing helps prevent postoperative respiratory complications.

81. A 30-month-old male is being admitted with asthma. To decrease the stress of hospitalization for the toddler, the nurse should:

    1. Explain procedures and routines.
    2. Encourage contact with children of the same age.
    3. Provide for privacy.
    4. Encourage rooming-in.

    1. No. You can explain procedures, but given a choice, this is not the best answer. This becomes a more appropriate stress reducing technique when as the child matures into school age and adolescence.

    2. The peer group is not the major support for the toddler. This would be a more successful plan with the school age or adolescent client.

    3. Incorrect. Adolescence is the age in which stress may be reduced by providing privacy in order for them to cope more effectively.

    4. Right! Rooming-in is the most effective means of providing emotional support for the toddler. The family's presence provides a sense of security that will increase the child's ability to cope in an unfamiliar environment. This is well supported by nursing research.

82. A client taking lithium is discharged. After five days, she tells the nurse that she is still having difficulty with hyperactivity. She asks how long it will take for her lithium to be effective. The best explanation by the nurse is:

    1. "Each person is different. Lithium usually takes one to two weeks to be effective."
    2. "We are monitoring your blood level to see when it is in the therapeutic range. At that point your manifestations should be controlled."
    3. "You should see an immediate improvement. I will call your psychiatrist so she can increase your dose."
    4. "You will begin to see some improvement when your blood level reaches the therapeutic range, but it still may be a while before your manifestations are controlled."

    1. This is a possibility, because it is a true statement, but there is a better answer. Read the other options.

    2. This is not a true statement. Manifestations only begin to remit after the blood level reaches the therapeutic range. It can take up to two weeks for the client to achieve maximum effect.

    3. This statement is not correct. Lithium dosage is prescribed based on the client's blood level, not clinical manifestations.

    4. Correct. There is a lag between the time when the lithium level reaches the normal range and the manic episode is under control. The length of time this takes varies among clients.

83. The nurse finds an elderly client standing in a puddle of water in the hallway of the unit. The nurse does not know this client. What is the nurse's initial action?

    1. Ask the client for her name and room number.
    2. Wipe up the water until the floor is completely dry.
    3. Call the supervisor for assistance in identifying the client.
    4. Have the client wait in the lounge until security arrives.

    1. Wrong. The issue in this question is the puddle of water on the floor. The water on the floor threatens the safety of the client and others on the unit. After the nurse ensures safety, the client can be identified and assisted back to the correct room.

    2. Very good! The issue in this question is the

puddle of water on the floor. The water on the floor threatens the safety of the client and others on the unit. The nurse's first action should be to alleviate the safety hazard by wiping up the water.

> **PRIORITY ALERT!** *Maslow's Hierarchy of Needs indicates that when no physiological need exists, safety needs should receive priority. Note: the word "water" in the question is repeated in this option. The test-taking strategy of looking for similar words in the question would identify this option as a possible answer.*

3. *Wrong! The issue in this question is the puddle of water on the floor. The water on the floor threatens the safety of the client and others on the unit. After the nurse ensures safety, the client can be identified and assisted back to the correct room.*

4. *No. The issue in this question is the puddle of water on the floor. The water on the floor threatens the safety of the client and others on the unit. Asking the client to wait in the lounge until security arrives does not assure safety. Someone may still slip on the puddle of water and injure themselves.*

84. **After a series of nine ECT treatments, a client reports that his depressive manifestations are gone. However, he does complain of short-term memory loss. The initial nursing action is to:**

1. Report the problem immediately to his psychiatrist.
2. Encourage him to ventilate his feelings about the problem.
3. Explain that this memory loss is only temporary, and his memory will return to normal in four to eight weeks.
4. Tell him that this is a side effect of the treatment, and he can expect his memory to return to normal in five to ten days.

1. *The nurse should chart this manifestation, but it does not need to be reported immediately to the psychiatrist because it is an expected outcome of the ECT treatments.*

2. *This action is not incorrect, but it is not the initial nursing action because the client has not been given some important information about his memory problems.*

3. **Correct. *Research indicates that short-term memory problems are temporary outcomes of ECT treatment. While the length of time the client has these memory problems differs among individuals, it is a temporary effect that usually does not last longer than two months.***

4. *This response is only partially true. Temporary memory problems are a common side effect of ECT. The length of time the client experiences these memory problems differs among individuals but*

it most often lasts for a longer period of time than five to 10 days.

85. **When caring for elderly clients who are treated with antidepressant medication, the nurse knows that:**

1. They will probably require a higher doses of medication than a younger person.
2. Psychotherapy and medication together are usually more effective than either alone in treating elderly depressed clients.
3. Antidepressant medications are not usually tolerated well by elderly clients because of their many side effects.
4. Antidepressants are expensive medications, and the potential results may not be worth their cost.

1. *This is not true. Elderly persons, and other clients with coexisting medical problems, are treated with LOWER doses of antidepressants.*

2. **Correct. *Treatment that includes both psychotherapy and antidepressant medication is usually more effective in treating elderly clients with clinical depression than either modality is when used alone.***

3. *Not the correct choice. Elderly clients are more sensitive to the side effects of antidepressants. The elderly also are more likely to be taking other drugs for medical problems which could lead to drug interactions. Nevertheless, elders can still be effectively treated with antidepressants when their responses to the drug treatment are monitored closely. Select again.*

4. *This is not true. Treatment with antidepressants, when combined with psychotherapy, is an effective way to treat depression in the elderly. With proper treatment, the depressed elderly can be helped and can live fulfilling lives.*

86. **Although most depressed clients do not attempt suicide, an estimated 80% of persons with depression do have suicidal thoughts. In caring for an elderly widower with agitated depression who has trouble sleeping, the nurse considers that his risk of suicide is:**

1. No different than for any other depressed client.
2. Lower than that of an elderly man who has never married.
3. Quite low.
4. Extremely high.

1. *Wrong. An elderly client with agitated depression has a higher risk of suicide than that of most other groups of depressed clients. This is especially true for clients who have persistent insomnia.*

2. *Wrong. Elderly men who have never married have a lower risk of suicide than those who have been widowed, separated, or divorced.*

3. *Wrong. There are several factors that identify this client as at high risk for suicide. Select the correct option, and review the rationale.*

4. ***You are right. Elderly widowers with agitated depression are one of the groups with the highest risk for suicide. Persistent insomnia in this client is an additional risk factor. The nursing care plan should reflect that this client is at high risk for suicide.***

87. **A 30-year-old single man who works as a computer analyst is admitted to the hospital with a diagnosis of bipolar depression, acute manic episode. When taking a nursing history, the nurse would identify which information that would support this diagnosis?**

    1. He describes himself as a "loner" with a history of being withdrawn and aloof in relationships.
    2. His paternal grandfather had mood swings all his life and died in a mental institution.
    3. He had a similar episode when in college. He dropped out of school without finishing his degree, and his friends say he was never the same again.
    4. His parents were divorced when he was a young child.

    1. *This is not correct. Most manic clients have had successful relationships and are quite sociable with many acquaintances. In contrast, schizophrenic clients are more likely to be described as aloof and withdrawn.*
    2. ***Correct. Most manic clients come from a family where a close relative also suffered from a unipolar or bipolar disorder. The theory that genetic factors are involved in the occurrence of manic-depressive illness results from this observation.***
    3. *Ninety percent of manic clients have periods of normal or near normal behavior between manic episodes. Most clients do not experience chronic deterioration after an acute episode of illness.*
    4. *There is no evidence that a divorce in the family causes manic illness. This is not the correct option.*

88. **Before administering lithium, the nurse checks the client's latest lab report for her serum lithium level and notes a level of 1.2 mEq/L. What is the best action for the nurse to take next?**

    1. Administer the next prescribed dose of lithium.
    2. Suggest the blood test be repeated.
    3. Withhold the next dose of lithium and notify the psychiatrist of the lab results.
    4. Ask the client how she is feeling, to identify any untoward effects.

    1. *Although the lithium level is within the therapeutic range, it is at the very top of the range. This action is a possibility, but it could be unsafe. Read the other options to see if there is a better choice.*
    2. *This action could be appropriate, but it is not the best action for the nurse to take next. Read the other options.*
    3. *This is not correct. The lithium level is still within the normal range, so withholding the lithium is not an appropriate nursing action.*
    4. ***Correct! A lithium level of 1.2 mEq/L is at the top of the therapeutic range. Before the nurse can safely give the next dose, the client can be assessed for any signs of lithium toxicity. If the client has none, give the medication as prescribed.***

89. **When a client's mother comes to visit, the client does not acknowledge her greeting and lies down on her bed, curling up into the fetal position. After talking with the client's mother, the nurse returns to the client's room. The client is still lying in a fetal position. What action by the nurse would be most therapeutic at this time?**

    1. Ask the client to get up and put away the clothing her mother has brought in.
    2. Ask the client why she responded to her mother that way.
    3. Sit in a chair next to the bed and ask the client to talk about what happened when her mother visited.
    4. Explain unit expectations about how visitors are to be treated.

    1. *This is not correct. The nurse is avoiding the client's response to her mother's visit by switching the focus to another task. The nurse is not conveying that she/he is a trustworthy person to help the client with her recovery, because she/he is not dealing with issues as they come up during the day.*
    2. *This is not correct. The nurse is attempting to gather data in order to do an assessment of what transpired. However, the client will most likely not be able or willing to respond to a direct question that is phrased in this manner. In asking "why" questions, the nurse is requiring an explanation, which is characteristic of an authority figure and is not therapeutic in the nurse-client relationship. "Why" questions may also make the client feel intimidated.*
    3. ***Correct. The nurse is being available to talk about the situation that just occurred. The nurse is doing this in a way that does not put further pressure on the client. If the client is not able to talk about her mother's visit, the nurse should say that she/he will stay with her for a few more minutes and they can sit quietly without talking. This further action will convey***

that the nurse is willing to accept the client as she is and begin to establish the basis for a therapeutic relationship.

4. *This is not correct. In discussing unit rules instead of helping the client deal with her feelings about her mother's visit, the nurse is addressing an inappropriate issue. The issue in this question is the client's response to her mother's visit.*

90. **A depressed client has not bathed or changed her clothes during the two days she has been on the psychiatric unit. When the nurse suggests that she take a shower, the client states an emphatic "No!" and turns her back to the nurse. What is the best action for the nurse to take initially?**

1. Withdraw and return at a later time.
2. Question the client about her resistance to showering.
3. Get another staff member to help get the client into the shower.
4. Tell her she will be much more acceptable to other people on the unit if she cleans up and changes her clothes.

1. *Correct. The nurse should withdraw to avoid a power struggle with the client. Later, the nurse can return and offer to help her gather together the things she will need and gently lead her to the shower. This directive approach does not require a decision on the part of the client, so she is more likely to cooperate with the nurse.*
2. *This is not correct. The client's behavior indicates her anxiety level has increased. She will probably not be able to explain her resistance to showering.*
3. *Wrong. If two staff members overpower the client, they will destroy any trust she may have started to develop with the staff and will further undermining her feelings of self-worth. This is not the correct option.*
4. *This is not correct. This response would cause harm to the client's self-esteem and self-worth. Try again.*

91. **The nurse is caring for a client who is mourning a recent loss. The nurse understands that it is inaccurate to state that mourning:**

1. Is a normal response to loss.
2. Functions to free the individual from an attachment to the lost object so that future relationships can be established.
3. Is accompanied by a growing realization that the loss has occurred.
4. Occurs only in humans.

1. *Wrong choice. The process of mourning or grieving is a normal response to a loss. This is a true*

statement, so it isn't the correct option in this question with a negative response stem.

2. *Wrong choice. The ultimate goal of mourning is to free the individual from too close an attachment to the lost object and permits the person to move on and establish new relationships. This is a true statement, so it isn't the correct option in this question with a negative response stem.*
3. *Wrong choice. The initial phase of the grief process is usually shock and denial. This is followed by a growing realization that the loss has occurred. This is a true statement, so it isn't the correct option in this question with a negative response stem.*
4. *Good work! This option is NOT a true statement. Mourning occurs in animals other than humans, particularly those that form individual attachments, such as primates and household pets.*

92. **After her first night in the hospital, a depressed client complains of feeling too tired to get out of bed in the morning. In planning how to deal with this therapeutically, the nurse is guided by the knowledge that:**

1. Helping to mobilize the client physically will also help to improve her emotional state.
2. Most people do require more rest when they are depressed.
3. It is best to wait until the client indicates that she is ready to participate in structured activities.
4. Encouraging the client to get up and come out on the ward will only increase her feelings of worthlessness and guilt.

1. *Correct. Mobilizing persons who are depressed helps to convey that it is possible to change, and thus counters feelings of hopelessness. Also, activity helps shift the client's preoccupation with self to interests in the outside world.*
2. *This is not correct. Persons who are depressed lack energy and often sleep excessively, but the sleep and rest are not restorative, as they would be for the nondepressed person.*
3. *Depressed persons are reluctant to initiate any activity on their own. This cannot be the correct option.*
4. *This option is not a true statement! Try another option.*

93. **The nurse learns that a depressed client is an expert at crewel embroidery. The nurse asks the client if she will teach her crewel work. Which of the following is the best rationale for this nursing intervention?**

1. To assess the client's ability to communicate clearly.
2. To distract the client from thinking about her problems.

3. To reinforce the client's identity as a homemaker.
4. To use the client's strengths to build self-esteem.

1. *Wrong. Depression may interfere with a person's willingness to communicate, but it is not primarily a communication disorder.*
2. *Engaging a depressed person in a productive task is one way to interrupt or limit the amount of time spent focusing on negative evaluations of him or herself. There is a better option, however.*
3. *Wrong. There is no data to support this as the client's occupation or identity. Do not "read into" the question. Try again.*
4. ***Correct. The nurse is attempting to reinforce the client's self-worth by providing an opportunity for the client to succeed at a task that earns positive feedback from the nurse.***

94. The nurse tells the client that a catheter must be inserted to collect a urine specimen. The client pulls the covers to her neck. She glances at the open door and says, "Someone might see me out there!" At this time, the best nursing action is to:

1. Explain the procedure to the client.
2. Obtain some assistance, since the client does not appear to be comfortable and may be resistant to the procedure.
3. Close the door and assure the client that you will cover her as much as possible during the procedure.
4. Gather all of the needed equipment before starting the procedure.

1. *Explaining the procedure is an appropriate nursing action, but it doesn't address the client's concern. Try again.*
2. *Although the client exhibits concern about privacy, the case situation does not indicate that she will be uncooperative. Do not "read into" the question! The client is communicating non-verbally to the nurse and indicating a concern for privacy. The nurse should respond therapeutically and address the client's concern. Try again.*
3. ***Very good! The client has expressed her concern for privacy. The nurse uses both verbal and nonverbal communication to respond therapeutically, addressing the client's concern.***
4. *This is an appropriate nursing action, but it does not address the client's concern. Try again.*

95. A client is admitted to the hospital with abdominal pain. She overhears her doctor and nurse discussing cancer of the liver. Later, she says to her nurse, "Having cancer of the liver must be a terrible thing." Which of the following nursing responses is most helpful?

1. "Yes, it is a terrible disease."
2. "What made you think about cancer of the liver?"
3. "Any kind of cancer is terrible, but you can't live without a liver."
4. "Yes, it is. A client on this floor has it, and it's sad for everyone."

1. *This response is a factual statement, but it doesn't encourage further communication between the nurse and the client. The client has an obvious concern or she wouldn't have mentioned the subject. Her need for more information should be addressed by the nurse.*
2. ***Correct! This question clarifies for the nurse why the client is concerned about cancer of the liver. The case situation tells you that the client overheard her doctor and nurse talking about a client. The client may think that the conversation concerned her. This response by the nurse enhances therapeutic communication through clarification.***

STRATEGY ALERT! Note that the phrase "cancer of the liver" appears in both the question and this option. This is a clue that this might be the correct answer.

3. *This response by the nurse does not identify or clarify why the client is talking about this particular illness. The nurse needs more information, and this response deters the client from pursuing this topic any further.*
4. *This response does not address the client in the question. It addresses the other client and "everyone" who is sad. This response can also be interpreted as a breach in confidentiality for the client who has the cancer. Therefore, this is an inappropriate response.*

96. The nurse is teaching a client about self breast exams when the client states that she doesn't understand why she is being taught this since she doesn't plan on doing it anyway. The best nursing response is:

1. "The self breast exam is taught to women to detect any lumps or changes in the breast which can be an early sign of cancer, and early treatment has a higher rate of cure."
2. "You're right. If you don't plan on doing the exam, then I don't need to show you how to do it."
3. "If you don't plan on doing the exam yourself, then you should have your doctor do it at your annual check up."
4. "It is your body, and you have the right to do whatever you choose."

1. ***Correct! This response by the nurse gives the client information concerning the rationale for self breast exams. This response provides information that will allow the client to make***

an informed choice. The communication strategy is to give information.

> **STRATEGY ALERT!** Note that Options 2 and 4 are similar: they both support the client's decision not to do the self exams. Similar distractors should be eliminated.

2. *This response implies that the nurse has become defensive, which is a block to communication because it also places the client on the defensive. This approach does not promote therapeutic communication.*

3. *Having a physician perform an exam annually is a good validation action but it should not replace monthly self exams. This is not an appropriate response, since it does not address the need for regular breast exams to detect early changes and implies that this is an acceptable recommendation. It does not provide for further explanation of the client's statement.*

4. *Although this is true statement and clients should have choices concerning their health care, the choices should be informed choices. This client has made a decision without the benefit of an explanation of the rationale for the intervention. This response does not encourage any further communication and is not therapeutic.*

97. **A daughter has come to take her mother home from the hospital after a colostomy. The daughter tells the nurse that she doesn't know how she is going to care for her mother's colostomy. The nurse's most helpful response to the daughter is:**

1. "Your mother can take care of her colostomy without difficulty."
2. "What part of your mother's care are you concerned about?"
3. "A home health nurse will be stopping by tomorrow. If you have any questions, you can ask her."
4. "It is quite simple. I'll make sure that her colostomy bag is clean before she leaves."

1. *This may be a true statement, but it does not allow the client to express her concerns. The daughter is the client in this question, and the nurse's response should always be therapeutic for the client. Try again.*

2. ***Excellent! The daughter is the client in this question. This response is therapeutic for the daughter because it uses the communication tool of clarification to allow her to express her concerns.***

3. *The daughter is the client in this question, and the nurse's response should be therapeutic for the client. This response uses the communication block of putting the client's concerns "on hold," and is*

not therapeutic for the client. This cannot be the best response. Try again.

4. *The daughter is the client in this question, and the nurse's response should be therapeutic for the client. This response uses the communication block of false reassurance. It is not therapeutic because it fails to address the client's concerns. Make another choice.*

98. **A client is scheduled for a mastectomy in the morning. Her daughter says to the nurse, "I should call my brother and sister and have them here in the morning, just in case something goes wrong." The most helpful nursing response is:**

1. To ask the mother if she would like her children there in the morning.
2. To suggest to the daughter that she ask her mother how she feels about that.
3. To say to the daughter, "If your brother and sister want to be here, they are welcome."
4. To ask the daughter what she knows about her mother's surgery and diagnosis.

1. *Wrong! Although the mother is the person with the health care problem, the client in the question is her daughter. The nursing response should be addressed to the daughter.*

2. *Wrong! The daughter is the client in this question. This response is not therapeutic for the daughter because it does not address her concern about her mother's impending surgery.*

3. *Wrong. The daughter is the client in this question. This response is not therapeutic because it focuses on the needs of the brothers and sisters, not on the daughter's concerns about her mother's surgery. This response might also appear to the daughter to validate her fears about the surgery. This option cannot be the answer.*

4. ***You are correct. The daughter is the client in this question, and the nurse is addressing the daughter's needs by clarifying the daughter's understanding of her mother's health problems. This response is therapeutic for the daughter.***

99. **A disruptive 10-year-old child is having difficulty interacting with other children on the unit. Which nursing action would be best initially?**

1. Have a unit conference with other staff members and discuss strategies to solve the problem.
2. Talk to the child about the behavior that is causing the problem and identify possible solutions.
3. Tell the other children to stop teasing the client and to observe for changes in the client's behavior.
4. Tell the client's mother that she needs to talk to her son about his disruptive behavior.

1. *No, try again. The client in this question is the child, and the issue is disruptive behavior. This option is only indirectly related to the client. This is not the best option.*
2. ***You are correct. Since the child is the client in this question, the correct answer must be related to him. This option deals directly with the issue of the client's behavior.***
3. *The client in this question is the child, not the other children on the unit. The answer should be related to the client. Also, "telling" the other children what to do about the problem is characteristic of an authority figure and is not therapeutic in the nurse-client relationship. The nurse's response must be therapeutic for the client.*
4. *Wrong. This option focuses on inappropriate person, the client's mother. Also, "telling" the client's mother what she "needs" to do is characteristic of an authority figure and is not therapeutic in the nurse-client relationship.*

100. **A client is paralyzed from the waist down. He is to be up in a chair three times a day. What is the best nursing approach when transferring the client from a bed into a wheelchair?**

1. Place the wheelchair close to the foot of the bed.
2. Utilize the principles of body mechanics while providing a safe transfer for the client.
3. Slide the client to the edge of the bed, keeping the nurse's back straight and using a rocking motion to pull the client.

4. Place the nurse's arms under the client's axillae from the back of the client.

1. *This is not correct. The wheelchair should be placed as close to the position of the client's buttocks as possible for a safe and easy transfer. The wheelchair should not be placed at the foot of the bed.*
2. ***Very good! The nurse is in control of his or her own body and the client's movement during the transfer. Providing for the safety of the client, and utilizing the principles of body mechanics to provide safety for the nurse and the client, is the best nursing approach.***

> **TEST-TAKING TIP:** Options 3 and 4 describe specific actions that are correct in transferring a client, but Option 2 is the best option because it is a more comprehensive or global statement of the correct nursing approach.

3. *Almost. This is an appropriate nursing action, which addresses the safety of the nurse and client. Positioning the client near the edge of the bed will reduce the energy required to move the client to the wheelchair, and the nurse's back will be protected by using leg and arm muscles to move the client to the edge of the bed. There is another option, however, that better describes the best nursing approach in transferring this client.*
4. *Almost. This is a correct action, which helps provide for the nurse's and the client's safety. Supporting the upper portion of the client's body helps to place the weight of the client over the nurse's center of gravity. There is another option, however, that better describes the best nursing approach in transferring this client.*

NCLEX-PN

Test 4

NCLEX-PN TEST 4

1. A client has recently received albuterol (Ventolin) for an asthma attack. Which finding by the nurse indicates a side effect of albuterol?

    1. A heart rate of 110.
    2. A blood pressure of 100\52.
    3. Fine basilar crackles.
    4. Capillary refill of greater than five seconds.

2. The nurse is caring for a client who is receiving a glucocorticoid. In order to detect electrolyte imbalance caused by steroid use, the nurse would be alert for:

    1. Muscle weakness and lethargy.
    2. Itching and red scaly patches.
    3. Poor skin turgor and sticky mucous membranes.
    4. Tremors and nervousness.

3. A client is treated for a major depression with nortriptyline (Pamelor) 150 mg. Which of the following statements by the client indicates that she needs further instruction about this drug?

    1. "I'm glad this medicine helps me. My husband and I would like to start our family as soon as possible."
    2. "If I should feel hopeless and suicidal again, I have the telephone number of my therapist to call for help."
    3. "I plan to see my psychiatrist regularly. She told me if I continue to do well, I can probably stop taking my medication in nine to 12 months."
    4. "I hope I will not have to continue taking medicine forever. I guess I'll have to see how I do."

4. The nurse should advise a client taking rifampin (Rifadin) for treatment of tuberculosis to avoid:

    1. Antacids containing magnesium.
    2. Aspirin products.
    3. Over-the-counter cold products.
    4. Alcoholic beverages.

5. A client is hospitalized for gastrointestinal bleeding. He is given temazepam (Restoril) at bedtime to help him sleep. What nursing action is indicated immediately following his dose?

    1. Raise the side rails on his bed and tell him to use his call light to summon the nurse if he has to get up during the night.
    2. Keep a padded tongue blade at the bedside and observe for seizures.

    3. Monitor his blood pressure and respirations.
    4. Observe and record his sleep patterns.

6. A client is treated in the emergency room for a panic attack. Thirty minutes after receiving diazepam (Valium), he tells the nurse that he is feeling much calmer. "I can't believe how scared I was. I will do anything to avoid having another panic attack." The most helpful nursing measure is to:

    1. Advise him to admit himself to the psychiatric unit, where he can have a comprehensive evaluation in a protected setting.
    2. Suggest to him that he reduce the amount of stress in his life.
    3. Make an appointment for outpatient psychotherapy to receive help with any emotional issues that might be responsible for his panic attacks.
    4. Tell him he can always return to the emergency room if he should have another panic attack.

7. A physician orders a body magnetic resonance imaging (MRI) for diagnostic purposes. It would be most important for the nurse to tell the client that the procedure:

    1. Takes 15 to 30 minutes.
    2. Involves injection of a contrast dye.
    3. Is painless, except for the discomfort of lying still.
    4. Uses only small amounts of radiation.

8. A 42-year-old female is admitted with right-sided weakness and slurred speech. About which diagnostic tests should the nurse be prepared to instruct the client/family?

    1. EEG and MRI.
    2. Angiography and EMG.
    3. PET and pneumoencephalogram.
    4. CT scan and lumbar puncture.

9. The nurse is preparing client teaching for a 56-year-old client who is being discharged after a simple mastectomy. The client will begin radiation therapy as an outpatient tomorrow. Which of the following instructions given by the nurse would be directed at maintaining skin integrity?

    1. Wear a good support bra and use ice for any swelling.
    2. Use of a heating pad is contraindicated.
    3. Skin breakdown is common and should be treated with antibiotic ointment.
    4. Keep skin lubricated to prevent dryness.

10. In dealing with a client with obsessive-compulsive disorder who engages in ritualistic behaviors centering around cleansing his mouth of offensive odors, the nurse would first:

   1. Confront the client about the senseless nature of the ritualistic behaviors.
   2. Set strict limits on the behaviors so the client can better conform to the unit rules and schedules.
   3. Isolate the client for a period of time to lower his anxiety about offending others.
   4. Plan the client's schedule to allow extra time to perform the rituals to keep his anxiety within manageable levels.

11. Two weeks after a client started taking amitriptyline (Elavil), she reported that she was sleeping better and her appetite had improved. She said, however, that she still felt hopeless and sad. In response to this statement, the best nursing action is to:

   1. Notify her physician so that she can be switched to another drug.
   2. Ask her physician to increase her dose of Elavil.
   3. Explain that antidepressants often take three to four weeks to be fully effective.
   4. Chart her complaints in the nursing notes.

12. A discharged client will continue taking lithium and will be seen in the clinic on a regular basis after discharge. The nurse understands that, as a possible result of long-term lithium therapy, the client is at risk for developing:

   1. Hyperthyroidism.
   2. Hypoglycemia.
   3. Impaired kidney function.
   4. Gall stones.

13. A discharged client will continue taking lithium and will be seen in the clinic on a regular basis after discharge. The nurse understands that lithium toxicity could occur if the client:

   1. Fasts.
   2. Engages in mild exercise.
   3. Increases her sodium intake.
   4. Receives carbamazepine (Tegretol) therapy.

14. An anorexic client tells the nurse that she thinks too much fuss is being made about what she eats. "I have plenty of energy and get all A's in school. I do not think I am too thin. Look, my hips are fat." What is the most appropriate nursing response to her statement?

   1. "You say your hips look fat to you, but you seem very thin to me."
   2. "Let's go over to the mirror so you can see how thin you really are."
   3. "You are such a bright girl. I don't understand

how you can do this to yourself."
   4. "You would be much more attractive if you were not so skinny."

15. A postoperative client is to ambulate for the first time after surgery. The nurse understands that which of the following would be an unsafe action?

   1. Have the client get up and sit in the chair next to the bed.
   2. Have the client sit on the edge of the bed with his feet down for a few minutes before he starts to ambulate.
   3. Have the client stand at the side of the bed for a few minutes before taking his first steps.
   4. Encourage the client to try to walk straight ahead while you assist him with his walking.

16. When transporting a client, the nurse should:

   1. Always use a stretcher.
   2. Push the stretcher very quickly so the client does not become chilled during the transport.
   3. Never cover a client with a blanket, since it can get caught in the wheels.
   4. Use the safety rails or straps that are available on the equipment.

17. A client in a long-term care facility has been given a cane to assist her with ambulation. In caring for this client, which of the following would be an unsafe nursing action?

   1. Inspect the rubber tip often and replace it if appears to be worn.
   2. Place the cane on the side of the weak leg.
   3. Position the cane to support and balance the client with decreased strength in one of the lower extremities.
   4. Keep the cane within easy reach when sleeping or sitting.

18. The nurse discovers that the wrong medication was given to a confused client who answered to the name stated upon entering the room. The physician is notified and states that the medication that the client received will not harm him and nothing needs to be done. The priority nursing action after notifying the physician is:

   1. Apologize to the client involved.
   2. Make out an incident report documenting the occurrence.
   3. Try to avoid being responsible for administering medications again, since this could have been terrible situation.
   4. Realize that everyone makes mistakes, and continue to administer the rest of the medications to the other clients.

19. The nurse is preparing medications for administration in a pediatric unit. Of the following nursing actions, which would be inappropriate?

    1. Prepare medications for one client at a time.
    2. Calculate correct drug dosage.
    3. Open unit dose tablets and place medications in medication cup.
    4. Avoid touching tablets or capsules with the hands.

20. The nurse is preparing to administer medication to a client who is scheduled to receive his insulin at 8:00 a.m. The best nursing approach is to:

    1. Read the label three times.
    2. Check the client's identification bracelet.
    3. Administer the correct medication to the right client.
    4. Check the dosage prescribed.

21. The nurse finds an elderly client with her IV pulled out, standing next to her bed, with the side rails in the up position. The client is confused, does not have an identification bracelet on, and cannot remember her name. What should the nurse do first?

    1. Help the client into bed, and remind her to call the nurse when she wants to get out of bed.
    2. Help the client into bed, and then restart the IV.
    3. Place a restraining vest on the client.
    4. Put an identification bracelet on the client and help her back to bed.

22. The most important nursing goal for a client who is admitted with an acute attack of ulcerative colitis is to:

    1. Provide emotional support.
    2. Prevent skin breakdown.
    3. Maintain fluid and electrolyte balance.
    4. Promote physical rest.

23. A client returns from surgery for a lung resection due to cancer. Of the following postoperative orders, which is the nurse's highest priority?

    1. Oxygen per mask at six liters per minute.
    2. Change dressings as needed.
    3. Vital signs every hour.
    4. Cough and deep breathe every two hours.

24. A client is scheduled for surgery and asks the nurse if she can put on some makeup before going to surgery. The best response by the nurse is:

    1. "Only a light application of makeup is allowed."
    2. "Hospital policy states that all makeup must be removed before surgery."
    3. "I will check with the charge nurse to find out the regulations."

    4. "Makeup will interfere with the ability to see your skin color during surgery."

25. A client is in the hospital and has weakness on her left side because of a stroke. She becomes upset when eating, because liquids drool out of her mouth on her weak side. What nursing intervention would be most appropriate?

    1. Provide only pureed and solid foods to prevent drooling, so the client will not become upset.
    2. Have a member of the family assist with the client's feedings.
    3. Teach the client how to drink fluids on the unaffected side to prevent drooling.
    4. Have the client use a syringe to squirt liquids into the back of her mouth.

26. The nurse knows that in caring for a client with second and third degree burns of the head, neck and chest, the greatest initial complication is caused by:

    1. Infection.
    2. Airway obstruction.
    3. Fluid imbalance.
    4. Paralytic ileus.

27. To administer a Mantoux test for tuberculosis the nurse:

    1. Inserts the needle with the bevel up.
    2. Administers 0.1 ml of PPD on the outer surface of the arm.
    3. Uses a 21 or 22 gauge needle.
    4. Massages the area after administration of the medication.

28. A client has a tracheostomy tube in place following a complete laryngectomy. To properly suction the client's tracheostomy tube, the nurse would:

    1. Apply suction for 10 to 15 seconds while withdrawing the catheter.
    2. Hyperoxygenate for several deep breaths with the Ambu bag after each procedure.
    3. Maintain clean equipment at all times while suctioning.
    4. Suction the oral cavity prior to suctioning the tracheostomy tube.

29. Which statement written by a laryngectomy client preparing for discharge would indicate to the nurse that he needs further teaching?

    1. "I'll remember to buy non-aerosol products for personal grooming."
    2. "I sure will miss taking showers from now on."
    3. "Giving up swimming won't bother me, since I never learned how in the first place."
    4. "I never thought that belching could be transferred into speech, but I'm learning quickly."

30. Which statement, if made by a client with varicose veins, indicates to the nurse that the client has accurate understanding of the application and use of anti-embolic stockings?

    1. "I won't take them off until I go to bed at night."
    2. "I'll put them on in the morning after I've taken my daily walk."
    3. "I know that they should feel tight when I put them on."
    4. "I'm glad I can cross my legs now since I'll have these stockings on."

31. Which understanding expressed by a male client who is HIV positive indicates to the nurse that he needs further teaching?

    1. He won't donate blood anymore.
    2. He's glad that his newly prescribed drug, zidovudine (Retrovir), will prevent him from developing AIDS.
    3. He'll use a latex condom whenever he has sex.
    4. He's planning to attend a seminar on stress reduction next week.

32. An elderly client is in a nursing home and confined to bed. What is the most important nursing action that will prevent skin breakdown and decubitus ulcers?

    1. Massage all bony prominences with lotion.
    2. Keep the skin clean and dry.
    3. Turn the client at least every two hours.
    4. Place an egg crate mattress on the bed.

33. Which nursing action is contraindicated for a client with an indwelling Foley catheter?

    1. Instill sterile distilled water in the catheter.
    2. Use minimal pressure to clear the catheter of clots or mucous plugs.
    3. Use sterile equipment for irrigation.
    4. Use the flow of gravity for return of the irrigant.

34. A client has been diagnosed with iron deficiency anemia. When teaching the client about her diet, which foods should be identified by the nurse as good sources of iron?

    1. Fresh fruits.
    2. Milk and cheese.
    3. Organ meats.
    4. Whole grain breads.

35. While caring for the client with an IV, it is most important for the nurse to:

    1. Report any signs of infection to the charge nurse.
    2. Record the condition of the IV site and the rate of infusion, and report any unusual findings.
    3. Record intravenous intake.
    4. Ask the client if the IV site is painful or tender.

36. The nurse is informed during report that a postoperative client has not voided for eight hours. The initial nursing action would be to:

    1. Assist the client to the bathroom.
    2. Place the client on a bed pan and pour warm water over her perineum.
    3. Palpate and percuss the client's bladder.
    4. Catheterize the client.

37. A 78-year-old client has been in the hospital for a week on bed rest. She complains of elbow pain. The best nursing action is to:

    1. Place elbow pads on the client.
    2. Examine the elbow.
    3. Call the physician for an order for pain medication.
    4. Reposition the client so that she is more comfortable.

38. After complaining of severe chest pain for the last hour, a client is admitted to the ICU with an acute myocardial infarction. The nurse knows that the results of the cardiac enzyme studies will help determine the:

    1. Degree of damage to the myocardium.
    2. Location of the myocardial infarction.
    3. Size of the myocardial infarction.
    4. Coexistence of pulmonary congestion.

39. Six days after a craniotomy, which complaint by the client would the nurse assess as a possible early manifestation of a complication?

    1. He wants to leave the hospital.
    2. He feels nauseated.
    3. He has a slight headache.
    4. He is extremely sleepy.

40. A 22-year-old client sustained a T4 spinal cord injury. While doing morning assessments four weeks post-injury, the nurse discovers that the client's BP is 280/140 and he is complaining of nasal stuffiness and a severe, pounding headache. The first nursing action is:

    1. Sit the client upright.
    2. Call the nurse in charge.
    3. Check the client's bladder for distension.
    4. Administer the prescribed antihypertensive.

41. A client was admitted for a severe episode of gastrointestinal bleeding. Which statement by the client indicates to the nurse a need for further instruction?

   1. "If my arthritis bothers me, I'll take acetaminophen (Tylenol)."
   2. "It's a good thing I gave up drinking five years ago."
   3. "It will sure be good to have my morning coffee."
   4. "I'll take my cimetidine (Tagamet) before I eat and at bed time."

42. An elderly client is experiencing a decrease in his white blood cell count and is placed on protective precautions for infection. Which of the following comments by the client indicate to the nurse that he understands his condition and the precautions?

   1. "I have never been so aware that germs are everywhere around us."
   2. "I didn't realize that I am so contagious that I need a private room."
   3. "Everyone who touches me washes their hands like I am really contaminated."
   4. "I might make my sister's baby sick, so I told her not to visit."

43. A client is scheduled for left below-the-knee amputation in the morning. Before surgery, the preoperative teaching plan included deep breathing and coughing. In evaluating the effectiveness of preoperative teaching, the nurse should ask the client:

   1. "Do you understand what we have just discussed about deep breathing and coughing?"
   2. "Do you think that you will need to have a sedative to help you sleep tonight?"
   3. "Will you demonstrate for me the correct method of deep breathing and coughing?"
   4. "Do you have any questions concerning your scheduled surgical procedure?"

44. A client is seen in the emergency room for abdominal pain, and is scheduled for emergency surgery. In preparing to do the client's preoperative teaching, the nurse knows that it is most important to:

   1. Explain of the hospital billing process for clients receiving surgery.
   2. Teach deep breathing and coughing with abdominal splinting.
   3. Obtain the surgical consent.
   4. Explain where the incision will be and how much drainage to expect on the dressing after surgery.

45. A 21-year-old client is admitted to the hospital because of extreme weight loss. It is noted on the admission assessment that the client believes that she is overweight at 88 pounds. In planning the care for this client, the nurse should first:

   1. Assess the client's nutritional status.
   2. Obtain a psychiatric consult.
   3. Plan a therapeutic diet for the client.
   4. Talk to the family members to find out more about the client's self-concept.

46. A client has a nasogastric tube in place following abdominal surgery. Which nursing action would be contraindicated when planning the care for a client with a nasogastric tube?

   1. Attach the nasogastric tube to high suction.
   2. Provide frequent oral hygiene.
   3. Measure the amount of drainage from the nasogastric tube.
   4. Attach the nasogastric tube to the client's gown in order to prevent pulling at the insertion site.

47. A client has been incontinent of loose stool and is complaining of a painful perineum. The most appropriate initial nursing action is to:

   1. Notify the physician to obtain an order for the loose stools.
   2. Check the client's perineum.
   3. Turn the client every two hours.
   4. Increase the client's fluid intake to prevent dehydration.

48. A client is admitted to the hospital in respiratory distress. The doctor orders oxygen per mask and the client to be placed in high Fowler's position. Which nursing action is most important for this client?

   1. Support and align the hands with the forearms.
   2. Use handrolls.
   3. Raise the head of the bed to allow for greater lung expansion.
   4. Support the feet at right angles to the lower legs.

49. A diabetic is admitted and placed on bedrest because of suspected gangrene of her left great toe. At this time the initial nursing action is to:

   1. Apply heel protectors.
   2. Place a sheepskin under the client.
   3. Assess hydration and nutritional status.
   4. Turn the client every two hours.

50. A client was treated four weeks ago for streptococcal pharyngitis and is seeking treatment for recurrent manifestations. The nurse understands that the most likely cause of the client's recurring manifestations is:
    1. Enlarged cervical lymph node involvement.
    2. Failure to complete his oral antibiotic therapy.
    3. Contact with his coworkers.
    4. Failure to change his toothbrush.

51. A 50-year-old client is a heavy smoker and is admitted with newly diagnosed COPD, chronic bronchitis, and left lower lobe pneumonia. Which nursing measure will receive the highest priority?

    1. Facilitate O_2 and CO_2 exchange.
    2. Teach the importance of cessation of smoking.
    3. Allay his fears about his illness.
    4. Encourage adequate fluid intake.

52. A client is three days postoperative after abdominal surgery. The nurse notes thick yellow drainage from the wound. The nurse would document this type of drainage as:

    1. Serous.
    2. Purulent.
    3. Serosanguineous.
    4. Sanguineous.

53. A 75-year-old man is a psychiatric client taking lithium for a bipolar disorder. The nurse knows that elderly clients:

    1. Cannot be safely treated with lithium.
    2. Take the same dosage of lithium as younger adults.
    3. Treated with lithium have a therapeutic range of 0.6-0.8 mEq/L.
    4. Treated with lithium have a therapeutic range of 0.6-1.4 mEq/L.

54. A client is admitted to the abuse treatment unit for a heroin addiction. On the client's third day in the hospital, a friend visits in the evening. The nurse notices that the client seems much more relaxed after his friend leaves. The client says that the worst of his withdrawal manifestations from heroin seem to be over. At this time, what action by the nurse would be best?

    1. Obtain a urine specimen to send for a drug screen.
    2. Congratulate him for staying with the program.
    3. Ask about his relationship with his friend, to evaluate whether the friend could be a good source of emotional support.
    4. Continue to assess his withdrawal manifestations.

55. The best approach for the nurse to take initially with a client who has severe anxiety is to:

    1. Move the person to a calm, non-stimulating environment.
    2. Encourage expression of feelings without attempting to modify defensive behavior.
    3. Reduce the client's level of anxiety by offering medication.
    4. Suggest that the client engage in some automatic behavior, such as pacing, to reduce his anxiety level.

56. Which of the following actions would the nurse do first for a client in panic?

    1. Determine the source of his anxiety by asking the client to describe the events before the anxiety occurred.
    2. Provide privacy for the client by moving him to a quiet area away from other people, and leaving him alone so he can regain control.
    3. Help the client describe his feelings, to begin to diagnose the problem as anxiety.
    4. Provide a sense of safety and security by remaining with the client, speaking in a calm manner and offering sedation if needed.

57. The psychiatrist orders tranylcypromine (Parnate) for a depressed client who has not responded to tricyclics. In preparing client teaching about diet, the nurse knows that the client may safely select:

    1. Beer and red wine.
    2. Cheddar cheese and sausage.
    3. Cottage cheese and canned peaches.
    4. Liver and Italian green beans.

58. A 66-year-old man is an outpatient taking tricyclic antidepressants. The client's wife telephones the clinic and tells the nurse that she has just found her husband lying unconscious and an empty bottle of his medication on the nightstand. The nurse's instructions to the wife are guided by the knowledge that overdoses of tricyclic antidepressants are:

    1. Medical emergencies.
    2. Serious but rarely fatal.
    3. Dangerous for clients in poor health.
    4. Easily treated by inducing vomiting.

59. A manic client is readmitted to the hospital. After two weeks, her lithium level is within the therapeutic range and she no longer has manic manifestations. Before discharge, what information should the nurse give to the client about her diet when taking lithium?

    1. Sodium intake should be restricted.
    2. Fluid intake should be restricted to 1000 cc per day.
    3. An adequate daily intake of sodium and fluids should be maintained.

4. Sodium and fluid intake should be increased.

60. **A client's psychiatrist orders fluphenazine (Prolixin) 10 mg b.i.d. Before the first dose, the client asks the nurse what the medicine is supposed to do. What response by the nurse would be most therapeutic for a suspicious client?**

    1. "It will help you feel less anxious."
    2. "It is to help make your thinking clearer and decrease your fears."
    3. "This medication will help you maintain self-control."
    4. "This medication will help you get better."

61. **The wife of an alcoholic client says to the nurse, "I told my husband I would leave him if he did not get into treatment. Now that he is here, I feel differently. What can I do to help him?" The most therapeutic nursing response is:**

    1. "You should attend an Al-Anon meeting. The group can teach you how best to help him stay sober."
    2. "You have already done a great deal by getting him to come into treatment. Now it is up to him to make the best use of his time here."
    3. "Are you feeling some responsibility for his drinking?"
    4. "Tell me more about the kind of help you feel you are able to provide at this time."

62. **During heroin withdrawal, a client complains continuously to the nursing staff about his discomfort. One day the nurse overhears a nursing assistant say to the client, "You brought these problems on yourself by taking drugs. What did you think would happen when you continued to use heroin?" Which of the following comments to the nursing assistant would be most helpful?**

    1. "Your comments were inappropriate. I will have to report this to the supervisor."
    2. "Weren't you a bit hard on this client? He is having a great deal of discomfort."
    3. "This client is getting on all our nerves."
    4. "I overheard you speaking with the client and I thought your comment about his causing his own problems was inappropriate. You have worked well with other addicted clients. What is different about this man?"

63. **A 32-year-old married woman is treated in the emergency room for a broken arm. She tells the nurse that her husband accidentally hit her during an argument. Which of the following approaches is most appropriate when responding to her comment?**

    1. Convey concern and ask the client to describe how her injury occurred.

2. Ask the client how the couple usually solve their conflicts.
3. Point out that no person has a right to physically harm another human being, even during an argument.
4. Inform the client that spouse abuse is illegal, and there are legal and social services available to her.

64. **A rape victim says to the nurse, "I feel so humiliated. I don't want anyone to know what happened to me." What is the most therapeutic nursing response?**

    1. "This is a normal feeling after what has happened to you."
    2. "You should not be so hard on yourself, it was not your fault."
    3. "Are you saying that you are fearful about what others will think? Let's talk about that feeling."
    4. "Are you afraid people will blame you for what has happened?"

65. **The nurse is assisting a frail elderly client to eat. The client begins to choke and indicates to the nurse that she cannot talk. The first nursing action is to:**

    1. Perform the Heimlich maneuver to obtain a patent airway.
    2. Begin mouth to mouth resuscitation.
    3. Place an oxygen mask on the client.
    4. Go to the nurses' station to get some help.

66. **While changing a surgical dressing, the nurse notes green, foul-smelling drainage at the incision site. Another postoperative client is sharing the same room with this client. The most appropriate nursing action is to:**

    1. Place the client with the drainage in a private room.
    2. Institute drainage and secretion precautions.
    3. Move the other client to another room.
    4. Place the client in strict isolation until the organism has been cultured and identified.

67. **When administering ear drops with a dropper, which nursing action best prevents contamination of the bottle of medication?**

    1. Thorough hand washing prior to preparing the medication.
    2. Hold the dropper with the tip above the ear canal.
    3. Wash the client's ear prior to instilling the medication.
    4. Only fill the dropper with the prescribed number of drops.

68. The nurse is preparing to transfer a client from a bed to a chair. To avoid back injury to the nurse, the correct technique is to:

    1. Bend at the waist while maintaining a wide stance, lift the client to a standing position, and then pivot the client toward the chair.
    2. Have the client lock his or her hands around the nurse's neck, so that the client will feel more secure during the transfer.
    3. Place the bed in an elevated position so that the client's hips are at the same level as the nurse's hip, resulting in the center of gravity being the same for both individuals.
    4. Bend at the knees, while maintaining a wide stance and straight back, with the client's hands on the nurse's shoulders and the nurse's hands at the client's axillae.

69. The nurse would demonstrate a good understanding of safe body mechanics by avoiding which of the following actions?

    1. Move muscles quickly, using short tugs in order to avoid muscle fatigue.
    2. Use the longest and strongest muscles of the body whenever possible.
    3. Lean toward objects being pushed, such as a stretcher.
    4. Carry objects close to the body without touching your clothing.

70. After admission to the hospital with pulmonary emphysema, the client is extremely short of breath and is receiving oxygen per nasal cannula. The essential nursing action for this client receiving oxygen therapy is to:

    1. Make sure the client is receiving at least six liters per minute to alleviate his respiratory distress.
    2. Provide low oxygen percentages to prevent respiratory arrest.
    3. Provide oral hygiene.
    4. Clean the nostrils around the cannula as needed.

71. A client has just begun receiving magnesium sulfate for treatment of preterm labor. Which nursing assessment will have the least priority in this client?

    1. Maternal respirations.
    2. Uterine contractions.
    3. Urinary output.
    4. Maternal temperature.

72. A client is admitted to the labor unit with a diagnosis of complete placenta previa. She asks the nurse what will happen when she goes into labor. The best nursing response is:

    1. "We will monitor you and your fetus very carefully to pick up any problems early."
    2. "We will have several units of blood on hand in case you have bleeding at the time of delivery."
    3. "Once the fetal head drops into the pelvis there will be pressure on the placenta and bleeding should be minimal."
    4. "A cesarean section will be done prior to the onset of labor."

73. The nursing action that plays the greatest role in prevention of postpartum infections is:

    1. Administration of antibiotics on time.
    2. Daily bathing of all clients.
    3. Frequent hand washing.
    4. Routine postpartum assessment for manifestations of infection.

74. The nurse is completing an admission physical exam on a newborn infant and notices that his color has become pale and that he is experiencing nasal flaring, which was not evident before. What should the nurse do first?

    1. Report these findings to the RN immediately.
    2. Place the baby in or under a heat source.
    3. Do a chemstix on the infant.
    4. Give the baby the first feeding one hour early.

75. An antepartum client with insulin dependent diabetes comes to the emergency room at 28 weeks gestation because her blood sugars have been elevated. A serum blood sugar is 428. The resident orders 25 units of NPH insulin and an IV with glucose to be given stat. What should the nurse do first?

    1. Notify the RN to start the IV before giving the ordered insulin.
    2. Give the insulin and then notify the RN to start the IV.
    3. Question the large dose of insulin.
    4. Question the type of insulin ordered.

76. An antepartum client has hydramnios at 35 weeks gestation. Based upon this diagnosis, the nurse should anticipate:

    1. Decreased maternal weight gain.
    2. Abnormal swallowing mechanism in the fetus.
    3. Kidney defects in the fetus.
    4. Fundal height less than expected for gestational age.

77. The nurse is caring for a 19-year-old client who had a spontaneous abortion at nine weeks gestation. The nurse walks into the client's room and finds her crying uncontrollably. Which of the following statements by the nurse is a therapeutic response to the client's emotional needs?

1. "You are young and will have other children."
2. "When a pregnancy ends in spontaneous abortion, there is often something wrong with the fetus."
3. "It is hard to deal with losing a pregnancy. I have a number for a local support group for women who experience pregnancy loss."
4. "The best thing for you is to go home and try again."

78. The nurse in the family planning clinic is explaining birth control options to an 18-year-old man. He tells the nurse that his 16-year-old girlfriend recently had an abortion and asks the nurse about the advisability of using condoms. In responding to the client, the nurse understands that the primary advantage of condoms as a method of birth control is:

    1. The cost.
    2. The availability.
    3. Protection from AIDS.
    4. Low failure rate.

79. Which of the following foods should the nurse teach the client to include in a daily diet to minimize the most critical electrolyte loss when taking furosemide (Lasix)?

    1. Grains.
    2. Milk.
    3. Red meats.
    4. Dried fruits.

80. In assessing a postpartum client, the nurse knows that which finding would indicate that the methylergonovine maleate (Methergine) was effective?

    1. A rise in blood pressure.
    2. An increase in lochia.
    3. A firm fundus.
    4. Absent breast discomfort.

81. In providing nursing care to a 30-year-old client following an abdominal hysterectomy, which of the following will receive priority?

    1. Administration of estrogen to prevent manifestations of menopause.
    2. Maintenance of bedrest for the first 24 hours to prevent an increase in vaginal bleeding.
    3. Frequent assessment for bleeding on the dressing and the peripad.
    4. Foley catheter in place for two to three weeks to prevent pressure on the surgery site.

82. An infant is admitted for surgery on an inguinal hernia. Which observation would the nurse interpret as indicating the need for immediate surgery?

    1. A change in the character of stools.

2. Inability to reduce the hernia following a diaper change.
3. Decreasing frequency of voiding.
4. Temperature of 102° F.

83. When planning diversionary activities for the child in the acute phase of rheumatic fever, it is helpful for the nurse to understand that the physician will most likely order:

    1. Bedrest.
    2. Ambulate t.i.d.
    3. Activity as tolerated.
    4. Muscle strengthening exercises.

84. An infant is born with a myelomeningocele and is placed in the pediatric unit awaiting surgery. Which activity has the highest priority in the nurse's plan of care?

    1. Maintain skin integrity.
    2. Provide family with genetic counseling information.
    3. Monitor infant's temperature frequently.
    4. Maintain IV site.

85. A new order is written for ear drops on a three-year-old child. Which nursing action has the lowest priority in preparation for this procedure?

    1. Anticipate the need for assistance to restrain.
    2. Check the child's name bracelet, before administration.
    3. Explain the purpose of the medication to the child.
    4. Check which ear is to receive the drops prior to administration.

86. An infant had her first MMR injection yesterday. Today the baby has a fever of 100° F, and the area around the injection site is warm and tender. What is the priority nursing action?

    1. Report this immediately to the RN.
    2. Hot pack the warm area.
    3. Increase the frequency of observations of the site.
    4. Document this information on the chart.

87. A newly diagnosed six-year-old diabetic is distressed after his insulin injection. The nurse knows that which play activity would be most therapeutic in helping the child deal with his injection?

    1. A video game.
    2. A needleless syringe and a doll.
    3. Read a story to him about a child with diabetes.
    4. A supervised playtime in the playroom.

88. In caring for a preschooler who is being admitted the evening before surgery, the nurse knows that which

activity is least appropriate for reducing the stress of hospitalization?

1. Explaining the surgical procedure.
2. Playing "surgery" with cap and masks.
3. Showing her the call light and bathroom.
4. Having her mother undress her.

89. The nurse is caring for a child admitted with a possible diagnosis of celiac disease. The nurse knows that which other disease causes stools that resemble the stools with celiac disease?

1. Cystic fibrosis.
2. Hirschsprung disease.
3. Intussusception.
4. Crohn's.

90. In caring for a child undergoing diagnostic tests, the nurse knows that which tests would be most helpful to aid in the diagnosis of pediatric leukemia?

1. Blood test by venipuncture.
2. Blood culture.
3. Lumbar puncture.
4. Bone marrow aspiration.

91. A four-year-old is visiting his brother who is critically ill and may be dying. In talking with this young visitor, the nurse is aware that he would be least likely to believe that death is:

1. Like going to sleep.
2. The result of magic.
3. Permanent and lasting.
4. The result of a wish.

92. Anticipatory guidance is given to the parents of a 10-year-old girl. The nurse knows that understanding of this information would be demonstrated by the parents if they say they will reinforce:

1. Sex education and self breast exam.
2. The need for increased caloric intake.
3. The child's increasing need for sleep.
4. Fewer dental visits are needed.

93. A child is admitted from the emergency room with a fractured radius. The injury has been splinted. The nurse understands that the expected result of this is:

1. Reduced edema in extremity.
2. Reduction of the fracture.
3. Callus formation at fracture site.
4. Reduced pain.

94. The nurse teaches the mother to have syrup of ipecac on hand in case of accidental poisoning. The nurse wants the mother to know when to give ipecac. The mother should be able to state that the correct situation in which to give ipecac is:

1. Only upon direction of the poison control center.
2. If the label information on the poison says to induce vomiting.
3. When the poison was taken within the last two hours.
4. By specific age guidelines, followed by one full glass of water.

95. A client is being discharged following bilateral vein ligation and stripping. While doing discharge planning, the nurse knows that the most important instruction to give the client is to:

1. Wear slacks and opaque hose regularly for cosmetic reasons.
2. Purchase and wear above-the-knee support hose only.
3. Join a local diet center and lose weight.
4. Elevate legs above the heart level four times a day for 15-20 minutes.

96. The nurse is planning discharge teaching for a client following abdominal surgery. Which of the following instructions about changing dressings in the home would the nurse consider most appropriate?

1. The appropriate opening of bandages to maintain their sterility.
2. Information about proper aseptic technique.
3. Proper gloving technique.
4. Information about good hand washing technique.

97. A client who has right-sided weakness needs to be transferred from his bed to a wheel chair. In transferring the client, the nurse must remember to:

1. Keep the client at arm's length while transferring him.
2. Bend at the waist to get down to his level.
3. Maintain a straight back and bend at the knees.
4. Attempt to transfer the client alone, before determining that help is needed.

98. When obtaining a urine specimen from an indwelling catheter for culture and sensitivity, the nurse should:

1. Empty the drainage bag from the urometer port.
2. Wear sterile gloves.
3. Cleanse the entry site prior to inserting the needle.
4. Drain the bag and wait for a fresh urine sample to send from the drainage bag.

99.   A three-year-old is being admitted with nephrotic syn-
       drome. In considering the possible roommates for this
       client, the nurse would most appropriately select:

       1.   A 16-year-old postoperative following a ruptured
             appendix.
       2.   An eight-year-old with leukemia.
       3.   A toddler with rheumatic fever.
       4.   No roommate, because isolation is required.

100.   A confused elderly client is found wandering around
       the ward wearing a bathrobe and cotton socks. He also
       is bumping into walls as he walks. What is the priority
       nursing action?

       1.   Take the client's shoes to him and assist him in
             putting them on.
       2.   Accompany the client to his room and obtain a
             baseline assessment.
       3.   Ask the client to return to his room and rest until
             he feels better.
       4.   Tell the client to be careful of any wet spots on the
             floor.

NOTES

NCLEX-RN

Test 4

Questions with Rationales

NCLEX-PN TEST 4 WITH RATIONALES

1.   A client has recently received albuterol (Ventolin) for an asthma attack. Which finding by the nurse indicates a side effect of albuterol (Ventolin)?

   1.   A heart rate of 110.
   2.   A blood pressure of 100\52.
   3.   Fine basilar crackles.
   4.   Capillary refill of greater than five seconds.

   1.   *Great! You remembered that albuterol is a beta agonist, which means that it stimulates the sympathetic nervous system. One of the effects of this stimulation is an increased heart rate.*
   2.   *No, this would not be due to albuterol. Albuterol is a beta agonist and, therefore, increases cardiac output. It is unlikely that an increased cardiac output would cause low blood pressure — think about it!*
   3.   *No, this would not be due to albuterol. Crackles at the bases of the lungs occur when small airways are reinflated. Crackles are common in pneumonia and in bedridden clients. While crackles are a sign of airway disease, they are not a result of bronchodilator treatment.*
   4.   *No, this would not be due to albuterol. Poor capillary refill indicates poor tissue perfusion. Albuterol is primarily a beta agonist and has little effect on alpha receptors.*

2.   The nurse is caring for a client who is receiving a glucocorticoid. In order to detect electrolyte imbalance caused by steroid use, the nurse would be alert for:

   1.   Muscle weakness and lethargy.
   2.   Itching and red scaly patches.
   3.   Poor skin turgor and sticky mucous membranes.
   4.   Tremors and nervousness.

   1.   *Good for you! Not only did you remember that steroid use can cause hypokalemia, you also know the classic signs of hypokalemia.*
   2.   *No. Some allergic reactions may cause itching, but this is not a sign of an electrolyte imbalance. You need to review your electrolytes.*
   3.   *No. These are signs of dehydration. Glucocorticoids, however, cause sodium and water retention, not loss. Think again about which electrolyte is excreted in glucocorticoid therapy.*
   4.   *Tremors and nervousness are side effects of beta agonists or sympathetic stimulation, not glucocorticoids. You're on the wrong drug!*

3.   A client is treated for a major depression with nortriptyline (Pamelor) 150 mg. Which of the following statements by the client indicates that she needs further instruction about this drug?

   1.   "I'm glad this medicine helps me. My husband and I would like to start our family as soon as possible."
   2.   "If I should feel hopeless and suicidal again, I have the telephone number of my therapist to call for help."
   3.   "I plan to see my psychiatrist regularly. She told me if I continue to do well, I can probably stop taking my medication in nine to 12 months."
   4.   "I hope I will not have to continue taking medicine forever. I guess I'll have to see how I do."

   1.   *Yes, the client needs further instruction! Tricyclic antidepressants should be avoided during pregnancy, especially during the first trimester, because they are associated with fetal anomalies.*
   2.   *No, this statement by the client is correct. Since 60% of depressed persons experience suicidal thoughts, each hospitalized client should have a plan for obtaining help if these thoughts recur after discharge. The client's statement indicates that she has a good plan to follow, which the nurse should reinforce. The stem asks for the statement that indicates a knowledge deficit. Try again.*
   3.   *This is not the correct option. The client correctly understands that most clients remain on their antidepressant for nine to 12 months after recovering from a episode of depression. A rebound depression can occur if the medication is discontinued too soon. The client's statement is appropriate, so it does not indicate a need for further instruction.*
   4.   *No, this is not the correct option. This is a realistic statement that does not indicate a need for further instruction. An estimated 15% of clients with depressive illness develop chronic or recurring manifestations of depression. Clients should remain under the care of a mental health professional after hospital discharge so their condition can be monitored. The stem asks for the statement that indicates a knowledge deficit. Read the options again.*

4.   The nurse should advise a client taking rifampin (Rifadin) for treatment of tuberculosis to avoid:

   1.   Antacids containing magnesium.
   2.   Aspirin products.

3. Over-the-counter cold products.
4. Alcoholic beverages.

1. *Incorrect. Rifadin should be taken on an empty stomach but, if GI irritation occurs, the client may need to take the drug with food or an antacid. Try again.*
2. *No. There is no contraindication for taking aspirin products while the client is on Rifadin. Choose another option.*
3. *Incorrect choice. Clients may take over-the-counter cold preparations if necessary. Try again.*
4. ***Good choice! Clients should be advised to avoid alcoholic beverages while taking Rifadin because alcohol may increase the risk of hepatotoxicity and increase the rate of Rifadin metabolism. Dosage adjustment may be necessary.***

5. **A client is hospitalized for gastrointestinal bleeding. He is given temazepam (Restoril) at bedtime to help him sleep. What nursing action is indicated immediately following his dose?**

1. Raise the side rails on his bed and tell him to use his call light to summon the nurse if he has to get up during the night.
2. Keep a padded tongue blade at the bedside and observe for seizures.
3. Monitor his blood pressure and respirations.
4. Observe and record his sleep patterns.

1. ***Correct. Restoril is a benzodiazepine that is often prescribed to induce sleep. Ataxia and dizziness are common side effects. The bedrails of a hospitalized client should be raised and instructions given to call for assistance before getting up during the night, to prevent falling and the risk of injuries.***
2. *This is not correct. Seizures are associated with withdrawal from prolonged use of high doses of benzodiazepines. They are not a side effect of Restoril when taken for nighttime sedation on a short-term basis.*
3. *This is not correct. Depressed blood pressure and respirations are associated with intravenous administration of benzodiazepines, such as Valium, which may be given IV to manage delirium tremens (DTs). They are not a side effect of Restoril when taken for nighttime sedation on a short-term basis.*
4. *This is not correct. The nurse should observe and record his sleep patterns, but this is not an "immediate" (priority) action.*

6. **A client is treated in the emergency room for a panic attack. Thirty minutes after receiving diazepam (Valium), he tells the nurse that he is feeling much calmer. "I**

can't believe how scared I was. I will do anything to avoid having another panic attack." The most helpful nursing measure is to:

1. Advise him to admit himself to the psychiatric unit, where he can have a comprehensive evaluation in a protected setting.
2. Suggest to him that he reduce the amount of stress in his life.
3. Make an appointment for outpatient psychotherapy to receive help with any emotional issues that might be responsible for his panic attacks.
4. Tell him he can always return to the emergency room if he should have another panic attack.

1. *This is incorrect. There is no data to support his need for inpatient treatment. Panic disorder is usually treated in an outpatient setting.*
2. *This is not the best option for this question because stress reduction alone will not prevent future panic attacks. Look again to select a better option.*
3. ***Excellent! Panic attacks occur when the individual's defense mechanisms fail to contain his anxiety. Psychotherapy will help him learn to identify and resolve his emotional issues and conflicts and thereby prevent future panic attacks.***
4. *Wrong! This is not a helpful comment, because the client wants to prevent future panic attacks.*

7. **A physician orders a body magnetic resonance imaging (MRI) for diagnostic purposes. It would be most important for the nurse to tell the client that the procedure:**

1. Takes 15 to 30 minutes.
2. Involves injection of a contrast dye.
3. Is painless, except for the discomfort of lying still.
4. Uses only small amounts of radiation.

1. *Incorrect. This procedure will take 60 to 90 minutes for body imagery. Try again.*
2. *No, the standard examination does not require contrast dye. This is a noninvasive procedure. Choose another option.*
3. ***Correct! No discomfort is felt during the test. A tingling sensation may be felt in metal fillings, and the client may experience discomfort from remaining motionless, but there is no pain.***
4. *Wrong. MRI does not require ionizing radiation. Select again.*

8. **A 42-year-old female is admitted with right-sided weakness and slurred speech. About which diagnostic tests**

should the nurse be prepared to instruct the client/family?

1. EEG and MRI.
2. Angiography and EMG.
3. PET and pneumoencephalogram.
4. CT scan and lumbar puncture.

1. *No, incorrect. An EEG is not initially utilized. The EEG would be abnormal, but it doesn't provide specific information about the type and amount of damage. This information is most useful in diagnosis of seizure disorders. Try again.*
2. *Incorrect. EMG is electromyography, which measures muscle potentials. Although cerebral angiography will detect cerebrovascular disorders, it is not usually used initially. Try again.*
3. *PET would be appropriate, but the pneumoencephalogram would not be appropriate. A pneumoencephalogram is an x-ray of the cerebral ventricles. While it is useful in the diagnosis of cerebral malformations, it is very painful. Try again.*
4. ***You are correct! The CT scan may show areas of hematoma or infarct, with distortion or shift of ventricles. The lumbar puncture may be useful if there is a subarachnoid hemorrhage.***

9. The nurse is preparing client teaching for a 56-year-old client who is being discharged after a simple mastectomy. The client will begin radiation therapy as an outpatient tomorrow. Which of the following instructions given by the nurse would be directed at maintaining skin integrity?

1. Wear a good support bra and use ice for any swelling.
2. Use of a heating pad is contraindicated.
3. Skin breakdown is common and should be treated with antibiotic ointment.
4. Keep skin lubricated to prevent dryness.

1. *No, both of these measures are contraindicated as they may cause increased irritation. Try again.*
2. ***Terrific! This is the only true statement and should help avoid tissue damage. Radiated tissue becomes thinner and may lack tissue receptors that normally would alert the client to a potential burn.***
3. *Incorrect. Skin breakdown may occur, but ointments should be used only with specific instructions from the physician responsible for the radiation therapy. Select another option.*
4. *Not correct. This implies that creams should be used routinely. Discharge instructions should state that the skin is to be kept clean and dry.*

10. In dealing with a client with obsessive-compulsive disorder who engages in ritualistic behaviors centering around cleansing his mouth of offensive odors, the nurse would first:

1. Confront the client about the senseless nature of the ritualistic behaviors.
2. Set strict limits on the behaviors so the client can better conform to the unit rules and schedules.
3. Isolate the client for a period of time to lower his anxiety about offending others.
4. Plan the client's schedule to allow extra time to perform the rituals to keep his anxiety within manageable levels.

1. *Wrong! Most clients with rituals recognize the senselessness of their behaviors, but they cannot control them, so this is not the correct option.*
2. *Strict limit setting will increase the client's anxiety, especially when he is first beginning treatment. This is not correct.*
3. *This client isolates himself from others because he fears that his mouth odors are offensive to others. Isolating him will further reinforce these irrational thoughts. This is not correct.*
4. ***Correct. It is important that sufficient time be allotted for the client to perform his rituals early in his treatment. This will help him keep his anxiety level manageable.***

11. Two weeks after a client started taking amitriptyline (Elavil), she reported that she was sleeping better and her appetite had improved. She said, however, that she still felt hopeless and sad. In response to this statement, the best nursing action is to:

1. Notify her physician so that she can be switched to another drug.
2. Ask her physician to increase her dose of Elavil.
3. Explain that antidepressants often take three to four weeks to be fully effective.
4. Chart her complaints in the nursing notes.

1. *This is not correct. Although the client's physician will want to know how she is responding to her medication, this is not the best option. Her antidepressant most likely will not be changed if she is experiencing some improvement in her target manifestations. Note also that this action does not deal with client education, which is the issue raised in this question. Try to identify an option that describes a better choice.*
2. *This is a possibility, but it is not the best nursing action because it does not deal with client education, which is the issue raised in this question. Look at the other options and identify a better choice.*
3. ***Correct. Tricyclic antidepressants have a lag***

time of three to four weeks for before the client will experience significant improvement. The client has only taken her medication for two weeks, so she still has manifestations of a depressed mood, even though her sleep patterns and appetite have improved. This nursing action responds to the issue of client education, which is the issue in this question.

4. *This is an appropriate action, but it is not the best option because it does not address client education, which is the issue in this question.*

12. A discharged client will continue taking lithium and will be seen in the clinic on a regular basis after discharge. The nurse understands that, as a possible result of long-term lithium therapy, the client is at risk for developing:

    1. Hyperthyroidism.
    2. Hypoglycemia.
    3. Impaired kidney function.
    4. Gall stones.

    1. *This is not correct. Hypothyroidism is a risk of long-term lithium therapy, not hyperthyroidism.*
    2. *This is not correct. Long-term lithium therapy is associated with diabetes insipidus, but not diabetes mellitus or hypoglycemia. Read the options again to identify the correct answer.*
    3. ***Excellent! A major risk of long-term lithium therapy is impairment of the ability of the kidneys to concentrate urine, which can progress to nephrogenic diabetes insipidus. Good work!***
    4. *This is not correct. Long-term lithium therapy is not associated with gall bladder disease.*

13. A discharged client will continue taking lithium and will be seen in the clinic on a regular basis after discharge. The nurse understands that lithium toxicity could occur if the client:

    1. Fasts.
    2. Engages in mild exercise.
    3. Increases her sodium intake.
    4. Receives carbamazepine (Tegretol) therapy.

    1. ***Correct. Crash dieting or fasting can lead to lithium toxicity because alterations in the sodium and electrolyte balance can cause blood levels of lithium to rise.***
    2. *Wrong. Mild exercise would not lead to lithium toxicity. Most clients are able to engage in strenuous exercise without difficulty, but they should take care to replace any sodium that has been lost through profuse sweating.*
    3. *Wrong. Increasing sodium intake will lead to excretion of lithium and a drop in lithium level. If the lithium level should drop below the therapeutic*

range, the client may have a relapse of her bipolar disorder.

4. *Wrong. Tegretol is an anticonvulsant that is used to treat acute mania and prevent future manic episodes. It is most often used alone in clients who cannot take lithium. When given with lithium, it has to be closely monitored because the combination can produce manifestations of neurotoxicity in the client. It is not, however, associated with a dose-related lithium toxicity.*

14. An anorexic client tells the nurse that she thinks too much fuss is being made about what she eats. "I have plenty of energy and get all A's in school. I do not think I am too thin. Look, my hips are fat." What is the most appropriate nursing response to her statement?

    1. "You say your hips look fat to you, but you seem very thin to me."
    2. "Let's go over to the mirror so you can see how thin you really are."
    3. "You are such a bright girl. I don't understand how you can do this to yourself."
    4. "You would be much more attractive if you were not so skinny."

    1. ***Correct. The client's perception of her body image is distorted. The nurse can be most therapeutic by responding to her statement in a factual, nonjudgmental way that does not support her distorted body image.***
    2. *Incorrect. The client's perception of her body is distorted. Looking in the mirror will not change her problem with body image. There is a better option.*
    3. *Incorrect. This statement by the nurse is demeaning and shows a lack of understanding about the client's problem.*
    4. *Incorrect. This statement by the nurse is not therapeutic because it is harmful to the client's self-esteem. The client's perception of her body image is distorted.*

15. A postoperative client is to ambulate for the first time after surgery. The nurse understands that which of the following would be an unsafe action?

    1. Have the client get up and sit in the chair next to the bed.
    2. Have the client sit on the edge of the bed with his feet down for a few minutes before he starts to ambulate.
    3. Have the client stand at the side of the bed for a few minutes before taking his first steps.
    4. Encourage the client to try to walk straight ahead while you assist him with his walking.

1. **This is the correct response since you are looking for an unsafe action. If a client is to ambulate, placing him in a chair next to the bed does not meet the requirements for preparing for ambulation.**

2. *Wrong choice! Having the client sit at the edge of the bed with his feet dangling allows assessment of the client for weakness and dizziness, which, if present, would place the client at increased risk of falling. This is a correct action, but the question asks you to select an UNSAFE option.*

3. *Wrong choice! Having the client stand at the edge of the bed allows for assessment of the client's tolerance of this activity. He is still close to the bed, so if he becomes faint or weak he can easily be assisted back to bed. This is not the correct answer, however, because the question is asking for an UNSAFE action.*

4. **A client should be assisted during the initial ambulation following surgery so that assessment can be made of the client's tolerance to this activity. You are, however, looking for an UNSAFE action. Make another choice.**

16. **When transporting a client, the nurse should:**

1. Always use a stretcher.
2. Push the stretcher very quickly so the client does not become chilled during the transport.
3. Never cover a client with a blanket, since it can get caught in the wheels.
4. Use the safety rails or straps that are available on the equipment.

1. *This option is incorrect because a stretcher is not always necessary for transport; a wheelchair may be used safely in many cases.*

2. *Incorrect. The stretcher should not be pushed quickly. This may increase the client's anxiety and does not provide for safe transport.*

3. *Incorrect. The client should be covered to provide warmth and privacy. Tucking in the edges of the blanket will prevent the blanket from getting caught in the wheels of the stretcher.*

4. **You are right! Straps and belts are provided for the client's safety and should be used to prevent falls.**

17. **A client in a long-term care facility has been given a cane to assist her with ambulation. In caring for this client, which of the following would be an unsafe nursing action?**

1. Inspect the rubber tip often and replace it if appears to be worn.
2. Place the cane on the side of the weak leg.
3. Position the cane to support and balance the client with decreased strength in one of the lower extremities.

4. Keep the cane within easy reach when sleeping or sitting.

1. *Wrong choice. This is a correct action, but you are looking for an option that is UNSAFE. A cane that does not have a good rubber tip on it places the client at risk for falling, since the wood or metal on the bottom of the cane can cause it to slip on the floor.*

2. **Good, you have identified the unsafe action! The cane should be placed on the strong side of the client. Since weight is placed on the cane at the same time that it is placed on the weakened extremity, the body weight will be divided equally between the cane and the weakened leg.**

3. *Wrong choice. You are looking for an option that is UNSAFE. The client must have some strength in the affected extremity, or a cane will not provide enough support to allow for ambulation.*

4. *Wrong choice. You are looking for an UNSAFE action. If a cane is needed for ambulation, then it should be kept within the client's reach in order to prevent falling while trying to locate the cane.*

18. **The nurse discovers that the wrong medication was given to a confused client who answered to the name stated upon entering the room. The physician is notified and states that the medication that the client received will not harm him and nothing needs to be done. The priority nursing action after notifying the physician is:**

1. Apologize to the client involved.
2. Make out an incident report documenting the occurrence.
3. Try to avoid being responsible for administering medications again, since this could have been terrible situation.
4. Realize that everyone makes mistakes, and continue to administer the rest of the medications to the other clients.

1. *No. Since the client is confused, he will not know what the apology is about. This action may make the nurse feel better but will not be of any value to the client.*

2. **Best choice! An incident report should be initiated whenever an error is made involving a client. If an adverse effect results and the caregiver needs to remember the events at a later date, the documentation will be available to refresh the memory. The incident reports are also used for statistical purposes in determining the types of incidents that occur. They help administrators to recognize when a particular problem occurs and to help in problem solving to prevent reoccurrences.**

3. *No. Refusing to administer any more medications is not realistic or practical. Although the outcome could have been terrible, accepting responsibility for the error and learning from the situation is important. What is the nurse's next action?*

4. *Wrong choice. Although no one is perfect, the fact that the error was made should be acknowledged through documentation. The error may have been made because of understaffing or a variety of other factors that need to be addressed by administration. The error may have been carelessness on the part of the caregiver, which may be a pattern of behavior that needs to be changed for safe client care.*

19. **The nurse is preparing medications for administration in a pediatric unit. Of the following nursing actions, which would be inappropriate?**

   1. Prepare medications for one client at a time.
   2. Calculate correct drug dosage.
   3. Open unit dose tablets and place medications in medication cup.
   4. Avoid touching tablets or capsules with the hands.

   1. *Wrong choice, this action is correct. Preparing medications for one client at a time helps prevent preparation errors such as inadvertently placing one client's medication into another client's medication cup. You are looking for the option that is INAPPROPRIATE.*

   2. *Wrong choice, this action is correct. Calculation of drug dosage should be done prior to administration, when the information from the drug label is readily available. You are looking for the option that is INAPPROPRIATE.*

   3. **Good work! You have identified the inappropriate action. Unit dose medications should remain in their wrappers to maintain cleanliness, to better identify the medication and to avoid waste if the medication is not given.**

   4. *Wrong choice, this action is correct. Using aseptic technique maintains cleanliness of the medications and prevents possible absorption through contact with the nurse's skin. You are looking for the option that is INAPPROPRIATE.*

20. **The nurse is preparing to administer medication to a client who is scheduled to receive his insulin at 8:00 a.m. The best nursing approach is to:**

   1. Read the label three times.
   2. Check the client's identification bracelet.
   3. Administer the correct medication to the right client.
   4. Check the dosage prescribed.

   1. *Sorry, wrong choice. Checking the label is important in preparing the correct medication, but this is not the BEST nursing approach. Read all the options before selecting the best one!*

   2. *Sorry, wrong choice. Checking the client's identification is important in ensuring that the medication is administered to the right client, but this is not the BEST nursing approach. Read all the options before selecting the best one!*

   3. **Very good! Administering the right medication to the right client is the "best nursing approach" because it includes the correct concepts in all of the other options.**

   4. *Sorry, wrong choice. Checking the prescribed dosage assists in administering the correct medication, but this is not the BEST nursing approach.*

   > **TEST-TAKING TIP:** *When two or more of the options are possible answers, look for a more global option that includes the same concepts.*

21. **The nurse finds an elderly client with her IV pulled out, standing next to her bed, with the side rails in the up position. The client is confused, does not have an identification bracelet on, and cannot remember her name. What should the nurse do first?**

   1. Help the client into bed, and remind her to call the nurse when she wants to get out of bed.
   2. Help the client into bed, and then restart the IV.
   3. Place a restraining vest on the client.
   4. Put an identification bracelet on the client and help her back to bed.

   1. *Reminding a confused client to use a call light is not an appropriate nursing action. The case scenario tells you that the client cannot remember her name, so she will probably not remember to use a call light. Since a physiological need is not identified in this question, the safety of the client is the most important nursing consideration at this time. Which priority setting guideline will you use in this question? Make another choice.*

   2. *The case scenario does not tell you whether the IV has life saving medications or fluids infusing, so you cannot assume that the IV is a physiological need. Do not "read into" the question! Since a physiological need is not identified, the safety of the client is the most important nursing consideration at this time. Make another choice. Which priority setting guideline will you use in this question?*

   3. **Excellent! The case scenario tells you that the client got out of a bed that had the side rails up. This is an unsafe situation, since the client is at risk of falling. Such an injury can be life-**

threatening. Placing a restraining vest on the client will provide for her safety. Good work!

4. *The client's lack of an identification bracelet is an important safety concern. The case scenario, however, tells you that the client got out of a bed that had the side rails up. This is an unsafe situation, since the client is at risk for falling. Such an injury can be life-threatening. After the immediate physical safety of the client is assured, an identification bracelet can be obtained. Try again. Which priority setting guideline will you use in this question?*

22. **The most important nursing goal for a client who is admitted with an acute attack of ulcerative colitis is to:**

1. Provide emotional support.
2. Prevent skin breakdown.
3. Maintain fluid and electrolyte balance.
4. Promote physical rest.

1. *No. Emotional support is necessary, but physiological needs must be the priority in the acute stage.*
2. *Incorrect, because skin breakdown can more successfully be prevented if the client's fluid and electrolyte balance is maintained.*
3. **Correct! Problems related to fluid and electrolyte balance can affect all systems. The goal would be to treat imbalances.**
4. *Incorrect. Rest promotes a decreased metabolic rate but it is not sufficient to counteract problems resulting from fluid and electrolyte imbalances.*

23. **A client returns from surgery for a lung resection due to cancer. Of the following postoperative orders, which is the nurse's highest priority?**

1. Oxygen per mask at six liters per minute.
2. Change dressings as needed.
3. Vital signs every hour.
4. Cough and deep breathe every two hours.

1. **Very good. The postoperative client may need supplemental oxygen in order to maintain normal blood oxygen levels as a result of the surgery and anesthesia.**
2. *Changing the dressings provides the nurse with information concerning the amount and type of drainage that the client is having. However, this is not the priority postoperative action. Try again.*
3. *Assessing vital signs provides information related to the present status of the client. In specifying the "hourly" assessment of vital signs, this order is an implementation order. This option does not follow the nursing process as the priority setting guideline! Notice that one of the options identifies a basic physiological need. Make another choice.*
4. *Coughing and deep breathing helps prevent postoperative respiratory complications. This nursing*

action is an appropriate intervention to prevent a potential problem. However, it is not the first priority in this question. Look for an option that identifies a basic physiological need.

24. **A client is scheduled for surgery and asks the nurse if she can put on some makeup before going to surgery. The best response by the nurse is:**

1. "Only a light application of makeup is allowed."
2. "Hospital policy states that all makeup must be removed before surgery."
3. "I will check with the charge nurse to find out the regulations."
4. "Makeup will interfere with the ability to see your skin color during surgery."

1. *Incorrect! Makeup of any kind masks the color of the skin or nails. Assessment of the circulatory system is monitored by observing the color of the skin, nails and mucosa.*
2. *Wrong. Using hospital policy as an explanation is not very helpful. It does not answer the question being asked. Using hospital policy for an answer is "passing the buck." Clients deserve a better explanation.*
3. *The nurse should know this information. With this response, the nurse is "passing the buck".*
4. **Congratulations! Makeup colors the skin and masks the ability to assess circulatory status. Before surgery, all makeup must be removed, including any colored nail polish.**

25. **A client is in the hospital and has weakness on her left side because of a stroke. She becomes upset when eating, because liquids drool out of her mouth on her weak side. What nursing intervention would be most appropriate?**

1. Provide only pureed and solid foods to prevent drooling, so the client will not become upset.
2. Have a member of the family assist with the client's feedings.
3. Teach the client how to drink fluids on the unaffected side to prevent drooling.
4. Have the client use a syringe to squirt liquids into the back of her mouth.

1. *Wrong! Eliminating liquids from the client's diet is inappropriate, since fluids are a basic physiological need.*
2. *Wrong! This option does not solve the problem of the drooling fluids and does not promote independence in this client.*
3. **Correct! This action promotes independence and addresses the problem of drooling. The client still has control over swallowing and tongue motion on the unaffected side, which will address her concerns. This question re-**

flects the implementation phase of the nursing process.

4. *Although this may help eliminate some drooling, it does not promote normalcy during eating, which can result in a decrease in self-esteem.*

26. **The nurse knows that in caring for a client with second and third degree burns of the head, neck and chest, the greatest initial complication is caused by:**

    1. Infection.
    2. Airway obstruction.
    3. Fluid imbalance.
    4. Paralytic ileus.

    1. *Incorrect. Although it is necessary to prevent infection throughout burn treatment, a patent airway is the priority.*
    2. **Good choice! Burns in this area may involve damage to the pulmonary tree, resulting in severe respiratory difficulty.**
    3. *Incorrect. Although adequate fluid replacement is necessary for cellular and organ function, initially, a patent airway is the priority.*
    4. *Incorrect. During the acute phase, paralytic ileus may occur, requiring nasogastric suction. It does not, however, take precedence over a patent airway.*

27. **To administer a Mantoux test for tuberculosis the nurse:**

    1. Inserts the needle with the bevel up.
    2. Administers 0.1 ml of PPD on the outer surface of the arm.
    3. Uses a 21 or 22 gauge needle.
    4. Massages the area after administration of the medication.

    1. **Correct. The tuberculin syringe should be held close to the skin, so that the hub of the needle touches it as the needle is introduced, bevel up. This reduces the needle angle at the skin surface and facilitates the injection of tuberculin just beneath the surface of the skin, in order to form a wheal.**
    2. *No. The dosage listed is correct, but the injection is made on the inner aspect of the forearm. Choose again.*
    3. *Incorrect. A tuberculin syringe with a 26 or 27 gauge needle must be used. Try again.*
    4. *No, the area should not be massaged after an intradermal injection. A wheal should form for accurate determination of a skin reaction within 48 to 72 hours.*

28. **A client has a tracheostomy tube in place following a complete laryngectomy. To properly suction the client's**

tracheostomy tube, the nurse would:

1. Apply suction for 10 to 15 seconds while withdrawing the catheter.
2. Hyperoxygenate for several deep breaths with the Ambu bag after each procedure.
3. Maintain clean equipment at all times while suctioning.
4. Suction the oral cavity prior to suctioning the tracheostomy tube.

1. **Correct choice! The client can become hypoxic and develop dysrhythmias if suctioning is performed for more than 15 seconds at a time.**
2. *Incorrect. The client should be hyperoxygenated for several deep breaths with an Ambu bag both before and after the procedure. Make another selection.*
3. *No! All equipment that comes into direct contact with the client's lower airway must be sterile to prevent overwhelming pulmonary and systemic infections. Try again.*
4. *No. Remember that the basic principle of asepsis is clean to dirty. The sterile trachea should be suctioned prior to the mouth.*

29. **Which statement written by a laryngectomy client preparing for discharge would indicate to the nurse that he needs further teaching?**

    1. "I'll remember to buy non-aerosol products for personal grooming."
    2. "I sure will miss taking showers from now on."
    3. "Giving up swimming won't bother me, since I never learned how in the first place."
    4. "I never thought that belching could be transferred into speech, but I'm learning quickly."

    1. *No, the client is correct when he writes this. Clients with a tracheostomy should avoid using aerosol products, which could accidentally be inhaled. He understands his teaching.*
    2. **Good, you have found the incorrect statement. Clients with a tracheostomy can shower or take a tub bath, as long as care is taken to avoid aspirating water into the opening. The client will need to have his teaching reinforced to include this important fact.**
    3. *No, the client is correct when he writes this. Clients with a tracheostomy should be told to avoid swimming. Remember the risk of aspiration through the opening! This client understands the information given to him.*
    4. *No, this can be an accurate statement made by a tracheostomy client who is learning esophageal speech. Air is swallowed and then moved quickly back up through the esophagus. Clients learn to coordinate lip and tongue movements with the sound produced by the air passing over vibrating folds of the esophagus. Choose another option.*

30. **Which statement, if made by a client with varicose veins, indicates to the nurse that the client has accurate understanding of the application and use of anti-embolic stockings?**

1. "I won't take them off until I go to bed at night."
2. "I'll put them on in the morning after I've taken my daily walk."
3. "I know that they should feel tight when I put them on."
4. "I'm glad I can cross my legs now since I'll have these stockings on."

1. *No, the client should remove the stockings at least every eight hours for 30-45 minutes. Otherwise, they should remain on the legs.*
2. *Incorrect. Anti-embolic stockings should be applied in the morning before the legs have been dependent. If the client is ambulatory prior to applying the stockings, then he/she should lie on a flat surface with the legs elevated for five to 10 minutes before applying the stockings. This prevents trapping blood in the extremities.*
3. **Yes, this statement is correct. The stockings should feel tight but not constrictive to the extremities. If the stockings feel too tight or if there is numbness in the feet or toes, they should not be worn and, instead, returned for a better fitting pair.**
4. *No! The client must avoid activities that contribute to occluded blood flow, such as crossing the legs, keeping legs in a dependent position, and prolonged standing or sitting.*

31. **Which understanding expressed by a male client who is HIV positive indicates to the nurse that he needs further teaching?**

1. He won't donate blood anymore.
2. He's glad that his newly prescribed drug, zidovudine (Retrovir), will prevent him from developing AIDS.
3. He'll use a latex condom whenever he has sex.
4. He's planning to attend a seminar on stress reduction next week.

1. *Incorrect choice, this understanding is accurate and does not indicate a need for further teaching. HIV is transmitted by contact with blood or blood products, by sexual contact, and from mother to fetus. Clients who are HIV positive should never donate blood.*
2. **Correct choice! This understanding is not accurate and would require further teaching on the nurse's part. Retrovir is given to help prevent the HIV from replicating. It improves the status of the immune system and helps decrease the number and severity of opportu-**

nistic infections. It will NOT prevent the client from developing AIDS.
3. *Incorrect choice, this understanding is accurate and does not indicate a need for further teaching. The client should use a latex condom, ideally one lubricated with a spermicide containing nonoxynol-9, for intercourse.*
4. *Incorrect choice, this understanding is accurate and does not indicate a need for further teaching. Stress reduction will help the HIV positive client. There is a proven connection between stress and the immune system. Maintaining a healthy body and immune system with adequate sleep, good nutrition, and appropriate exercise are important components of deterring progression to full-blown AIDS.*

32. **An elderly client is in a nursing home and confined to bed. What is the most important nursing action that will prevent skin breakdown and decubitus ulcers?**

1. Massage all bony prominences with lotion.
2. Keep the skin clean and dry.
3. Turn the client at least every two hours.
4. Place an egg crate mattress on the bed.

1. *This is not the best choice. Massage of the bony prominences helps in preventing skin breakdown, but massage alone will not eliminate breakdown if the client is left in one position for long periods of time.*
2. *This is not the best choice. Clean, dry skin is helpful in the prevention of skin breakdown. Nevertheless, if the client has clean dry skin and is not moved frequently, skin breakdown still will occur.*
3. **This is the best choice. Turning the client frequently is the most important nursing intervention. This measure alternates the areas where the pressure of the mattress decreases circulation and tends to cause skin breakdown. This question reflects the planning phase of the nursing process.**
4. *This is not the best choice. An egg crate mattress will help alleviate some of pressure on the skin, but the client must be turned in order to eliminate pressure at a particular site.*

33. **Which nursing action is contraindicated for a client with an indwelling Foley catheter?**

1. Instill sterile distilled water in the catheter.
2. Use minimal pressure to clear the catheter of clots or mucous plugs.
3. Use sterile equipment for irrigation.
4. Use the flow of gravity for return of the irrigant.

1. **Great job! Sterile solution is necessary. However, distilled water is hypotonic and may be absorbed by body tissues. Sterile normal saline is the solution of choice, since it is the most similar to normal body tissue fluid.**

> **TEST-TAKING TIP:** This option is different from the other three and is an incorrect action. Note that this planning question has a negative response stem.

2. *Wrong choice! Minimal pressure is used to clear clots, in order to avoid trauma to the bladder tissue. The option offers a correct statement but it is not the correct selection because this question has a negative response stem.*

3. *Wrong choice! The bladder is a sterile cavity, and any procedure that introduces foreign substances into it should utilize surgical asepsis. This option is a correct statement. However, this question has a false response stem.*

4. *Wrong choice. The option correctly states that the irrigant should be allowed to return by the flow of gravity. Negative pressure or suction can cause injury to bladder tissue. However, this question has a false response stem, so this is a wrong choice. Try again!*

34. **A client has been diagnosed with iron deficiency anemia. When teaching the client about her diet, which foods should be identified by the nurse as good sources of iron?**

    1. Fresh fruits.
    2. Milk and cheese.
    3. Organ meats.
    4. Whole grain breads.

    1. *Wrong! Fruits provide the body with a rich source of Vitamins A and C; this client is deficient in iron.*
    2. *Wrong. Dairy products are good sources of high quality complete protein, not iron.*
    3. **Right choice! A diet rich in organ meats provides iron, which is what the client needs to improve her anemia.**
    4. *Wrong. Whole grain breads are rich in carbohydrates and dietary fiber, not iron.*

35. **While caring for the client with an IV, it is most important for the nurse to:**

    1. Report any signs of infection to the charge nurse.
    2. Record the condition of the IV site and the rate of infusion, and report any unusual findings.
    3. Record intravenous intake.
    4. Ask the client if the IV site is painful or tender.

    1. *This is an appropriate nursing action, since the charge nurse may need to contact the physician to provide orders to alleviate the problem. However, this is not the best option. Read the other options, and try again.*
    2. **Good work! Observing the site and infusion**

rate is part of providing safe care to the client receiving intravenous therapy. **This option is the most comprehensive and includes the ideas in the other options.**

3. *This action is standard care for the client receiving intravenous therapy and is a possible choice. However, this is not the best option. Read the other options, and try again.*

4. *This action is part of assessing the site for possible infiltration or phlebitis. This is an appropriate action, but there is a better choice. Try again.*

36. **The nurse is informed during report that a postoperative client has not voided for eight hours. The initial nursing action would be to:**

    1. Assist the client to the bathroom.
    2. Place the client on a bed pan and pour warm water over her perineum.
    3. Palpate and percuss the client's bladder.
    4. Catheterize the client.

    1. *Assisting the client to the bathroom may be helpful if the client needs to urinate. This information needs to be obtained before action is taken. Make another choice.*
    2. *Placing the client on a bed pan is not always conducive to urinating. If the client is allowed out of bed, sitting on the toilet while pouring warm water over the perineum can help the client to void. However, this is not the priority action. The client should have the need and an urge to void before this intervention is implemented. Make another choice.*
    3. **Very good! Assessing the client's bladder provides information concerning the need to void. This is the priority action and the only option that provides for assessment of the client.**
    4. *Catheterizing the client should only be done after it has been determined that the client has a full bladder and is unable to void. The nurse must use assessment first. Make another choice.*

37. **A 78-year-old client has been in the hospital for a week on bed rest. She complains of elbow pain. The best nursing action is to:**

    1. Place elbow pads on the client.
    2. Examine the elbow.
    3. Call the physician for an order for pain medication.
    4. Reposition the client so that she is more comfortable.

    1. *Since the case scenario does not tell you what is causing the elbow pain, you cannot assume that it is related to pressure or skin breakdown. More information must be obtained by the nurse before*

implementing any actions. Try again.

2. **Very good! Examining the elbow is an assessment of the client's complaint. The nurse does not know enough about the elbow pain or its probable cause. The elbows can be assessed for redness, swelling, or joint pain. Then, after assessing the problem, the nurse can analyze the situation and develop a plan of care and implement the appropriate nursing interventions.**

3. *Calling the physician at this time is not appropriate! The nurse does not know enough about the elbow pain or what is causing it. After obtaining further information, the nurse may not need to notify the physician if nursing interventions will alleviate the problem. If the physician must be notified, the nurse needs to gather the information that the physician will need to analyze the problem and order appropriate medical treatment.*

4. *Repositioning the client provides for the client's comfort. However, the nurse does not know what is causing the pain. Repositioning the client should not precede the nurse's investigation of the client's complaint of pain. The nursing process requires that assessment be performed before planning or implementing any other nursing action, because those actions must be based on information obtained during the assessment. Choose another option!*

38. After complaining of severe chest pain for the last hour, a client is admitted to the ICU with an acute myocardial infarction. The nurse knows that the results of the cardiac enzyme studies will help determine the:

1. Degree of damage to the myocardium.
2. Location of the myocardial infarction.
3. Size of the myocardial infarction.
4. Coexistence of pulmonary congestion.

1. **Good choice! Cardiac enzyme studies are checked on admission, and then daily for several days, because their degree of elevation can reflect the degree of damage to the myocardium.**

2. *Wrong. The location of the myocardial infarction is determined by ECG findings.*

3. *Incorrect. The size of the infarction can be determined through a PET Scan, which is a noninvasive method of assessing the infarct.*

4. *Incorrect. This can be a complication of myocardial infarction. Enzyme studies do not reflect coexistence of pulmonary congestion.*

39. Six days after a craniotomy, which complaint by the client would the nurse assess as a possible early manifestation of a complication?

1. He wants to leave the hospital.
2. He feels nauseated.
3. He has a slight headache.
4. He is extremely sleepy.

1. *Incorrect. This is a normal response for anyone recovering from surgery.*

2. *Incorrect. Vomiting may occur infrequently with increased intracranial pressure, but it is not accompanied by nausea.*

3. *Incorrect. This is considered normal post craniotomy. If a headache becomes intense, it may be indicative of increased intracranial pressure.*

4. **Good work! Excessive lethargy is an early manifestation of increased intracranial pressure, which can be a complication of cranial surgery.**

40. A 22-year-old client sustained a T4 spinal cord injury. While doing morning assessments four weeks post-injury, the nurse discovers that the client's BP is 280/140 and he is complaining of nasal stuffiness and a severe, pounding headache. The first nursing action is:

1. Sit the client upright.
2. Call the nurse in charge.
3. Check the client's bladder for distension.
4. Administer the prescribed antihypertensive.

1. **Correct choice! Since autonomic hyperreflexia is a medical emergency, the first action is to lower the BP. By sitting the client upright, compensatory orthostatic hypotension is used to lower the blood pressure.**

2. *Wrong choice. Calling the charge nurse is important after nursing measures have been initiated to lower the blood pressure.*

3. *Wrong choice. This should be done to assess the cause of hyperreflexia, but the first goal is to lower the blood pressure and, ultimately, to prevent stroke.*

4. *No, not at this time! Orthostatic hypotension will provide the same results initially. Antihypertensives are used if non-pharmacologic methods are unsuccessful.*

41. A client was admitted for a severe episode of gastrointestinal bleeding. Which statement by the client indicates to the nurse a need for further instruction?

1. "If my arthritis bothers me, I'll take acetaminophen (Tylenol)."
2. "It's a good thing I gave up drinking five years ago."
3. "It will sure be good to have my morning coffee."
4. "I'll take my cimetidine (Tagamet) before I eat and at bed time."

1. *This is a correct statement because Tylenol is appropriate. An aspirin-related drug would be con-*

traindicated because it causes GI bleeding. This option is a distractor, because this question has a false response stem. The answer will be a statement that indicates that the client does not understand how to care for his health problem.

2. This is a correct statement and a distractor. The client understands that he should avoid alcohol, which stimulates the GI tract. This question has a false response stem, so the answer will be a statement that indicates that the client does not understand how to care for his health problem.

3. **Coffee stimulates the GI tract and should be avoided. This response shows that the client "needs further instruction." Very good!**

4. The client is correctly taking Tagamet before eating and at bedtime. Tagamet is used in treatment of peptic ulcers to inhibit the secretion of histamine. This is a true statement and a distractor, since this question has a false response stem. The answer will be a statement that indicates to the nurse that the client does not understand how to care for his health problem.

42. **An elderly client is experiencing a decrease in his white blood cell count and is placed on protective precautions for infection. Which of the following comments by the client indicate to the nurse that he understands his condition and the precautions?**

1. "I have never been so aware that germs are everywhere around us."
2. "I didn't realize that I am so contagious that I need a private room."
3. "Everyone who touches me washes their hands like I am really contaminated."
4. "I might make my sister's baby sick, so I told her not to visit."

1. **Correct. This comment is the answer, because it indicates an understanding of the need for precautions.**

2. This is not the answer. The client's condition is not contagious. Protective precautions are implemented to protect the client from infection, not to prevent the spread of a contagious disease. This comment indicates that the client does not understand his condition or the need for precautions.

3. The client is not contaminated with a contagious disease. Strict hand washing is done to protect the client from infection. This comment indicates that the client does not understand his condition or the need for precautions. This is not the answer.

4. The client's condition is not contagious. The sister and her baby are not at risk for developing an illness as a result of visiting the client. This comment indicates that the client does not understand his condition or the need for precautions. Select again.

43. **A client is scheduled for left below-the-knee amputation in the morning. Before surgery, the preoperative teaching plan included deep breathing and coughing. In evaluating the effectiveness of preoperative teaching, the nurse should ask the client:**

1. "Do you understand what we have just discussed about deep breathing and coughing?"
2. "Do you think that you will need to have a sedative to help you sleep tonight?"
3. "Will you demonstrate for me the correct method of deep breathing and coughing?"
4. "Do you have any questions concerning your scheduled surgical procedure?"

1. Not the best option! This question asks the client about the content of the preoperative teaching in the form of a closed question, which requires only a "yes" or "no" answer. The client could answer "yes" regardless of the true state of his understanding. This is not the best question to ask.

2. Wrong choice. The test question asked you to select a question that the nurse should ask to evaluate preoperative teaching. In this option, the nurse is asking about the need for a sedative, not about the client's understanding of preoperative teaching. Although the question is an appropriate question for the nurse to ask at this time, it is not the correct answer because it does not relate to the issue in the question.

3. **Excellent! This question asks the client about the content of the preoperative teaching. In addition, the question requests a return demonstration of deep breathing and coughing. If the preoperative teaching has been effective, the client will be able to do the return demonstration. If additional teaching is required, the client will be unable to do the return demonstration properly. This is the best question for evaluating the effectiveness of preoperative teaching.**

4. Wrong choice. This question is an appropriate question for the nurse to ask at this time. It is not the correct answer, however, because the stem of this test question asks you to select a question that the nurse should ask to evaluate preoperative teaching. Here, the nurse is asking about the client's understanding of the surgical procedure. The client's questions concerning the surgical procedure should be referred to the doctor.

44. **A client is seen in the emergency room for abdominal pain, and is scheduled for emergency surgery. In preparing to do the client's preoperative teaching, the nurse knows that it is most important to:**

1. Explain of the hospital billing process for clients receiving surgery.
2. Teach deep breathing and coughing with abdomi-

nal splinting.
3. Obtain the surgical consent.
4. Explain where the incision will be and how much drainage to expect on the dressing after surgery.

1. Wrong. Explaining this process to the client is informative, but it is not appropriate prior to emergency surgery. This option does not address the issue in the question, which is preoperative teaching. Make another choice.

2. Excellent! Any client having abdominal surgery should be taught deep breathing and coughing.

3. Wrong. Obtaining the surgical consent is not a part of preoperative teaching, which is the issue in this question. Make another choice.

4. Wrong. There is not enough information to permit the nurse to explain the location of the incision and amount of drainage. There is another option that is more important in preoperative teaching. Try again.

45. **A 21-year-old client is admitted to the hospital because of extreme weight loss. It is noted on the admission assessment that the client believes that she is overweight at 88 pounds. In planning the care for this client, the nurse should first:**

1. Assess the client's nutritional status.
2. Obtain a psychiatric consult.
3. Plan a therapeutic diet for the client.
4. Talk to the family members to find out more about the client's self-concept.

*1. **Excellent! The client's nutritional status should receive first priority, because nutrition is a basic physiological need. If the client's nutritional needs are not met, the situation may be life-threatening.***

2. Wrong choice. Obtaining a psychiatric consult may be an appropriate intervention, but with only the information given in this case scenario, it would not take priority at this time. Make another selection.

3. Wrong choice. The client will need adequate nutrition. You are correct in identifying nutrition as a basic physiological need and a high priority. However, planning nursing interventions should come after one of the other options in this question. Make another selection.

4. Wrong choice. Obtaining further information from the family may be appropriate, but it is not the priority action in this situation. Make another selection.

46. **A client has a nasogastric tube in place following abdominal surgery. Which nursing action would be con-**

traindicated when planning the care for a client with a nasogastric tube?

1. Attach the nasogastric tube to high suction.
2. Provide frequent oral hygiene.
3. Measure the amount of drainage from the nasogastric tube.
4. Attach the nasogastric tube to the client's gown in order to prevent pulling at the insertion site.

*1. **Excellent! The amount of suction is determined by the physician and should be a part of the medical plan that is implemented by the nurse. This is not an independent nursing action. This incorrect action is the correct answer, because this planning question has a false response stem and asks for an action that would be contraindicated.***

2. Wrong choice, this action is appropriate. Frequent oral hygiene provides comfort for the client, since the mucous membranes of a client with a nasogastric tube in place can become dry and uncomfortable. The question asks for an INAPPROPRIATE action.

3. Wrong choice, this action is appropriate. Drainage from a nasogastric tube should be measured, since it represents a fluid loss for the client. This needs to be considered by the physician when determining fluid replacement therapy. The question asks for an INAPPROPRIATE action.

4. Wrong choice, this action is appropriate. A nasogastric tube that is not secured can cause irritation to the nares as a result of the tube being pulled and caught on the bed or other equipment. The tube also can be accidentally dislodged if not properly secured. The question asks for an INAPPROPRIATE action.

47. **A client has been incontinent of loose stool and is complaining of a painful perineum. The most appropriate initial nursing action is to:**

1. Notify the physician to obtain an order for the loose stools.
2. Check the client's perineum.
3. Turn the client every two hours.
4. Increase the client's fluid intake to prevent dehydration.

1. Informing the physician is a possibility, but this action does not address the client's concern. The issue in the question is perineal pain. This is the client's concern. Also, note that this option is an implementation action. The key word in this question is "initial." The nurse should always assess first! Make another choice.

2. Excellent! This option addresses the client's concern, which is the painful perineum. This is

the issue in the question. This option is also the best because it is an assessment action. The nurse should always assess first!

3. *Turning an immobilized client every two hours will help prevent skin breakdown but it does not address the issue of the question, which is the perineal pain. Try again.*

4. *Preventing dehydration is important for the client with loose stools. Although this is the client's medical diagnosis, it is not the issue this question. The issue is perineal pain, which is the subject of the client's complaint. Make another choice.*

48. A client is admitted to the hospital in respiratory distress. The doctor orders oxygen per mask and the client to be placed in high Fowler's position. Which nursing action is most important for this client?

1. Support and align the hands with the forearms.
2. Use handrolls.
3. Raise the head of the bed to allow for greater lung expansion.
4. Support the feet at right angles to the lower legs.

1. *Supporting and aligning the hands prevents potential contractures of the wrist. This option does not address the issue in the question, which is respiratory distress. Try again.*

2. *Handrolls aid in preventing contractures by maintaining the fingers and thumbs in a functional position. This option does not address the issue in the question, which is respiratory distress. Try again.*

3. ***Good! The elevation of the head of the bed allows for greater lung expansion and decreased respiratory effort. This option correctly addresses the issue in the question, which is respiratory distress.***

4. *Supporting the feet prevents foot drop and contractures at the ankle. This option does not address the issue in the question, which is respiratory distress. Try again.*

49. A diabetic is admitted and placed on bedrest because of suspected gangrene of her left great toe. At this time the initial nursing action is to:

1. Apply heel protectors.
2. Place a sheepskin under the client.
3. Assess hydration and nutritional status.
4. Turn the client every two hours.

1. *Application of heel protectors is an appropriate nursing intervention. It helps prevent pressure sores. However, this is not the most appropriate INITIAL nursing intervention.*

2. *A sheepskin helps absorb moisture, which can contribute to skin breakdown. This is an appropri-*

ate action. However, this is not the most appropriate INITIAL nursing intervention.

3. ***Excellent! The nutritional status and hydration of the client is directly related to the potential for skin breakdown. This option is the only assessment action. The other options are all appropriate and relevant, but they are implementation actions. The nurse should always assess first. The key word in this question is "initial."***

4. *Turning the client frequently prevents skin breakdown. However, this is not the most appropriate INITIAL nursing intervention.*

50. A client was treated four weeks ago for streptococcal pharyngitis and is seeking treatment for recurrent manifestations. The nurse understands that the most likely cause of the client's recurring manifestations is:

1. Enlarged cervical lymph node involvement.
2. Failure to complete his oral antibiotic therapy.
3. Contact with his coworkers.
4. Failure to change his toothbrush.

1. *Wrong choice. This is a clinical manifestation of strep, not a cause, and it would not necessarily only occur now.*

2. ***Good choice! Strep usually resolves within five to seven days even without antibiotic therapy, yet this is the best answer since non-suppurative complications, such as recurrence, result when the full course of antibiotic therapy is not completed.***

3. *Incorrect choice, because the type of contact is not specified. Contact must be airborne. This distractor just says contact with co-workers.*

4. *Wrong choice. This is recommended to all clients, yet is not the best answer. The client will resolve his illness, even if he doesn't change his toothbrush.*

51. A 50-year-old client is a heavy smoker and is admitted with newly diagnosed COPD, chronic bronchitis, and left lower lobe pneumonia. Which nursing measure will receive the highest priority?

1. Facilitate O_2 and CO_2 exchange.
2. Teach the importance of cessation of smoking.
3. Allay his fears about his illness.
4. Encourage adequate fluid intake.

1. ***Correct! Without a patent airway, none of the other distractors would matter.***

2. *Sorry, this is not the highest priority. This is important, yet the client may not be ready to quit. He must have the desire to quit. Try to identify an immediate physiological need of the client.*

3. *Wrong choice. Although this is important, it is not the priority. The client's fear is very real, and will be well founded if his airway is not maintained. Try to identify an immediate physiological need.*

4. *Wrong! Encouraging fluids may be contraindicated. Try to identify an immediate physiological need.*

52. A client is three days postoperative after abdominal surgery. The nurse notes thick yellow drainage from the wound. The nurse would document this type of drainage as:

1. Serous.
2. Purulent.
3. Serosanguineous.
4. Sanguineous.

l. *No, serous describes clear, watery plasma.*

2. *Correct, purulent describes thick yellow, green or brown drainage.*

3. *No, serosanguineous describes pale, very watery drainage.*

4. *No, sanguineous indicates fresh bleeding.*

53. A 75-year-old man is a psychiatric client taking lithium for a bipolar disorder. The nurse knows that elderly clients:

1. Cannot be safely treated with lithium.
2. Take the same dosage of lithium as younger adults.
3. Treated with lithium have a therapeutic range of 0.6-0.8 mEq/L.
4. Treated with lithium have a therapeutic range of 0.6-1.4 mEq/L.

1. *Incorrect. Elderly clients who do not have cardiovascular problems or other medical problems that would be contraindications, can be treated safely with lithium.*

2. *Incorrect. In general, elderly clients are treated with lower doses of lithium. The dose is determined by the serum levels, so some elders may take the same dosage as younger adults. This is not the answer.*

3. *Correct. The therapeutic range for elderly clients is narrower, with 0.8 mEq/L as the upper level. This is because elderly clients, or clients with medical illness, may develop manifestations of neurotoxicity such as confusion and disorientation.*

4. *This is incorrect! 1.4 mEq/L is too high for the upper limit. Elderly clients, or clients with medical illness, are at risk for manifestations of neurotoxicity such as confusion and disorientation.*

54. A client is admitted to the abuse treatment unit for a heroin addiction. On the client's third day in the hospital,

a friend visits in the evening. The nurse notices that the client seems much more relaxed after his friend leaves. The client says that the worst of his withdrawal manifestations from heroin seem to be over. At this time, what action by the nurse would be best?

1. Obtain a urine specimen to send for a drug screen.
2. Congratulate him for staying with the program.
3. Ask about his relationship with his friend, to evaluate whether the friend could be a good source of emotional support.
4. Continue to assess his withdrawal manifestations.

1. *Correct. A drug screen should be done when the nurse observes that the client's withdrawal manifestations dramatically improve, especially when the withdrawal syndrome has not run its full course. In the case of opioids, including heroin, this is seven to 10 days.*

2. *This is not correct. The nursing priority is to assess the reason for this client's improvement.*

3. *The issue in this question is the sudden improvement in withdrawal manifestations. The nurse needs to accurately assess the reason for this client's improvement, since the withdrawal syndrome has not run its full course.*

4. *The issue in this question is the sudden improvement in withdrawal manifestations. The nurse needs to accurately assess the reason for this client's improvement, since the withdrawal syndrome has not run its full course.*

55. The best approach for the nurse to take initially with a client who has severe anxiety is to:

1. Move the person to a calm, non-stimulating environment.
2. Encourage expression of feelings without attempting to modify defensive behavior.
3. Reduce the client's level of anxiety by offering medication.
4. Suggest that the client engage in some automatic behavior, such as pacing, to reduce his anxiety level.

1. *This might be a good intervention, but this is not the best initial nursing action. Try again!*

2. *Correct. The nurse should encourage the client to further communicate by being available and listening in a nonjudgmental manner. The initial goal is to support the client's defenses to help him gain more control over his anxiety.*

3. *Wrong! Medication is indicated for panic levels of anxiety. Clients with a severe level of anxiety can be helped without medication.*

4. *This might be a good intervention, but this is not the*

best initial nursing action. There is a better option.

56. **Which of the following actions would the nurse do first for a client in panic?**

1. Determine the source of his anxiety by asking the client to describe the events before the anxiety occurred.
2. Provide privacy for the client by moving him to a quiet area away from other people, and leaving him alone so he can regain control.
3. Help the client describe his feelings, to begin to diagnose the problem as anxiety.
4. Provide a sense of safety and security by remaining with the client, speaking in a calm manner and offering sedation if needed.

1. *Incorrect! Assisting the client to determine the source of his anxiety is appropriate in mild to moderate levels of anxiety, but the client with a panic level of anxiety needs immediate relief from his overwhelming feelings.*
2. *Incorrect option! A client in panic should not be left alone.*
3. *Incorrect! The client in panic will not be able to deal coherently with his feelings until his level of anxiety is lowered.*
4. ***Correct. The initial goal for a client in panic is to obtain relief. Staying with the client, speaking in a calm manner and offering sedation are the best initial actions for the nurse.***

57. **The psychiatrist orders tranylcypromine (Parnate) for a depressed client who has not responded to tricyclics. In preparing client teaching about diet, the nurse knows that the client may safely select:**

1. Beer and red wine.
2. Cheddar cheese and sausage.
3. Cottage cheese and canned peaches.
4. Liver and Italian green beans.

1. *Wrong. Beer and red wine must be avoided by a client on tranylcypromine. You are looking for something that will be SAFE for the client to consume.*
2. *Wrong. Cheddar, other aged cheeses, sausage, and other cured or aged meats should all be avoided by this client.*
3. ***Correct. Cottage cheese and cream cheese are two cheeses that can be safely eaten because they are not aged. Also, most fresh and canned fruits are allowed. Good work!***
4. *Wrong. Liver and Italian green beans (fava beans) should be avoided.*

58. **A 66-year-old man is an outpatient taking tricyclic antidepressants. The client's wife telephones the clinic and tells the nurse that she has just found her husband lying unconscious and an empty bottle of his medication on**

the nightstand. The nurse's instructions to the wife are guided by the knowledge that overdoses of tricyclic antidepressants are:

1. Medical emergencies.
2. Serious but rarely fatal.
3. Dangerous for clients in poor health.
4. Easily treated by inducing vomiting.

1. ***Correct! Tricyclics are among the most dangerous substances available when taken in overdose. Emergency medical attention and hospitalization should be sought for any client who has overdosed, regardless of the amount ingested. Serious, life-threatening manifestations can develop over the three to five days following the overdose.***
2. *This option is not a true statement. Tricyclics are extremely dangerous and often fatal if emergency medical care is not obtained.*
3. *This is not a true statement because overdoses are equally dangerous for all clients, regardless of their health status.*
4. *Although the ingested drug should be removed by gastric lavage or emesis, overdoses require additional medical treatment, including close electrocardiographic monitoring. This cannot be the best answer to the question.*

59. **A manic client is readmitted to the hospital. After two weeks, her lithium level is within the therapeutic range and she no longer has manic manifestations. Before discharge, what information should the nurse give to the client about her diet when taking lithium?**

1. Sodium intake should be restricted.
2. Fluid intake should be restricted to 1000 cc per day.
3. An adequate daily intake of sodium and fluids should be maintained.
4. Sodium and fluid intake should be increased.

1. *Incorrect. Restricting sodium intake would cause the lithium level to rise, leading to a state of toxicity. A loss of sodium through profuse sweating, vomiting, or diarrhea would also lead to toxicity.*
2. *Incorrect. Clients on lithium should drink six to eight glasses of water a day to maintain a normal state of hydration. This cannot be the correct answer.*
3. ***Correct. Clients should be cautioned to maintain consistent intakes of sodium and fluids to avoid developing lithium toxicity. If they should become physically ill, they should notify their psychiatrist at once.***
4. *Incorrect. Increasing sodium or fluid intake would lower the lithium. If the level should drop below*

the therapeutic range, the client might relapse.

60. **A client's psychiatrist orders fluphenazine (Prolixin) 10 mg b.i.d. Before the first dose, the client asks the nurse what the medicine is supposed to do. What response by the nurse would be most therapeutic for a suspicious client?**

1. "It will help you feel less anxious."
2. "It is to help make your thinking clearer and decrease your fears."
3. "This medication will help you maintain self-control."
4. "This medication will help you get better."

1. *This is not a true statement. Antipsychotics are often sedating, but that is not their primary mode of action.*
2. **Correct. The primary reasons for prescribing antipsychotics for clients with problems like this is to improve their thought processes and control delusional thoughts and hallucinations. This is an accurate and truthful statement so it is the best response for the nurse to make.**
3. *This statement is true, but it is not the best response to this client's question.*
4. *This statement is true, but it does not specifically answer the client's question. It also could be interpreted as patronizing by the client. There is a better option.*

61. **The wife of an alcoholic client says to the nurse, "I told my husband I would leave him if he did not get into treatment. Now that he is here, I feel differently. What can I do to help him?" The most therapeutic nursing response is:**

1. "You should attend an Al-Anon meeting. The group can teach you how best to help him stay sober."
2. "You have already done a great deal by getting him to come into treatment. Now it is up to him to make the best use of his time here."
3. "Are you feeling some responsibility for his drinking?"
4. "Tell me more about the kind of help you feel you are able to provide at this time."

1. *In this response, the nurse is giving advice, which is not therapeutic. In addition, the nurse is inaccurately describing the Al-Anon program. Al-Anon provides information to family members on enabling behaviors and how to cope more effectively with the person who drinks, but the Al-Anon program emphasizes that the decision to stay sober rests with the alcoholic. Al-Anon members are encouraged to focus more closely on meeting their own needs and*

less on those of the alcoholic.
2. *This response is not therapeutic, because it implies that there is no further role for the wife, and overlooks the wife's need for help in dealing more effectively with her husband's behaviors. Alcoholism is identified as a "family disease," because each member is affected by the drinking behavior. Most programs include the family in aspects of the treatment process.*
3. *This is not a therapeutic response. It asks for a "yes" or "no" answer and it addresses an inappropriate issue. The wife did not present any information to indicate that she felt responsible for her husband's drinking. A therapeutic response would address the issue raised by the client.*
4. **Excellent! The wife is the client in this question. This response will help the wife clarify what assistance she can realistically provide without sacrificing her own needs in the process.**

62. **During heroin withdrawal, a client complains continuously to the nursing staff about his discomfort. One day the nurse overhears a nursing assistant say to the client, "You brought these problems on yourself by taking drugs. What did you think would happen when you continued to use heroin?" Which of the following comments to the nursing assistant would be most helpful?**

1. "Your comments were inappropriate. I will have to report this to the supervisor."
2. "Weren't you a bit hard on this client? He is having a great deal of discomfort."
3. "This client is getting on all our nerves."
4. "I overheard you speaking with the client and I thought your comment about his causing his own problems was inappropriate. You have worked well with other addicted clients. What is different about this man?"

1. *This is not correct. The nurse is responsible for supervising the nursing assistant's work and for dealing directly with him on matters that concern the care of clients. If the nurse and the nursing assistant are not able to resolve the issue, then the nursing supervisor may need to be approached for consultation.*
2. *This is not the most constructive approach. The nurse's comment will not help the nursing assistant explore his own behavior so that he could deal more constructively with this client in the future.*
3. *This is not correct. This statement ignores the nursing assistant's inappropriate comment to the client.*
4. **Correct. The nurse is giving specific feedback about what was observed. The nurse also intervenes to focus the nursing assistant on his behavior in a way that could help him gain**

insight into his behavior and deal more constructively with this client in the future.

63. A 32-year-old married woman is treated in the emergency room for a broken arm. She tells the nurse that her husband accidentally hit her during an argument. Which of the following approaches is most appropriate when responding to her comment?

1. Convey concern and ask the client to describe how her injury occurred.
2. Ask the client how the couple usually solve their conflicts.
3. Point out that no person has a right to physically harm another human being, even during an argument.
4. Inform the client that spouse abuse is illegal, and there are legal and social services available to her.

1. *Correct. Conveying acceptance and concern is critical to establishing a trusting relationship in which the client feels secure in disclosing pertinent information and participating in treatment. Asking the client to describe how the incident occurred is a good way to begin the process of building trust.*
2. *This approach fails to address the issue of the client's "accidental" injury. What is the nurse's initial goal, and how can the nurse establish a therapeutic relationship with this client, who is probably fearful?*
3. *The client has stated that the injury was accidental. This statement (while true) implies that it was not an accident and thus argues with the client's statement to the nurse. This approach by the nurse will not help the nurse to establish a trusting relationship with the client. The client is probably experiencing fear. What is the nurse's initial goal?*
4. *This is a true statement, but it will not help the nurse to establish a therapeutic relationship with the client. The client, instead of identifying the issue as "spouse abuse," has told the nurse that the injury was accidental. The client is probably experiencing fear. What is the nurse's initial goal?*

64. A rape victim says to the nurse, "I feel so humiliated. I don't want anyone to know what happened to me." What is the most therapeutic nursing response?

1. "This is a normal feeling after what has happened to you."
2. "You should not be so hard on yourself, it was not your fault."
3. "Are you saying that you are fearful about what others will think? Let's talk about that feeling."
4. "Are you afraid people will blame you for what has happened?"

1. *This is not therapeutic. This response devalues the client's feelings and does not encourage the client to continue to express her feelings, a key component of crisis intervention work. Instead, this response may be perceived by the client as demeaning and condescending. Look for a response that uses a communication tool.*
2. *In this response, the nurse blocks further communication with the client by giving advice. The nurse is cutting off further exploration by the client of her feelings, which is an important element of crisis intervention. Look for a response that uses a communication tool.*
3. *Correct. The nurse is reflecting the feeling expressed by the client and encouraging her to explore her feelings and thoughts more fully, so she and the nurse can do a more complete assessment.*
4. *Although this question may look like an attempt at clarification, the feeling of humiliation expressed by the client is not the same as the fear of blame suggested by the nurse. This question by the nurse also invites a "yes/no" answer and thus does not effectively encourage further exploration by the client of her feelings. This is not a helpful response by the nurse.*

65. The nurse is assisting a frail elderly client to eat. The client begins to choke and indicates to the nurse that she cannot talk. The first nursing action is to:

1. Perform the Heimlich maneuver to obtain a patent airway.
2. Begin mouth to mouth resuscitation.
3. Place an oxygen mask on the client.
4. Go to the nurses' station to get some help.

1. *You are correct! The client is beginning to choke, which is a life-threatening situation. Performing the Heimlich maneuver on this client may alleviate the obstruction and provide the client with a patent airway.*
2. *Because the client does not have a patent airway and is conscious, mouth to mouth resuscitation is an inappropriate first nursing action. Try again.*
3. *Oxygenation correctly identifies a physiological need in this question. However, administering oxygen to a client who does not have a patent airway is inappropriate. There is no access for air exchange, so the oxygen is of no value to this client. Make another choice.*
4. *Leaving a client who is in distress is very inappropriate! If immediate nursing measures are ineffective, help can be summoned without leaving the client. The nurse can summon help by calling out, using the call system, or using the emergency call system. Make another choice.*

66. While changing a surgical dressing, the nurse notes green, foul-smelling drainage at the incision site. Another postoperative client is sharing the same room with this client. The most appropriate nursing action is to:

1. Place the client with the drainage in a private room.
2. Institute drainage and secretion precautions.
3. Move the other client to another room.
4. Place the client in strict isolation until the organism has been cultured and identified.

1. This action is not necessary. A client with a wound infection does not need a private room. However, the integrity of the other client in the room needs to be taken into consideration. The nurse should institute measures that will meet the basic needs of both clients. Try again.

2. Very good! Implementing drainage and secretion precautions protects not only the client with the wound infection, but other clients and the nurse as well. This option meets the physiological needs of all of the people mentioned in the case scenario by maintaining their physiological integrity in preventing the spread of infection.

3. Moving the other client is not appropriate in the care of a client with a wound infection. Other, less drastic nursing measures can be instituted that will meet the basic needs of both clients. Make another choice.

4. Placing the client in strict isolation is not an appropriate nursing action for a client with a wound infection. Strict isolation is used to prevent the transmission of highly communicable diseases. A wound infection is not considered to be highly communicable. Other nursing measures can be instituted to prevent possible spread of the infection. Make another choice.

67. When administering ear drops with a dropper, which nursing action best prevents contamination of the bottle of medication?

1. Thorough hand washing prior to preparing the medication.
2. Hold the dropper with the tip above the ear canal.
3. Wash the client's ear prior to instilling the medication.
4. Only fill the dropper with the prescribed number of drops.

1. This is not the best option. Hands should be washed before preparing any medication; but the tip of the dropper should not come in contact with the hands.

2. Yes! Holding the dropper above the ear canal prevents the tip of the dropper from touching the ear. Touching the dropper tip to the skin will contaminate the end of the dropper, which will contaminate the solution when the dropper is placed in the bottle.

3. The ear may be cleansed if dried secretions or drainage will interfere with absorption of the medication, but this action will not protect the bottle of solution from contamination.

4. This is not correct. It is difficult to determine how many drops are available in every size of dropper. Instead, the dropper should be filled with sufficient medication to ensure that enough drops are available for use at the time of instillation. Even if it were possible to predetermine the number of drops, this would not protect the bottle of solution from contamination.

68. The nurse is preparing to transfer a client from a bed to a chair. To avoid back injury to the nurse, the correct technique is to:

1. Bend at the waist while maintaining a wide stance, lift the client to a standing position, and then pivot the client toward the chair.
2. Have the client lock his or her hands around the nurse's neck, so that the client will feel more secure during the transfer.
3. Place the bed in an elevated position so that the client's hips are at the same level as the nurse's hip, resulting in the center of gravity being the same for both individuals.
4. Bend at the knees, while maintaining a wide stance and straight back, with the client's hands on the nurse's shoulders and the nurse's hands at the client's axillae.

1. Wrong. Bending at the waist places strain on the small lower back muscles, which are prone to injury. Try again!

2. Wrong. If the client's hands are locked around the nurse's neck and then the client starts to fall, all of the client's weight is placed on the cervical vertebrae of the nurse, which can result in a serious injury. The client's hands should rest on the shoulders of the nurse. Make another selection.

3. Wrong. The bed should be in the low position, which provides a place for the client to sit if he is unable to stand. With the bed elevated, once the client attempts to stand, the client cannot sit back down on the bed if he becomes weak or faint. If the client begins to fall, the nurse is at risk for back injury in attempting to prevent the fall. Try again!

4. That's right! Bending at the knees results in the use of the large muscles of the legs. Keeping the back straight avoids using the small, easily

injured back muscles. When the client's hands rest on the nurse's shoulders, this provides security for the client. Placing the hands under the axillae of the client avoids placing pressure on the chest, which can be uncomfortable for the client.

69. **The nurse would demonstrate a good understanding of safe body mechanics by avoiding which of the following actions?**

    1. Move muscles quickly, using short tugs in order to avoid muscle fatigue.
    2. Use the longest and strongest muscles of the body whenever possible.
    3. Lean toward objects being pushed, such as a stretcher.
    4. Carry objects close to the body without touching your clothing.

    1. *This is the correct answer, because the question is asking you to select an action to AVOID. Jerky movements produce increased strain on muscles and are usually uncomfortable for the client.*
    2. *Wrong choice! The longest, strongest muscles are less likely to become injured than the small muscles. This is a correct action, but the question is asking you to select an option to AVOID. Make another selection.*
    3. *Wrong choice! Body weight adds force to muscle action when pushing any object. This is a correct action, but the question is asking you to select an option to AVOID. Make another selection.*
    4. *Wrong choice! When objects are close to the body, the line of gravity is within the body's base of support, which improves balance and reduces strain on the arm muscles. This is a correct action, but the question is asking you to select an option to AVOID. Make another selection.*

70. **After admission to the hospital with pulmonary emphysema, the client is extremely short of breath and is receiving oxygen per nasal cannula. The essential nursing action for this client receiving oxygen therapy is to:**

    1. Make sure the client is receiving at least six liters per minute to alleviate his respiratory distress.
    2. Provide low oxygen percentages to prevent respiratory arrest.
    3. Provide oral hygiene.
    4. Clean the nostrils around the cannula as needed.

    1. *This is an inappropriate action for a client who has emphysema. High levels of oxygen can cause respiratory distress.*
    2. *Very good. This is the most important nursing action for this client, because it provides for his safety.*

    3. *This is an appropriate nursing action. However, it is not the most important action.*
    4. *This is an appropriate nursing action, but it is not the most important action.*

71. **A client has just begun receiving magnesium sulfate for treatment of preterm labor. Which nursing assessment will have the least priority in this client?**

    1. Maternal respirations.
    2. Uterine contractions.
    3. Urinary output.
    4. Maternal temperature.

    1. *No, maternal respirations are an important assessment because magnesium sulfate may result in respiratory depression.*
    2. *Incorrect. When magnesium sulfate is used to treat preterm labor, assessment of contractions is very important to evaluate if it is working.*
    3. *No, urinary output is very important because magnesium sulfate is excreted through the kidneys.*
    4. *Right! Maternal temperature is really not a priority in the preterm labor, unless the client's membranes have been ruptured for more than 24 hours.*

    > **TEST-TAKING TIP:** The case scenario does not state that the client has PROM. Be careful not to "read into" a test question!

72. **A client is admitted to the labor unit with a diagnosis of complete placenta previa. She asks the nurse what will happen when she goes into labor. The best nursing response is:**

    1. "We will monitor you and your fetus very carefully to pick up any problems early."
    2. "We will have several units of blood on hand in case you have bleeding at the time of delivery."
    3. "Once the fetal head drops into the pelvis there will be pressure on the placenta and bleeding should be minimal."
    4. "A cesarean section will be done prior to the onset of labor."

    1. *Wrong. Complete previa means the placenta is completely covering the cervix. Any time the cervix changes, there will be vaginal bleeding. This client must be delivered by cesarean section.*
    2. *Wrong. This statement in itself is correct, but it does not reply to the client's questions about labor.*
    3. *No, this statement relates to a marginal placenta previa. With a complete previa the fetal head cannot drop into the pelvis because the area is covered by the placenta.*
    4. *Correct. The client with a total or complete previa must be delivered by cesarean section.*

73. **The nursing action that plays the greatest role in prevention of postpartum infections is:**

    1. Administration of antibiotics on time.
    2. Daily bathing of all clients.
    3. Frequent hand washing.
    4. Routine postpartum assessment for manifestations of infection.

    1. *No, giving the antibiotics on time will not always prevent infections if aseptic technique is not followed.*
    2. *This is not correct. Daily bathing promotes client comfort but does not necessarily prevent infections.*
    3. ***Yes! Yes! Yes! Frequent hand washing is the simplest and single most effective way to prevent the spread of bacteria that cause infections.***
    4. *No, assessing the client for manifestations of infection will result in early detection but serves no part in prevention.*

74. **The nurse is completing an admission physical exam on a newborn infant and notices that his color has become pale and that he is experiencing nasal flaring, which was not evident before. What should the nurse do first?**

    1. Report these findings to the RN immediately.
    2. Place the baby in or under a heat source.
    3. Do a chemstix on the infant.
    4. Give the baby the first feeding one hour early.

    1. *Wrong. While you are assessing a newborn, he often is exposed to hypothermia. This is easily corrected by warming the infant. In fact, it is best prevented by doing all assessments under a radiant heater.*
    2. ***Good choice. Simply warming this baby will quite likely resolve these changes.***
    3. *No, these are not manifestations of hypoglycemia. When the blood sugar is low, the infant will be jittery.*
    4. *Wrong. The only reason to feed a baby early would be a low blood sugar. This baby is cold, not hypoglycemic.*

75. **An antepartum client with insulin dependent diabetes comes to the emergency room at 28 weeks gestation because her blood sugars have been elevated. A serum blood sugar is 428. The resident orders 25 units of NPH insulin and an IV with glucose to be given STAT. What should the nurse do first?**

    1. Notify the RN to start the IV before giving the or-

dered insulin.
    2. Give the insulin and then notify the RN to start the IV.
    3. Question the large dose of insulin.
    4. Question the type of insulin ordered.

    1. *Wrong. This client has a very high blood sugar and needs a rapid acting insulin immediately to prevent ketoacidosis. The ordered insulin is intermediate acting.*
    2. *Incorrect. NPH insulin will take one to four hours to be effective. The client needs a short acting insulin.*
    3. *Wrong. It is not the dosage that should be questioned, but the type of insulin.*
    4. ***Correct. The client needs a short acting insulin immediately. The resident ordered the wrong type of insulin.***

76. **An antepartum client has hydramnios at 35 weeks gestation. Based upon this diagnosis, the nurse should anticipate:**

    1. Decreased maternal weight gain.
    2. Abnormal swallowing mechanism in the fetus.
    3. Kidney defects in the fetus.
    4. Fundal height less than expected for gestational age.

    1. *Wrong. Hydramnios means an excess amount of amniotic fluid, which would result in an increase in weight gain, not a decrease.*
    2. ***Correct. Hydramnios is associated with fetal malformations that affect fetal swallowing, and neurologic disorders in which fetal meninges are exposed in the amniotic cavity. Two examples of these are tracheoesophageal fistula and anencephaly.***
    3. *No, kidney defects or absent kidneys are associated with too little amniotic fluid (oligohydramnios).*
    4. *Incorrect. If the amniotic fluid is excessive, the fundal height will be much greater than expected for the gestational age.*

77. **The nurse is caring for a 19-year-old client who had a spontaneous abortion at nine weeks gestation. The nurse walks into the client's room and finds her crying uncontrollably. Which of the following statements by the nurse is a therapeutic response to the client's emotional needs?**

    1. "You are young and will have other children."
    2. "When a pregnancy ends in spontaneous abortion, there is often something wrong with the fetus."
    3. "It is hard to deal with losing a pregnancy. I have a number for a local support group for women who experience pregnancy loss."
    4. "The best thing for you is to go home and try again."

    1. *Wrong. This statement ignores the fact that the client is upset and grieving for the child she just lost.*

2. *Wrong. Although this is a correct statement, the client is not comforted by the fact that the fetus she was carrying had something wrong with it. When and if she ever conceives again, she will worry about whether that fetus also has something wrong with it. This response by the nurse is not empathetic and is not therapeutic for the client.*

3. **Correct. The client who experiences spontaneous abortion rarely remains hospitalized more than a few hours. She needs to know there is someone she can call who will be understanding of her feelings and provide needed support. This response by the nurse uses the therapeutic communication tool of empathy and provides helpful information for the client, who is upset and grieving for the child she just lost.**

4. *Wrong! The grieving period following a spontaneous abortion usually lasts six to 24 months. Repeat pregnancy should be delayed until the client is able to come to terms with her loss. This response by the nurse is not therapeutic because it does not address the client's feelings of grief, and because giving advice is not therapeutic.*

78. **The nurse in the family planning clinic is explaining birth control options to an 18-year-old man. He tells the nurse that his 16-year-old girlfriend recently had an abortion and asks the nurse about the advisability of using condoms. In responding to the client, the nurse understands that the primary advantage of condoms as a method of birth control is:**

1. The cost.
2. The availability.
3. Protection from AIDS.
4. Low failure rate.

1. *No, the low cost is a "plus," but not the most important advantage.*
2. *No, the availability makes condoms easy to purchase but is not the primary advantage.*
3. **Good choice! Regular use of latex condoms is the most effective method, other than abstinence, to prevent the spread of most sexually transmitted diseases, including AIDS.**
4. *No, there are other methods that have a lower failure rate than condoms in preventing pregnancy. Using condoms along with spermicides will decrease the number of failures.*

79. **Which of the following foods should the nurse teach the client to include in a daily diet to minimize the most critical electrolyte loss when taking furosemide (Lasix)?**

1. Grains.
2. Milk.
3. Red meats.
4. Dried fruits.

1. *Incorrect. Grains, which are high in fiber and iron, would not be indicated to prevent electrolyte loss. Choose again.*
2. *Wrong choice. Milk, high in calcium and Vitamin D, would not correct the major electrolyte lost by the administration of Lasix.*
3. *Absolutely not. Red meats are high in fat and cholesterol (lean meats are iron-rich). This protein product would not affect the electrolyte loss caused by Lasix.*
4. **Yes! Dried fruits, avocados, broccoli, cantaloupe, grapefruit, lima and navy beans, oranges, nuts, bananas, peaches, potatoes, prunes, spinach, and tomatoes are potassium-rich foods. You remembered that Lasix causes the loss of potassium, along with the loss of sodium, chloride, magnesium, and calcium. Good job!**

80. **In assessing a postpartum client, the nurse knows that which finding would indicate that the methylergonovine maleate (Methergine) was effective?**

1. A rise in blood pressure.
2. An increase in lochia.
3. A firm fundus.
4. Absent breast discomfort.

1. *Wrong. A rise in blood pressure is a side effect of the drug, not a desired effect.*
2. *No. An increase in lochia may occur after a dose of Methergine because of the increase in uterine contractions, but that is not a desired effect.*
3. **Correct. Methergine is an oxytocic drug that is given to promote uterine contractions.**
4. *No, Methergine has no effect on breast discomfort.*

81. **In providing nursing care to a 30-year-old client following an abdominal hysterectomy, which of the following will receive priority?**

1. Administration of estrogen to prevent manifestations of menopause.
2. Maintenance of bedrest for the first 24 hours to prevent an increase in vaginal bleeding.
3. Frequent assessment for bleeding on the dressing and the peripad.
4. Foley catheter in place for two to three weeks to prevent pressure on the surgery site.

1. *Wrong. When a hysterectomy is done on a 30-year-old client it cannot be assumed that the ovaries were removed. In most cases the ovaries are not removed unless the woman is near menopause or at risk for ovarian cancer.*
2. *Wrong. A hysterectomy is like any other major surgery. Early ambulation is an important action in preventing postoperative complications.*

3. *Correct. Careful assessment of blood loss is an important part of care following a hysterectomy. Even though the uterus has been removed, the client will have vaginal bleeding. Increase in vaginal bleeding could be a major cause for concern.*

4. *No, early postoperative removal of the Foley catheter is usually indicated unless reconstructive surgery is done at the same time as the hysterectomy.*

82. **An infant is admitted for surgery on an inguinal hernia. Which observation would the nurse interpret as indicating the need for immediate surgery?**

1. A change in the character of stools.
2. Inability to reduce the hernia following a diaper change.
3. Decreasing frequency of voiding.
4. Temperature of 102° F.

1. *You got it right! This may indicate that there is an obstruction and the intestine is strangulated. This is considered a surgical emergency.*
2. *No, this child was admitted for surgery of the hernia. This is not an unusual finding in the scenario given. Select again.*
3. *Incorrect. The urinary tract is not directly affected by a weakness in the musculature. Choose again.*
4. *Incorrect. An elevated temperature would not indicate the need for surgery. In fact, most of the time this is a contraindication for surgery, unless there were additional manifestations of a rupture or abscess. Select another option.*

83. **When planning diversionary activities for the child in the acute phase of rheumatic fever, it is helpful for the nurse to understand that the physician will most likely order:**

1. Bedrest.
2. Ambulate t.i.d.
3. Activity as tolerated.
4. Muscle strengthening exercises.

1. *Yes, this is correct. Bedrest and minimal exertion are the expected orders to prevent complications during the acute phase.*
2. *Incorrect. The key to the correct answer is in the diagnosis and the phase of the illness. Try again.*
3. *No, this would not be considered safe at this point in the disease process. Choose again.*
4. *Incorrect. Reread the question, looking at the stage of the disease.*

84. **An infant is born with a myelomeningocele and is placed in the pediatric unit awaiting surgery. Which activity has**

the highest priority in the nurse's plan of care?

1. Maintain skin integrity.
2. Provide family with genetic counseling information.
3. Monitor infant's temperature frequently.
4. Maintain IV site.

1. *Right! The infant is at great risk for meningitis because the meninges are exposed until repair is complete. This action has high priority because it is a primary preventative activity.*
2. *No, this is the lowest priority during the preoperative phase of care. Select again.*
3. *No, this is not the highest priority. Can you identify an activity that is a more important part of care for this client than a monitoring activity?*
4. *Not the most important priority of care. The site can be restarted if it does come out. Make another selection.*

85. **A new order is written for ear drops on a three-year-old child. Which nursing action has the lowest priority in preparation for this procedure?**

1. Anticipate the need for assistance to restrain.
2. Check the child's name bracelet, before administration.
3. Explain the purpose of the medication to the child.
4. Check which ear is to receive the drops prior to administration.

1. *No, this is not a low priority. You may very well need help to prevent injury to the child and to correctly instill the medication. Select again.*
2. *No, this is not a low priority! Checking the name bracelet is always a high priority for drug administration. Select again.*
3. *Correct. Even though you want to have an informed client, this isn't the highest priority — especially since this child is three years old and does not have the cognitive ability to understand the reason for the medication. Safety is more important.*

> **TEST-TAKING TIP:** *When selecting priority actions, remember Maslow's Hierarchy of Needs. If you cannot identify a physiological need, look for a safety issue.*

4. *No, this is not a low priority. The client has two ears and the nurse must be certain that the medication is administered in the proper ear, or both! Try another selection.*

86. **An infant had her first MMR injection yesterday. Today the baby has a fever of 100° F, and the area around the injection site is warm and tender. What is the priority nursing action?**

1. Report this immediately to the RN.
2. Hot pack the warm area.
3. Increase the frequency of observations of the site.
4. Document this information on the chart.

1. *No, the RN does not need to know this at this time. You were asked to prioritize; this is not the best answer.*
2. *Incorrect, since this area is already showing signs of increased blood supply and irritation. Hot packs would also require a specific order. Select again.*
3. *Not the best answer. What further information do you expect to gain from increasing site observations? Try again.*
4. ***Good! You realized that this was within normal expectations for the day following the injection, and that the temperature and warmth at the site are the signs of a mild response. It is always appropriate to document assessment findings.***

87. **A newly diagnosed six-year-old diabetic is distressed after his insulin injection. The nurse knows that which play activity would be most therapeutic in helping the child deal with his injection?**

1. A video game.
2. A needleless syringe and a doll.
3. Read a story to him about a child with diabetes.
4. A supervised playtime in the playroom.

1. *No, the question asks "which is the most therapeutic." Look for an activity that is more than a distraction from the pain of the injection.*
2. ***Yes! This is a therapeutic activity, since it will allow the child to act out feelings of anger and helplessness.***
3. *Not the best answer, because it does not allow working out the feelings that the child is unable to verbalize at the age of six. Make another choice.*
4. *Incorrect. This would be correct if the stem had asked you to select a reward for the child's cooperation, but it does not qualify as a therapeutic activity. Look for a response that will help the child deal with the source of his distress. Select again.*

88. **In caring for a preschooler who is being admitted the evening before surgery, the nurse knows that which activity is least appropriate for reducing the stress of hospitalization?**

1. Explaining the surgical procedure.
2. Playing "surgery" with cap and masks.
3. Showing her the call light and bathroom.
4. Having her mother undress her.

1. ***Good work. The evening before surgery is too early to explain the procedure to a***

preschooler.
2. *Wrong choice, this action is an appropriate stress-reducing activity. Play is practice/learning for young children, and this will help prepare the child for the experience of surgery. Select another option.*
3. *Wrong choice, this action is an appropriate stress-reducing activity. The purpose of this nursing action is to increase the client's feelings of security and control, and to provide a safe environment for the client. Choose again.*
4. *Wrong choice, this action is an appropriate stress-reducing activity. The child will feel safe and more comfortable in this "foreign" environment. Also, the mother will feel more capable of nurturing her child. Select again.*

89. **The nurse is caring for a child admitted with a possible diagnosis of celiac disease. The nurse knows that which other disease causes stools that resemble the stools with celiac disease?**

1. Cystic fibrosis.
2. Hirschsprung disease.
3. Intussusception.
4. Crohn's.

1. ***Good work! Steatorrhea, which is bulky, frothy, foul smelling stools, characterize both of these disorders. You need to remember the differences in pathology of these two diseases.***
2. *Wrong. Due to the aganglionic portion of intestine, the stools in Hirschsprung disease are constipated or absent. Make another choice.*
3. *Wrong. The stools in intussusception are red-currant-jelly, due to the mucous and blood. Abdominal pain and spasms are also part of the clinical picture. Choose another option.*
4. *Wrong. The typical stools of children with Crohn's are frequent, watery and diarrheal in consistency. Occult bleeding is also common. Select another option.*

90. **In caring for a child undergoing diagnostic tests, the nurse knows that which tests would be most helpful to aid in the diagnosis of pediatric leukemia?**

1. Blood test by venipuncture.
2. Blood culture.
3. Lumbar puncture.
4. Bone marrow aspiration.

1. *Wrong. Although the presence of blast cells in the CBC will be suspicious of leukemia, this does not provide a definite diagnosis. You are on the right track. Select again.*
2. *Incorrect. This test will be used when infection is suspected, not leukemia.*
3. *Incorrect. A lumbar puncture is used to obtain cerebral spinal fluid. This will be done if the defini-*

tive test for leukemia is positive. The lumbar puncture will tell if there is central nervous system involvement. Choose again.

   4.   ***Good work! Leukemia is a primarily cancer of the blood marrow. A large number of immature white cells are found, and a decreased number of RBCs, platelets, and granulocytes.***

91.   A four-year-old is visiting his brother who is critically ill and may be dying. In talking with this young visitor, the nurse is aware that he would be least likely to believe that death is:

   1.   Like going to sleep.
   2.   The result of magic.
   3.   Permanent and lasting.
   4.   The result of a wish.

   1.   *Wrong choice. Children may frequently make this comparison, since they have little experience with death. This may make it frightening for a preschooler. Select again.*
   2.   *Wrong choice. A child this age may see death as the result of magic, since it is not well understood. Choose again.*
   3.   ***Right. Four-year-olds have difficulty understanding the concept of time and are therefore not likely to believe that death is permanent.***
   4.   *Wrong choice. Preschoolers do believe that their thoughts and wishes can make things happen, since they are egocentric. This is one reason why the death of a family member can be very difficult for a child this age. Select again.*

92.   Anticipatory guidance is given to the parents of a 10-year-old girl. The nurse knows that understanding of this information would be demonstrated by the parents if they say they will reinforce:

   1.   Sex education and self breast exam.
   2.   The need for increased caloric intake.
   3.   The child's increasing need for sleep.
   4.   Fewer dental visits are needed.

   1.   ***Great! This is correct. "Anticipatory guidance" means family/client teaching about the next developmental stage. Since puberty is usually attained between 10 and 12 for females, the most important information is about her developing sexual body.***
   2.   *Incorrect. The most important nutritional information at this age is the need for increased sources of iron. Try another option.*
   3.   *No, sleep requirements diminish from birth to adulthood. This is mainly due to the maturing*

body's ability to get into REM sleep more quickly. Select again.

   4.   *Definitely not! Although permanent teeth are in by this age, this is all the more reason to have regular check-ups and good oral hygiene, which includes brushing and flossing. These habits will help the child keep these teeth for a lifetime. Choose again.*

93.   A child is admitted from the emergency room with a fractured radius. The injury has been splinted. The nurse understands that the expected result of this is:

   1.   Reduced edema in extremity.
   2.   Reduction of the fracture.
   3.   Callus formation at fracture site.
   4.   Reduced pain.

   1.   *Incorrect. Reduction of edema will not happen immediately and is more dependent upon elevation. Try again.*
   2.   *Incorrect. Splinting is the immobilization of the broken fragments. That's all it does. Select another option.*
   3.   *No, callus is the stage of healing where new bone is being formed. Choose again.*
   4.   ***Correct! Splinting is the immobilization of the broken fragments. Pain should decrease after immobilization, since most of the pain related to fractures is from soft tissue trauma.***

94.   The nurse teaches the mother to have syrup of ipecac on hand in case of accidental poisoning. The nurse wants the mother to know when to give ipecac. The mother should be able to state that the correct situation in which to give ipecac is:

   1.   Only upon direction of the poison control center.
   2.   If the label information on the poison says to induce vomiting.
   3.   When the poison was taken within the last two hours.
   4.   By specific age guidelines, followed by one full glass of water.

   1.   ***Great! You picked the correct answer. Although you teach the mother to have the ipecac on hand, she should not give it unless the poison center directs her to give it. Remind her to have the poison control center's phone number where she can easily find it in an emergency.***
   2.   *No, the mother should be taught to consult poison control. Studies have shown that many packaging directions are incorrect. Choose again.*
   3.   *No, time alone is not the deciding factor in the decision to induce vomiting. Pick another option.*
   4.   *No, age is not the deciding factor in the decision to induce vomiting. This could result in potentially*

dangerous outcomes. Reread the question and choose again.

95. A client is being discharged following bilateral vein ligation and stripping. While doing discharge planning, the nurse knows that the most important instruction to give the client is to:

    1. Wear slacks and opaque hose regularly for cosmetic reasons.
    2. Purchase and wear above-the-knee support hose only.
    3. Join a local diet center and lose weight.
    4. Elevate legs above the heart level four times a day for 15-20 minutes.

    1. Incorrect. This certainly can be suggested, but is not necessary.
    2. Incorrect, because above the knee support hose will cause pressure in the popliteal area. Below-the-knee hose are recommended.
    3. Incorrect. The client must be ready to lose weight. The nurse's responsibility includes teaching proper nutrition, not suggesting that the client join a diet center to learn proper nutrition.
    4. Yes! This position is necessary to decrease venous hydrostatic pressure, reduce stasis, and relieve manifestations.

96. The nurse is planning discharge teaching for a client following abdominal surgery. Which of the following instructions about changing dressings in the home would the nurse consider most appropriate?

    1. The appropriate opening of bandages to maintain their sterility.
    2. Information about proper aseptic technique.
    3. Proper gloving technique.
    4. Information about good hand washing technique.

    1. Incorrect. The client is at risk for the transmission of microorganisms that may cause infection. However, very often the home environment does not lend itself to the practice of aseptic technique, so the nurse must help the client improvise with the resources available.
    2. Incorrect. The client is at risk for the transmission of microorganisms that may cause an infection. However, very often the home environment does not lend itself to the practice of aseptic technique, so the nurse must help the client improvise with the resources available.
    3. Incorrect. The client is at risk for the transmission of microorganisms that may cause an infection. However, very often the home environment does not lend itself to the practice of aseptic technique, so the nurse must help the client improvise with the resources available.

    4. Correct! The client is at risk for the transmission of microorganisms that may cause an infection. The home environment may not lend itself to the entire practice of aseptic technique, so the nurse must help the client improvise with the resources available. Hand washing is the most important and most basic technique in preventing and controlling the transmission of pathogens and it should be practiced in every case.

97. A client who has right-sided weakness needs to be transferred from his bed to a wheel chair. In transferring the client, the nurse must remember to:

    1. Keep the client at arm's length while transferring him.
    2. Bend at the waist to get down to his level.
    3. Maintain a straight back and bend at the knees.
    4. Attempt to transfer the client alone, before determining that help is needed.

    1. This is incorrect. When lifting an object or a client, it is important to hold the object or person close to the body, where the base of support is.
    2. The nurse should not bend at the waist, since all of the client's weight will be placed on the back muscle and possibly cause injury to the nurse.
    3. Excellent. A straight back usually limits the amount of weight that is placed on the back muscles. Good body mechanics are essential in preventing injury to the nurse.
    4. If a client or object appears to be too heavy for one person, the nurse should always get help first rather than attempting the lift alone and risk a back injury.

98. When obtaining a urine specimen from an indwelling catheter for culture and sensitivity, the nurse should:

    1. Empty the drainage bag from the urometer port.
    2. Wear sterile gloves.
    3. Cleanse the entry site prior to inserting the needle.
    4. Drain the bag and wait for a fresh urine sample to send from the drainage bag.

    1. Incorrect, try again. The urometer port can only be used to obtain a non-sterile specimen. You cannot obtain a urine culture and sensitivity from this port.
    2. Incorrect. Sterile gloves are unnecessary when obtaining a specimen for culture and sensitivity since the nurse does not disrupt the closed system except with a sterile needle.
    3. Excellent choice! Disinfecting the needle insertion site removes or destroys any microorganisms on the surface of the catheter, thereby avoiding contamination of the needle and entrance of microorganisms into the catheter.

4. Incorrect. Urine obtained from the drainage bag is unsterile because the bag contains microorganisms. Urine from the drainage bag cannot be used for culture and sensitivity.

99. **A three-year-old is being admitted with nephrotic syndrome. In considering the possible roommates for this client, the nurse would most appropriately select:**

1. A 16-year-old postoperative following a ruptured appendix.
2. An eight-year-old with leukemia.
3. A toddler with rheumatic fever.
4. No roommate, because isolation is required.

1. Wrong. The child with nephrotic syndrome is at risk for infection.

2. **Right. This child is not infectious, which is important because a child with nephrotic syndrome is at risk for infection. The roommates may have nothing in common, but the potential for infection is a high priority nursing diagnosis for this admission.**

3. No, this isn't the best choice, since the child with rheumatic fever may still be infectious from the original causative organism.

4. No, it is not necessary to place this child on isolation. Try again.

100. **A confused elderly client is found wandering around the ward wearing a bathrobe and cotton socks. He also is bumping into walls as he walks. What is the priority nursing action?**

1. Take the client's shoes to him and assist him in putting them on.
2. Accompany the client to his room and obtain a baseline assessment.
3. Ask the client to return to his room and rest until he feels better.
4. Tell the client to be careful of any wet spots on the floor.

1. Wrong. In this option, the nurse fails to ensure the client's immediate safety. He is at risk of falling because of ambulating in stocking feet and bumping into walls. This option does not address the issue of the client's bumping into walls at all. Try again.

2. **Excellent! The nurse ensures the client's safety by accompanying him to his room. Assessment is also essential because the client's bumping into walls suggests that oxygenation problems may be interfering with the client's balance and level of consciousness. Good work!**

3. Wrong. In this option, the nurse fails to ensure the client's immediate safety. Also, the nurse does not know that the client feels ill or will feel better later. The nurse needs more information.

4. The question does not tell you anything about wet spots on the floor, and this option does not address the issue of the client's bumping into walls. The nurse must act to provide for the client's immediate safety and the nurse needs more information to determine the cause of the client's behavior.

NOTES

NCLEX-PN

Test 5

NCLEX-PN TEST 5

1. A client has been taking phenytoin (Dilantin) for several years for her epilepsy. She has recently married and wants to start a family. What information should the nurse give her about her medication usage?

    1. Epilepsy should not interfere with her pregnancy or medicine regime.
    2. She will have to be careful about her weight gain while on Dilantin.
    3. There is an increased incidence of birth defects born to mothers who use anticonvulsants.
    4. She will need to increase her dose of Dilantin during her pregnancy.

2. A 51-year-old man is admitted to an alcohol treatment unit. His wife reports that he has been drinking daily for 20 years and recently lost his driver's license for driving while intoxicated. During the admission interview, the client tells the nurse that he is only there because his wife has threatened to leave him if he does not get treatment. He states, "I only have one drink after work each evening." What is the most appropriate nursing response?

    1. "What is your definition of one drink?"
    2. "Are you feeling angry with your wife for insisting you get treatment?"
    3. "If you only have one drink, how did you get a DWI?"
    4. "Do you use any other drugs besides alcohol?"

3. In caring for abused children, the nurse understands that sexual abuse of children:

    1. Is significantly less common than physical abuse and neglect.
    2. Is usually perpetrated by strangers.
    3. Is often repeated from generation to generation.
    4. Occurs primarily in poor and disenfranchised segments of society.

4. In caring for a client who is a victim of spousal abuse, the nurse is guided by the knowledge that:

    1. Although the media tend to report lurid stories of spousal abuse, wife beating is a relatively rare occurrence in modern society.
    2. Most battered women are eager to leave the abusive spouse, and will do so when appropriate social, financial, and legal services are available to them.

    3. Both partners usually accept responsibility for spousal abuse, because they each participate in the cycle of anger that precedes an incident of battering.
    4. The risk of homicide is greatest when the battered spouse leaves the abusive partner or tells him she is thinking of ending the relationship.

5. The 19-year-old son of well-to-do parents is admitted to the psychiatric hospital, under court order, with a diagnosis of antisocial personality disorder. He was arrested with two friends for stealing a car, driving it for several hours, and then pushing it over a cliff. If the diagnosis is correct, the nurse can most realistically expect him to display:

    1. Remorse for stealing and destroying the car.
    2. Anger and rage with the police and court for hospitalizing him against his will.
    3. Withdrawal from others because of shame over his recent actions.
    4. Little responsibility or concern for the predicament he is in.

6. The nurse learns that an obsessive-compulsive client brushes his tongue several times a day, and has developed several ulcerations on it. His nursing care plan should have as its highest initial priority:

    1. The client will eliminate his brushing and mouth care rituals.
    2. The client will verbalize the underlying cause of his behavior.
    3. The client will seek out the nurse when he is feeling anxious.
    4. The client will re-establish healthy tissue in his mouth and tongue.

7. A client on a psychiatric unit is very suspicious of the nursing staff and of other clients. Her nurse would like to establish a therapeutic relationship with her. Which nursing action would promote doing this?

    1. Avoid pressuring the client by waiting for her to initiate interactions with the nurse.
    2. Approach the client frequently during the day for brief interactions.
    3. Set aside a specific time each day to spend with the client.
    4. Approach the client in a friendly manner offering to disclose some personal information so she will

feel she knows the nurse better.

8. **An elderly client is admitted to a long-term care facility. Which of the following nursing measures would be most important in planning his care?**

   1. An explanation of the roles of the registered nurse, practical nurse and the nursing assistant.
   2. An understanding of his routine for his own care at home.
   3. An assessment of his mobility.
   4. An introduction to his health care team members.

9. **A client with a diagnosis of borderline personality disorder has become attached to one of her nurses. One day her favorite nurse phones in sick. When the client is given this news, she goes into her room, breaks a bottle of cologne, and scratches her arm with a jagged piece of glass. After providing first aid, what is the next most therapeutic nursing action in relation to the client's behavior?**

   1. Institute suicide precautions.
   2. Help the client connect her thoughts and feelings to her acting-out behavior.
   3. Telephone the client's favorite nurse to talk with the client.
   4. Permit the client to remain in her room alone to compose herself.

10. **A client with a diagnosis of borderline personality disorder purposely cut herself with a piece of glass when she learned that her favorite nurse had called in sick. The client's favorite nurse returns to the unit and meets with the client to discuss the incident when she cut herself. How can the nurse best prevent future incidents of self-mutilating behavior in this client?**

    1. Emphasize that self-destructive behavior is not acceptable and obtain a written contract from the client stating that she will not harm herself.
    2. Ask the client to make a promise that she will discuss any self-destructive feelings she may have with a staff member.
    3. Assign a staff member to supervise the client's whereabouts at all times.
    4. Point out to the client that she is making increasingly unrealistic demands on the nurse and other staff members.

11. **In caring for rape victims, the nurse knows that rape survivors:**

    1. May experience the hospital and police procedures as further violations of their privacy and integrity.
    2. Usually recover from any emotional manifesta-

tions within a year after the rape.
    3. Rarely require the assistance of rape crisis programs.
    4. May have provoked the attack by being seductive, if they appear calm after the attack.

12. **The nurse diagnoses a client as experiencing rape-trauma syndrome. The client agrees to meet with a clinical nurse specialist for crisis intervention therapy. The primary purpose of crisis intervention is to:**

    1. Assist the client to recognize and gain insight into her feelings.
    2. Help the client learn how her current problems relate to unresolved earlier childhood conflicts and traumas.
    3. Provide long-term therapy to resolve the emotional issues connected with this current event.
    4. Prevent the development of serious psychiatric manifestations.

13. **A client asks the nurse to telephone her husband and ask him if he remembered to pick up his suit at the cleaners. The nurse knows that her husband died five years before. The best nursing response is:**

    1. "It may seem like your husband is still here, but he died five years ago."
    2. "You miss your husband a lot, don't you? It must seem like he's almost here with you."
    3. "You've forgotten that your husband is dead, haven't you?"
    4. "Don't worry. Your husband will remember to pick up his cleaning."

14. **An 84-year-old married man is admitted from his home to a skilled nursing facility with a diagnosis of Alzheimer's disease. While speaking with the admitting nurse, his wife begins to cry and says, "I never thought it would come to this. I feel so guilty bringing him here." Which nursing response is best?**

    1. "You have done all you could. We will take good care of him here."
    2. "This has been a difficult time for you. Let's find a quiet place where we can talk."
    3. "Admitting your husband was the right decision. He requires more care then you can provide at home."
    4. "What are you feeling guilty about?"

15. **A 77-year-old client was hospitalized for observation falling when he was walking for exercise. He is to ambulate for the first time since his fall. He tells the nurse that he is afraid to get up. The most helpful nursing response is:**

1. "There is nothing to be afraid of. The doctor wouldn't have written the order if he didn't think that you were ready."
2. "Tell me what concerns you about getting up today."
3. "I will have another person here to help you when you get up."
4. "Are you afraid of falling again?"

16. **The nurse enters a client's room. The client's son tells the nurse, "You people can't do anything right. Ever since my father was admitted to this hospital, it has been one mistake after another. I am taking him out of here before you kill him." The appropriate response to the son is:**

1. "You feel that your father is not being well taken care of?"
2. "We have the best intentions for the clients."
3. "I'll get the supervisor for you."
4. "Your father hasn't complained about the care. What specifically is the problem?"

17. **A client has been told by the doctor that he has cancer and that it has advanced so far that treatment will not help. When the nurse comes to help him with his bath, he says to the nurse, "I'm not an invalid, you know! I can take care of myself. Get out and leave me alone." How should the nurse respond?**

1. "I know that you are not an invalid. However, I was trying to help you."
2. "It sounds to me like you are angry about something. Did somebody do something wrong?"
3. "You are pretty upset. Let's talk about it."
4. "I'll just set up this equipment for you to bathe and come back later when you're not so angry."

18. **The nurse tells a client that the doctor has ordered an intravenous line to be started. The client appears to be upset but says nothing. What should the nurse say?**

1. "Do you have any questions about the procedure?"
2. "The doctor wants you to have antibiotics, and this method eliminates getting frequent injections."
3. "What is there about this procedure that concerns you?"
4. "It only hurts a little bit. It'll be over before you know it."

19. **A client tells the nurse that his name is not spelled right on his identification bracelet. The nurse should:**

1. Tell the client that as long as his medical record numbers are correct, the mistake is not a problem.
2. Ask the client for the correct spelling and change his medical records.
3. Notify the admitting office of the error and obtain a correct identification bracelet for the client.
4. Notify the physician.

20. **The nurse is to administer an intramuscular injection. The most important action by the nurse to prevent introduction of the medication into the venous system is to:**

1. Inject the medication slowly to allow for slow absorption.
2. Insert the needle at a 45-degree angle where there are fewer blood vessels.
3. Use the Z track method of injection.
4. Aspirate the drug after insertion of needle.

21. **The nurse is caring for an elderly client who is often unsteady while walking. Which nursing measure is most important in providing for the safety of such a client?**

1. Wipe up spills immediately.
2. Make crutches or canes available for the elderly clients.
3. Raise the side rails on the bed.
4. Assist all elderly clients when ambulating.

22. **When collecting a urine specimen for a routine urinalysis, which of the following nursing actions is the most important?**

1. Label the container with the client's room number.
2. Check the identification of the client.
3. Do not use gloves when handling a urine specimen.
4. Instruct the client to put the specimen on the counter at the nurses' station for pick up.

23. **A client is admitted to the hospital for evaluation of inadequate circulation to her lower extremities. The doctor orders a tub bath at the client's request. In assisting the client with her bath, which action would be unsafe?**

1. Place a rubber mat on the bottom of the tub.
2. Fill the tub approximately half full.
3. When the client steps into the tub, ask her if the water is the right temperature for her.
4. Obtain all of the supplies necessary for the bath and place them within easy reach of the client.

24. **A client is to be up in a chair three times a day. He is paralyzed from the waist down. What is the best nursing approach when transferring this client from a bed into a wheel chair?**

1. Place the wheel chair close to the foot of the bed.
2. Utilize the principles of body mechanics while providing a safe transfer for the client.
3. Slide the client to the edge of the bed, keeping the nurse's back straight and using a rocking motion to pull the client.
4. Place the nurse's arms under the client's axillae from the back of the client.

25. **Of the following information, which should be recorded first in the client's record by the nurse admitting the client?**

    1. The client's vital signs.
    2. The plan that was developed for the care of the client while in the hospital.
    3. Nursing actions performed for the client.
    4. Assessment of the client.

26. **While preparing to give a morning medication, the first nursing action is to:**

    1. Read the label.
    2. Check for the right dose.
    3. Wash hands.
    4. Check for the right time.

27. **The client is very confused and combative. The physician orders the client to be placed in a jacket restraint and wrist restraints. In order to prevent injury to the client with restraints, the most important nursing action is to:**

    1. Explain the procedure and reason for the restraints to the client and the family.
    2. Remove the restraints and observe the extremities for circulation at least every four hours.
    3. Tell the client that if he is more cooperative the restraints will not be necessary.
    4. Document the use of restraints in the chart.

28. **A client is in the intensive care unit and is in a coma as a result of a head injury. The most important nursing action in performing mouth care on this client is to:**

    1. Turn the client to her side before starting mouth care.
    2. Use a soft toothbrush.
    3. Use a mouth bite to keep her mouth open.
    4. Wear gloves.

29. **Restraints may be used to immobilize a client, or the client's extremity. The nurse understands that it is inconsistent with proper restraint functionality to use a restraint to:**

    1. Prevent a client from pulling out an IV or other type of therapy.

    2. Reduce the risk to all elderly clients from falling out of bed or off a chair.
    3. Prevent removal of life support equipment.
    4. Prevent injury to health care personnel by combative clients.

30. **A client has just been admitted to the hospital. In showing the client how to use the call system, the nurse understands that which of the following statements is incorrect?**

    1. The call system allows the client to signal for help.
    2. The call system should be limited to use in emergencies.
    3. The client should be able to reach the call button easily.
    4. The client should be taught how to use the call system.

31. **An ambulatory client is being readied for bed. The nursing action that promotes safety for this client is:**

    1. Turning off all of the lights to help promote sleep and rest.
    2. Instructing the client in the use of the call bell.
    3. Putting the side rail up.
    4. Placing the bed in the high position.

32. **An infant with AIDS is being prepared for discharge. The nurse is instructing the grandmother, who will care for the infant, in methods of home care. Which statement, made by the grandmother, represents the greatest hazard to successful home maintenance?**

    1. "I know that hand washing is an important preventive measure."
    2. "I'll use disposable diapers, discarding them in separate plastic bags."
    3. "Blood spills should be washed up immediately with hot soapy water."
    4. "Gloves should be worn by whomever changes the baby's diapers."

33. **While preparing to give a client a bed bath, which nursing action is appropriate?**

    1. Place the bed in the lowest position.
    2. Expose the top side of the body and wash and dry quickly; then do the same on the posterior side.
    3. Gather all of the articles necessary for the bath and place them within easy reach of the nurse during the bath.
    4. Use firm, scrubbing strokes to remove dirt and bacteria.

34. **While getting an elderly client, who is very weak, out of bed, the best nursing approach is:**

1. Locking the wheels of the bed.
2. Placing the equipment in such a way as to provide the safest transfer that is possible for the client.
3. Aligning the wheel chair as close to the bed as possible, to prevent the client from falling to the floor.
4. Removing the wheel chair's leg support on the side closest to the bed.

35. **A client is to receive an IM injection of penicillin (Wycillin). In preparing this medication, the best nursing approach is to:**

1. Use a sterile syringe and needle.
2. Provide for the safety of the client by using the proper equipment and aseptic technique.
3. Prepare the skin site with an antiseptic swab, moving from the center of the site outward.
4. Prevent contamination of the needle by not allowing it to touch any contaminated surfaces.

36. **A client is entering menopause and is identified as at risk for osteoporosis. In instructing this client in preventive measures, the nurse knows that osteoporosis is best prevented in the menopausal woman by:**

1. Avoidance of all exercise.
2. Estrogen replacement therapy.
3. Drinking one glass of red wine daily.
4. Limiting calcium intake.

37. **A client, admitted with hypertension, is taking furosemide (Lasix) 40 mg. PO twice a day. Which of the following interventions, if included in the plan of care by the nurse, would require further clarification?**

1. Daily weights before breakfast.
2. Monitor intake and output.
3. Orthostatic blood pressure checks every eight hours.
4. Limit fluid intake to 1ml. in 24 hours.

38. **The nurse is caring for a client on the second postoperative day following a cesarean section for a breech. She has a vertical incision into the abdomen. She asks if she will need to have a cesarean birth with her future pregnancies. What is the nurse's best reply?**

1. "I will need to check your operative record before I can answer that."
2. "Because your incision is classical, future labor could be unsafe."
3. "As long as you your next baby comes head first, you can safely deliver vaginally."
4. "It is impossible to predict at this time. Let's wait until the next pregnancy occurs."

39. **When the nurse assesses a client on the first postpartum day, the findings are: fundus firm, one fingerbreadth below and to the right of the umbilicus, lochia rubra with small clots, temperature 99.2° F, pulse rate 52. The appropriate nursing action is to:**

1. Report the lochia to the charge nurse.
2. Report the temperature to the charge nurse.
3. Report the pulse rate to the charge nurse.
4. Ask the client when she last voided.

40. **The nurse caring for a client in the first hour following delivery is having difficulty taking her blood pressure because the client is shaking uncontrollably. What nursing intervention is indicated at this time?**

1. Call the charge nurse immediately to come in to assess the client.
2. Give the client a warm blanket.
3. Check to be sure there is a padded tongue blade readily available.
4. Take the client's temperature immediately.

41. **When meperidine (Demerol) is given to a laboring woman, the nurse should be prepared to treat:**

1. Maternal hyperventilation.
2. Neonatal depression.
3. Maternal hypertension.
4. Neonatal hypoglycemia.

42. **While caring for the client who is having an induction of labor with oxytocin (Pitocin), which nursing assessment is indicated?**

1. Blood pressure every five minutes.
2. Maternal temperature every hour.
3. Maternal contraction pattern every hour.
4. Continuous fetal heart rate monitoring.

43. **In the first hours postpartum, which behavior would the nurse expect to see in a new mother?**

1. Upset because her lunch is late.
2. Asking many questions about infant care.
3. Eagerly unwrapping the baby and attempting to engage the baby in play.
4. Confidently providing all infant care.

44. **The nurse should know the recommended frequency for mammogram testing is:**

1. Yearly for all females over age 20.
2. Baseline at puberty, every two years thereafter until age 50, and then yearly.
3. At least every two years between ages 40-49.
4. Baseline at age 25, then yearly thereafter.

45. The nurse knows that which of the following statements by a client warrants further teaching about self breast exam (SBE)?

    1. "SBE is very important for early detection of breast cancer."
    2. "As long as I have a mammogram every year, SBE is not necessary."
    3. "I will do SBE each month on the last day of my menses."
    4. "Comparing one breast against the other is part of regular SBE."

46. The nurse is teaching a client how to take her basal body temperature (BBT) as a method of birth control. Which statement by the client indicates to the nurse that further teaching is needed?

    1. "I will take my temperature every morning before I get out of bed."
    2. "When my body temperature rises, it means I should not have intercourse for the next three days."
    3. "It is important that I do not shake the thermometer in the morning before I take my temperature."
    4. "I will get a BBT thermometer to take my temperature."

47. A 10-month-old is admitted following a febrile seizure. The mother is very upset because of the seizure. What information should the nurse provide to the mother?

    1. This will probably never happen again.
    2. Febrile seizures are a lifelong disorder.
    3. The seizure is related to fever and can be treated.
    4. An anticonvulsant, perhaps phenobarbital, will be ordered to prevent further seizures.

48. In determining the care for a child admitted with a probable diagnosis of Hirschsprung disease (megacolon), the nurse would plan to prepare the child for:

    1. A barium enema.
    2. A sweat chloride test.
    3. A flat plate of the abdomen.
    4. Occult blood in stool specimen.

49. The day after abdominal surgery, a 10-year-old girl is lying quietly in bed when the nurse makes rounds. The last rounds were made four hours ago, and she was last medicated six hours ago. At this time, the nurse should first:

    1. Encourage her to turn, cough, and deep breathe.
    2. Assess the need for pain medication.

    3. Ambulate her to the door.
    4. Ask her if she is hungry, and provide fluids.

50. Which nursing intervention would be the most helpful in prevention of a stress ulcer related to a burn in a three-year-old child?

    1. Instruct on relaxation exercises.
    2. Administer cimetidine (Tagamet) as ordered.
    3. Administer meperidine (Demerol) as ordered.
    4. Initiate a bland diet.

51. A child is in Buck's traction. To prevent complications, the nurse should:

    1. Clean pin sites every shift as ordered.
    2. Encourage foods that are high in calcium.
    3. Provide small meals with high fiber.
    4. Limit range of motion in all extremities.

52. A BRAT diet is prescribed for a child with gastroenteritis. Which food should be removed by the nurse from the child's tray?

    1. Ice cream.
    2. Popsicle.
    3. Banana.
    4. Applesauce.

53. The nurse knows that which of the following behaviors would indicate regression in a hospitalized five-year-old?

    1. Bedwetting several times a day.
    2. Crying when mother leaves.
    3. Eating only food from home.
    4. Wanting his teddy bear for bedtime.

54. The nurse is evaluating the degree of bonding between a mother and her infant, who has been hospitalized for a high bilirubin. To collect this data the nurse would:

    1. Ask the mother how she feels about her baby.
    2. Provide a cot so that the mother can stay with the infant.
    3. Observe the mother feeding the infant.
    4. Find out if the pregnancy of this infant was planned.

55. A child is admitted with suspected Reye's syndrome. The parents tell the nurse that he was sick a week before this admission. The nurse knows that which of the following diseases would influence the child's present condition?

    1. Rheumatic fever.
    2. Diphtheria.

3.   Chicken pox.
4.   Bacterial meningitis.

56.   **A two-year-old is admitted with laryngotracheal bronchitis and is placed in a cool mist tent. The direct result of the mist tent that the nurse would expect to observe is:**

1.   Improved hydration.
2.   Decreased stridor.
3.   Diminished output.
4.   Normal temperature.

57.   **A six-week-old is returned from the operating room after repair of a pyloric stenosis. What data would the nurse most depend on for evaluating this client's need for pain control?**

1.   Physiologic responses.
2.   Behavioral changes.
3.   Response to medication.
4.   Mother's assessment.

58.   **The nurse teaches the newborn's mother to speak to the baby while making eye contact. If this is done, the nurse can expect that the child will display:**

1.   Decreased crying.
2.   Improved fine motor skills.
3.   Diminished extrusion reflex.
4.   Increased social behaviors.

59.   **A nine-year-old girl is admitted with asthma. In planning her care, the nurse should anticipate that the child will prefer to:**

1.   Play with another girl her age.
2.   Be with older girls.
3.   Associate with small groups of boys and girls.
4.   Have male companions.

60.   **Which of the following statements made by a client indicate the need for further teaching regarding a scheduled arthroscopy of the knee?**

1.   "I know the doctor will be looking at the joint to check for cartilage damage."
2.   "I'll have to limit my exercising for a few weeks after this procedure."
3.   "I hope the incision heals quickly with those staples in place."
4.   "I know that I'll have to keep my knee straight and elevated to reduce the swelling after the surgery."

61.   **CPR has been initiated on a client in the emergency room. Which finding by the nurse would indicate effective cardiac compressions?**

1.   An EKG pattern with each compression.
2.   Compression depth of 1 1/2 to 2 inches.
3.   A palpable femoral pulse during each compression.
4.   Pupils changing from pinpoint to dilated.

62.   **Following a colostomy, a client and his wife have been taught to perform a colostomy irrigation. Which behavior by the client would best indicate readiness for discharge?**

1.   The client's wife verbalizes all steps in the irrigation procedure.
2.   The client performs the irrigation following written instructions.
3.   The client and his wife attend all classes given about colostomy care.
4.   The client asks appropriate questions about irrigations.

63.   **The client returns with a Foley catheter after surgery. In providing catheter care, which is the best nursing approach?**

1.   Preventing infection and maintaining a patent catheter and drainage system.
2.   Keeping the collection bag above the level of the bladder.
3.   Using soap and water to clean the perineal area.
4.   Maintaining a closed system without any kinks in the tubing.

64.   **An elderly client is admitted to the hospital for prostatic hypertrophy. The nurse places the bed in the low position and puts the call light within easy reach. He is scheduled to have surgery in the morning. The most important nursing action during the admission of this client is to:**

1.   Explain the surgical procedure to the client and family.
2.   Explain to the client how to use his call light if he needs the nurse.
3.   Tell the client and his family about visiting regulations.
4.   Teach the client how to deep breathe and cough.

65.   **A client who is incontinent of stool has been placed on a bowel training program. The nurse understands that the goal of bowel training is to:**

1.   Prevent soiling of the bed.
2.   Prevent cancer of the colon.
3.   Prevent loose stools.
4.   Provide the client with control over his bowels.

66. **A client is scheduled for surgery on his bowel. The doctor orders a cleansing enema for the morning of surgery. The best nursing approach is to:**

    1. Wear gloves to insert the tubing.
    2. Use universal precautions and provide comfort measures to help the client relax during the procedure.
    3. Lubricate the tubing well prior to insertion.
    4. Position the client on his side and drape the client for warmth and privacy.

67. **A client is hospitalized for a closed reduction of a fractured femur and application of a cast. A vital nursing action in the care of this client is to:**

    1. Perform neurovascular checks of the extremities.
    2. Use the palms of the hands when moving an extremity with a wet cast.
    3. Provide an instrument for the client to scratch the itching areas of skin under the cast.
    4. Petal the edges of the cast to provide smooth edges.

68. **A client is admitted to the hospital for cataract surgery of the left eye. The physician has ordered eye drops to be administered to both eyes at frequent intervals prior to surgery. Which nursing action is most appropriate?**

    1. Use aseptic technique and avoid dropping the medication onto the cornea.
    2. Gently wash away any crust along the eyelid margin with warm water.
    3. Have the client look up toward the ceiling prior to instillation of drops.
    4. Drop prescribed number of drops into the conjunctival sac.

69. **A client, who says she has the flu, is seen in the clinic with complaints of vomiting, diarrhea, headache, and dizziness. The nurse takes her vital signs and obtains the following: Blood pressure of 198/110, pulse of 82, respirations of 24 and temperature of 100.8° F. The nurse should immediately report which finding?**

    1. Complaints of vomiting.
    2. Complaints of diarrhea.
    3. Complaints of headache and dizziness.
    4. Temperature of 100.8° F.

70. **A client shows the nurse the result of his recent tuberculin skin test. The site is red and swollen. The nurse interprets this as:**

    1. The client has active tuberculosis.
    2. The client has a history of tuberculosis.
    3. The tubercle bacillus is in the active pulmonary stage.

4. The client has had contact with the tubercle bacillus.

71. **The nurse is caring for a client who had abdominal surgery two days ago. The nurse should be most concerned about which finding?**

    1. A urinary drainage bag with 100 ccs of straw colored urine.
    2. A wound dressing with thick light green drainage.
    3. A blood pressure reading of 98/66.
    4. Shallow respirations, with a rate of 30.

72. **An elderly client is discharged from the hospital after treatment for poor circulation to her lower extremities. The nurse would consider it an indication that discharge teaching was unsuccessful if the client:**

    1. Puts on stockings with elastic tops and tells the nurse that she does not like other kinds of hosiery.
    2. Tells the nurse that she will get a thermometer to measure the temperature of the bath water.
    3. Asks her husband to take her sandals home, and bring a pair of shoes to the hospital for her to wear home.
    4. The client tells the nurse that she is going to have to remember to keep her legs uncrossed.

73. **A client, age 63, is being discharged after insertion of a pacemaker for a persistent dysrhythmia. Which statement by the client indicates the need for further teaching by the nurse?**

    1. "I know that I have to check my pulse every day, preferably in the morning."
    2. "I sure will miss being able to continue with my bowling league. I guess I'll take up walking as a sport!"
    3. "I'll stay away from my microwave oven so that it doesn't interfere with my pacemaker."
    4. "If I start having any palpitations or dizziness, I'll call my doctor right away."

74. **A client diagnosed with urolithiasis is advised to follow a low calcium diet after his pathology report reveals calcium oxalate stones. Which menu selection by the client indicates to the nurse the need for further teaching?**

    1. Hamburger, baked potato, squash.
    2. Shrimp, scalloped potatoes, broccoli.
    3. Chicken, wild rice, green beans.
    4. Roast pork, whipped potatoes, carrots.

75. **A 72-year-old client was admitted to the hospital for pneumonia. He is receiving oxygen at six liters per mask. In obtaining his vital signs, it would be inappro-**

priate for the nurse to:

1. Take an axillary temperature.
2. Listen to his lungs when counting respirations.
3. Listen to an apical heart rate.
4. Take an oral temperature.

76. **The client is admitted with anorexia nervosa. A nasogastric tube is to be inserted. In preparing the client for this procedure, what would the nurse do first?**

1. Assist the client to a sitting position.
2. Explain the procedure to the client.
3. If the client has dentures, make sure that they are in place in the client's mouth.
4. Have a stethoscope available to listen for proper placement.

77. **A client fell at home and fractured her hip. She is to have surgery in the morning. In preparing the client for surgery, it is outside the scope of the nurse's responsibilities to:**

1. Assess the health status of the client.
2. Explain the operative procedure and any risks that may be involved with the procedure.
3. Determine that the history, physical, and specific laboratory tests have been ordered or completed according to hospital protocol.
4. Determine that a signed surgical consent form is completed.

78. **A client is scheduled for an abdominal hysterectomy. In order to prevent pneumonia from developing postoperatively, the most important nursing action is:**

1. Teach the client how to deep breathe and cough before surgery.
2. Inform the client that even though she will have pain after surgery, she will have to move from side to side in bed.
3. Tell the client that if she does not ambulate soon after surgery that there is a good chance that she may develop complications.
4. Tell the client that it is very important that she deep breathe and cough often after surgery to prevent complications.

79. **An obese client has been placed on a high protein, low calorie diet by his physician. It would be most important for the nurse to explain to the client:**

1. That he will have to change his eating habits.
2. The importance of exercise when dieting.
3. What types of foods are permitted on a low calorie, high protein diet.
4. That if he doesn't stay on this diet he will continue to gain weight.

80. **In obtaining a blood pressure measurement, the most appropriate nursing action is to:**

1. Obtain the proper equipment, place the client in a comfortable position, and record the appropriate information in the client's chart.
2. Measure the client's arm, if you are uncertain of the size of cuff to use.
3. Have the client recline or sit comfortably in a chair with the forearm at the level of the heart.
4. Document the measurement, which extremity was used, and the position that the client was in during the measurement.

81. **A client has just returned to her room after abdominal surgery. She has a nasogastric tube in place and a drain attached to a HemoVac. The Foley catheter is draining clear yellow urine. The nurse understands the reason for maintaining the side rails in the raised position is to:**

1. Prevent the urine collection bag and tubing from getting tangled up in the side rails when the client is turned in bed.
2. Prevent the client from falling out of bed after receiving an anesthetic.
3. Provide a place to attach the nasogastric tubing to prevent it from being dislodged.
4. Attach the call light so it is within easy reach.

82. **An elderly client was admitted to the hospital with a cerebrovascular accident with left-sided paralysis. He is placed on an air mattress. The nurse explains to the family that the purpose of frequently turning this client is to:**

1. Prevent sensory deprivation by varying what the client sees in his environment.
2. Prevent skin breakdown, which is a common problem in the elderly.
3. Prevent stasis of blood in the lower extremities.
4. Increase blood supply to the affected side.

83. **In caring for elderly clients the nurse understands that the aging process generally results in:**

1. A decline in physiological and sensory systems of the body.
2. A decreased skin resilience.
3. A diminished hearing acuity.
4. An absence of sexual interest and activity.

84. **A client had a cholecystectomy three days ago. Which diet modification would the nurse include in the client's plan of care?**

1. Low fat diet, gradually progressing to moderate fat if tolerated.

2. Low sodium, low fat diet.
3. Elimination of red meat.
4. Elimination of dairy products.

85. **Nursing care of the client with glomerulonephritis includes administering:**

1. Antibiotics, corticosteroids and anticoagulants.
2. Vitamin K and hypoglycemic agents.
3. Immunoglobulins and antibiotics.
4. Vasodilators and cardiotonic glycosides.

86. **Nursing management of the client with Addison's disease, who is experiencing Addisonian crisis, includes which nursing action?**

1. Maintain the restriction of fluids.
2. Encourage a low protein, low carbohydrate diet.
3. Teach effective daily exercises.
4. Weigh the client daily and monitor intake and output.

87. **An elderly client tripped on some stairs and injured her right hip. She underwent a total hip replacement. In caring for this client in the immediate postoperative period, the nurse knows it would be inappropriate to:**

1. Maintain immobilization of the right hip.
2. Encourage fluid intake to prevent dehydration.
3. Observe for signs of thrombus formation.
4. Perform all of the client's personal care activities.

88. **A client is being prepared for an MRI (Magnetic Resonance Imaging) of the spinal column. Prior to the procedure, the nurse should instruct the client to:**

1. Remain as motionless as possible during the procedure.
2. Refrain from eating.
3. Request a sleeping pill.
4. Take an enema.

89. **The nurse is teaching a class on diabetes mellitus. The nurse explains that differences between childhood and adult onset diabetes mellitus include:**

1. Insulin therapy is frequently used in childhood diabetes, and oral hypoglycemic drugs often are used in the management of adult onset diabetes.
2. The onset in childhood diabetes is insidious, while the onset in an adult diabetes is rapid.
3. The use of dietary treatment for childhood diabetes is adequate, while it is inadequate for treatment of adult onset diabetes.
4. The incidence of hypoglycemia and ketoacidosis is infrequent in children and more common with adult onset diabetes.

90. **A client is scheduled for a colostomy after being diagnosed with cancer of the large intestine. The nurse should begin client teaching:**

1. Postoperatively, after the pain has subsided, when the client will be better able to concentrate.
2. Postoperatively, after meeting with the ostomy nurse.
3. When the client demonstrates an interest in learning about the ostomy.
4. Preoperatively, to involve the client in his care and give him a sense of control over his life.

91. **The physician requests a stool specimen for culture, for an alert and ambulatory client. The nurse would give which directions to the client for proper stool collection?**

1. Restrict food and liquids the night before the collection.
2. Maintain a sterile procedure.
3. Require the collection of specimens on three consecutive days.
4. Retrieve from the toilet with sterile gloves and then place in the container.

92. **The nurse is to prepare a client for a proctosigmoidoscopy. The proper position for this client is the:**

1. Left lateral (left side) or knee chest.
2. Right lateral (right side).
3. Dorsal recumbent position (back-lying).
4. Prone position (abdomen).

93. **A client is hospitalized for gastrointestinal bleeding and is being treated with temazepam (Restoril). After the client's physician examines him, the nurse notes the physician has written an order for the client to begin taking amitriptyline (Elavil). Which action by the nurse is best initially?**

1. Revise his medication schedule so that Elavil is administered during the day and the Restoril at night.
2. Monitor the client's vital signs closely.
3. Question the physician about administering both Elavil and Restoril to the client.
4. Assess the client for manifestations of depression.

94. **A client is taking erythromycin delayed-release capsules (Eryc) for a urinary tract infection. By the fourth day of a 10-day treatment, he tells the nurse he's fine now and will keep the remainder of his medicine for another infection. The appropriate nursing response is:**

1. "Good idea, you will save lots of money that way."
2. "You should always take the full course of antibiotics because it is still possible for many of the bacteria to be in your urinary tract."
3. "Take at least one more day of medication."
4. "That would really be a stupid thing to do."

95. **On the third day of amoxicillin (Amoxil) therapy, a client develops diarrhea. The nurse should instruct the client to:**

    1. Stop taking the drug, as this is an indication of toxicity.
    2. Contact her physician about treatment of the diarrhea.
    3. Drink extra liquids to compensate for the fluid lost in the diarrhea.
    4. Take an over-the-counter antidiarrheal agent according to package directions.

96. **In order to minimize the most common side effect of tetracycline therapy, the nurse should instruct the client to:**

    1. Drink at least 2000 ml of fluid a day.
    2. Take the medicine with a full glass of water.
    3. Take the medicine with milk or an antacid.
    4. Increase the intake of high fiber foods and roughage.

97. **A client is taking propranolol (Inderal) for hypertension. The nurse reviewing the client's history knows that the use of Inderal may be contraindicated by:**

    1. "Smoker's" cough.
    2. Sinusitis.
    3. Asthma
    4. Hay fever.

98. **A client diagnosed with emphysema is being prepared for discharge. Which nursing measure would be most beneficial for improving his gas exchange?**

    1. Teaching home oxygen therapy at five liters/minute.
    2. Encouraging him to take slow, deep breaths.
    3. Demonstrating the proper technique for chest breathing.
    4. Teaching him pursed lip breathing.

99. **The client is being discharged after diagnosis of a peptic ulcer. To help to decrease acid secretions in the stomach, the nurse should instruct the client to:**

    1. Increase intake of milk and cream products.
    2. Limit alcohol consumption.
    3. Avoid high fiber foods.
    4. Eat a bland diet; decaffeinated coffee only.

100. **A four-year-old is admitted to the hospital with croup. When the mother comes to visit the next day, she finds the nurse changing the bedding after the client has wet the bed. The mother says, "He never wets the bed at home. I am so embarrassed." Which nursing response is most helpful to the mother?**

    1. "I know this can really be embarrassing, but I have kids myself, so I understand and it doesn't bother me."
    2. "It is not uncommon for children to regress during a hospitalization. His toileting skills will return when he is feeling better."
    3. "It's probably due to the medication we are giving him for his infection."
    4. "I plan to discuss your child's incontinency with the physician, as this may require further investigation."

NOTES

NCLEX-PN

Test 5

Questions with Rationales

NCLEX-PN TEST 5 WITH RATIONALES

1. A client has been taking phenytoin (Dilantin) for several years for her epilepsy. She has recently married and wants to start a family. What information should the nurse give her about her medication usage?

   1. Epilepsy should not interfere with her pregnancy or medicine regime.
   2. She will have to be careful about her weight gain while on Dilantin.
   3. There is an increased incidence of birth defects born to mothers who use anticonvulsants.
   4. She will need to increase her dose of Dilantin during her pregnancy.

   1. *This is incorrect. There is evidence that pregnant women who take Dilantin have a greater risk for infants with birth defects. Choose again.*
   2. *Wrong! Dilantin has no bearing on weight gain. Try again.*
   3. **Correct! Birth defects are more common when the mother uses Dilantin, and this needs to be communicated to the client.**
   4. *This is incorrect. Dilantin would not be increased, due to the greater likelihood of birth defects.*

2. A 51-year-old man is admitted to an alcohol treatment unit. His wife reports that he has been drinking daily for 20 years and recently lost his driver's license for driving while intoxicated. During the admission interview, the client tells the nurse that he is only there because his wife has threatened to leave him if he does not get treatment. He states, "I only have one drink after work each evening." What is the most appropriate nursing response?

   1. "What is your definition of one drink?"
   2. "Are you feeling angry with your wife for insisting you get treatment?"
   3. "If you only have one drink, how did you get a DWI?"
   4. "Do you use any other drugs besides alcohol?"

   1. **Correct. Estimating the client's alcohol consumption is necessary to determine how best to manage his withdrawal. The admitting nurse must ask the details of his alcohol use, including what he drinks, how much, how often, and whether he abuses other substances besides alcohol. Some individuals could define one drink as a 12-ounce glass of bourbon.**
   2. *This is not an inappropriate question to ask this client, who is denying that he needs treatment,*

   but the client's feelings about his wife are not the issue in this question. The nurse needs to respond to the client's statement, and obtain additional information needed to determine how best to manage his withdrawal. Try again.
   3. *This response is not professional! With this question, the nurse is requiring an explanation, which is not therapeutic. This question would most likely elicit a defensive or argumentative response from the client, who denies that he has a drinking problem.*
   4. *This is a good question to ask while taking a substance abuse history, but it is not the best response at this time. The nurse should respond to the client's statement.*

3. In caring for abused children, the nurse understands that sexual abuse of children:

   1. Is significantly less common than physical abuse and neglect.
   2. Is usually perpetrated by strangers.
   3. Is often repeated from generation to generation.
   4. Occurs primarily in poor and disenfranchised segments of society.

   1. *This is not a true statement. Reports of cases of sexual abuse are increasing, with an estimated one million children per year sexually abused. The rate of sexual abuse is similar to that of other types of abuse in children.*
   2. *This is not true. Sexual abuse is most often perpetrated by family members or other adults who know the child well.*
   3. **Correct. Sexual abuse of children occurs in families with long-standing relationship problems. Often there has been a multigenerational pattern of abuse on both sides of the family.**
   4. *This is not correct. Sexual abuse of children occurs throughout all segments of society, and is not associated with any particular socioeconomic or ethnic group.*

4. In caring for a client who is a victim of spousal abuse, the nurse is guided by the knowledge that:

   1. Although the media tend to report lurid stories of spousal abuse, wife beating is a relatively rare occurrence in modern society.
   2. Most battered women are eager to leave the abusive spouse, and will do so when appropriate social, financial, and legal services are available to them.

3. Both partners usually accept responsibility for spousal abuse, because they each participate in the cycle of anger that precedes an incident of battering.

4. The risk of homicide is greatest when the battered spouse leaves the abusive partner or tells him she is thinking of ending the relationship.

1. This is not accurate. It is estimated that each year about six million wives are abused by their husbands in this country. Domestic homicide (the murder of one spouse by the other) accounts for 15 to 20 percent of all homicides.

2. This is not accurate. Most battered wives have ambivalent feelings about their domestic situation. Loyalty and affection may often sustain the hope that things will get better. Women who are emotionally and financially dependent on their spouses may be reluctant to leave the relationship, especially if they also have dependent children.

3. This is not accurate. Abusers tend to refuse to accept responsibility for their actions by blaming the victims, and many abused wives accept blame for the abuse because of their low self-esteem.

4. Correct. Spouses who are battered are in high risk situations that become worse when they threaten to leave, because the violence is part of a system of coercive control. Nursing intervention consists of helping to empower the victim, by assisting her to explore her options and mobilize any needed support services, so that when she leaves the abusive situation she can do so safely.

5. The 19-year-old son of well-to-do parents is admitted to the psychiatric hospital, under court order, with a diagnosis of antisocial personality disorder. He was arrested with two friends for stealing a car, driving it for several hours, and then pushing it over a cliff. If the diagnosis is correct, the nurse can most realistically expect him to display:

1. Remorse for stealing and destroying the car.
2. Anger and rage with the police and court for hospitalizing him against his will.
3. Withdrawal from others because of shame over his recent actions.
4. Little responsibility or concern for the predicament he is in.

1. This is not correct. Clients with antisocial behavior usually display a sense of entitlement, and rarely express any remorse for their illegal or unethical actions.

2. This is a possibility, but it is not the correct option.

Clients with antisocial behavior rarely seek psychiatric treatment of their own volition. Most hospitalizations result from the client choosing treatment over incarceration in jail. There is a better answer, keep looking!

3. This is not correct. Clients with antisocial behavior do not view their own behavior objectively, and rarely experience any anxiety or guilt over their actions.

4. Correct. The most common response of clients with antisocial behavior is a lack of concern about their situation, as well as an absence of sensitivity to the feelings of persons they may have harmed.

6. The nurse learns that an obsessive-compulsive client brushes his tongue several times a day, and has developed several ulcerations on it. His nursing care plan should have as its highest initial priority:

1. The client will eliminate his brushing and mouth care rituals.
2. The client will verbalize the underlying cause of his behavior.
3. The client will seek out the nurse when he is feeling anxious.
4. The client will re-establish healthy tissue in his mouth and tongue.

1. This is not correct. This option is the goal of his treatment, but it is not the highest initial priority.

2. This goal may or may not be appropriate, as behavioral methods will most likely be used to treat his problems. This is not the correct response, however, because it is not the highest initial priority.

3. This is an appropriate goal, but is not the highest initial priority for his care.

4. Correct. Restoring physiological integrity is the highest initial priority for this client. This will be done while working on the long-term goal of decreasing the mouth care rituals.

7. A client on a psychiatric unit is very suspicious of the nursing staff and of other clients. Her nurse would like to establish a therapeutic relationship with her. Which nursing action would promote doing this?

1. Avoid pressuring the client by waiting for her to initiate interactions with the nurse.
2. Approach the client frequently during the day for brief interactions.
3. Set aside a specific time each day to spend with the client.
4. Approach the client in a friendly manner offering to disclose some personal information so she will feel she knows the nurse better.

1. *The nurse is not demonstrating trustworthiness by waiting for the client to initiate the interaction. This is not correct.*
2. *This approach might be effective. However, there is a better option.*
3. **Correct. To promote a therapeutic relationship, it is best to set aside a specific time for the nurse and client to meet together. It is also important that the nurse be consistent in order to earn the client's trust.**
4. *This approach is promoting a social relationship and is not appropriate if the nurse's goal is to form a therapeutic relationship.*

8. **An elderly client is admitted to a long-term care facility. Which of the following nursing measures would be most important in planning his care?**

   1. An explanation of the roles of the registered nurse, practical nurse and the nursing assistant.
   2. An understanding of his routine for his own care at home.
   3. An assessment of his mobility.
   4. An introduction to his health care team members.

   1. *The question focuses on the most important nursing measure. Explanations to the client are necessary to help the client feel comfortable in the new surroundings, however, this is not the most important action. Try again!*
   2. **Congratulations! This is a difficult question! It is most important that the nurse find out and understand the client's routines at home so that these routines may be integrated in his present care. The goal of the nurse is to create a safe environment for the client. Following pre-existing routines will help the client feel more secure and less threatened. This question requires the ability to plan nursing care for an elderly client.**
   3. *This is a good choice, but not the best answer. Very close! The ability of the client to move and care for himself is important. However, this is not the most important measure. Try again!*
   4. *Like Option 1, this option involves giving information to the client about the health care team. Since these options are similar, both are incorrect. The question focuses on the most important nursing measure. Although introducing the client to members of the health care team is important to help the client feel safe and comfortable in his new surroundings, it is not the most important action. Try again!*

9. **A client with a diagnosis of borderline personality disorder has become attached to one of her nurses. One day her favorite nurse phones in sick. When the client**

is given this news, she goes into her room, breaks a bottle of cologne, and scratches her arm with a jagged piece of glass. After providing first aid, what is the next most therapeutic nursing action in relation to the client's behavior?

1. Institute suicide precautions.
2. Help the client connect her thoughts and feelings to her acting-out behavior.
3. Telephone the client's favorite nurse to talk with the client.
4. Permit the client to remain in her room alone to compose herself.

1. *This may be appropriate, but it is not the most therapeutic nursing action.*
2. **Correct. The most therapeutic nursing action is to help the client verbalize the feelings she had prior to cutting herself, and begin to connect these feelings to her acting-out behavior. This is an important first step in learning to control impulsive behavior.**
3. *This is not correct. The client's clinging behavior with her favorite nurse is preventing her from establishing supportive relationships with other staff members and clients on the unit.*
4. *Most clients with borderline behaviors are not able to tolerate being alone, and will experience chronic feelings of emptiness or boredom when alone. This cannot be the correct option.*

10. **A client with a diagnosis of borderline personality disorder purposely cut herself with a piece of glass when she learned that her favorite nurse had called in sick. The client's favorite nurse returns to the unit and meets with the client to discuss the incident when she cut herself. How can the nurse best prevent future incidents of self-mutilating behavior in this client?**

    1. Emphasize that self-destructive behavior is not acceptable and obtain a written contract from the client stating that she will not harm herself.
    2. Ask the client to make a promise that she will discuss any self-destructive feelings she may have with a staff member.
    3. Assign a staff member to supervise the client's whereabouts at all times.
    4. Point out to the client that she is making increasingly unrealistic demands on the nurse and other staff members.

    1. **Correct. This conveys in the strongest way the staff's stand against self-destructive behavior. The staff will provide the external controls needed to prevent acting-out behavior until the client develops sufficient internal control.**
    2. *This is a true statement, but it is not the best option. Identify the option that provides even greater*

protection against self-destructive behavior.

3. *This is not correct. While this action may be desirable with a highly suicidal client, it is not used with the client who impulsively acts out feelings, because it does not help the client develop better self-control.*

4. *This is not correct because this action is not therapeutic. The client requires the staff's assistance to learn to control her acting-out behavior.*

11. In caring for rape victims, the nurse knows that rape survivors:

1. May experience the hospital and police procedures as further violations of their privacy and integrity.
2. Usually recover from any emotional manifestations within a year after the rape.
3. Rarely require the assistance of rape crisis programs.
4. May have provoked the attack by being seductive, if they appear calm after the attack.

1. *Correct. The process of questioning the rape victim and the physical examination after the rape is often experienced by the victim as a second violent intrusion.*

2. *This is not a true statement. Follow-up studies indicate that those victims who fully recover from the emotional aftermath of a sexual assault commonly take four to six years to resolve their psychological manifestations.*

3. *This is not a true statement. Rape crisis programs offer many valuable services, including counseling and support immediately after the attack, legal advice, and support group services to aid in long-term recovery.*

4. *This is not a true statement. Although many victims are visibly upset after a rape, about half may appear calm on the surface. The nurse should be aware of the common myths and misconceptions about rape that could interfere with the nurse's ability to provide effective care to rape victims.*

12. The nurse diagnoses a client as experiencing rape-trauma syndrome. The client agrees to meet with a clinical nurse specialist for crisis intervention therapy. The primary purpose of crisis intervention is to:

1. Assist the client to recognize and gain insight into her feelings.
2. Help the client learn how her current problems relate to unresolved earlier childhood conflicts and traumas.
3. Provide long-term therapy to resolve the emotional issues connected with this current event.
4. Prevent the development of serious psychiatric manifestations.

1. *This statement of the primary purpose of crisis intervention is incomplete. Read all the options before selecting the best one!*

2. *This is not a true statement. Crisis intervention focuses on the client's current situation and her responses to it. It does not focus on her early childhood, or events that occurred prior to the crisis situation.*

3. *This is not correct. Crisis intervention is brief, time-limited treatment that focuses on the current crisis situation.*

4. *Correct. The focus of crisis intervention therapy is the client's current crisis situation and her emotional responses to it. Its purpose is to prevent the development of future mental health problems.*

13. A client asks the nurse to telephone her husband and ask him if he remembered to pick up his suit at the cleaners. The nurse knows that her husband died five years before. The best nursing response is:

1. "It may seem like your husband is still here, but he died five years ago."
2. "You miss your husband a lot, don't you? It must seem like he's almost here with you."
3. "You've forgotten that your husband is dead, haven't you?"
4. "Don't worry. Your husband will remember to pick up his cleaning."

1. *This response is an attempt to orient the client to reality, but it does not address the client's feelings.*

2. *Correct. This nursing response validates the client's feelings and acknowledges her experience. This is the best option because the nurse is responding to the feelings underlying the client's comment, instead of the disordered content. This response uses the therapeutic communication tool of empathy.*

3. *This is not correct because the nurse responds only to the content in the client's statement, and indicates no empathy for how the client is feeling.*

4. *This is not correct. The nurse should not reinforce the client's belief that her husband is still alive.*

14. An 84-year-old married man is admitted from his home to a skilled nursing facility with a diagnosis of Alzheimer's disease. While speaking with the admitting nurse, his wife begins to cry and says, "I never thought it would come to this. I feel so guilty bringing him here." Which nursing response is best?

1. "You have done all you could. We will take good care of him here."
2. "This has been a difficult time for you. Let's find a quiet place where we can talk."

3. "Admitting your husband was the right decision. He requires more care then you can provide at home."
4. "What are you feeling guilty about?"

1. *This statement is not the best nursing response because it uses a form of false reassurance. The nurse is assuming the wife did all she could, but the nurse does not know that this is true. The nurse is also referring to an inappropriate issue — the quality of care at the skilled nursing facility. The client in this question is the wife, and the issue is her feelings of guilt. The nursing goal is to help the wife deal with her feelings so she will be able to support her husband with his adjustment to the nursing home.*
2. **Correct. The nurse acknowledges the wife's feelings and offers an availability to assist her with them. The nursing goal is to help the wife deal with her feelings so she will be able to support her husband with his adjustment to the nursing home.**
3. *This is not the best option. The nurse is giving advice instead of helping the wife to deal constructively with her feelings.*
4. *This is not correct. The wife has told the nurse that she feels guilty about admitting her husband to the long-term care facility. Asking this question indicates that the nurse either has not listened or is not sensitive to the wife's feelings.*

15. **A 77-year-old client was hospitalized for observation falling when he was walking for exercise. He is to ambulate for the first time since his fall. He tells the nurse that he is afraid to get up. The most helpful nursing response is:**

1. "There is nothing to be afraid of. The doctor wouldn't have written the order if he didn't think that you were ready."
2. "Tell me what concerns you about getting up today."
3. "I will have another person here to help you when you get up."
4. "Are you afraid of falling again?"

1. *Wrong choice. This response does not facilitate a response from the client. It contradicts and devalues his feelings, and it focuses on an inappropriate person (the doctor) and an inappropriate issue (the doctor's order). It also offers false reassurance, since the nurse has not clarified why the client is afraid to get up. A therapeutic response focuses on the client's feelings.*
2. **Excellent! This nursing response focuses therapeutically on the "here and now" and on the client's feelings. It gives value to the**

client's statement by directly addressing it and clarifying what the client is feeling concerning ambulating.
3. *This response may not address the client's concerns, since the nurse does not know why the client is afraid. Clarification is necessary before the nurse can plan to meet the client's needs. This response focuses on the nurse's action, not on the client's feelings and that is not therapeutic.*
4. *Wrong. Communication theory states that clarification is an important aspect of effective communication. Simple "yes/no" questions are not very therapeutic, either, because the client can answer the question with just a "yes" or "no".*

16. **The nurse enters a client's room. The client's son tells the nurse, "You people can't do anything right. Ever since my father was admitted to this hospital, it has been one mistake after another. I am taking him out of here before you kill him." The appropriate response to the son is:**

1. "You feel that your father is not being well taken care of?"
2. "We have the best intentions for the clients."
3. "I'll get the supervisor for you."
4. "Your father hasn't complained about the care. What specifically is the problem?"

1. **Excellent! This response uses the communication tool of restatement. It focuses on the client's issue, and it encourages the son to express his concerns to the nurse. The nurse needs more information from the client before problem-solving can occur. This response also focuses therapeutically on the "here and now".**
2. *Incorrect. This response is a defensive remark by the nurse, which is a communication block. This response implies that whatever is bothering the son cannot be valid, and this response may escalate the situation. A therapeutic response would encourage the son to tell the nurse why he feels upset concerning his father's care.*
3. *This response puts the feelings of the son on hold by asking him to wait until the supervisor arrives. Therapeutic communication addresses the "here and now," and does not "pass the buck" to another person. Indeed, the supervisor may become involved, but the best response by the nurse is to address the client's immediate needs.*
4. *This response focuses on the father, but the son is the one with the concerns. It implies that the son's feelings cannot be valid since his father has not voiced any complaints. This is not a therapeutic nursing response and it contains the communication blocks of not addressing the client and devaluing his feelings.*

17. A client has been told by the doctor that he has cancer and that it has advanced so far that treatment will not help. When the nurse comes to help him with his bath, he says to the nurse, "I'm not an invalid, you know! I can take care of myself. Get out and leave me alone." How should the nurse respond?

   1. "I know that you are not an invalid. However, I was trying to help you."
   2. "It sounds to me like you are angry about something. Did somebody do something wrong?"
   3. "You are pretty upset. Let's talk about it."
   4. "I'll just set up this equipment for you to bathe and come back later when you're not so angry."

   1. *This is an incorrect option because this response is defensive and focuses on the nurse, not on the client.*
   2. *This option assumes that the client is angry. By asking if "somebody" did something wrong, it focuses on "somebody" else instead of focusing on the client's feelings.*
   3. ***Good choice! This option addresses the emotional state of the client by stating that he is upset. The communication tool of clarification is used to promote therapeutic communication, which focuses on the client's feelings.***
   4. *This option does not promote any communication with the client. It implies that his behavior is inappropriate and that the nurse is not willing to deal with it.*

18. The nurse tells a client that the doctor has ordered an intravenous line to be started. The client appears to be upset but says nothing. What should the nurse say?

   1. "Do you have any questions about the procedure?"
   2. "The doctor wants you to have antibiotics, and this method eliminates getting frequent injections."
   3. "What is there about this procedure that concerns you?"
   4. "It only hurts a little bit. It'll be over before you know it."

   1. *Wrong. This response focuses on the procedure, not on the client's feelings.*
   2. *Wrong. This response focuses on an inappropriate person (the doctor) and on an inappropriate issue (antibiotics by injection). This is a block to communication, since the client's feelings aren't addressed.*
   3. ***Excellent choice! This response uses the communication tool of clarification and inquires about the client's concerns, in a way that indicates the nurse is willing to talk with the client about both the procedure and the client's feelings.***
   4. *This option is incorrect. An intravenous puncture*

hurts more than a little bit. This communication block is identified as false reassurance.

19. A client tells the nurse that his name is not spelled right on his identification bracelet. The nurse should:

   1. Tell the client that as long as his medical record numbers are correct, the mistake is not a problem.
   2. Ask the client for the correct spelling and change his medical records.
   3. Notify the admitting office of the error and obtain a correct identification bracelet for the client.
   4. Notify the physician.

   1. *No. The client's identification bracelet should be corrected. It is possible that his name also appears incorrectly in his medical chart and other hospital records as well, and these records will have to be checked. Try again.*
   2. *The client's records will have to be corrected. However, this is not the correct procedure, since the hospital has other records in addition to the chart. The client's identification bracelet should also be corrected. Try again.*
   3. ***Good choice! The admitting office must be informed of the error, and the client's identification bracelet should show his name correctly.***
   4. *The spelling of the client's name is not a medical problem. This in an inappropriate nursing action. The stem asks for a true statement. Make another choice.*

20. The nurse is to administer an intramuscular injection. The most important action by the nurse to prevent introduction of the medication into the venous system is to:

   1. Inject the medication slowly to allow for slow absorption.
   2. Insert the needle at a 45-degree angle where there are fewer blood vessels.
   3. Use the Z track method of injection.
   4. Aspirate the drug after insertion of needle.

   1. *No. Injecting the medication slowly decreases trauma at the site and minimizes discomfort for the client. It does not prevent medication from entering the venous system.*

   TEST-TAKING TIP: *This is an appropriate nursing action, but this action does not address the issue in the question. What is the question asking?*

   2. *No. An intramuscular injection is administered at a 90-degree angle. A subcutaneous injection is administered at a 45-degree angle. Neither position will prevent the medication from entering the venous system.*
   3. *Wrong. The Z track method is used for irritating*

medications. It does not prevent medication from entering the venous system.

> **TEST-TAKING TIP:** This may be an appropriate nursing action, but this action does not address the issue in the question. What is the question asking? The question does not indicate that the medication is irritating. Be careful not to "read into" the question!

4. *Right! The drug is aspirated to determine if any blood is in the syringe. If blood is seen, the medication will enter the venous system if it is injected. Many intramuscular medications are not safe for intravenous administration.*

21. **The nurse is caring for an elderly client who is often unsteady while walking. Which nursing measure is most important in providing for the safety of such a client?**

    1. Wipe up spills immediately.
    2. Make crutches or canes available for the elderly clients.
    3. Raise the side rails on the bed.
    4. Assist all elderly clients when ambulating.

    1. *You are correct! Wiping up spills immediately to prevent slipping on wet floors is an important safety intervention, and the best choice in this test question.*

> **TEST-TAKING TIP:** Options 2 and 4 involve assistance to the client while walking. Neither of these similar distractors is the answer.

    2. *Not every elderly client needs assistance or crutches when ambulating! This is not correct.*
    3. *No! This client, although unsteady when walking, is ambulatory. This action is inappropriate because the client is at risk of falling by attempting to climb over the rail. This would not be safe for the client. Look for an option that provides for the client's safety while ambulating.*
    4. *Not all elderly clients need help while walking. The nurse should avoid judgments of this kind.*

22. **When collecting a urine specimen for a routine urinalysis, which of the following nursing actions is the most important?**

    1. Label the container with the client's room number.
    2. Check the identification of the client.
    3. Do not use gloves when handling a urine specimen.
    4. Instruct the client to put the specimen on the counter at the nurses' station for pick up.

    1. *This is not the most important measure, and it is not sufficient for identifying the specimen.*
    2. *Yes, you are correct! In order to avoid errors, the most important thing to do is to identify the client. Then, after the client is identified, the next action is to make sure the specimen*

label has the client's name and room number.
    3. *This is not correct. Gloves should be worn when handling any specimen.*
    4. *No! The nurse should take the specimen container to the dirty utility room.*

23. **A client is admitted to the hospital for evaluation of inadequate circulation to her lower extremities. The doctor orders a tub bath at the client's request. In assisting the client with her bath, which action would be unsafe?**

    1. Place a rubber mat on the bottom of the tub.
    2. Fill the tub approximately half full.
    3. When the client steps into the tub, ask her if the water is the right temperature for her.
    4. Obtain all of the supplies necessary for the bath and place them within easy reach of the client.

    1. *A rubber mat helps prevent slipping on a slippery tub bottom. This is an appropriate intervention. This question has a false response stem, however, so you are looking for an option that represents an action the nurse should NOT do. Try again.*
    2. *Since water is displaced when the client sits in the tub, filling the tub about half full will prevent the water from running over, which could result in a fall from water on the floor. This is an appropriate nursing action. This question has a false response stem, however, so you are looking for an option that represents an action the nurse should NOT do. Try again.*
    3. *Very good, you have identified the unsafe action! This question has a false response stem, and this correct answer is something the nurse should NOT do. For the safety and comfort of the client, the nurse should regulate the water temperature to between 105-110° F. A client with poor circulation in the lower extremities will not be able to accurately detect feelings of hot and cold when they step into a tub.*
    4. *The equipment should be available to the client, within easy reach. Safety is a concern here, as the client may slip and fall trying to reach the equipment. This question has a false response stem, however, so you are looking for an option that represents an action the nurse should NOT do. Try again.*

24. **A client is to be up in a chair three times a day. He is paralyzed from the waist down. What is the best nursing approach when transferring this client from a bed into a wheel chair?**

    1. Place the wheel chair close to the foot of the bed.
    2. Utilize the principles of body mechanics while providing a safe transfer for the client.

3. Slide the client to the edge of the bed, keeping the nurse's back straight and using a rocking motion to pull the client.
4. Place the nurse's arms under the client's axillae from the back of the client.

1. *This is not correct. The wheel chair should be placed as close as possible to the position of the client's buttocks, for a safe and easy transfer. The wheel chair should not be placed at the foot of the bed. Try again.*
2. ***Very good! The nurse is in control of the nurse's own body and the client's movement during the transfer. Providing for the safety of the client, and utilizing the principles of body mechanics to provide safety for the nurse and the client, is the best nursing approach.***
3. *This is an appropriate nursing action, which addresses the safety of the nurse and client. Positioning the client near the edge of the bed will reduce the energy required to move the client to the wheel chair, and the nurse's back will be protected by using leg and arm muscles to move the client to the edge of the bed. There is another option, however, that better describes the best nursing approach for transferring this client. Read all the options before you select the best one! Try again.*
4. *This is a correct action, which helps provide for the nurse's and the client's safety. Supporting the upper portion of the client's body helps to place the weight of the client over the nurse's center of gravity. There is another option, however, that better describes the best nursing approach in transferring this client. Read all the options before you select the best one! Make another choice.*

25. **Of the following information, which should be recorded first in the client's record by the nurse admitting the client?**

1. The client's vital signs.
2. The plan that was developed for the care of the client while in the hospital.
3. Nursing actions performed for the client.
4. Assessment of the client.

1. *The client's vital signs should be recorded in the client's record in order to document that the nurse assessed the client's condition on admission. This is an appropriate nursing action and a possible answer, but it is not the best option. Read all the options before you select your answer! Try again.*
2. *The plan of care should be documented. A plan cannot be developed, however, until the nurse finds out more about the client. Try again.*
3. *Nursing actions are documented as the plan of care is implemented. Since the case scenario tells*

you that the client is being admitted, the nursing process requires that the nurse gather data and develop a plan before implementing actions. Make another choice.
4. ***Excellent! The nurse should document the findings on assessment in order to provide information concerning the status of the client on admission.***

26. **While preparing to give a morning medication, the first nursing action is to:**

1. Read the label.
2. Check for the right dose.
3. Wash hands.
4. Check for the right time.

1. *This is an important part of avoiding medication errors. However, it is not the first thing that the nurse should do.*
2. *It is important to have the right dose to prevent over or under dosing the client. However, this is not the first step in preparing medications.*
3. ***Excellent! Hand washing is the first action prior to performing any procedure.***
4. *The time for administration of the medication is very important, but this is not the first thing that the nurse should do.*

27. **The client is very confused and combative. The physician orders the client to be placed in a jacket restraint and wrist restraints. In order to prevent injury to the client with restraints, the most important nursing action is to:**

1. Explain the procedure and reason for the restraints to the client and the family.
2. Remove the restraints and observe the extremities for circulation at least every four hours.
3. Tell the client that if he is more cooperative the restraints will not be necessary.
4. Document the use of restraints in the chart.

1. *This is an important part of nursing care. However, this action will not prevent injury to the client. This is not the answer.*
2. ***Very good. This nursing action will help prevent nerve and musculoskeletal injuries to the client as a result of poor circulation caused by the restraints.***
3. *The case scenario tells you that the client is confused. Giving him this choice is inappropriate.*
4. *Documentation of the use of restraints and the client's behavior that warranted their use for the client's safety is very important. However, this action will not prevent injury to the client. This is not the answer.*

28. A client is in the intensive care unit and is in a coma as a result of a head injury. The most important nursing action in performing mouth care on this client is to:

1. Turn the client to her side before starting mouth care.
2. Use a soft toothbrush.
3. Use a mouth bite to keep her mouth open.
4. Wear gloves.

*1. **Very good! Turning the client on her side is the most important intervention, since it will help prevent aspiration of the fluids used for cleaning the mouth.***

2. A soft toothbrush is preferred, but this is not the most important action in this procedure.

3. This intervention is helpful while cleaning the mouth, but this is not the most important action in this procedure.

4. The nurse should wear gloves, but this is not the most important action in this procedure.

29. Restraints may be used to immobilize a client, or the client's extremity. The nurse understands that it is inconsistent with proper restraint functionality to use a restraint to:

1. Prevent a client from pulling out an IV or other type of therapy.
2. Reduce the risk to all elderly clients from falling out of bed or off a chair.
3. Prevent removal of life support equipment.
4. Prevent injury to health care personnel by combative clients.

1. Wrong. A confused client may pull out an IV or nasogastric tube because of discomfort or inability to understand the purpose of the therapy.

*2. **Very good! This option implies that ALL elderly clients should be restrained in order to reduce the risk of falls. Many elderly clients can care for themselves without falling. Each individual should be assessed for risk to fall.***

TEST-TAKING TIP: Absolute words like "all," "every," and "always," or "none" or "never," are hints that a statement may be false. This question has a false response stem, so this false statement is the answer.

3. Wrong. Some clients may become combative or confused while on life support systems and may cause life support systems to become dislodged.

TEST-TAKING TIP: This question has a false response stem and is asking you to identify the option that is NOT an objective for using restraints on a client.

4. Incorrect. Occasionally a client can become com-

bative, and restraints can be the only means of protecting the health care worker while providing care.

30. A client has just been admitted to the hospital. In showing the client how to use the call system, the nurse understands that which of the following statements is incorrect?

1. The call system allows the client to signal for help.
2. The call system should be limited to use in emergencies.
3. The client should be able to reach the call button easily.
4. The client should be taught how to use the call system.

1. This statement is correct, but it is not the right answer. It is necessary for the safety and well-being of the client to be able to signal for help when needed. The question asks you to select an option that is NOT a true statement about the call system.

*2. **Right! This statement is an incorrect statement about the use of the call system, and is the answer to this question, which has a false response stem. The call system should be used whenever a client needs help, not only in emergencies. For the safety and well-being of the client, the client should be instructed how to use the system, and should be able to reach it easily and safely.***

3. This statement is correct, but it is not the answer. It is necessary for the safety and well-being of the client to be able to reach the call bell easily. The question asks you to select an option that is NOT a true statement about the call system.

4. This is a correct statement about the call system. It is necessary for the safety and well-being of the client to teach the client to use the call system. This question asks you to select an option that is not a true statement about the call system.

31. An ambulatory client is being readied for bed. The nursing action that promotes safety for this client is:

1. Turning off all of the lights to help promote sleep and rest.
2. Instructing the client in the use of the call bell.
3. Putting the side rail up.
4. Placing the bed in the high position.

1. Don't turn off all the lights! A small light should remain on in the event that the client wakes up to go to the bathroom or for some other reason, and becomes disoriented to place.

*2. **Right! The client should be instructed in the use of the call bell in the event that help is needed.***

3. Putting the side rails up on a client that is ambula-

tory could cause a fall if the client attempted to climb over them to get out of bed.

4. *A client who is ambulatory should have the bed in a low position to prevent a fall when getting out of bed.*

32. An infant with AIDS is being prepared for discharge. The nurse is instructing the grandmother, who will care for the infant, in methods of home care. Which statement, made by the grandmother, represents the greatest hazard to successful home maintenance?

1. "I know that hand washing is an important preventive measure."
2. "I'll use disposable diapers, discarding them in separate plastic bags."
3. "Blood spills should be washed up immediately with hot soapy water."
4. "Gloves should be worn by whomever changes the baby's diapers."

1. *No, this statement by grandmother indicates an good understanding of transmission of the disease and of the role of hand washing in preventing the spread of infection to the client and to the family. You are looking for an INCORRECT statement. Try again.*

2. *No, this statement by grandmother indicates an good understanding of an acceptable method of infection control. Any items that cannot be disposed of in the toilet should be kept in a closed plastic bag until trash disposal. You are looking for an INCORRECT statement. Try again.*

3. **Correct. This is an inadequate method of cleaning blood or potentially contaminated body substances. Bleach solution should be used and gloves worn whenever coming in contact with blood products. This INCORRECT statement by the grandmother is the correct answer to this question, which has a false response stem.**

4. *No, this statement by grandmother indicates an good understanding of transmission of the disease and one important action in preventing the spread of infection to the client and to the family. Gloves should be worn by anyone when changing the diaper of a child who has tested HIV positive or has the AIDS virus, because blood and body fluids are a means of disease transmission. You are looking for an INCORRECT statement. Try again.*

33. While preparing to give a client a bed bath, which nursing action is appropriate?

1. Place the bed in the lowest position.
2. Expose the top side of the body and wash and dry

quickly; then do the same on the posterior side.
3. Gather all of the articles necessary for the bath and place them within easy reach of the nurse during the bath.
4. Use firm, scrubbing strokes to remove dirt and bacteria.

1. *This is an incorrect action, the question has a true response stem. The bed should be placed in a high position to prevent back strain in the nurse. Try again.*

2. *This is an incorrect action, and the question has a true response stem. Each area of the body should be exposed, washed, and dried separately to avoid chilling the client and to provide privacy. Try again.*

3. **Very good! This question has a true response stem. This is the only option with a correct statement about what the nurse should do to facilitate bathing the client.**

4. *This is an incorrect action, and the question has a true response stem. The strokes should be firm but gentle — not "scrubbing" — to avoid injuring the skin. Make another choice.*

34. While getting an elderly client, who is very weak, out of bed, the best nursing approach is:

1. Locking the wheels of the bed.
2. Placing the equipment in such a way as to provide the safest transfer that is possible for the client.
3. Aligning the wheel chair as close to the bed as possible, to prevent the client from falling to the floor.
4. Removing the wheel chair's leg support on the side closest to the bed.

1. *The wheels of the bed should be in the locked position to prevent it from moving. There is another option that is a more comprehensive statement of the best nursing approach. Read all of the options before selecting the best one! Try again.*

2. **Good work! This option is the best because it emphasizes assuring the client's safety and is a comprehensive statement about the initial nursing approach in transferring a client.**

3. *This is an appropriate action that provides for the client's safety. There is another option that is a more comprehensive statement of the best nursing approach. Read all of the options before selecting the best one! Try again.*

4. *This an appropriate action, since it provides unobstructed access to the wheel chair. This is not the best answer, however, there is another option that is a more comprehensive statement of the best nursing approach. Try again!*

35. A client is to receive an IM injection of penicillin

(Wycillin). In preparing this medication, the best nursing approach is to:

1. Use a sterile syringe and needle.
2. Provide for the safety of the client by using the proper equipment and aseptic technique.
3. Prepare the skin site with an antiseptic swab, moving from the center of the site outward.
4. Prevent contamination of the needle by not allowing it to touch any contaminated surfaces.

1. *A sterile syringe and needle is standard equipment for an IM injection of a medication. This is an appropriate nursing action. However, this not the best option. Read all the options and make another choice.*
2. ***Excellent! The safety of the client is the most important consideration. This choice includes that idea as well as aseptic technique and equipment. It is a comprehensive statement of the best nursing approach.***
3. *Swabbing the skin site with an antiseptic is an appropriate nursing action for an IM injection. However, this not the best option. Read all the options and make another choice.*
4. *Preventing contamination is important. A contaminated needle can cause an infection at the injection site. This is a correct nursing action. However, this not the best option. Read all the options and make another choice.*

36. **A client is entering menopause and is identified as at risk for osteoporosis. In instructing this client in preventive measures, the nurse knows that osteoporosis is best prevented in the menopausal woman by:**

1. Avoidance of all exercise.
2. Estrogen replacement therapy.
3. Drinking one glass of red wine daily.
4. Limiting calcium intake.

1. *No! In fact, exercise is suggested as a means to prevent osteoporosis.*
2. ***Correct. The administration of estrogen to menopausal women has been proven effective in the prevention of osteoporosis.***
3. *No, this is not recommended! It is suggested that women at risk for osteoporosis eliminate alcohol, caffeine and smoking from their lifestyle.*
4. *No! On the contrary, a diet high in calcium is recommended for women a risk for osteoporosis.*

37. **A client, admitted with hypertension, is taking furosemide (Lasix) 40 mg. PO twice a day. Which of the following interventions, if included in the plan of care by the nurse, would require further clarification?**

1. Daily weights before breakfast.
2. Monitor intake and output.
3. Orthostatic blood pressure checks every eight hours.
4. Limit fluid intake to 1ml. in 24 hours.

1. *Wrong. This intervention would be appropriate for the client's plan of care because of the need to monitor for fluid volume deficits which can be caused by Lasix. Remember that daily weights are the best indicators of fluid balance (a gain or loss of 1 kg. is equal to a gain or loss of 1 liter of fluid).*
2. *Incorrect. Monitoring intake and output would be important for the client on furosemide therapy. Recall that this drug is a very potent diuretic that can easily cause dehydration.*
3. *No. It would be wise to make this assessment because Lasix can cause orthostatic hypotension. The client is cautioned to make position changes slowly to minimize the incidence of orthostatic hypotension, which can result from hypovolemia.*
4. *Correct option. This intervention would need to be discussed further. Lasix, a potent diuretic, can frequently cause dehydration. Limiting a client's fluid intake may contribute to this problem; therefore, this would not be a safe nursing measure.*

38. **The nurse is caring for a client on the second postoperative day following a cesarean section for a breech. She has a vertical incision into the abdomen. She asks if she will need to have a cesarean birth with her future pregnancies. What is the nurse's best reply?**

1. "I will need to check your operative record before I can answer that."
2. "Because your incision is classical, future labor could be unsafe."
3. "As long as you your next baby comes head first, you can safely deliver vaginally."
4. "It is impossible to predict at this time. Let's wait until the next pregnancy occurs."

1. ***Correct. The direction of the skin incision has no relationship to the uterine incision. Before you can answer her question, you must check to be sure the incision into the uterus is low transverse. This information will be on the operating room record.***
2. *Wrong! The direction of the skin incision has no relationship to the uterine incision.*
3. *Wrong! You cannot tell the client this until you have verified that the uterine incision is low transverse. The direction of the skin incision has no relationship to the uterine incision.*
4. *Wrong! The client has an indication for cesarean section with subsequent pregnancies but may deliver vaginally as long as the uterine scar is low transverse. This information is reassuring to the postoperative client.*

39.   When the nurse assesses a client on the first postpartum day, the findings are: fundus firm, one fingerbreadth below and to the right of the umbilicus, lochia rubra with small clots, temperature 99.2° F, pulse rate 52. The appropriate nursing action is to:

1.   Report the lochia to the charge nurse.
2.   Report the temperature to the charge nurse.
3.   Report the pulse rate to the charge nurse.
4.   Ask the client when she last voided.

1.   *No, this is a normal lochia for the first day postpartum.*
2.   *Wrong. Elevation in temperature in the first 24 hours after delivery is related to the exertion and dehydration of labor. It is not a cause for concern unless it goes above 100.4° F.*
3.   *Incorrect. Maternal bradycardia is commonly seen in the first six to 10 days postpartum.*
4.   **Correct. Because the muscles supporting the uterus have been stretched over the pregnancy months, it is easily displaced when the bladder is full. Normally the fundus should be found firm at midline.**

40.   The nurse caring for a client in the first hour following delivery is having difficulty taking her blood pressure because the client is shaking uncontrollably. What nursing intervention is indicated at this time?

1.   Call the charge nurse immediately to come in to assess the client.
2.   Give the client a warm blanket.
3.   Check to be sure there is a padded tongue blade readily available.
4.   Take the client's temperature immediately.

1.   *Wrong. Many mothers experience a shaking chill after delivery. It may be related to neurologic response or to vasomotor changes. The charge nurse does not need to be alerted at this time.*
2.   **Correct. Many mothers experience a shaking chill after delivery. It may be related to neurologic response or to vasomotor changes. Providing warmth to the client at this time seems to alleviate the chills.**
3.   *Incorrect. These postpartum chills are not related to seizure activity.*
4.   *This action is unnecessary in response to the client's chills. When these chills occur within the first few hours after delivery there is no cause for concern. Late in the puerperium, chills may be related to fever and warrant further evaluation.*

41.   When meperidine (Demerol) is given to a laboring woman, the nurse should be prepared to treat:

1.   Maternal hyperventilation.
2.   Neonatal depression.
3.   Maternal hypertension.
4.   Neonatal hypoglycemia.

1.   *Wrong. The laboring woman who receives Demerol should be assessed for respiratory depression, manifested by slow respiratory rate.*
2.   **Good work! Whenever the laboring mother receives Demerol, there is a risk of neonatal depression usually reflected in low APGAR scores. The risk is greatest when the birth occurs within two to three hours after maternal administration.**
3.   *No. Maternal hypotension is commonly seen following administration of Demerol.*
4.   *Wrong. The administration of Demerol to the laboring woman has no effect on the neonate's blood sugar.*

42.   While caring for the client who is having an induction of labor with oxytocin (Pitocin), which nursing assessment is indicated?

1.   Blood pressure every five minutes.
2.   Maternal temperature every hour.
3.   Maternal contraction pattern every hour.
4.   Continuous fetal heart rate monitoring.

1.   *No, fluctuations in blood pressure are not related to oxytocin administration. Routine monitoring, usually every 30 to 60 minutes, is indicated.*
2.   *Wrong. Maternal temperature changes are associated with prolonged ruptured membranes (greater than 24 hours), not oxytocin administration.*
3.   *Wrong. When the mother is receiving oxytocin during labor, the contractions need to be monitored continuously, using the fetal monitor.*
4.   **Very good! Whenever oxytocin is administered to an antepartum client, the fetal monitor must be used to continuously monitor the fetal heart rate and maternal contractions.**

43.   In the first hours postpartum, which behavior would the nurse expect to see in a new mother?

1.   Upset because her lunch is late.
2.   Asking many questions about infant care.
3.   Eagerly unwrapping the baby and attempting to engage the baby in play.
4.   Confidently providing all infant care.

1.   **Correct. Immediately after delivery the new mother focuses primarily on her own needs. Food and sleep are often her main concern.**
2.   *Wrong. The mother needs to meet her own needs before she can focus on her newborn's needs.*

3. *Incorrect. A new mother will touch her baby gently in the first days, often with fingertip touch.*
4. *Wrong. The client often is unsure and tentative in providing care in the first days. As she adjusts to her role as new mother, she gains confidence in her caregiving abilities.*

44.   The nurse should know the recommended frequency for mammogram testing is:

1. Yearly for all females over age 20.
2. Baseline at puberty, every two years thereafter until age 50, and then yearly.
3. At least every two years between ages 40-49.
4. Baseline at age 25, then yearly thereafter.

1. *No, this scheduling is begun at too early an age and done too often. Rarely are mammograms begun prior to age 35 to 40.*
2. *Wrong. There is very little reason to do a baseline mammogram prior to age 35.*
3. **Good choice. The baseline is suggested between age 35 to 40, repeated every one to two years between ages 40-49, and yearly after age 50.**
4. *No, this is too early and too frequent a schedule.*

45.   The nurse knows that which of the following statements by a client warrants further teaching about self breast exam (SBE)?

1. "SBE is very important for early detection of breast cancer."
2. "As long as I have a mammogram every year, SBE is not necessary."
3. "I will do SBE each month on the last day of my menses."
4. "Comparing one breast against the other is part of regular SBE."

1. *No, the client understands correctly. SBE has been proven to be one of the best methods for early detection of breast masses. You are looking for an INCORRECT statement that indicates the client needs further teaching.*
2. **Correct, this statement indicates that the client needs further teaching. Mammography is a useful tool but it cannot replace SBE in detection of breast masses. Up to 15% of early stage breast cancers detected by SBE are not detected by mammogram.**
3. *No, the client understands correctly. This describes the correct timing for monthly SBE. You are looking for an INCORRECT statement that indicates the client needs further teaching.*
4. *No, the client understands correctly. The comparison of both breasts is part of SBE procedure. You are looking for an INCORRECT statement that in-*

dicates the client needs further teaching.

46.   The nurse is teaching a client how to take her basal body temperature (BBT) as a method of birth control. Which statement by the client indicates to the nurse that further teaching is needed?

1. "I will take my temperature every morning before I get out of bed."
2. "When my body temperature rises, it means I should not have intercourse for the next three days."
3. "It is important that I do not shake the thermometer in the morning before I take my temperature."
4. "I will get a BBT thermometer to take my temperature."

1. *No, this statement is correct and reflects a good understanding for the correct method to assess BBT. You are looking for an INCORRECT statement that indicates the client needs further teaching.*
2. **Good! This statement indicates that the client has not understood the principles of BBT. To use BBT for the purpose of birth control, the woman needs to predict ovulation in subsequent months. The client's BBT rises following ovulation. If the client has intercourse on the days prior to the temperature rise, pregnancy could result because sperm is capable of fertilization for up to 72 hours.**
3. *No, this statement is correct and reflects the correct procedure for assessing BBT. Shaking the thermometer down could affect the BBT. You are looking for an INCORRECT statement that indicates the client needs further teaching.*
4. *No, use of a special thermometer is suggested to provide a more accurate record of degrees. A BBT measures 0.1 degree markings. You are looking for an INCORRECT statement that indicates the client needs further teaching.*

47.   A 10-month-old is admitted following a febrile seizure. The mother is very upset because of the seizure. What information should the nurse provide to the mother?

1. This will probably never happen again.
2. Febrile seizures are a lifelong disorder.
3. The seizure is related to fever and can be treated.
4. An anticonvulsant, perhaps phenobarbital, will be ordered to prevent further seizures.

1. *This is untrue. Although a febrile seizure may never reoccur, it would not be appropriate to make this assumption. Once the child has had a febrile seizure, he is likely to have another if the stimuli for febrile seizures occur again. Choose another option.*

2. *Not true! The tendency is usually outgrown by about five years of age. Select again.*

3. **Yes, febrile seizures occur due to fevers in children who are neurologically immature. Children are treated with aspirin, acetaminophen (Tylenol), and sponging. Most children outgrow this tendency by five years of age.**

4. *Incorrect. Although phenobarbital may be prescribed for some children with febrile seizures, this is not included in all treatment plans.*

48. **In determining the care for a child admitted with a probable diagnosis of Hirschsprung disease (megacolon), the nurse would plan to prepare the child for:**

1. A barium enema.
2. A sweat chloride test.
3. A flat plate of the abdomen.
4. Occult blood in stool specimen.

1. **Correct. A barium enema is one of the tests that may be performed to see the bowel, which is distorted from stool. It may also be a nonsurgical approach to management of this disease.**
2. *Incorrect. This is the test used to diagnose cystic fibrosis, not Hirschsprung disease. Try again.*
3. *Wrong choice. A flat plate of the abdomen may show distention, but it would not be considered diagnostic of megacolon. Make another choice.*
4. *Incorrect, since bleeding is not a manifestation of this disorder. Choose again.*

49. **The day after abdominal surgery, a 10-year-old girl is lying quietly in bed when the nurse makes rounds. The last rounds were made four hours ago, and she was last medicated six hours ago. At this time, the nurse should first:**

1. Encourage her to turn, cough, and deep breathe.
2. Assess the need for pain medication.
3. Ambulate her to the door.
4. Ask her if she is hungry, and provide fluids.

1. *Wrong. Although this is part of thorough postoperative care, you have missed an important piece of assessment data in the question. Reread the question and make another selection.*
2. **Correct. A child lying quietly, medicated six hours ago, who is one day postoperative, is very probably in pain. Children at this age are apt to lie motionless to prevent pain. They may not request pain medication for fear of needles. Before any other nursing care is provided, the nurse should complete an assessment of pain and medicate the child. Ambulating and deep breathing will be better tolerated with pain relief.**
3. *Ambulating is not the priority, given the informa-*

tion in the question. Try again.

4. *Incorrect. Although fluids are important to the postoperative client, this is not the priority of care. You do not have enough information to know if oral intake is appropriate on the first day. Make another selection.*

50. **Which nursing intervention would be the most helpful in prevention of a stress ulcer related to a burn in a three-year-old child?**

1. Instruct on relaxation exercises.
2. Administer cimetidine (Tagamet) as ordered.
3. Administer meperidine (Demerol) as ordered.
4. Initiate a bland diet.

1. *No, look at the age of the child! Teaching relaxation would only be appropriate in an older child. Select again.*
2. **Excellent! Tagamet is an anti-ulcer medication and can be used for prophylaxis in burn clients.**
3. *Wrong choice. Demerol may be given to this child, but for pain — not to prevent the ulcer. Select again.*
4. *No. Bland diets are rarely ordered for children, since they are not as appetizing. Usually, the child is allowed to eat anything they like while ill. This is a principle that is applied to most hospitalized children. Choose again.*

51. **A child is in Buck's traction. To prevent complications, the nurse should:**

1. Clean pin sites every shift as ordered.
2. Encourage foods that are high in calcium.
3. Provide small meals with high fiber.
4. Limit range of motion in all extremities.

1. *No, there are no pins with Buck's traction. This is skin traction. Select again.*
2. *Wrong. There is a chance of the client developing renal calculi with excess calcium. The nurse should encourage only the daily requirement for age. Select another choice.*
3. **This is correct. Since appetite may be diminished due to decreased activity, the fiber will reduce the chance of constipation.**
4. *No, only the affected extremity should be restricted. Choose again.*

52. **A BRAT diet is prescribed for a child with gastroenteritis. Which food should be removed by the nurse from the child's tray?**

1. Ice cream.
2. Popsicle.
3. Banana.
4. Applesauce.

1. *Right answer! Ice cream is a dairy product and should be eliminated from a BRAT (banana, rice, apple, and tea) diet, which is low-fat, low-residue, and non-dairy. It is used in treatment of gastroenteritis.*

2. *No, it is OK to let the child eat a Popsicle, because clear fluids are allowed on a BRAT diet. Dehydration is the major cause of hospitalization in the child with gastroenteritis.*

3. *No, the "B" in BRAT stands for bananas, so this should be on the tray. Try another option.*

4. *No, the "A" in BRAT stands for applesauce, so this should be on the tray. Make another selection.*

53. **The nurse knows that which of the following behaviors would indicate regression in a hospitalized five-year-old?**

1. Bedwetting several times a day.
2. Crying when mother leaves.
3. Eating only food from home.
4. Wanting his teddy bear for bedtime.

1. *Correct. You would expect a five-year-old to be toilet trained. Incontinence is a commonly seen sign of regression in young children.*

2. *No, this is not a sign of regression for this child. Separation anxiety is seen in children between the ages of six months and five years. This is within normal for this child's age. Make another choice.*

3. *No, this is not a sign of regression. Children frequently do not eat foods that are different. Sick children particularly do not make changes in their dietary habits. Try again.*

4. *No, this is not a sign of regression. Many young children are attached to a familiar object from home, which is referred to as a transitional object. Select again.*

54. **The nurse is evaluating the degree of bonding between a mother and her infant, who has been hospitalized for a high bilirubin. To collect this data the nurse would:**

1. Ask the mother how she feels about her baby.
2. Provide a cot so that the mother can stay with the infant.
3. Observe the mother feeding the infant.
4. Find out if the pregnancy of this infant was planned.

1. *No, this would not be the best way to gather objective information. This will provide subjective information. Try again.*

2. *Go back and reread the question. What is the issue in the question? This action may encourage bonding, but it doesn't evaluate bonding.*

3. *Good answer! Observation is the best way to gather objective data. In this situation you are looking for the mother's ability to com-*

fort, stimulate, and meet her infant's needs.

4. *No, this will not provide information about actual bonding. If this was an unplanned pregnancy, it would be at high risk for a lack of bonding, during the prenatal period. Try again, but first reread this question.*

55. **A child is admitted with suspected Reye's syndrome. The parents tell the nurse that he was sick a week before this admission. The nurse knows that which of the following diseases would influence the child's present condition?**

1. Rheumatic fever.
2. Diphtheria.
3. Chicken pox.
4. Bacterial meningitis.

1. *No, rheumatic fever is not associated with Reye's syndrome. Make another choice.*

2. *No, diphtheria is not associated with Reye's syndrome. Select again.*

3. *Yes! Varicella (chicken pox) is one of the viral illnesses that may predispose a child to Reye's syndrome.*

4. *No, Reye's syndrome is not associated with bacterial illness. Choose again.*

56. **A two-year-old is admitted with laryngotracheal bronchitis and is placed in a cool mist tent. The direct result of the mist tent that the nurse would expect to observe is:**

1. Improved hydration.
2. Decreased stridor.
3. Diminished output.
4. Normal temperature.

1. *Incorrect. You're probably thinking that mist is water, that water increases hydration, and mist tents can be very damp inside. However, any real improvement in hydration can only be brought about by increased P.O. or IV fluids. Try again.*

2. *Yes. This is the best response because the purpose of cool mist tent is to decrease the respiratory effort. Respirations should become easier and the rate decreased.*

3. *Incorrect. Children with laryngotracheal bronchitis may have diminished output, but this would be a manifestation of the disease, not a result of the treatment. Choose again.*

4. *No, this is not a direct result of the mist tent. It may occur as a secondary effect because the environment is cool. Unless the child's hydration is adequate, the fever will not disappear. Choose again.*

57. **A six-week-old is returned from the operating room after repair of a pyloric stenosis. What data would the**

nurse most depend on for evaluating this client's need for pain control?

1. Physiologic responses.
2. Behavioral changes.
3. Response to medication.
4. Mother's assessment.

1. *No, changes in vital signs are considered a secondary source of information about pain in infants. Select another option.*
2. **Correct. The primary source of information about pain should be observations of the infant's behavior. Stiffening, crying, and withdrawal are the primary ways that a pre-verbal child demonstrates pain.**
3. *Wrong. Perhaps you misread the question. Although the nurse should always assess the effect of the pain medication once given, the issue in the question is how to tell when to give the medication in this client. Try again.*
4. *No, recent research says that parental assessment is not a reliable source of an infant's pain experience. Choose again.*

58. **The nurse teaches the newborn's mother to speak to the baby while making eye contact. If this is done, the nurse can expect that the child will display:**

1. Decreased crying.
2. Improved fine motor skills.
3. Diminished extrusion reflex.
4. Increased social behaviors.

1. *No, the amount of crying is not directly related to the eye contact and interaction with the mother. A hungry or exhausted infant will continue to cry. Select again.*
2. *Incorrect. Fine motor skills are improved with practice. This is not one of the first skills developed, since reflexes must first fade before fine motor skills can develop.*
3. *Oops, you forgot what this is. The extrusion reflex is pushing the food out of the mouth with the tongue. This is very strong in the newborn and begins to fade in the second six months of life. Select again.*
4. **Correct. This is the purpose of teaching the mother to make eye contact while holding and talking to the infant. The infant's social smile should be seen at about two months of age.**

59. **A nine-year-old girl is admitted with asthma. In planning her care, the nurse should anticipate that the child will prefer to:**

1. Play with another girl her age.
2. Be with older girls.

3. Associate with small groups of boys and girls.
4. Have male companions.

1. **Correct! The school age child is in the latent psychosexual stage according to Freud, and would feel most comfortable with a peer of the same age and sex.**
2. *No, this isn't the school age child's group of choice. Think about the activities that children of this age enjoy; this may help you know who they would be most comfortable with socially.*
3. *Incorrect. Younger children will socialize in this way, not really caring if the companions are male or female. Try again.*
4. *Incorrect. This would be way ahead of this child's psychosexual developmental stage. Adolescents, not school age children, prefer gender opposites. Make another choice.*

60. **Which of the following statements made by a client indicate the need for further teaching regarding a scheduled arthroscopy of the knee?**

1. "I know the doctor will be looking at the joint to check for cartilage damage."
2. "I'll have to limit my exercising for a few weeks after this procedure."
3. "I hope the incision heals quickly with those staples in place."
4. "I know that I'll have to keep my knee straight and elevated to reduce the swelling after the surgery."

1. *No, this is a correct statement. The arthroscopy is done to visualize the joint, including the synovium, articular surfaces, and joint structures. Choose an option that reflects the client's lack of knowledge.*
2. *No, this is a true statement by the client. The client is advised to limit activity following the procedure. Look for a statement that would indicate lack of knowledge about this procedure.*
3. **You're right! An arthroscopy only involves puncture wounds with no need for staples following completion of this procedure. On occasion, a suture may be needed after insertion of the large-bore needle, but it's not standard procedure.**
4. *No, this is correct understanding of post-procedure activity. These measures will help to reduce the swelling after the arthroscopy. Ice is also used for 24 hours afterwards. Choose an option that reflects the client's lack of knowledge.*

61. **CPR has been initiated on a client in the emergency room. Which finding by the nurse would indicate effective cardiac compressions?**

1. An EKG pattern with each compression.
2. Compression depth of 1 1/2 to 2 inches.

3. A palpable femoral pulse during each compression.
4. Pupils changing from pinpoint to dilated.

1. *No, the EKG only indicates an electrical impulse and does not guarantee that there is contraction of the myocardium. There will be an electrical pattern generated by any movement of the chest wall by the compressor.*
2. *Incorrect. This is the correct technique, but this is not an evaluation of effective compression. Try again.*
3. **Absolutely! The nurse should place several fingers on the femoral pulse during artificial compressions. If a pulse is generated with the compression, it is considered effective in circulating blood.**
4. *No, this is backwards! If the pupils change from pinpoint to dilated, this would indicate that the brain is not receiving adequate oxygen due to inadequate ventilations or compressions. Select again.*

62. **Following a colostomy, a client and his wife have been taught to perform a colostomy irrigation. Which behavior by the client would best indicate readiness for discharge?**

1. The client's wife verbalizes all steps in the irrigation procedure.
2. The client performs the irrigation following written instructions.
3. The client and his wife attend all classes given about colostomy care.
4. The client asks appropriate questions about irrigations.

1. *No, not the best response. Consider teaching/learning theory and how learning is best evaluated.*
2. **Yes, this is right. The client has demonstrated ability to perform the skill using the instructions that he will have when he is at home.**
3. *Sounded good, but this doesn't prove competence in the skill. Choose again.*
4. *No. This demonstrates involvement and effort, but not skill in the procedure. Select again.*

63. **The client returns with a Foley catheter after surgery. In providing catheter care, which is the best nursing approach?**

1. Preventing infection and maintaining a patent catheter and drainage system.
2. Keeping the collection bag above the level of the bladder.
3. Using soap and water to clean the perineal area.
4. Maintaining a closed system without any kinks in the tubing.

1. **Very good! This is a comprehensive statement of the best nursing approach in caring for a postoperative client with a catheter. Taking nursing measures to prevent infection will protect the client from the most common complication in catheter care. Maintaining a patent catheter and drainage system will assure drainage of urine and prevent back flow of urine into the bladder.**
2. *This is wrong! The collection bag must be kept below the level of the bladder to prevent back flow of urine into the bladder. Try again.*
3. *Wrong choice. Keeping the perineum clean helps reduce the possibility of infection. This option is a possible answer, however, there is another statement that is a more comprehensive or global statement of the best nursing approach.*
4. *Wrong choice. Preventing kinks and keeping the system closed are specific nursing actions that help to prevent infection and maintain patency of the system. These are appropriate nursing actions, and this option is a possible answer. However, this is not the best option. Look for another option that includes these actions.*

64. **An elderly client is admitted to the hospital for prostatic hypertrophy. The nurse places the bed in the low position and puts the call light within easy reach. He is scheduled to have surgery in the morning. The most important nursing action during the admission of this client is to:**

1. Explain the surgical procedure to the client and family.
2. Explain to the client how to use his call light if he needs the nurse.
3. Tell the client and his family about visiting regulations.
4. Teach the client how to deep breathe and cough.

1. *Wrong. It is the physician's responsibility to explain the surgical procedure to the client. This is not a nursing action. Try again.*
2. **Very good. Explaining the use of the call light provides for the client's safety.**
3. *Wrong choice. Knowledge of visiting hours is important, however, the key word in the stem is "most." This is not the most important nursing action during admission. Read the other options, looking for an option that represents a higher priority.*
4. *Deep breathing and coughing should be taught prior to surgery. However, teaching it at the time of admission is inappropriate and overwhelming for an 88-year-old client. Try again.*

65. **A client who is incontinent of stool has been placed on**

a bowel training program. The nurse understands that the goal of bowel training is to:

1. Prevent soiling of the bed.
2. Prevent cancer of the colon.
3. Prevent loose stools.
4. Provide the client with control over his bowels.

1. *Wrong choice. Bowel training will help the client to avoid soiling of the bed, but preventing soiling of the bed is not the goal of bowel training. Try again.*
2. *No, bowel training does not prevent cancer. Make another choice.*
3. *No, loose stools cannot be prevented by bowel training. Try again.*
4. ***Very good. The bowel training provides the client with the ability to control bowel elimination.***

66. **A client is scheduled for surgery on his bowel. The doctor orders a cleansing enema for the morning of surgery. The best nursing approach is to:**

1. Wear gloves to insert the tubing.
2. Use universal precautions and provide comfort measures to help the client relax during the procedure.
3. Lubricate the tubing well prior to insertion.
4. Position the client on his side and drape the client for warmth and privacy.

1. *Gloves should be worn to prevent contamination. This is a correct nursing action. However, there is a better statement of the best nursing approach. Try again.*
2. ***Very good. This is a comprehensive statement of the best nursing approach. Using universal precautions and providing comfort measures will prevent contamination and provide for the well-being of the client.***
3. *Lubricating the tube provides for the safety and comfort of the client by facilitating insertion. However, there is a better statement of the most appropriate nursing approach. Try again.*
4. *Positioning and privacy are important aspects of administering an enema. However, there is a better statement of the most appropriate nursing intervention. Try again.*

67. **A client is hospitalized for a closed reduction of a fractured femur and application of a cast. A vital nursing action in the care of this client is to:**

1. Perform neurovascular checks of the extremities.
2. Use the palms of the hands when moving an extremity with a wet cast.

3. Provide an instrument for the client to scratch the itching areas of skin under the cast.
4. Petal the edges of the cast to provide smooth edges.

1. ***Excellent! This is an important aspect of care for the client with a fracture. Circulation can become compromised and cause nerve and tissue damage. This action is more "vital" than the other three options.***
2. *Using palms rather than fingertips on a wet cast can avoid indentations in the cast that might result in pressure areas inside the cast. This is an appropriate nursing action, but not the most important or "vital" action. Read all the options, and make another choice.*
3. *This is not an appropriate nursing action! Scratching under the cast can cause injury to the skin and potential infection. Try again.*
4. *Petaling the edges of the cast should be done to prevent injury to the skin caused by uneven edges of the cast. This is an appropriate nursing action, but it is not the most important or "vital" action. This answer is also similar to another choice in that it concerns care of the cast. Make another choice.*

68. **A client is admitted to the hospital for cataract surgery of the left eye. The physician has ordered eye drops to be administered to both eyes at frequent intervals prior to surgery. Which nursing action is most appropriate?**

1. Use aseptic technique and avoid dropping the medication onto the cornea.
2. Gently wash away any crust along the eyelid margin with warm water.
3. Have the client look up toward the ceiling prior to instillation of drops.
4. Drop prescribed number of drops into the conjunctival sac.

1. ***Excellent! Aseptic technique is always used when you are administering medications. The cornea is very sensitive to anything applied to it and dropping medication onto it should be avoided.***
2. *Cleansing of the eyelid provides a clean area for instillation of the drops. This is an appropriate nursing action but it is not the best choice. Read the other options and try to identify the best option.*
3. *Having the client look up protects the cornea from the drops landing on it. This is an appropriate nursing action but it is not the best choice. Read the other options and try to identify the best option.*
4. *The drops should be instilled into the conjunctival sac to avoid placement on the cornea, which is very sensitive. This is an appropriate nursing action but it is not the best choice. Read the other options and try to identify the best option.*

69. A client, who says she has the flu, is seen in the clinic with complaints of vomiting, diarrhea, headache, and dizziness. The nurse takes her vital signs and obtains the following: Blood pressure of 198/110, pulse of 82, respirations of 24 and temperature of 100.8° F. The nurse should immediately report which finding?

1. Complaints of vomiting.
2. Complaints of diarrhea.
3. Complaints of headache and dizziness.
4. Temperature of 100.8° F.

1. *Wrong choice. Vomiting is a manifestation that should be evaluated with further assessment of signs of dehydration and weight loss. This option identifies the physiological needs of hydration and nutrition. However, all of the options in this question address physiological needs! Which need is most immediate for the client? Make another choice.*

2. *Wrong choice. Diarrhea is a manifestation that should be evaluated with further assessment of signs of dehydration and weight loss. Diarrhea may also have several different causes that may need to be explored, depending on the severity of the problem. The severity is not indicated in the case situation. This option identifies the physiological needs of hydration and nutrition. However, all of the options in this question address physiological needs. Make another choice.*

3. **Excellent! The complaints of headache and dizziness are very important manifestations for a client with a blood pressure of 198/110, since they may indicate poor circulation to the brain. This can be life-threatening to the client, and should receive immediate attention.**

4. *Wrong choice. An elevated temperature identifies a physiological need of the client. However, this temperature elevation is not a threat to the client's safety. Since all of the options are physiological needs, the need that most threatens the client's life or well-being is the most important. Make another choice.*

70. A client shows the nurse the result of his recent tuberculin skin test. The site is red and swollen. The nurse interprets this as:

1. The client has active tuberculosis.
2. The client has a history of tuberculosis.
3. The tubercle bacillus is in the active pulmonary stage.
4. The client has had contact with the tubercle bacillus.

1. *Wrong. A skin test that shows a marked change indicates that the client was exposed to the tu-*

bercle bacillus. A positive chest x-ray and a positive sputum for the acid-fast bacillus would indicate active tuberculosis.

2. *Wrong. A positive tuberculin skin test means that they have been exposed to the bacillus. This does not indicate that they have had tuberculosis.*

3. *Wrong. A positive skin test does not indicate an active lesion. Further tests are necessary to diagnose active tuberculosis. Note that Options 1 and 3 are similar distractors.*

4. **Yes! A marked reaction to the skin test indicates exposure to the tubercle bacillus. This question requires an understanding of what a positive reaction to the tuberculin skin test indicates.**

71. The nurse is caring for a client who had abdominal surgery two days ago. The nurse should be most concerned about which finding?

1. A urinary drainage bag with 100 ccs of straw colored urine.
2. A wound dressing with thick light green drainage.
3. A blood pressure reading of 98/66.
4. Shallow respirations, with a rate of 30.

1. *Wrong choice. The amount of urine in the drainage bag does not provide any useful data, since the clinical situation does not include a time frame for measuring the client's output. More information is needed.*

2. **Good choice! Thick light green drainage is indicative of an infection and should be reported to the physician immediately. The stem of the question requires analysis of the data by the nurse. This option also addresses a client safety issue, which requires an immediate response by the nurse.**

3. *Wrong choice. Since baseline data is not provided in the question, the nurse cannot determine whether or not the blood pressure reading is normal for this client. Further assessment is needed.*

4. *Wrong choice. Shallow respirations are not unusual for the client who has undergone abdominal surgery. Although the nurse needs to address this issue by having the client deep breathe and cough, it is not the priority action.*

72. An elderly client is discharged from the hospital after treatment for poor circulation to her lower extremities. The nurse would consider it an indication that discharge teaching was unsuccessful if the client:

1. Puts on stockings with elastic tops and tells the nurse that she does not like other kinds of hosiery.
2. Tells the nurse that she will get a thermometer to measure the temperature of the bath water.

3. Asks her husband to take her sandals home, and bring a pair of shoes to the hospital for her to wear home.
4. The client tells the nurse that she is going to have to remember to keep her legs uncrossed.

1. ***Good, you identified the incorrect action by the client! Elastic tops on stockings decrease circulation and should be avoided by clients with circulation problems. This action and statement by the client indicates that the client is not motivated to care for her health care needs.***
2. *Wrong choice, this action by the client would be appropriate. A client who has poor circulation has a decreased sense of temperature. This statement indicates that the client has successfully learned what the nurse taught her. Because this question has a false response stem, this option cannot be the correct answer. Try again.*
3. *Wrong choice, this action by the client is appropriate. Clients with poor circulation need to wear shoes that protect their feet from injury. This action by the client indicates to the nurse that learning has taken place. Because this question has a false response stem, this option cannot be the correct answer. Try again.*
4. *Wrong choice, this action by the client is appropriate. Crossing the legs at the knees impairs circulation and should be avoided by the client. This action by the client indicates to the nurse that the client does understand the discharge instructions. Because this question has a false response stem, this option cannot be the correct answer. Make another choice.*

73. **A client, age 63, is being discharged after insertion of a pacemaker for a persistent dysrhythmia. Which statement by the client indicates the need for further teaching by the nurse?**

1. "I know that I have to check my pulse every day, preferably in the morning."
2. "I sure will miss being able to continue with my bowling league. I guess I'll take up walking as a sport!"
3. "I'll stay away from my microwave oven so that it doesn't interfere with my pacemaker."
4. "If I start having any palpitations or dizziness, I'll call my doctor right away."

1. *No, the client understands the need to check the pacemaker's functioning every day. A pulse rate significantly above or below the programmed rate should be reported to the physician. Make another selection.*
2. ***Good for you! You recognized that the client does not have correct information regarding his participation in sports. He should avoid***

all contact sports, but should be able to resume bowling without problems.
3. *No, the client is correct in making this statement. He should avoid microwave ovens, arc welders, and electrical generators as well as holding electrical equipment such as blow dryers next to his pacemaker. These activities may cause interference, place the pacemaker in a fixed mode or shut it off. Choose another option.*
4. *No, the client is correct when he knows to report any signs of decreased cardiac output, such as dizziness, fatigue, "palpitations," or dyspnea. Look for a statement that is incorrect.*

74. **A client diagnosed with urolithiasis is advised to follow a low calcium diet after his pathology report reveals calcium oxalate stones. Which menu selection by the client indicates to the nurse the need for further teaching?**

1. Hamburger, baked potato, squash.
2. Shrimp, scalloped potatoes, broccoli.
3. Chicken, wild rice, green beans.
4. Roast pork, whipped potatoes, carrots.

1. *No, this menu selection is low in calcium. The client would be correct in choosing this menu. Try again.*
2. ***Correct. This menu choice is inappropriate for this client. Shellfish, broccoli, and the milk and cheese used to make the scalloped potatoes are all high in calcium. The client would need further teaching if he chose these menu items.***
3. *No, this menu is low in calcium and would be acceptable. You are to select an option that is an inappropriate choice for this client.*
4. *Incorrect. These food items are acceptable on a low calcium diet. The client would not need further teaching with this menu selection. Choose another option.*

75. **A 72-year-old client was admitted to the hospital for pneumonia. He is receiving oxygen at six liters per mask. In obtaining his vital signs, it would be inappropriate for the nurse to:**

1. Take an axillary temperature.
2. Listen to his lungs when counting respirations.
3. Listen to an apical heart rate.
4. Take an oral temperature.

1. *Wrong choice. This is appropriate, since the oral temperature of a client receiving oxygen therapy via nasal cannula or mask is not a reliable measurement. The stem of the question asks for an inappropriate action.*
2. *Wrong choice, this is an appropriate action. The lungs should be auscultated because the client has pneumonia. The stem of the question asks for an*

inappropriate action.

3. *Wrong choice. Because of the client's age, auscultating an apical heart rate is important because it allows the nurse to assess for any abnormal heart sounds. This is an appropriate action, but this question asks for an inappropriate action.*

4. ***Very good! This is an inappropriate nursing action, since the oral temperature of a client receiving oxygen therapy via nasal cannula or mask is not a reliable measurement.***

76. **The client is admitted with anorexia nervosa. A nasogastric tube is to be inserted. In preparing the client for this procedure, what would the nurse do first?**

1. Assist the client to a sitting position.
2. Explain the procedure to the client.
3. If the client has dentures, make sure that they are in place in the client's mouth.
4. Have a stethoscope available to listen for proper placement.

1. *This is an appropriate position, but it is not the initial nursing approach. The word "first" is a key word in the stem of the question.*

2. ***Excellent! Informing the client reduces fear and is helpful in gaining the cooperation of the client, which is necessary for implementation of this procedure.***

3. *This is an incorrect statement. This procedure may induce gagging, and dentures may become dislodged and cause the client to choke. Dentures should be removed before this procedure.*

4. *The issue in the question is insertion of a nasogastric tube, and the stem asks for the first nursing action to prepare the client. Although a stethoscope is necessary to allow the nurse to hear air that might be instilled into the stomach, this measure does not prepare the client for the procedure.*

77. **A client fell at home and fractured her hip. She is to have surgery in the morning. In preparing the client for surgery, it is outside the scope of the nurse's responsibilities to:**

1. Assess the health status of the client.
2. Explain the operative procedure and any risks that may be involved with the procedure.
3. Determine that the history, physical, and specific laboratory tests have been ordered or completed according to hospital protocol.
4. Determine that a signed surgical consent form is completed.

1. *Wrong choice. Assessing health status is an expected standard of care for the preoperative client. The is not the correct option, however, be-*

cause this question has a false response stem.

2. ***Excellent! Explaining the procedure and risks is a physician responsibility. This is not a nursing responsibility. Since this question has a false response stem, this is the correct option to choose.***

3. *Wrong choice. This action is a nursing responsibility that is part of record keeping and helps assure the safety of the client. This is not the correct option, however, because the question has a false response stem.*

4. *Wrong choice. A signed surgical consent is necessary for this case situation. It is a nursing responsibility to assure that the signed consent form is on the client's chart prior to surgery. This true statement is not the answer, however, since this question has a false response stem.*

78. **A client is scheduled for an abdominal hysterectomy. In order to prevent pneumonia from developing postoperatively, the most important nursing action is:**

1. Teach the client how to deep breathe and cough before surgery.
2. Inform the client that even though she will have pain after surgery, she will have to move from side to side in bed.
3. Tell the client that if she does not ambulate soon after surgery that there is a good chance that she may develop complications.
4. Tell the client that it is very important that she deep breathe and cough often after surgery to prevent complications.

1. ***Very good. Teaching the client prior to surgery is the most important nursing action to prevent pneumonia from developing after surgery. Having the client practice before she has incisional pain increases compliance, since she will know how to perform.***

2. *This is a good distractor. This is a true statement, but it is not the most important nursing action and does not address pneumonia, which is the issue in the question.*

3. *This is a true statement, but it is not the most important nursing action and does not specifically address pneumonia, which is the issue in the question.*

4. *This option may appear to be similar to Option 1, but it does not teach the client how to accomplish this task. This is not the best option.*

79. **An obese client has been placed on a high protein, low calorie diet by his physician. It would be most important for the nurse to explain to the client:**

1. That he will have to change his eating habits.
2. The importance of exercise when dieting.
3. What types of foods are permitted on a low calorie, high protein diet.

4. That if he doesn't stay on this diet he will continue to gain weight.

1. *This statement may be true, but it does not provide much useful information for the client. Consider the other options before selecting the best one.*

2. *Exercise enhances the diet process by burning up calories. However, this option does not address the issue of the question, which is a high protein, low calorie diet. There also is no indication that exercise is included in this client's care plan. Do not "read into" the question! Try again.*

3. **Very good. Providing the client with knowledge concerning the types of foods that he can eat will help him to be more compliant.**

4. *Although this may be a true statement, it is nontherapeutic. Also, the nurse does not know that the client is gaining weight at this time. Do not "read into" the question! Try again.*

80. **In obtaining a blood pressure measurement, the most appropriate nursing action is to:**

1. Obtain the proper equipment, place the client in a comfortable position, and record the appropriate information in the client's chart.
2. Measure the client's arm, if you are uncertain of the size of cuff to use.
3. Have the client recline or sit comfortably in a chair with the forearm at the level of the heart.
4. Document the measurement, which extremity was used, and the position that the client was in during the measurement.

1. **Very good! This is a general or comprehensive statement about the correct procedure, and it includes the basic ideas that are found in the other options.**

2. *This option is a possibility. The correct size cuff is necessary in order to obtain a reliable measurement. However, this is not the best option. Try to restate the question in your own words. Read the other options and try again.*

3. *This is an appropriate nursing action. The client should be relaxed and comfortable for a reliable reading. However, this is not the best option. Try to restate the question in your own words. Read the other options and try again.*

4. *Documentation of these parameters is essential. However, this is not the best option. Try to restate the question in your own words. Read the other options and try again.*

81. **A client has just returned to her room after abdominal surgery. She has a nasogastric tube in place and a drain attached to a HemoVac. The Foley catheter is draining clear yellow urine. The nurse understands the reason for maintaining the side rails in the raised position is to:**

1. Prevent the urine collection bag and tubing from getting tangled up in the side rails when the client is turned in bed.
2. Prevent the client from falling out of bed after receiving an anesthetic.
3. Provide a place to attach the nasogastric tubing to prevent it from being dislodged.
4. Attach the call light so it is within easy reach.

1. *This option might be a possibility. However, the urine collection bag and tubing can be attached to the side rails even if the side rails are lowered, so this is not a reason for having the side rails up on the bed. Try again.*

2. **This is the correct answer. Post operative clients who have received anesthesia are usually very sleepy and not aware of their surroundings. The client may fall out of bed if the side rails are not raised. This is the best option because it provides for the safety of the client. Good work!**

3. *This option is false! It is an incorrect nursing action to attach the nasogastric tube to the side rail, because it may become dislodged when the side rail is lowered or raised.*

4. *This option might be a possibility. However, the call light can be attached to the side rail even if the side rails are lowered, so this is not the reason for maintaining the side rails in a raised position.*

82. **An elderly client was admitted to the hospital with a cerebrovascular accident with left-sided paralysis. He is placed on an air mattress. The nurse explains to the family that the purpose of frequently turning this client is to:**

1. Prevent sensory deprivation by varying what the client sees in his environment.
2. Prevent skin breakdown, which is a common problem in the elderly.
3. Prevent stasis of blood in the lower extremities.
4. Increase blood supply to the affected side.

1. *Wrong choice. Although this is accomplished by turning a client, it is not the best rationale for turning this client. Read the other options, and try to identify a better rationale.*

2. **Correct. The elderly have very thin, fragile skin, which breaks down very easily. Therefore, in order to prevent bed sores, the client should be turned every two hours.**

3. *No, turning the client does not prevent stasis of blood. Contraction of the muscles or support stockings are measures that help prevent stasis of blood in the lower extremities. This cannot be the answer.*

4. *Wrong choice. Although increased blood supply may reach the affected side by turning the client,*

this is not the best reason for turning this client. Read the other options, and try to identify a better rationale.

83.   In caring for elderly clients the nurse understands that the aging process generally results in:

1.   A decline in physiological and sensory systems of the body.
2.   A decreased skin resilience.
3.   A diminished hearing acuity.
4.   An absence of sexual interest and activity.

1.   Good! This is a general statement about the effects of aging.
2.   Wrong choice. Loss of skin resilience is a normal finding in the elderly, however, this is not the best option. Read the other options, and try to select the best one.
3.   Wrong choice. Many elderly clients experience some hearing loss, however, this is not the best option. Read the other options, and try to select the best one.
4.   This is not true! Sexual interest and activity does not cease in the elderly. Try again!

84.   A client had a cholecystectomy three days ago. Which diet modification would the nurse include in the client's plan of care?

1.   Low fat diet, gradually progressing to moderate fat if tolerated.
2.   Low sodium, low fat diet.
3.   Elimination of red meat.
4.   Elimination of dairy products.

1.   Correct. Low fat diet is prescribed postoperatively with a gradual introduction of moderately fatty foods on a maintenance basis.
2.   Incorrect. Sodium is not restricted following gallbladder surgery.
3.   Incorrect. Red meat does not have to be eliminated, though the diet should be restricted to lean meats.
4.   Incorrect. Dairy products do not have to be eliminated, though the diet should be limited to low fat dairy products.

85.   Nursing care of the client with glomerulonephritis includes the administration of:

1.   Antibiotics, corticosteroids and anticoagulants.
2.   Vitamin K and hypoglycemic agents.
3.   Immunoglobulins and antibiotics.
4.   Vasodilators and cardiotonic glycosides.

1.   Correct. These drugs are commonly prescribed for glomerulonephritis.
2.   Incorrect. Anticoagulants, not vitamin K, are indicated. Hypoglycemic agents are not generally pre-

scribed unless the client has non-insulin dependent diabetes. Try again.
3.   Incorrect. Immunoglobulins are not commonly prescribed for this condition. Try again.
4.   Incorrect. Vasodilators are not commonly prescribed, nor are cardiac glycosides. Try again.

86.   Nursing management of the client with Addison's disease, who is experiencing Addisonian crisis, includes which nursing action?

1.   Maintain the restriction of fluids.
2.   Encourage a low protein, low carbohydrate diet.
3.   Teach effective daily exercises.
4.   Weigh the client daily and monitor intake and output.

1.   Incorrect. Fluids are not restricted. Select another option.
2.   Incorrect. A high protein, high carbohydrate diet is prescribed to insure adequate caloric intake, because weight loss is common in Addisonian crisis. Select another option.
3.   Incorrect. Bedrest is generally prescribed to conserve energy. Select another option.
4.   Correct. GI disturbances are common, so it is important to weigh the client daily, monitor intake and output to detect dehydration, and monitor for hyperkalemia and hyponatremia.

87.   An elderly client tripped on some stairs and injured her right hip. She underwent a total hip replacement. In caring for this client in the immediate postoperative period, the nurse knows it would be inappropriate to:

1.   Maintain immobilization of the right hip.
2.   Encourage fluid intake to prevent dehydration.
3.   Observe for signs of thrombus formation.
4.   Perform all of the client's personal care activities.

1.   Wrong choice, this action is appropriate. The affected hip must be kept immobilized during the recuperative period.
2.   Wrong choice, this action is appropriate. Maintaining hydration postoperatively is important.
3.   Wrong choice, this action is appropriate. Observing for signs of possible thrombus formation is critical during the postoperative period.
4.   Correct. This would not be appropriate. The client should be encouraged to perform activities that permit independence, such as brushing hair and teeth, washing hands and face, and eating.

88.   A client is being prepared for an MRI (Magnetic Resonance Imaging) of the spinal column. Prior to the procedure, the nurse should instruct the client to:

1. Remain as motionless as possible during the procedure.
2. Refrain from eating.
3. Request a sleeping pill.
4. Take an enema.

*1. **Correct. It is important to remain motionless during the procedure, to decrease any interference.***
2. Incorrect. There are no food restrictions prior to the MRI.
3. Incorrect. Sometimes a sedative may be ordered if the client is very anxious, but a sleeping pill is not indicated.
4. Incorrect. This is not necessary prior to the MRI.

89. **The nurse is teaching a class on diabetes mellitus. The nurse explains that differences between childhood and adult onset diabetes mellitus include:**

1. Insulin therapy is frequently used in childhood diabetes, and oral hypoglycemic drugs often are used in the management of adult onset diabetes.
2. The onset in childhood diabetes is insidious, while the onset in an adult diabetes is rapid.
3. The use of dietary treatment for childhood diabetes is adequate, while it is inadequate for treatment of adult onset diabetes.
4. The incidence of hypoglycemia and ketoacidosis is infrequent in children and more common with adult onset diabetes.

*1. **Correct. Insulin is not produced by the Islets of Langerhans in childhood diabetes and therefore must be obtained exogenously. Oral hypo-glycemic agents are used in adult onset diabetes when some insulin can still be produced by the pancreas.***
2. Incorrect. There is a rapid onset of diabetes in children, compared to a slower onset in adults.
3. Incorrect. The use of dietary treatment is possible in one third of adult diabetics but is rarely adequate in childhood diabetes.
4. Incorrect. Hypoglycemia and ketoacidosis is common in children and less common in adults.

90. **A client is scheduled for a colostomy after being diagnosed with cancer of the large intestine. The nurse should begin client teaching:**

1. Postoperatively, after the pain has subsided, when the client will be better able to concentrate.
2. Postoperatively, after meeting with the ostomy nurse.
3. When the client demonstrates an interest in learning about the ostomy.
4. Preoperatively, to involve the client in his care and give him a sense of control over his life.

1. Incorrect. Teaching begins before the operation has occurred, not postoperatively.

> **TEST-TAKING TIP:** *This option is very similar to Option 2. Two options that use similar ideas are probably both wrong and can be ruled out as possible answers.*

2. Incorrect. Teaching begins before the operation, not postoperatively. Consultation with the ostomy nurse is also done preoperatively.

> **TEST-TAKING TIP:** *This option is very similar to Option 1. Two options that use similar ideas are probably both wrong and can be ruled out as possible answers.*

3. Incorrect. The client may be in denial, but the nurse has the responsibility to educate the client, using patience and empathy.
*4. **Correct. Teaching always begins in the preoperative period. Preparation of the client, mentally, emotionally, and physically, is one of the nurse's primary responsibilities.***

91. **The physician requests a stool specimen for culture, for an alert and ambulatory client. The nurse would give which directions to the client for proper stool collection?**

1. Restrict food and liquids the night before the collection.
2. Maintain a sterile procedure.
3. Require the collection of specimens on three consecutive days.
4. Retrieve from the toilet with sterile gloves and then place in the container.

1. Incorrect. There are no food or fluid restrictions involved in the collection of a stool specimen. Try again.
2. Incorrect. This is not possible. However, the client should use a procedure that will ensure that the specimen is not contaminated when transferred to the container.
*3. **Correct. This is normal procedure for a stool culture in order to detect pathogens of the gastrointestinal tract.***
4. No! The stool specimen should not be immersed in water, and certainly not in the toilet. It should be placed directly into the specimen container.

92. **The nurse is to prepare a client for a proctosigmoidoscopy. The proper position for this client is the:**

1. Left lateral (left side) or knee chest.
2. Right lateral (right side).
3. Dorsal recumbent position (back-lying).
4. Prone position (abdomen).

1. *Correct. The bowel is best visualized in this position.*
2. *Incorrect. This is not the position used for this procedure. Try again.*
3. *Incorrect. This position is ineffective and inappropriate for the endoscopic procedure, since the bowel cannot be accessed.*
4. *Incorrect. This is an ineffective and inappropriate position for the endoscopic procedure, since the knees need to be flexed for the bowel to be visualized.*

93. A client is hospitalized for gastrointestinal bleeding and is being treated with temazepam (Restoril). After the client's physician examines him, the nurse notes the physician has written an order for the client to begin taking amitriptyline (Elavil). Which action by the nurse is best initially?

1. Revise his medication schedule so that Elavil is administered during the day and the Restoril at night.
2. Monitor the client's vital signs closely.
3. Question the physician about administering both Elavil and Restoril to the client.
4. Assess the client for manifestations of depression.

1. *This is not correct. Elavil is a tricyclic antidepressant that is very sedating. It is often chosen for depressed clients who also have difficulty sleeping. There is a better option.*
2. *This is not the best option. The client's vital signs should be monitored when he is placed on Elavil because it may cause orthostatic hypotension. Review the choices to select a better one.*
3. *Correct. Benzodiazepines, such as Restoril, potentiate the effects of other central nervous system depressants, such as the tricyclic, Elavil. The nurse should question the safety of administering these two medications to the client.*
4. *This is an appropriate nursing action, but it is not the best initial action. Review the choices again and select the better action.*

94. A client is taking erythromycin delayed-release capsules (Eryc) for a urinary tract infection. By the fourth day of a 10-day treatment, he tells the nurse he's fine now and will keep the remainder of his medicine for another infection. The appropriate nursing response is:

1. "Good idea, you will save lots of money that way."
2. "You should always take the full course of antibiotics because it is still possible for many of the bacteria to be in your urinary tract."

3. "Take at least one more day of medication."
4. "That would really be a stupid thing to do."

1. *No! If the client only takes a few days of the medication, the bacteria that are left become sensitized to the antibiotic and may become resistant. When the bacteria start to grow again, the client will need more potent (and more expensive medications) to treat his infection.*
2. *This is the correct response. It is important to take the full course of medications unless there are untoward effects like severe diarrhea, or sensitivity reactions. Medications should not be shared or saved!*
3. *Wrong! Taking the medication for one more day would still allow bacterial resistance to develop and would not be beneficial.*
4. *No! This would not be a professional statement! Please read the options again.*

95. On the third day of amoxicillin (Amoxil) therapy, a client develops diarrhea. The nurse should instruct the client to:

1. Stop taking the drug, as this is an indication of toxicity.
2. Contact her physician about treatment of the diarrhea.
3. Drink extra liquids to compensate for the fluid lost in the diarrhea.
4. Take an over-the-counter antidiarrheal agent according to package directions.

1. *Incorrect. Diarrhea is an adverse reaction to Amoxil but not a toxic reaction. It's not an indication to stop taking the medication. Try another selection.*
2. *Good choice! Diarrhea is a frequent adverse GI reaction to amoxicillin therapy. It is advisable to contact the physician before adding any new drug to a treatment regimen, including over-the-counter antidiarrheal agents.*
3. *Sorry, this is not the best answer. Although drinking extra fluids is appropriate to prevent fluid volume deficit, the client needs intervention to control diarrhea and to prevent electrolyte depletion (especially potassium). Try again.*
4. *This is not sound judgment on the nurse's part. Clients should be cautioned about taking over-the-counter drugs without notifying their primary care giver. Try another option.*

96. In order to minimize the most common side effect of tetracycline therapy, the nurse should instruct the client to:

1. Drink at least 2000 ml of fluid a day.
2. Take the medicine with a full glass of water.

3. Take the medicine with milk or an antacid.
4. Increase the intake of high fiber foods and roughage.

1. Incorrect. Drinking extra fluids is basically a sound intervention, as most tetracyclines are excreted via the kidneys, but renal toxicity is most commonly seen in clients with preexisting renal insufficiency. It is not a common adverse reaction. Choose another option.

2. Correct! Tetracyclines should be taken with a full glass of water to prevent esophageal erosion and GI irritation, the most common complaint of clients taking this medication. Manifestations include nausea/vomiting, diarrhea, epigastric distress, and abdominal discomfort.

3. No! Tetracyclines should not be taken with milk or antacids because they decrease the drug's absorption.

4. This would not be a correct action, since constipation is not a side effect of tetracycline therapy. Make another selection.

97. A client is taking propranolol (Inderal) for hypertension. The nurse reviewing the client's history knows that the use of Inderal may be contraindicated by:

1. "Smoker's" cough.
2. Sinusitis.
3. Asthma
4. Hay fever.

1. Not the best choice. A "smoker's" cough can be due to many causes, some as minor as throat irritation, and some manifestations of much more serious conditions. The cause of the cough must be determined before any medications become contraindicated or treatments are undertaken. Because of this, this option is not the best answer.

2. This is not a contraindication. Sinusitis, usually due to allergies, does not contraindicate the use of Inderal. Inderal most probably will not affect the sinusitis either adversely or beneficially.

3. You are correct! Inderal can cause bronchospasm, because it blocks the sympathetic stimulation for smooth muscle relaxation. Asthma is characterized by secretion production and bronchospasm. Inderal is contraindicated.

4. Sorry, no. Inderal will not affect hay fever adversely or beneficially. A hay fever allergy is not indicative of a possible hypersensitivity to medications.

98. A client diagnosed with emphysema is being prepared for discharge. Which nursing measure would be most beneficial for improving his gas exchange?

1. Teaching home oxygen therapy at five liters/minute.
2. Encouraging him to take slow, deep breaths.
3. Demonstrating the proper technique for chest breathing.
4. Teaching him pursed lip breathing.

1. Incorrect! Remember that low concentrations of oxygen (1-2 liters/minute) are indicated for clients with COPD. Try again!

2. No, although this is an expected outcome, the nurse must teach the client how to achieve this effect. Make another selection.

3. No! The client with COPD should be taught diaphragmatic breathing, which helps to reduce the respiratory rate and increases alveolar ventilation. Choose another option.

4. Good choice! Pursed lip breathing slows expiration, prevents collapse of lung units, and helps the client to control the rate and depth of respirations.

99. The client is being discharged after diagnosis of a peptic ulcer. To help to decrease acid secretions in the stomach, the nurse should instruct the client to:

1. Increase intake of milk and cream products.
2. Limit alcohol consumption.
3. Avoid high fiber foods.
4. Eat a bland diet; decaffeinated coffee only.

1. No! Diets rich in milk and cream are potentially harmful because they're potent acid stimuli and, over a long period they increase serum lipids, which can lead to atherosclerosis. Choose another option.

2. Correct choice! Overstimulation by alcohol and coffee, including decaffeinated coffee, can cause oversecretion of gastric acids, leading to delayed healing.

3. There is no evidence to suggest that high fiber foods lead to oversecretion of gastric acids. The client should include some of these foods in his diet to prevent constipation. Select again.

4. There is little evidence to support the theory that bland diets are more beneficial than regular meals. Clients are encouraged to eat whatever agrees with them, but to avoid all forms of coffee during the early stages of ulcer healing because even decaffeinated coffee stimulates acid secretion.

100. A four-year-old is admitted to the hospital with croup. When the mother comes to visit the next day, she finds the nurse changing the bedding after the client has wet the bed. The mother says, "He never wets the bed at home. I am so embarrassed." Which nursing response is most helpful to the mother?

1. "I know this can really be embarrassing, but I have kids myself, so I understand and it doesn't bother me."
2. "It is not uncommon for children to regress during a hospitalization. His toileting skills will return when he is feeling better."
3. "It's probably due to the medication we are giving him for his infection."
4. "I plan to discuss your child's incontinency with the physician, as this may require further investigation."

1. *No. Even though you may have heard nurses say this, this is not therapeutic communication, since it offers no information about the source or treatment of the incontinency.*

2. **This is correct. A recently gained skill such as toilet training is often temporarily lost due to the stress of hospitalization. It is appropriate to reassure the mother that this is an expected behavior in young children and that continence will be regained when his health is regained.**

3. *Not true. The medications most likely to be administered for croup would be antibiotics and acetaminophen; neither have side effects of incontinency.*

4. *Not likely, with the information given. Are you reading into the question? Manifestations such as hematuria, abdominal pain, or pain during urination would be necessary to warrant follow-up from this one episode.*

NOTES

NCLEX-PN

Test 6

NCLEX-PN TEST 6

1. An 82-year-old client has oral candidiasis and is prescribed nystatin (Mycostatin) oral suspension. Which statement by the client indicates to the nurse that the client needs further teaching regarding the administration of Mycostatin?

   1. "I'll make sure to brush my teeth before taking a dose of this medicine."
   2. "I know that I should drink a full glass of water after each dose of medicine."
   3. "I'll keep the medicine in my mouth for several minutes before swallowing it."
   4. "I'll limit the amount of mouthwash I use from now on to decrease my chances of getting this fungal infection again."

2. In preparing to teach a client with glaucoma about the use of eye medication, the nurse knows that which information about the treatment of glaucoma is inaccurate?

   1. The drops should be instilled without touching the dropper to the eye.
   2. The medication must be stored at the proper temperature.
   3. Vision may become blurred after use, so the client needs to use caution.
   4. The medication is taken for 2-3 weeks and then discontinued.

3. A newly diagnosed diabetic is receiving instructions about dietary management of his disease. In providing information, the nurse is aware that the most important objective in the dietary management of diabetes mellitus is:

   1. Control of total calorie intake in order to attain or maintain ideal weight.
   2. An accurate distribution of calories from carbohydrates, protein, and fat.
   3. Weight reduction to reverse the hyperglycemia.
   4. Meeting energy needs while decreasing blood lipid levels.

4. A client is being treated with nystatin (Mycostatin) oral suspension for a candida oropharyngeal infection. The nurse should instruct the client to:

   1. Swallow the solution quickly, to avoid burning the throat.
   2. Take the medication with a glass of water.
   3. Swish the solution around in the mouth, then hold it there for as long as possible.
   4. Take the medication on an empty stomach.

5. A client has been diagnosed with tuberculosis. Isoniazid (INH) and rifampin (Rifadin) have been prescribed and the client asks the nurse how long he'll be taking the drugs. Which statement by the nurse is most accurate?

   1. "You'll need to stay on the medications for approximately three months, until the manifestations subside and your sputum culture is negative."
   2. "You'll need to take both medications for a year. It's important to follow the exact schedule set up by your physician."
   3. "You'll be taking both medications for six months, at which time the doctor will discontinue the rifampin and then you'll have another three months on just the INH."
   4. "You'll need to take both medications for approximately six to nine months, at which time there should be complete eradication of the disease."

6. A pediatric nurse suspects that a recently admitted child has been abused. He is three years old and has a dislocated shoulder and internal bleeding. Which observation would lead the nurse to suspect abuse of this client?

   1. The child's mother cried while describing the accident that caused her son's injuries, saying it was all her fault because she was talking on the telephone when it happened.
   2. The child's mother held him closely and comforted him while talking with the nurse.
   3. The child's mother gives an account of the accident that is not consistent with the injuries her son sustained.
   4. The child, while crying from time to time, cooperated with the examination.

7. In planning the initial care for client with an acute schizophrenic illness, the nurse should emphasize:

   1. Establishing a daily routine to promote orientation to the unit.
   2. Providing a variety of activities to keep the client focused on reality-based topics.
   3. Encouraging the client to enter into simple group activities.
   4. Assigning the same members of the nursing staff to work with the client each day.

8. As the nurse approaches a schizophrenic, paranoid type client, he says, "Back off. Leave me alone." He appears tense and is pacing rapidly. The best nursing response to his remark is:

1. "I can't leave you alone when you are this upset. Sit down and try to relax."
2. "Let's go to your room and you can tell me what is bothering you."
3. "I will keep my distance as long as you can control yourself. You appear quite angry and I'd like to know more about what is causing you to feel this way."
4. "I will leave you alone for a few minutes while you try to compose yourself."

9. A 45-year-old business executive was diagnosed with a gastric ulcer two years ago and was advised to scale down his activities and learn to relax. He is now returning to the HMO with increased epigastric pain. Upon questioning, he tells the nurse that he has been busier than ever. The most realistic short-term goal for dealing with stress that the nurse can suggest to this client is to:

1. Express his emotions more directly.
2. Decrease his workload.
3. Use relaxation techniques each day.
4. Decrease social activities.

10. The nurse refers a rape client to a support group in her community. The client asks how the support group can help her. In responding to the client, the nurse understands that which of the following is not consistent with the goals of this kind of support group?

1. Decreasing the client's feelings of isolation and shame through membership in a group.
2. Support for the client in regaining her positive self-esteem.
3. Examining the client's behavior and receiving useful feedback, in a safe place and from persons who understand what she has been through.
4. Learning better interpersonal skills through examination of the process that develops among the members of the support group.

11. In cases of suspected child abuse, the nurse's primary legal obligation is to:

1. Prevent the parents from taking the child home from the hospital until a full investigation has been completed.
2. Inform the physician of the nurse's suspicions, so the physician can order any x-ray or laboratory studies that may be warranted to document the abuse.
3. Contact the appropriate authorities, usually Child Protective Services, to file a report.
4. Notify the nursing supervisor, so that the hospital's

attorney can be contacted for legal counsel.

12. A 16-year-old, 5'4" high school student is admitted to an eating disorders program by her psychiatrist. She tells the admitting nurse she has lost 25 pounds over the past month and now weighs 85 pounds. In assessing the client, the nurse would identify which manifestations as early characteristics of anorexia nervosa?

1. Appetite loss, amenorrhea, bradycardia, loss of 15% of pre-illness body weight.
2. Appetite loss, amenorrhea, tachycardia, hyper- activity.
3. Tachycardia, insomnia, fear of obesity, bulimia.
4. Amenorrhea, bradycardia, disturbed body image, loss of 15% of pre-illness body weight.

13. The nurse realizes a typical characteristic of girls with anorexia nervosa is:

1. They fail to comply with their parents' wishes or societal expectations.
2. They exercise relentlessly.
3. They are truthful in reporting their eating habits.
4. They have problems with self-control.

14. In caring for a bulimic client, the nurse understands that in contrast to clients with anorexia nervosa, clients with bulimia characteristically:

1. Recognize that their eating behavior is abnormal.
2. Rarely suffer serious medical consequences.
3. Have positive feelings about their eating patterns.
4. Vomit or use laxatives after an eating binge, to purge the food.

15. Which activity would be most appropriate for the nurse to suggest to a manic client?

1. A daily walk on the hospital grounds.
2. Playing a computer game with another client.
3. Participation in a basketball game with other male clients.
4. Reading quietly in his room.

16. An 18-year-old client is hospitalized for treatment of severe depression. Because of the client's condition, which approach is most appropriate for the nurse to include in the client's plan of care?

1. Giving the client choices.
2. Spending time with the client.
3. Providing a chess game.
4. Encouraging decision-making.

17. An elderly client is admitted to the hospital with pneumonia. His daughter, who takes care of him at home, says to

the nurse, "I'm so glad he is here. You can take much better care of him than I can." What is the best nursing response to the daughter?

1. "We do have the equipment and people to take care of sick clients."
2. "It is not easy to care for the elderly. How do you manage?"
3. "Sir, your daughter takes good care of you at home, doesn't she?"
4. "Are you feeling guilty because your father has pneumonia?"

18. A client is to have a nasogastric tube inserted. The nurse explains the procedure to him and is about to begin the insertion, when the client says, "No way! You are not putting that hose down my throat. Get away from me." Which is the most appropriate nursing response?

1. "You have the right to refuse treatment. Why don't you talk to your doctor about it?"
2. "Something is upsetting you. Can you tell me what it is?"
3. "What do you feel about this 'hose'?"
4. "I would just get it over with, because you won't get better without this tube."

19. The nurse observes an elderly client trying to climb over the side rails of the bed. When placing a vest restraint on the client, the client's daughter says to the nurse, "My mother does not need to be tied down in bed. I've been caring for her for years, and she hasn't fallen out of bed yet." Which response is therapeutic for the daughter?

1. "I just saw your mother trying to climb over the side rails. Since I am concerned about her falling and hurting herself, I think this is best for her safety."
2. "Tell me how you managed to care for her at home."
3. "Hospital policy requires restraint vests on clients who are at risk for falling. I just saw your mother trying to climb over the rails. You don't want her to get hurt, do you?"
4. "The elderly may become confused in an unfamiliar place and do things they wouldn't do at home. It is difficult to see her restrained. While you are with her, the restraints can be off. Let me know when you are ready to leave."

20. A mother arrives at the emergency room with her child, who is wet, and the color of his skin is blue. She shouts to the nurse, "I think that I have killed my son. I wasn't watching him like I should have, and he fell in the pool." While the doctor and other nursing staff are providing care for the child, the nurse stays with the mother to obtain information. What is the most appropriate response by the nurse?

1. "These things happen. Don't blame yourself."
2. "You are right. A child should always be watched when he is playing near a pool."
3. "You didn't kill him. He is still alive. It is going to be all right."
4. "It must feel terrible to have something like this happen to your child."

21. The nurse is preparing to give an elderly client a bath. The client says to the nurse, "I don't think that I need a bath today. I just had one yesterday. My skin is going to get too dry. I bathe completely every other day at home." Which response by the nurse is best?

1. "My head nurse wants all of the clients bathed daily because it decreases the number of germs on your skin that cause infection. Would you like to talk to the head nurse about your concerns?"
2. "A bath can make you feel refreshed and make the day seem brighter. Don't you agree?"
3. "Would you like to compromise and just wash your face and hands today?"
4. "I heard you say that you didn't want a bath today."

22. A 15-year-old client is being seen in the family planning clinic. She says to the nurse that she is nervous and has never had a pelvic examination before. The best response by the nurse is:

1. "All you have to do is relax."
2. "It is only slightly uncomfortable."
3. "What part of the exam makes you nervous?"
4. "If you want birth control pills, then a pelvic exam is required."

23. The nurse finds an elderly client on bedrest standing next to her bed. The side rails are in the up position, and the client's IV is pulled out. The client is confused, does not have an identification bracelet on, and cannot remember her name. What should the nurse do first?

1. Help the client into bed, and remind her to call the nurse when she wants to get out of bed.
2. Help the client into bed, and then restart the IV.
3. Place a restraining vest on the client.
4. Put an identification bracelet on the client and help her back to bed.

24. The nurse must lift a heavy object that is found in the hallway. Which is the best approach for the nurse?

1. Lift the object at arm's length so all of the arm muscles are being used.
2. Bend from the waist, using a wide stance, so that

the leg muscles are used.

3. Maintain good body alignment and use the large muscles of the body while lifting the object.

4. Bend at the knees and use the large leg muscles when lifting the object.

25. In preparing a client for surgery, the preoperative checklist has been completed, and the nurse has just administered the preoperative injection. What would the nurse do next?

1. Take the client to the bathroom to void.
2. Dim the overhead and bedside lights.
3. Review deep breathing and coughing exercises.
4. Put the side rails up on both sides of the bed.

26. A mother watches the nurse in the pediatrics ward place her toddler in a highchair for a meal. After placing the client in the highchair, what nursing action would be most essential?

1. Pour a small amount of milk into the glass.
2. Ask the mother to feed the child.
3. Belt the child securely to the chair.
4. Cut the child's food into bite size pieces.

27. Which of the following actions reduces muscle strain for the nurse while making a bed?

1. Placing the bed in the low horizontal position.
2. Placing the bed in the high horizontal position.
3. Pulling all of the linen off from the foot of the bed.
4. Placing the bed in semi-Fowler's position.

28. A client is ambulating down the tile hallway in her stocking-covered feet. How should the nurse ensure the client's safety?

1. Remind the client to avoid any wet spots on the floor.
2. Tell the client that she should always wear slippers or shoes when ambulating.
3. Get the client's slippers and have her put them on.
4. No action is necessary, since the client has her feet covered.

29. A visitor asks the nurse about the client in the next room, who has metastatic cancer and cries out frequently. "That person must have a terrible disease. What is the matter with him?" The most appropriate response by the nurse is:

1. "That client has cancer and is quite uncomfortable."
2. "Mr. Jones is being kept as comfortable as possible."
3. "That person is quite uncomfortable. Does his crying out bother you?"

4. "I cannot reveal anything about his diagnosis. Why don't you ask his family when they visit? I'm sure they would appreciate your concern."

30. A client is very irritable at breakfast. When asked if there is a problem, the client states that he was unable to sleep because of noise made by the staff on the night shift. The best initial response by the nurse is:

1. "It must be very distressing to be unable to sleep at night. Would you like to take a nap this morning?"
2. "I'll report that to the supervisor."
3. "Maybe we can move you to a room further from the nurses' station when one of those rooms becomes available."
4. "Why don't you close your door at night? Sometimes the nurses make noise and don't realize it."

31. The physician has determined that a client is extremely dehydrated and in need of intravenous fluids. The client is confused, and has pulled out one intravenous catheter and caused another intravenous site to become infiltrated. The nurse restarts the IV in the client's left arm. An order for restraints is given. The best nursing action is to:

1. Apply a vest restraint and extremity restraints to ensure that the intravenous site will be protected.
2. Apply a restraint to the left arm.
3. Apply a restraint to the right arm.
4. Apply restraints to the right and left arms.

32. The physician has ordered extremity restraints for safety reasons for a confused, elderly client. After placing the client in extremity restraints, the priority nursing action is to:

1. Release each extremity every two hours for range of motion exercises.
2. Discuss the rationale for the restraints with the family members.
3. Reduce the client's distress by dimming the lights and closing the door.
4. Tie the restraints to the side rails using a half bow knot.

33. An elderly client requires extremity restraints for safety reasons. After applying restraints to the client's extremities, the nurse should consider which of the following as a priority action concerned with the client's safety?

1. Documenting the type of restraints applied to the client.
2. Explaining to family members the reason for the restraints.
3. Checking the restraints for circulatory adequacy once during each shift.

4. Observing the restrained extremities for color and pulses at least every hour.

34. **When giving a partial bath, which nursing action is inappropriate?**

    1. Arrange equipment and linen for easy access.
    2. Open the windows to let fresh air in.
    3. Pull the curtain for privacy.
    4. Rinse off all of the soap.

35. **While starting an intravenous infusion, the nurse's gloved hands get spotted with blood. The client has not been diagnosed with any organisms that are transmitted by way of the blood stream. The first action the nurse should take upon completion of the task is:**

    1. Remove the gloves carefully and follow with hand washing.
    2. Wash the gloved hands, and then throw the gloves away.
    3. Prepare an incident report so that this occurrence will be documented, in case a health care problem develops at a later date.
    4. Ask the client to have a blood test to determine if a bloodborne pathogen is present in the client's blood.

36. **A client is admitted to the hospital with active tuberculosis. She is placed in respiratory isolation and started on medication. A chest x-ray is ordered. While transporting the client to x-ray, the nurse should:**

    1. Wear a mask and gown for protection from the client's organisms.
    2. Have the client wear a mask and protect the wheel chair with a clean bath blanket or sheet.
    3. Have x-ray come to the client's room to do the x-ray.
    4. Take no special precautions.

37. **While the nurse is caring for a client, the intravenous tubing becomes disconnected from the intravenous catheter, resulting in the client's blood spilling onto the side of the bed and floor. The nurse knows that which solution is recommended for disinfection of blood spills?**

    1. Betadine solution.
    2. Alcohol.
    3. Soap and water.
    4. Sodium hypochlorite or chlorine bleach solution.

38. **While caring for a client receiving fluids using an IV pump that is plugged into an electrical outlet, which of the following is an inappropriate nursing action?**

    1. Palpate the client's IV site while resetting the pump for the next bag of IV solution.
    2. Assess the IV site.
    3. Change the tubing according to hospital protocol.
    4. Observe the pump for correct operation.

39. **The nurse notices a fire in the linen room. Which type of extinguisher should the nurse use?**

    1. Dry powder.
    2. Water.
    3. Dry chemical.
    4. Carbon dioxide.

40. **An antepartum client has an ultrasound exam at 14 weeks gestation because of increased fundal height. After she is told that she has a uterine fibroid, the client asks the nurse what will happen. In responding, the nurse is guided by the knowledge that, in pregnancy complicated with a uterine fibroid:**

    1. The fibroid should be removed soon, to prevent problems with fetal growth.
    2. The tumors usually shrink during pregnancy and rarely cause problems.
    3. The uterus may not contract properly at term because of the fibroid tumor.
    4. The fibroid will probably be removed following a cesarean birth.

41. **The nurse is caring for a 54-year-old client two hours following a modified radical mastectomy. Which nursing action receives the lowest priority?**

    1. Encouraging the client to talk about the surgery.
    2. Assessing vital signs.
    3. Auscultating lung and bowel sounds.
    4. Inspecting the dressing.

42. **The nurse is teaching a client about premenstrual syndrome (PMS). The nurse's teaching plan is guided by the knowledge that which intervention would have the least effect on the manifestations of PMS?**

    1. Decreasing or eliminating caffeine from the diet.
    2. Using stress reduction techniques.
    3. Involvement with support groups.
    4. Elimination of strenuous exercise programs.

43. **An antepartum client complains of frequent leg cramps. Which nursing intervention is indicated at this time?**

    1. Instruct the client to take calcium supplements.
    2. Instruct the client to do specific leg exercises to decrease the incidence of the cramps.
    3. Ask the client to write down her intake for two days.

4. Suggest that the client drink more milk to prevent the leg cramps.

44. **A client comes to the prenatal clinic early in pregnancy. She tells the nurse that she has lost 60 pounds over the last year on a 1200 calorie balanced diet. She is concerned about weight gain in this pregnancy and wants to limit her gain to 10 pounds. What is the nurse's best reply?**

    1. "Now that you're pregnant, you'll have to go off your diet."
    2. "You've done very well, however, sufficient weight gain is important to the developing fetus."
    3. "You can keep your caloric intake low by eating primarily proteins, which are good for the developing fetus."
    4. "As long as you eat properly in the first half of the pregnancy when most fetal development is occurring, you may decrease caloric intake in the later months."

45. **Following delivery, which of the following nursing actions should be done first to care for the newborn?**

    1. Stimulate the infant to cry.
    2. Dry the infant off and cover the head.
    3. Clear the respiratory tract.
    4. Instill silver nitrate into the eyes.

46. **An antepartum client is scheduled to have a blood test to check for alpha-fetoprotein (AFP) at 15 weeks gestation. The nurse understands that this test screens most effectively for the possibility of:**

    1. Spinal defects in the fetus.
    2. Chromosomal abnormalities in the fetus.
    3. Inborn errors of metabolism in the fetus.
    4. Maternal spinal cord defects.

47. **An antepartum client's blood work reveals: Rubella, negative; VDRL, negative; O positive; Coombs, negative. From these results, the nurse understands that which intervention is indicated at this time?**

    1. Discuss with the client the need for rubella vaccine after she delivers.
    2. The client needs to receive penicillin immediately.
    3. Blood work needs to be ordered for the father of the baby to check his Rh and type.
    4. The client needs to know that she will have frequent blood work to check for an incompatibility of her blood with the fetus.

48. **The nurse is monitoring the fetal heart rate of a laboring woman. The nurse's assessment is based on the**

knowledge that the normal baseline fetal heart rate is:

1. 100-150 beats per minute.
2. 110-160 beats per minute.
3. 120-160 beats per minute.
4. 120-170 beats per minute.

49. **The nurse is teaching an antepartum client about counting fetal movements. Which statement by the client demonstrates to the nurse that the client understands this procedure?**

    1. "I will count the times my fetus moves for a period of one hour at various times throughout a day."
    2. "I will call my doctor if my baby's movements increase considerably at any time."
    3. "I will count my baby's fetal movements after meals for 20 to 30 minutes."
    4. "It is normal for the fetus to have sleep times, so if I do not feel fetal movement early in the morning it's okay."

50. **A first time mother who is breast feeding tells the nurse she is concerned about whether her baby is receiving enough intake. Which is the best nursing assessment to use in evaluating the adequacy of hydration?**

    1. How often the baby cries.
    2. The number of wet diapers per day.
    3. The baby's skin turgor.
    4. The fit of the baby's clothes.

51. **In developing a plan to improve the self-image of an eight-year-old with asthma, the nurse should consider that:**

    1. The client is not able to understand the causes or limitations of chronic illness.
    2. The client's peers, parents, and teachers should be instructed in strategies for encouraging her.
    3. Teaching the client self-care skills will increase her sense of control.
    4. The client should be told about all potential long-term complications.

52. **A 10-year-old is overweight. He has no dietary restrictions. The nurse is helping him make out his menu. Which diet would the nurse plan to encourage?**

    1. A glass of whole milk, hot dog on a roll with pickles, and a candy bar.
    2. A glass of skim milk, baked fish sandwich on whole wheat roll with lettuce, and a medium apple.
    3. A glass of diet lemonade, hamburger and roll, medium orange and mashed potatoes.
    4. A salad plate of low fat cottage cheese, potato salad, and macaroni salad with a croissant and a glass of water.

53. The mother of a two-year-old who is hospitalized asks how she should handle her son's temper tantrums. The nurse should advise the mother to:

    1. Restrain the child physically.
    2. Ignore the behavior.
    3. Let the child know his temper tantrums are not acceptable.
    4. Play a game with him, or rock him quietly.

54. The nurse knows that instructions for the mother of a school age girl with pediculosis have been successful when the mother states:

    1. "My child must have a physician's note to return to school."
    2. "I will treat family members who have lice."
    3. "Before I put the shampoo on, I'll cut her hair."
    4. "All toys must be thrown out if they can't be dry cleaned or washed."

55. A five-month-old must undergo a spinal tap to rule out meningitis. The nurse who is planning to assist with the procedure should:

    1. Have several other nurses to help hold the infant.
    2. Position the child seated on the side of table.
    3. Hold chin to chest and knees to abdomen.
    4. Utilize a papoose board to restrain limbs.

56. A hospitalized eight-year-old is losing a game of checkers. He stands up and says, "I quit." The nurse understands that this behavior probably is:

    1. A personality change due to hospitalization.
    2. Immaturity for his age.
    3. A sign that this game is too hard for him.
    4. Normal for his social development.

57. The nurse knows that the observations most likely to be made on a child with celiac disease include:

    1. Pale, small arms, large belly.
    2. Periorbital edema and weight gain.
    3. Retractions, flushing, increased respirations.
    4. Diaphoresis and increased bowel sounds.

58. The nurse would interpret which finding as an indication that an infant's dehydration has been corrected?

    1. Weight gain of three ounces in 24 hours.
    2. Specific gravity of 1.028.
    3. Cool skin with tenting.
    4. Frequent stooling.

59. The nurse is evaluating the effectiveness of the teaching performed for the mother of a six-month-old who is teething. The nurse would consider the teaching to be successful if the mother:

    1. Provides the infant with a hard rubber toy to bite.
    2. Places aspirin against the erupting tooth.
    3. Rubs a topical anesthetic on the sensitive area.
    4. Places sherry and water mixture on gums at bedtime.

60. At nine months of age, an infant has been in the hospital four times for a total of 42 days. The nurse notices that the infant does not seem upset when her parents leave. The nurse would evaluate this behavior as:

    1. An infant with an easy temperament.
    2. A mature infant who is very secure.
    3. A strong attachment to the nurses.
    4. Experiencing detachment.

61. The nurse explains a bone marrow aspiration to a seven-year-old. Which response would the nurse interpret as indicating that the child understood the teaching?

    1. "I hope my headache won't be too bad."
    2. "The doctor will put me to sleep for a little while."
    3. "I'll have to lay on my belly while it's done."
    4. "My doctor will push on my chest, but it won't hurt."

62. In preparing a teaching plan for families about Reye's syndrome, the nurse knows that the most important part of the plan is:

    1. Avoiding the use of aspirin with children; only acetaminophen is safe.
    2. Treating all streptococcal infections immediately.
    3. Keeping the fever down with cool baths.
    4. Calling the child's doctor if a sick child is recovering and then becomes ill again.

63. The parents of a child with Hodgkin's lymphoma ask about their son's prognosis. The nurse's response should be based on the knowledge that Hodgkin's lymphoma:

    1. Is frequently a fatal disease.
    2. Is associated with excellent survival rates.
    3. Is associated with remissions that are usually short, and then manifestations return.
    4. Is completely unpredictable.

64. A client is being treated for an intracranial tumor. A CAT scan with contrast dye was ordered by the physician to determine if the tumor is shrinking. The client asks the nurse what to expect during the procedure. The most appropriate response by the nurse is:

1. "Just try to relax and go to sleep."
2. "It is important to remain still. You will be on your back on an x-ray table. Your head will be immobilized, and you will hear clicking sounds."
3. "The contrast dye will make you sleepy and may make your skin itch."
4. "Although the procedure may be uncomfortable, you have to do it because your physician ordered it."

65. When a contrast dye is used during a CAT scan, the nurse should observe the client for signs of an allergic reaction. Which finding would the nurse identify as indicating an allergic reaction to the dye?

    1. Flushed feeling.
    2. Nausea and vomiting.
    3. Headache.
    4. Dyspnea and urticaria.

66. The nurse has prepared a client for an MRI of the lower back to rule out a herniated disc. The nurse is aware that MRI procedures are generally contraindicated for clients who have a fear of:

    1. Closed spaces.
    2. Dark places.
    3. Immobilization.
    4. Needles.

67. The Tensilon test, used to diagnose myasthenia gravis, is administered intravenously and usually lasts about 15-30 minutes. If the client has myasthenia gravis, following administration of edrophonium chloride (Tensilon) the nurse would expect that muscle strength should:

    1. Stay the same.
    2. Decrease immediately.
    3. Improve immediately.
    4. Develop fasciculations.

68. To determining how much fluid the client loses during hemodialysis, the nurse measures the client's:

    1. Abdominal girth.
    2. Blood pressure.
    3. Ankle and calf measurements.
    4. Body weight.

69. In a client with Cushing's syndrome, which clinical manifestation(s) would the nurse expect to observe?

    1. Large extremities.
    2. Decreased body and facial hair.
    3. Moon face, truncal obesity, and hyperpigmentation.
    4. Muscle twitching, seizures.

70. A client has returned from the operating room following repair of the ligaments in his left knee. Upon awakening, he complains of severe pain. The physician has ordered morphine sulfate for the control of pain. Which assessment should be made by the nurse before administering the drug?

    1. Radial pulse rate.
    2. Blood pressure.
    3. Respiratory rate.
    4. Pulse pressure.

71. A client develops a fecal impaction. Before digital removal of the mass, what type of enema is usually given by the nurse to loosen the feces?

    1. Fleets.
    2. Oil retention.
    3. Soap suds.
    4. Tap water.

72. A nurse is caring for a client with a diagnosis of cancer of the colon. He is scheduled for a bowel resection in two days. Which order can the nurse expect to see included in his preoperative plan of care?

    1. NPO for three days prior to surgery.
    2. Administration of cleansing enemas.
    3. Administration of IV antibiotics as a bowel preparation.
    4. Instructions on colostomy irrigations.

73. A client just returned from the operating room, where he underwent a left-sided cardiac catheterization. One of the complications of this surgery can be an arterial embolus or thrombus in the affected limb. Which nursing action would be harmful in caring for this client?

    1. If ordered, administer a vasodilator to relieve painful constriction.
    2. Administer an anticoagulant as ordered, and monitor for signs of bleeding.
    3. Protect the affected limb from pressure, and maintain the limb at a level or slightly dependent position with respect to the heart.
    4. Massage the limb to promote circulation.

74. A client was admitted to the neurological unit of the hospital because of exacerbation of her multiple sclerosis. Her family asks the nurse what will happen, and how to deal with the client's emotional changes. The nurse would demonstrate an understanding of the family's emotional needs by:

    1. Encouraging the family to look on the bright side.
    2. Advising the family to overlook the client's mood

swings, since she really doesn't mean to be angry or depressed.

3. Providing the family with medical journals describing the latest research on multiple sclerosis.

4. Spending time listening to the family, and encouraging them to ventilate their feelings.

75. **A female client with a history of severe multiple sclerosis has requested a living will and has asked the nurse to witness it. The appropriate response is:**

1. "I would be honored to witness the will."
2. "I think your physician should witness the will."
3. "It would be a conflict of interest for me to witness the will, since I do not believe in living wills."
4. "I am unable to witness the will because of my professional relationship with you. Is there someone else you know who could do so?"

76. **A client with chronic osteoarthritis complains of discomfort when performing exercises prescribed by the physical therapist. Which response by the nurse is most appropriate?**

1. "The exercises will prevent pain."
2. "The exercises will prevent worsening of the disease."
3. "The exercises will help to maintain as near normal joint function as possible, as well as range of motion."
4. "The exercises will make you feel better."

77. **A client is to undergo cholecystosonography, which is the preferred method for detecting gallstones. The nurse explains to the client that this diagnostic evaluation of the gallbladder involves:**

1. X-ray of the abdomen.
2. Radioisotope imaging of the gallbladder.
3. Drinking an oral contrast medium.
4. Ultrasound imaging of the gallbladder and bile ducts.

78. **Acute renal failure usually follows direct injury to the kidneys or overwhelming physiologic stress such as burns, severe shock, or nephrotoxic drugs. Which manifestations would the nurse identify as inconsistent with a diagnosis of acute renal failure?**

1. Generalized edema.
2. Anorexia, nausea, and vomiting.
3. Irritability, restlessness, and headache.
4. Polyuria.

79. **A diabetic client with acute renal failure is receiving peritoneal dialysis, in addition to medication therapy. The nurse knows that a complication of peritoneal dialysis is:**

1. Hypoglycemia.
2. Metabolic acidosis.
3. Infection.
4. Hyponatremia.

80. **In explaining the treatment of peptic ulcers, the nurse would emphasize the need to avoid which substances that can aggravate a peptic ulcer?**

1. Smoking, coffee and tea.
2. Antacids.
3. Sedatives.
4. Bland diet.

81. **The doctor prescribes tube feedings for an elderly client who is hospitalized. The nurse understands that tube feedings may be prescribed when:**

1. The client is unable to swallow foods by mouth.
2. The client prefers this feeding method, since it is easier.
3. The client refuses to eat solid foods in the hospital because they contain meat and dairy products.
4. The family requests this method because it is more efficient.

82. **The nurse understands that a guaiac test detects microscopic particles in the feces of:**

1. Bile.
2. Lipid.
3. Bacteria.
4. Blood.

83. **In planning preoperative care for a client, the nurse is aware that obtaining legal, informed consent to perform surgery is the responsibility of:**

1. The nurse.
2. The surgeon.
3. The client's family physician.
4. The client.

84. **In writing the plan of care for a client with an ileostomy, the nurse states the need to protect the skin around the ileostomy stoma. The nurse's rationale for this client is based on the fact that:**

1. Friction causes irritation.
2. Urine causes skin excoriation.
3. Intestinal juices are irritating to the skin.
4. Organisms present on the skin can cause infection in the stoma.

85. **Which intervention would be most important for the nurse to include in the plan of care for a client with hepatitis B?**

1. Bedrest with bathroom privileges.
2. High calorie, high protein diet.
3. Force fluids to 3,000 ml in 24 hours.
4. Medicate for pain every three to four hours as needed.

86. **The nurse is caring for a male client, age 65, who has undergone a below-the-knee amputation because of persistent peripheral vascular disease (PVD). The orders are for wet to dry dressing changes b.i.d. The nurse knows that which dressing technique is the most appropriate?**

    1. Clean technique, using nonsterile gloves.
    2. Sterile technique, using sterile gloves.
    3. Sterile technique for the first week postoperatively, then clean technique.
    4. Mask, gown, and sterile gloves for all dressing changes.

87. **A young male client, age 11 years, sustained a broken tibia while playing football. The physician set the fracture in the operating room and applied a cast. The client returned to his room drowsy and complaining of mild pain. At this time, the nurse should:**

    1. Use a hair dryer to hasten the drying of the cast.
    2. Keep the casted leg in a flat position.
    3. Observe for signs of circulatory impairment, infection, swelling, and hemorrhage.
    4. Teach the client to keep his leg in contact with the floor while sitting.

88. **A client underwent a below-the-knee bilateral amputation of both lower extremities following a severe motor vehicle accident. On the first postoperative day, it is inappropriate for the nurse to:**

    1. Start range of motion exercises to both stumps.
    2. Encourage the client not to sit in any one position for prolonged periods of time.
    3. Elevate the stumps on a pillow.
    4. Apply compression bandages.

89. **A male client has developed right-sided heart failure. The nurse is aware that right-sided heart failure results in an increase in:**

    1. Central venous pressure (CVP).
    2. Blood pressure (BP).
    3. Pulse pressure.
    4. Intraocular pressure.

90. **Which characteristic is inconsistent with a client diagnosed with varicose veins?**

    1. Peripheral edema of the lower leg(s) that appears during the day, is aggravated by prolonged stand-

ing, and decreases or disappears during the night, when the client is sleeping.
    2. Reddish discoloration of the lower legs.
    3. Dryness and scaling over prominent varices.
    4. Ulcerations, including long-standing varicose ulcers.

91. **The nurse teaching a group of hypertensive clients about the prevention of arteriosclerosis is guided by the knowledge that a factor contributing to the development of arteriosclerosis is:**

    1. Hypotension.
    2. Elevated levels of high density lipoproteins (HDLs).
    3. Cholesterol levels less than 200 mg.
    4. Fat intake greater than 30% of daily calorie consumption.

92. **The nurse would select which infection control precautions as appropriate in caring for an AIDS client?**

    1. Strict isolation.
    2. Respiratory isolation.
    3. Contact isolation.
    4. Universal blood and body fluid precautions.

93. **In assessing a client, the nurse would recognize which manifestations or findings as consistent with AIDS?**

    1. Persistent fever, swollen glands, diarrhea, weight loss, and fatigue.
    2. Elevated hemoglobin level, increased urinary glucose, elevated BUN.
    3. Elevated BP, tachycardia, dyspnea, and edema.
    4. Hypotension, dehydration, and pallor in the nail beds, conjunctivae, lips, and skin.

94. **The nurse monitors a client who is taking digoxin (Lanoxin) for his heart condition. The nurse would interpret which manifestation as an indication that the client may be developing digitalis toxicity?**

    1. Polydipsia.
    2. Diplopia (double vision).
    3. Nausea and vomiting.
    4. Constipation.

95. **Before giving preoperative medication to a client going to surgery, the nurse must make sure that:**

    1. The client has an empty bladder.
    2. Vital signs are documented on the preoperative check list.
    3. Dentures are removed.
    4. The consent form has been signed.

96. **A client with advanced cirrhosis is admitted with bleeding esophageal varices. A Sengstaken-Blakemore tube**

has been inserted. In planning care for this client, the nurse knows that the primary purpose of the Sengstaken-Blakemore tube is to:

1. Coagulate the bleeding varices.
2. Prevent the aspiration of blood into the lungs.
3. Apply direct pressure to the bleeding varices.
4. Provide a means for removing blood from the stomach.

97. When planning care for the client receiving a narcotic antitussive, the nurse's main goal is to:

1. Deliver analgesia.
2. Provide intervals of rest.
3. Encourage productive coughing.
4. Suppress the cough center.

98. The nurse is assessing a young child with asthma in order to determine the usefulness of a metered dose inhaler. Which factor would the nurse assess as discouraging the use of the inhaler.

1. The child's inability to follow directions.
2. The family's poor financial situation.
3. The size of the medication particles.
4. The severity of the child's disease.

99. A client received discharge instructions regarding side effects of his kanamycin sulfate (Kantrex) therapy. Which of the following statements by the client indicates to the nurse the need for further teaching?

1. "I know I should drink extra fluids while taking this medicine — at least two quarts a day."
2. "I'll call the doctor if I notice any ringing in my ears or a change in my hearing."
3. "I won't forget to call the doctor's office to make an appointment for lab work, to check on the medication's blood level."
4. "I won't worry about slight numbness or tingling in my legs because I know it's just a side effect I have to live with while I'm on this medicine."

100. A client is diagnosed with active tuberculosis and is started on a treatment regimen of isoniazid (INH) and ethambutol (Myambutol). Which of the following manifestations would the nurse identify as demanding the discontinuation of ethambutol?

1. Anorexia, nausea/vomiting.
2. Loss of color discrimination.
3. Edema of feet and hands.
4. Red-orange discoloration to all body fluids.

NOTES

NCLEX-PN

Test 6

Questions with Rationales

NCLEX-PN TEST 6 WITH RATIONALES

1. An 82-year-old client has oral candidiasis and is prescribed nystatin (Mycostatin) oral suspension. Which statement by the client indicates to the nurse that the client needs further teaching regarding the administration of Mycostatin?

    1. "I'll make sure to brush my teeth before taking a dose of this medicine."
    2. "I know that I should drink a full glass of water after each dose of medicine."
    3. "I'll keep the medicine in my mouth for several minutes before swallowing it."
    4. "I'll limit the amount of mouthwash I use from now on to decrease my chances of getting this fungal infection again."

    1. *No, the client does understand the need for good oral hygiene prior to each medication dosage. You are asked to find a statement that indicates misunderstanding on the client's part.*
    2. ***Correct assessment. Nystatin produces a local antifungal effect. The client should not drink a glass of water after taking nystatin because the medication would be washed away from its site of action.***
    3. *This is exactly how the client should take nystatin oral suspension! It's obvious that he doesn't require any further teaching in this area. You are asked to find a statement that indicates misunderstanding on the client's part.*
    4. *No, the client is correct in his understanding that excessive use of mouthwash may alter flora and promote infection, especially in older clients. You are asked to find a statement that indicates misunderstanding on the client's part. Try again.*

2. In preparing to teach a client with glaucoma about the use of eye medication, the nurse knows that which information about the treatment of glaucoma is inaccurate?

    1. The drops should be instilled without touching the dropper to the eye.
    2. The medication must be stored at the proper temperature.
    3. Vision may become blurred after use, so the client needs to use caution.
    4. The medication is taken for 2-3 weeks and then discontinued.

    1. *Properly instilling eye drops is necessary to prevent infections, and to get the best results. This question has a negative response stem, so the correct option is one that is NOT accurate. Try*

    again.
    2. *This is a correct action. Eye medications must be stored properly, and some need refrigeration. This question has a negative response stem, so the correct option is one that is NOT accurate.*
    3. *No, this is true! Blurring of vision is very likely. If it happens, the client may fall or have an accident. Remember, this question has a negative response stem and is asking for a response that is NOT accurate.*
    4. ***Good work! This is the only statement that is inaccurate. Glaucoma medications will be taken for life.***

3. A newly diagnosed diabetic is receiving instructions about dietary management of his disease. In providing information, the nurse is aware that the most important objective in the dietary management of diabetes mellitus is:

    1. Control of total calorie intake in order to attain or maintain ideal weight.
    2. An accurate distribution of calories from carbohydrates, protein, and fat.
    3. Weight reduction to reverse the hyperglycemia.
    4. Meeting energy needs while decreasing blood lipid levels.

    1. ***Excellent! Success of this goal alone is often associated with reversal of the hyperglycemia in type II diabetic clients. In a young client with type I diabetes, priority should be given to providing a diet with enough calories to maintain normal growth and development.***
    2. *Although this is a focus of the diabetic meal plan, it is too limited in scope to be the major objective in the dietary treatment of diabetes. Try again.*
    3. *Incorrect. Weight reduction may be an effect of the dietary management of type II diabetes, but it's not the major goal for all clients. Some clients may be underweight at the onset of type I diabetes because of rapid weight loss from severe hyperglycemia. The goal for these clients may be to help them regain lost weight. Make another selection.*
    4. *Not the best choice. These are both goals for nutritional management of diabetes mellitus for selected clients, but they are not the most important objectives. Look for a more global response!*

4. A client is being treated with nystatin (Mycostatin) oral suspension for a candida oropharyngeal infection. The nurse should instruct the client to:

1. Swallow the solution quickly, to avoid burning the throat.
2. Take the medication with a glass of water.
3. Swish the solution around in the mouth, then hold it there for as long as possible.
4. Take the medication on an empty stomach.

1. *This is incorrect. Nystatin should not be swallowed quickly.*
2. *This is incorrect. Water will wash away the medication.*
3. **Good! The medication is not absorbed from the stomach. It provides a local anti-fungal effect, so it needs to be in contact with the fungus for as long as possible.**
4. *Incorrect. An empty stomach is not necessary.*

5. **A client has been diagnosed with tuberculosis. Isoniazid (INH) and rifampin (Rifadin) have been prescribed and the client asks the nurse how long he'll be taking the drugs. Which statement by the nurse is most accurate?**

1. "You'll need to stay on the medications for approximately three months, until the manifestations subside and your sputum culture is negative."
2. "You'll need to take both medications for a year. It's important to follow the exact schedule set up by your physician."
3. "You'll be taking both medications for six months, at which time the doctor will discontinue the rifampin and then you'll have another three months on just the INH."
4. "You'll need to take both medications for approximately six to nine months, at which time there should be complete eradication of the disease."

1. *Incorrect. Manifestations and positive sputum cultures usually disappear in 2-3 weeks after drug therapy is started. The client will be taking the combination medications for a longer period of time.*
2. *Incorrect. Clients on INH and ethambutol (Myambutol) will be taking the drugs for 18-24 months because ethambutol is bacteriostatic, not bacteriocidal. This prolonged treatment is usually not necessary when INH is used in conjunction with rifampin.*
3. *This is not a correct treatment protocol. Clients are directed to take both medications for the entire prescribed time period.*
4. **Correct. This is the standard treatment time period for INH and Rifadin. Both drugs are in the group of first-line antitubercular agents and are usually effective within the time frame of six to nine months.**

6. **A pediatric nurse suspects that a recently admitted child has been abused. He is three years old and has a dislocated shoulder and internal bleeding. Which ob-** servation would lead the nurse to suspect abuse of this client?

1. The child's mother cried while describing the accident that caused her son's injuries, saying it was all her fault because she was talking on the telephone when it happened.
2. The child's mother held him closely and comforted him while talking with the nurse.
3. The child's mother gives an account of the accident that is not consistent with the injuries her son sustained.
4. The child, while crying from time to time, cooperated with the examination.

1. *This is not a sign of abuse. Abusing parents usually do not admit that the child was abused, or assume responsibility for the injuries.*
2. *This is not a sign of abuse. Most parents who are abusive show little sympathy for their child's injuries and try to silence the child instead of comforting him or her.*
3. **Correct. Often the report of the accident given by the parent is not consistent with the injuries that were sustained. Also, the abusive parent often answers questions in an evasive or contradictory manner.**
4. *This is not a sign of abuse. Abused children are often wary of adults and of physical contact. Many times they also cry excessively or not at all during the physical examination.*

7. **In planning the initial care for client with an acute schizophrenic illness, the nurse should emphasize:**

1. Establishing a daily routine to promote orientation to the unit.
2. Providing a variety of activities to keep the client focused on reality-based topics.
3. Encouraging the client to enter into simple group activities.
4. Assigning the same members of the nursing staff to work with the client each day.

1. *A daily routine is important to help the client become adjusted to the unit, but this is not the most important nursing intervention for the client with an acute schizophrenic illness.*
2. *Initially, too much activity would overwhelm the acutely ill client. This is not the correct option.*
3. *This is not correct because the acutely ill client will become too anxious in group situations to cope with the demands of the activity.*
4. **Correct. Establishing trust is the primary initial goal for clients who are acutely ill with a schizophrenic disorder. This can best be achieved by assigning the same nursing staff members to work with her each day.**

8. As the nurse approaches a schizophrenic, paranoid type client, he says, "Back off. Leave me alone." He appears tense and is pacing rapidly. The best nursing response to his remark is:

    1. "I can't leave you alone when you are this upset. Sit down and try to relax."
    2. "Let's go to your room and you can tell me what is bothering you."
    3. "I will keep my distance as long as you can control yourself. You appear quite angry and I'd like to know more about what is causing you to feel this way."
    4. "I will leave you alone for a few minutes while you try to compose yourself."

    1. *This is not correct. The aggressive person is highly anxious and feeling out of control. He will not be able to sit quietly and relax.*
    2. *This is not correct. The nurse cannot discuss the client's concerns until the client first provides assurance that he is able to maintain self-control and not become violent.*
    3. **Correct. The nurse's first concern is to ensure safety. To avoid escalating the client's behavior, the nurse should stay at a comfortable distance and remain calm while stressing the importance of his maintaining control. Verbal intervention is the least restrictive form of action. If the client does not respond to verbal interventions, then more restrictive measures will have to be used.**
    4. *This is not correct. It is not safe to leave a potentially violent client alone.*

9. A 45-year-old business executive was diagnosed with a gastric ulcer two years ago and was advised to scale down his activities and learn to relax. He is now returning to the HMO with increased epigastric pain. Upon questioning, he tells the nurse that he has been busier than ever. The most realistic short-term goal for dealing with stress that the nurse can suggest to this client is to:

    1. Express his emotions more directly.
    2. Decrease his workload.
    3. Use relaxation techniques each day.
    4. Decrease social activities.

    1. *Incorrect choice! This goal is important, but it will take time to implement. The stem is looking for the best short-term goal.*
    2. *Incorrect! This is an important goal, but it is not the most realistic option.*
    3. **Correct. The nurse can demonstrate relaxation techniques and instruct him to begin performing them immediately. This is the most realistic short-term goal.**

    4. *This could be an important goal. However, if social activities are a form of relaxation for the client, this would not be a good goal for him. This is not the best option for this question.*

10. The nurse refers a rape client to a support group in her community. The client asks how the support group can help her. In responding to the client, the nurse understands that which of the following is not consistent with the goals of this kind of support group?

    1. Decreasing the client's feelings of isolation and shame through membership in a group.
    2. Support for the client in regaining her positive self-esteem.
    3. Examining the client's behavior and receiving useful feedback, in a safe place and from persons who understand what she has been through.
    4. Learning better interpersonal skills through examination of the process that develops among the members of the support group.

    1. *Support groups help members overcome the feeling that they must struggle alone with their common problem. Members usually feel acceptance and support from the other members. You are looking for something that is NOT a goal of a support group.*
    2. *Support groups help members regain their self-esteem and self-confidence. You are looking for something that is NOT a goal of a support group.*
    3. *Cohesiveness develops quickly in a support group because the members come to the group with a common problem. You are looking for something that is NOT a goal of a support group.*
    4. **Very good! Examination of the group process and how the individual members relate to one another is a goal of group psychotherapy. In contrast, the focus of support groups is primarily on discussing the members' common problem and how they are affected by it.**

11. In cases of suspected child abuse, the nurse's primary legal obligation is to:

    1. Prevent the parents from taking the child home from the hospital until a full investigation has been completed.
    2. Inform the physician of the nurse's suspicions, so the physician can order any x-ray or laboratory studies that may be warranted to document the abuse.
    3. Contact the appropriate authorities, usually Child Protective Services, to file a report.
    4. Notify the nursing supervisor, so that the hospital's attorney can be contacted for legal counsel.

1. No! The nurse cannot refuse to let the parents take a child from the hospital unless there is a court order to that effect. This action by the nurse would constitute false imprisonment.

2. The nurse is obligated to document what the nurse has witnessed, but not to gather any additional evidence. This is not the nurse's primary legal obligation.

3. Correct. Health professionals are mandated by laws in every state to report suspected cases of child abuse or neglect to the appropriate authorities, who will then conduct an investigation.

4. This may be appropriate, but this is not the specific responsibility of the nurse. Look for an option that identifies the needs of the client!

12. A 16-year-old, 5'4" high school student is admitted to an eating disorders program by her psychiatrist. She tells the admitting nurse she has lost 25 pounds over the past month and now weighs 85 pounds. In assessing the client, the nurse would identify which manifestations as early characteristics of anorexia nervosa?

1. Appetite loss, amenorrhea, bradycardia, loss of 15% of pre-illness body weight.
2. Appetite loss, amenorrhea, tachycardia, hyperactivity.
3. Tachycardia, insomnia, fear of obesity, bulimia.
4. Amenorrhea, bradycardia, disturbed body image, loss of 15% of pre-illness body weight.

1. Clients with anorexia usually experience amenorrhea, bradycardia, and loss of 15% of pre-illness body weight. Although they voluntarily refuse to eat, they do not typically experience appetite loss until they have been ill for a long time. Try another selection.

2. Clients with anorexia do experience amenorrhea and hyperactivity, but they do not experience tachycardia. Appetite loss does not occur until the late stages of the illness. Try again.

3. This is not the best option. Clients with anorexia do experience amenorrhea, and fear of obesity. They do not typically experience insomnia; and while many clients do have bulimia, many do not.

4. Correct. Amenorrhea, bradycardia, disturbed body image, and loss of 15% of pre-illness body weight are among the most common early manifestations in anorexic clients.

13. The nurse realizes a typical characteristic of girls with anorexia nervosa is:

1. They fail to comply with their parents' wishes or societal expectations.
2. They exercise relentlessly.

3. They are truthful in reporting their eating habits.
4. They have problems with self-control.

1. This is not correct. Girls with anorexia nervosa are often described as thoughtful, obedient at home, and excellent students.

2. Great choice! Many girls with anorexia nervosa participate in sports and other athletic activities. They also tend to exercise relentlessly in their efforts to lose more weight.

3. This is not correct. Clients with anorexia nervosa will often do whatever is necessary to continue losing weight, including lying to their parents and physicians about their eating patterns.

4. Wrong. Clients with anorexia nervosa do not have problems with self-control. They are most often preoccupied with compulsive over-control.

14. In caring for a bulimic client, the nurse understands that in contrast to clients with anorexia nervosa, clients with bulimia characteristically:

1. Recognize that their eating behavior is abnormal.
2. Rarely suffer serious medical consequences.
3. Have positive feelings about their eating patterns.
4. Vomit or use laxatives after an eating binge, to purge the food.

1. Correct. Bulimic clients are aware that their eating behavior is abnormal, and during binges fear that they won't be able to stop eating voluntarily. Anorexic clients typically deny that they have an eating disorder.

2. Wrong. Bulimia is associated with many medical problems, and some can become life-threatening. The most common problems are menstrual irregularities, enlarged parotid glands, dental caries, esophagitis, tears or rupture of the esophagus, hypokalemia, and aspiration pneumonia.

3. Wrong. Bulimics often suffer from depression and are self-critical and intensely ashamed of their eating behavior. In contrast, anorexics often express a sense of pride about their eating behavior and loss of weight.

4. Wrong. Both bulimic and anorexic clients terminate eating binges by self-induced vomiting or laxative use.

15. Which activity would be most appropriate for the nurse to suggest to a manic client?

1. A daily walk on the hospital grounds.
2. Playing a computer game with another client.
3. Participation in a basketball game with other male clients.
4. Reading quietly in his room.

1. *Correct. Physical exercise involving large motor skills is an appropriate way for him to work off excess energy and emotional tension.*
2. *This is not correct. Competitive games will tend to increase his anxiety and tension and therefore escalate his hyperactivity.*
3. *Incorrect response! Basketball games tend to be competitive and overly stimulating. This activity would escalate his hyperactive behavior.*
4. *This is not correct. Because mania is associated with a short attention span and high level of distractibility, the client usually is not able to sit and read quietly by himself.*

16. **An 18-year-old client is hospitalized for treatment of severe depression. Because of the client's condition, which approach is most appropriate for the nurse to include in the client's plan of care?**

1. Giving the client choices.
2. Spending time with the client.
3. Providing a chess game.
4. Encouraging decision-making.

1. *Wrong! Making choices is difficult for a depressed client.*

TEST-TAKING TIP: *Note that this option is similar to Option 4. Options that use the same idea should be eliminated, since neither of them can be the "best" option.*

2. *Yes! You made the right selection! Because depressed clients frequently have suicidal tendencies, the best nursing action for the client is to spend time with her. This will provide for her safety and promote her sense of self-esteem.*
3. *Try again. An intellectual game such as chess would not be a good activity for a depressed client. Non-intellectual activities such as latch hook or needle work would be a better choice. Read all of the other options, and then try to select the best one.*
4. *Try again! Decision-making is difficult for a depressed client.*

TEST-TAKING TIP: *Note that this option is similar to Option 1. Options that use the same idea should be eliminated, since neither of them can be the "best" option.*

17. **An elderly client is admitted to the hospital with pneumonia. His daughter, who takes care of him at home, says to the nurse, "I'm so glad he is here. You can take much better care of him than I can." What is the best nursing response to the daughter?**

1. "We do have the equipment and people to take care of sick clients."
2. "It is not easy to care for the elderly. How do you manage?"
3. "Sir, your daughter takes good care of you at home, doesn't she?"
4. "Are you feeling guilty because your father has pneumonia?"

1. *This response does not focus on the appropriate person (the daughter). This response also focuses on inappropriate issues concerning other people and hospital equipment. To be therapeutic, the nurse's response should focus on the daughter's feelings and concerns.*
2. *Very good! This response uses the communication tool of showing empathy, and asks for clarification of the statement made to the nurse.*

TEST-TAKING TIP: *Be sure to correctly identify the client in communication questions! The daughter is the client in this question, and the nurse's response should address her concerns. Note that Options 1 & 3 focus on inappropriate issues, and Option 4 implies to the client that she may be to blame for her father's pneumonia.*

3. *The daughter is the client in this communication question, and this response is not directed to her. Even though the father is the person with the medical problem, the daughter has addressed a comment to the nurse, and the nurse's response should be addressed to the daughter.*
4. *This response indirectly places blame on the daughter for her father's pneumonia. This type of a response can put the client on the defensive, which is not therapeutic.*

18. **A client is to have a nasogastric tube inserted. The nurse explains the procedure to him and is about to begin the insertion, when the client says, "No way! You are not putting that hose down my throat. Get away from me." Which is the most appropriate nursing response?**

1. "You have the right to refuse treatment. Why don't you talk to your doctor about it?"
2. "Something is upsetting you. Can you tell me what it is?"
3. "What do you feel about this 'hose'?"
4. "I would just get it over with, because you won't get better without this tube."

1. *Incorrect choice. The client does have the right to refuse treatment, but this is not the best response by the nurse. This response puts the client's feelings on hold, referring them to another person at a*

later time. This response blocks communication.

2. *Very good. This response addresses the client's feelings. It is more global than Option 3, which focuses only on the client's feelings about the nasogastric tube. This option uses the communication tool of clarification, which encourages communication by the client and helps the nurse assess the situation.*

3. *Wrong choice. This option asks for a response from the client concerning the hose. The nurse does not need information concerning the hose. The nurse needs information concerning the client's feelings about the whole situation.*

4. *Incorrect choice! In this response, the nurse is blocking communication by giving advice.*

19. The nurse observes an elderly client trying to climb over the side rails of the bed. When placing a vest restraint on the client, the client's daughter says to the nurse, "My mother does not need to be tied down in bed. I've been caring for her for years, and she hasn't fallen out of bed yet." Which response is therapeutic for the daughter?

1. "I just saw your mother trying to climb over the side rails. Since I am concerned about her falling and hurting herself, I think this is best for her safety."

2. "Tell me how you managed to care for her at home."

3. "Hospital policy requires restraint vests on clients who are at risk for falling. I just saw your mother trying to climb over the rails. You don't want her to get hurt, do you?"

4. "The elderly may become confused in an unfamiliar place and do things they wouldn't do at home. It is difficult to see her restrained. While you are with her, the restraints can be off. Let me know when you are ready to leave."

1. *Wrong. The client's safety is the issue in this question. Since the daughter and nurse are with her, she is not in immediate danger. It is important to note that the client in this test question is the daughter, and the nurse should address the daughter's concerns. This response focuses on safety and restraints, and not on the client's (the daughter's) concerns about her mother being tied down.*

2. *Wrong. This response does not focus on the issue in the question, which concerns the client's feelings about restraints being placed on her mother. This option may be appropriate later in the conversation, but is not the best initial response.*

3. *Wrong. This response implies that the daughter is not interested in her mother's safety and makes her defensive. It also focuses on hospital policy and not the daughter's concerns.*

4. *Excellent! This option focuses on the daughter's concerns and provides information and rationale for the restraints. It also provides for safety and offers a compromise to the daughter that addresses her concerns and gives her some control.*

20. A mother arrives at the emergency room with her child, who is wet, and the color of his skin is blue. She shouts to the nurse, "I think that I have killed my son. I wasn't watching him like I should have, and he fell in the pool." While the doctor and other nursing staff are providing care for the child, the nurse stays with the mother to obtain information. What is the most appropriate response by the nurse?

1. "These things happen. Don't blame yourself."

2. "You are right. A child should always be watched when he is playing near a pool."

3. "You didn't kill him. He is still alive. It is going to be all right."

4. "It must feel terrible to have something like this happen to your child."

1. *This response blocks communication by using a cliché when talking to the mother. It does not promote further effective communication from the client.*

2. *Wrong. This option implies that the mother was at fault by not supervising her child. It passes judgment and expresses the nurse's opinion about the situation. This is not a therapeutic response.*

3. *Not the best choice! The part of this option that makes it incorrect is the statement, "It is going to be all right." This statement offers false assurance, which is never appropriate when fostering therapeutic communication.*

4. *Very good. This option is an example of the nurse using empathy when responding to the client. This response lets the client know that the nurse is not blaming her for the accident and promotes further effective communication.*

21. The nurse is preparing to give an elderly client a bath. The client says to the nurse, "I don't think that I need a bath today. I just had one yesterday. My skin is going to get too dry. I bathe completely every other day at home." Which response by the nurse is best?

1. "My head nurse wants all of the clients bathed daily because it decreases the number of germs on your skin that cause infection. Would you like to talk to the head nurse about your concerns?"

2. "A bath can make you feel refreshed and make the day seem brighter. Don't you agree?"

3. "Would you like to compromise and just wash

your face and hands today?"

4. "I heard you say that you didn't want a bath today."

1. *Incorrect choice. This option blocks communication by "passing the buck" to the head nurse and by referring to an inappropriate issue (the head nurse's wishes and beliefs). The nurse should address the client's concerns.*

2. *Wrong. The client is concerned about dry skin, and this cliché does not address the client's concerns. It is an inappropriate response.*

3. **Excellent! Allowing the client to make a choice in her plan of care promotes a sense of independence and self-worth. The issue in this question is not a physiological need or a safety issue.**

4. *Not the best choice. Restatement is used to clarify and allow the client to express her feelings — but this client has already explained to the nurse why she doesn't want a bath. This tool is inappropriate in this question.*

22. **A 15-year-old client is being seen in the family planning clinic. She says to the nurse that she is nervous and has never had a pelvic examination before. The best response by the nurse is:**

1. "All you have to do is relax."
2. "It is only slightly uncomfortable."
3. "What part of the exam makes you nervous?"
4. "If you want birth control pills, then a pelvic exam is required."

1. *This statement does not address the client's concerns, and it blocks communication by using cliché and false reassurance. This cannot be the correct answer.*

2. *This response does not address the client's concerns and does not encourage further discussion. This option cannot be the answer.*

3. **Very good! This response recognizes the client's feelings. It also uses the tool of clarification to encourage the client to tell the nurse more about her concerns. This response is therapeutic.**

4. *This statement is true in its literal sense, but the nurse does not know if the client wants birth control pills. Do not "read into" the question! More importantly, however, the client might interpret this statement as expressing disapproval by the nurse. It is non-therapeutic for the nurse to express approval or disapproval. This response also fails to address the feelings that the client has shared with the nurse. This cannot be the answer!*

23. **The nurse finds an elderly client on bedrest standing next to her bed. The side rails are in the up position, and the client's IV is pulled out. The client is confused, does not have an identification bracelet on, and cannot remember her name. What should the nurse do first?**

1. Help the client into bed, and remind her to call the nurse when she wants to get out of bed.
2. Help the client into bed, and then restart the IV.
3. Place a restraining vest on the client.
4. Put an identification bracelet on the client and help her back to bed.

1. *Wrong. Reminding a confused client to use a call light is not an appropriate nursing action (the case situation tells you that the client cannot remember her name, so she will probably not remember to use a call light). Since a physiological need is not identified in this question, the safety of the client is the most important nursing consideration at this time. Try again.*

2. *Wrong. The case scenario does not tell you whether the IV has life-saving medications or fluids infusing, so you cannot assume that the IV is a physiological need. Do not "read into" the question! Since a physiological need is not identified, the safety of the client is the most important nursing consideration at this time. Try again.*

3. **Excellent! The case scenario tells you that a confused client on bedrest was found standing next to the bed with the side rails up. This is an unsafe situation, since the client was at risk of falling when she got out of the bed. Such an injury can be life-threatening. Placing a restraining vest on the client will provide for her safety. In fact, this is the only option that provides for the client's immediate safety.**

TEST-TAKING TIP: *Were you tempted to choose Option 2? The case situation does not tell you whether the IV has life-saving medications or fluids infusing, so you cannot assume that the IV is a physiological need. Do not "read into" the question!*

4. *The client's lack of an identification bracelet is an important safety concern. However, the case scenario tells you that the client got out of a bed that had the side rails up. This is an unsafe situation, since the client is at risk for falling. Such an injury can be life-threatening. After the immediate physical safety of the client is assured, an identification bracelet can be obtained.*

24. **The nurse must lift a heavy object that is found in the hallway. Which is the best approach for the nurse?**

1. Lift the object at arm's length so all of the arm muscles are being used.
2. Bend from the waist, using a wide stance, so that the leg muscles are used.
3. Maintain good body alignment and use the large muscles of the body while lifting the object.
4. Bend at the knees and use the large leg muscles when lifting the object.

1. Wrong. When lifting an object at arm's length, the muscles in the arm are stretched, which fatigues the muscles quickly. This position also results in poor balance, because the heavy object is outside the body's base of support.

2. Wrong. Bending from the waist results in the use of the small back muscles, which become stretched and easily injured.

3. **Right! Using good body alignment and large muscles provides a good base of support, which reduces back strain and helps maintain balance.**

> **TEST-TAKING TIP:** Note that this option includes or encompasses the correct idea in Option 4. Option 3 is more global, making it the best option.

4. Bending at the knees and using the large leg muscles to lift provides decreased risk for musculoskeletal strain. This is a correct action. However, one of the other options is a more global statement that includes this action, and is, therefore, the best option. Read the options again and try to identify the more global statement.

25. **In preparing a client for surgery, the preoperative checklist has been completed, and the nurse has just administered the preoperative injection. What would the nurse do next?**

1. Take the client to the bathroom to void.
2. Dim the overhead and bedside lights.
3. Review deep breathing and coughing exercises.
4. Put the side rails up on both sides of the bed.

1. The client should have voided before being given the injection. If he gets up now, he is at risk for falling. This is not correct.

2. This is an appropriate action, but it is not the priority at this time. The client is at risk to fall.

3. This action is an important part of preoperative teaching. However, this review is inappropriate at this time, because of the preoperative injection. The client is at risk to fall.

4. **Very good! The client is at risk of falling because of the injection. This action ensures the client's safety.**

26. **A mother watches the nurse in the pediatrics ward place her toddler in a highchair for a meal. After placing the client in the highchair, what nursing action would be most essential?**

1. Pour a small amount of milk into the glass.
2. Ask the mother to feed the child.
3. Belt the child securely to the chair.
4. Cut the child's food into bite size pieces.

1. This is an appropriate action. Never fill a glass or cup more than half full. However, this is not the most essential action initially.

2. This is an appropriate action. Toddlers have severe separation anxiety, and having mother feed the child will decrease their fear and increase their intake of food. However, this is not the most essential action initially.

3. **Very good! This is a prioritizing question, and the priority in this case scenario is safety. The nurse should assess this potentially unsafe situation and make the appropriate changes to provide a safe environment. The toddler is at immediate risk of falling.**

4. This is an appropriate action. A toddler should always have small pieces of food that can be picked up with the fingers. However, this is not the most essential action initially.

27. **Which of the following actions reduces muscle strain for the nurse while making a bed?**

1. Placing the bed in the low horizontal position.
2. Placing the bed in the high horizontal position.
3. Pulling all of the linen off from the foot of the bed.
4. Placing the bed in semi-Fowler's position.

1. Placing the bed in the low position causes the nurse to bend over, which places strain on the back muscles. Try again.

2. **This is correct. Placing the bed in the high position reduces the amount of bending by the nurse, thereby reducing the amount of musculoskeletal strain.**

3. Linens should be loosened all around the bed to prevent tugging on the linen, which places strain on the musculoskeletal system. Try again.

4. This is not correct. Making the bed while it is in semi-Fowler's position will cause the nurse to reach while making the head of the bed, which places strain on the musculoskeletal system. It will also cause the linen to pull out when the bed is placed in the horizontal position. Try again.

28. **A client is ambulating down the tile hallway in her stocking-covered feet. How should the nurse ensure the client's safety?**

1. Remind the client to avoid any wet spots on the floor.
2. Tell the client that she should always wear slippers or shoes when ambulating.
3. Get the client's slippers and have her put them on.
4. No action is necessary, since the client has her feet covered.

1. Although telling the client to avoid wet spots may help to prevent a fall, it is not the priority nursing

action. Stocking feet are very slippery on a tile floor, and this situation needs to be addressed first.

2. The client should be instructed in proper footwear to avoid falling. This action alone, however, will not prevent this client from slipping on the tile floor.

3. **You're right! Making sure that slippers or shoes are worn by the client is the priority action, since it addresses immediately the problem of slipping on the tile floor.**

4. This option is incorrect. The client should have footwear that protects the client from slipping and falling.

29. **A visitor asks the nurse about the client in the next room, who has metastatic cancer and cries out frequently. "That person must have a terrible disease. What is the matter with him?" The most appropriate response by the nurse is:**

1. "That client has cancer and is quite uncomfortable."
2. "Mr. Jones is being kept as comfortable as possible."
3. "That person is quite uncomfortable. Does his crying out bother you?"
4. "I cannot reveal anything about his diagnosis. Why don't you ask his family when they visit? I'm sure they would appreciate your concern."

1. Wrong! Identifying the client in the next room and revealing his diagnosis is an invasion of the client's privacy.

2. Wrong! Identifying the client in the next room by name is a breach of confidentiality. Make another choice.

3. **Correct! This option states the obvious and focuses on the client's feelings, rather than on confidential information concerning the uncomfortable person.**

4. This option does not address the immediate concern of the client, and it ignores the family's right to privacy. Make another selection.

30. **A client is very irritable at breakfast. When asked if there is a problem, the client states that he was unable to sleep because of noise made by the staff on the night shift. The best initial response by the nurse is:**

1. "It must be very distressing to be unable to sleep at night. Would you like to take a nap this morning?"
2. "I'll report that to the supervisor."
3. "Maybe we can move you to a room further from the nurses' station when one of those rooms becomes available."
4. "Why don't you close your door at night? Sometimes the nurses make noise and don't realize it."

1. **Excellent! Addressing the client's feelings is the first action by the nurse. This response lets the client know that his feelings are important and need to be addressed. This response also addresses the client's need for sleep. Sleep-deprived clients are at risk for injury related to decreased judgment, slower response time, and slower reflexes.**

2. Although reporting the situation to the supervisor may be appropriate, this response by the nurse is not therapeutic because it does not address the client's feelings or the problem of sleep deprivation, and passes the buck to the supervisor.

3. Moving the client when a room becomes available does not address the client's present problem of sleep deprivation. Sleep-deprived clients are at risk for injury related to decreased judgment, slower response time, and slower reflexes.

4. This response is not therapeutic, because it is defensive and attempts to provide justification for the noise. The client, for safety and health reasons, has the right to uninterrupted sleep if the physician's orders don't require that the client be awakened during the night.

31. **The physician has determined that a client is extremely dehydrated and in need of intravenous fluids. The client is confused, and has pulled out one intravenous catheter and caused another intravenous site to become infiltrated. The nurse restarts the IV in the client's left arm. An order for restraints is given. The best nursing action is to:**

1. Apply a vest restraint and extremity restraints to ensure that the intravenous site will be protected.
2. Apply a restraint to the left arm.
3. Apply a restraint to the right arm.
4. Apply restraints to the right and left arms.

1. This option completely restrains the client. The clinical situation indicates that only the intravenous site is in need of being protected. This is an example of over-restraining a client, and is inappropriate.

2. Restraining the left arm allows the client to reach the intravenous site with the right hand. The intravenous site is not protected.

3. Even though the right hand is restrained, the client can move the left hand over to the right side, which will allow the client to disturb the intravenous site. Make another choice.

4. **This is correct. Applying restraints to both upper extremities provides protection for the intravenous site. The client does not have the opportunity to disturb the site.**

32. **The physician has ordered extremity restraints for safety reasons for a confused, elderly client. After placing the**

client in extremity restraints, the priority nursing action is to:

1. Release each extremity every two hours for range of motion exercises.
2. Discuss the rationale for the restraints with the family members.
3. Reduce the client's distress by dimming the lights and closing the door.
4. Tie the restraints to the side rails using a half bow knot.

1. *This is the priority action, because the client with restraints is at risk of circulatory problems and possible permanent injury. Releasing the extremity for range of motion exercises addresses this risk, and allows the nurse to assess for possible injury from the restraints.*
2. *While it would be important to discuss the use of restraints with the family, it is not a priority action. Actions that ensure the safety of the client take priority.*
3. *The nurse should never isolate a restrained client by turning the lights off and closing the door. The client's distress might be increased. It is also important to visually check on a restrained client frequently.*
4. *The half bow knot is correct, but tying the restraints to the side rails is incorrect. The restraints are tied to the bed frame. Because part of this option is incorrect, this cannot be the correct answer.*

33. **An elderly client requires extremity restraints for safety reasons. After applying restraints to the client's extremities, the nurse should consider which of the following as a priority action concerned with the client's safety?**

1. Documenting the type of restraints applied to the client.
2. Explaining to family members the reason for the restraints.
3. Checking the restraints for circulatory adequacy once during each shift.
4. Observing the restrained extremities for color and pulses at least every hour.

1. *Wrong. The application of and reason for the restraints should be documented in order to help protect the nurse from possible assault and battery charges; however, this option is not a priority action concerned with the client's safety.*
2. *Wrong. Greater understanding and cooperation can be obtained from the family if they are given an explanation for the restraints placed on a client. This is not the most important action, however, because it does not directly address the safety of*

the client.
3. *This is not correct. Extremity restraints should be checked at least every hour. Allowing eight hours between checks can result in permanent damage to the client if circulation has been compromised, and the restraints are too tight or improperly applied.*
4. ***Right! This option is the priority action concerned with the client's safety. Observing the extremities for pulses and color allows the nurse to assess the potential for injury to the client that can be caused by the restraints.***

34. **When giving a partial bath, which nursing action is inappropriate?**

1. Arrange equipment and linen for easy access.
2. Open the windows to let fresh air in.
3. Pull the curtain for privacy.
4. Rinse off all of the soap.

1. *This action results in less disorganization of the bath for the client. However, this question has a false response stem. The correct answer will be something that the nurse should NOT do.*
2. ***Very good! Although fresh air is important, it is not appropriate to open the windows during a bath, since this can cause chilling of the client. This INAPPROPRIATE action is the correct option because the question has a false response stem.***
3. *Privacy is an important issue in care of the client. However, this question has a false response stem. The correct answer will be something that the nurse should NOT do.*
4. *Rinsing off all of the soap is important in order to avoid irritation and dry skin, which is more prone to skin breakdown. However, this question has a false response stem. The correct answer will be something that the nurse should NOT do.*

35. **While starting an intravenous infusion, the nurse's gloved hands get spotted with blood. The client has not been diagnosed with any organisms that are transmitted by way of the blood stream. The first action the nurse should take upon completion of the task is:**

1. Remove the gloves carefully and follow with hand washing.
2. Wash the gloved hands, and then throw the gloves away.
3. Prepare an incident report so that this occurrence will be documented, in case a health care problem develops at a later date.
4. Ask the client to have a blood test to determine if a bloodborne pathogen is present in the client's blood.

1. Very good. Universal precautions require the use of gloves and hand washing in the care of all clients. This response addresses the issue in the question.

2. Washing the gloves while still on the nurse's hands does not result in clean hands for the nurse. Hand washing is still required for infection control. Make another choice.

3. Unless there is a break in the nurse's skin, there is no need for an incident report or further investigation. Try again.

4. This is not a nursing action. If there is a concern about transmission of a disease, the nurse should follow the hospital protocol. Try again.

36. A client is admitted to the hospital with active tuberculosis. She is placed in respiratory isolation and started on medication. A chest x-ray is ordered. While transporting the client to x-ray, the nurse should:

1. Wear a mask and gown for protection from the client's organisms.
2. Have the client wear a mask and protect the wheel chair with a clean bath blanket or sheet.
3. Have x-ray come to the client's room to do the x-ray.
4. Take no special precautions.

1. When a client with a communicable disease is being transported to another department in the hospital, it is important to protect everyone that the client may come in contact with — not just the nurse! Try again.

2. Very good! This answer addresses what the nurse should do while transporting the client, to provide protection for anyone who may come in contact with the client.

3. The case scenario does not state that a portable x-ray was ordered. The stem of the question specifically asks what the nurse should do while transporting the client to x-ray. This option does not address the issue in the question! Try again.

4. The case scenario states that the client is in respiratory isolation, which indicates that something should be done to prevent the spread of the disease to others in the hospital. Make another choice.

37. While the nurse is caring for a client, the intravenous tubing becomes disconnected from the intravenous catheter, resulting in the client's blood spilling onto the side of the bed and floor. The nurse knows that which solution is recommended for disinfection of blood spills?

1. Betadine solution.
2. Alcohol.
3. Soap and water.
4. Sodium hypochlorite or chlorine bleach solution.

1. Wrong! Betadine solution is used for disinfecting skin and is effective after being allowed to dry on the skin surface. It is not appropriate to apply to objects because it stains surfaces with which it comes in contact.

2. Wrong! Alcohol is a skin disinfectant. It has not been found to destroy the HIV virus, therefore, it is not effective for blood spills.

3. Wrong! Soap and water emulsifies dirt for easy removal of the dirt, but it is not a disinfectant.

4. Correct! Chlorine acts as a disinfectant and is recommended for cleansing objects. It is recommended for blood spills because it is effective in killing the HIV virus, which can be found in body fluids such as blood.

38. While caring for a client receiving fluids using an IV pump that is plugged into an electrical outlet, which of the following is an inappropriate nursing action?

1. Palpate the client's IV site while resetting the pump for the next bag of IV solution.
2. Assess the IV site.
3. Change the tubing according to hospital protocol.
4. Observe the pump for correct operation.

1. Excellent! You have identified an incorrect action. The client should never be touched at the same time that a piece of electrical equipment is being handled. If there were any electrical current leakage from the pump, it would transfer from the nurse to the client.

2. This is a correct nursing action. Assessing an IV site for signs of phlebitis or infection should be done on a regular basis. The question asked you to identify an INAPPROPRIATE action, however, so this cannot be the correct answer.

3. This is a correct nursing action. Whatever protocol the hospital uses should be carefully followed. The question asked you to identify an INAPPROPRIATE action, however, so this cannot be the correct answer.

4. This is a correct nursing action. The pump should be observed to determine if it is operating correctly. The question asked you to identify an INAPPROPRIATE action, however, so this cannot be the correct answer.

39. The nurse notices a fire in the linen room. Which type of extinguisher should the nurse use?

1. Dry powder.
2. Water.
3. Dry chemical.
4. Carbon dioxide.

1. Wrong. Dry powder is used for metal fires. To review the proper uses of the other types of fire extinguishers, select each option number and read the rationale.

2. *Correct! Water may be used on Class A fires, which involve paper, wood or cloth. A soda and acid extinguisher may also be used for this type of fire. To review the proper uses of the other types of fire extinguishers, select each option number and read the rationale.*

3. *Wrong. Dry chemical extinguishers are appropriate for Type C fires, which involve electrical equipment, or Type D fires, which involve combustible metals. To review the proper uses of the other types of fire extinguishers, select each option number and read the rationale.*

4. *Incorrect! A carbon dioxide extinguisher is appropriate for Type B fires, which involve flammable liquids and gases. To review the proper uses of the other types of fire extinguishers, select each option number and read the rationale.*

40. **An antepartum client has an ultrasound exam at 14 weeks gestation because of increased fundal height. After she is told that she has a uterine fibroid, the client asks the nurse what will happen. In responding, the nurse is guided by the knowledge that, in pregnancy complicated with a uterine fibroid:**

1. The fibroid should be removed soon, to prevent problems with fetal growth.
2. The tumors usually shrink during pregnancy and rarely cause problems.
3. The uterus may not contract properly at term because of the fibroid tumor.
4. The fibroid will probably be removed following a cesarean birth.

1. *Wrong. Opening the uterus at this time would be very dangerous to the fetus.*
2. *No, pregnancy does not affect the growth rate. These tumors rarely shrink, except after menopause.*
3. *Correct. The presence of the fibroid in the uterus often interferes with the ability of the uterus to contract. Cesarean section is often indicated.*
4. *Wrong. Because of the increased blood supply to the uterus at the time of pregnancy, removal of the fibroid at this time would place the client at high risk for hemorrhage.*

41. **The nurse is caring for a 54-year-old client two hours following a modified radical mastectomy. Which nursing action receives the lowest priority?**

1. Encouraging the client to talk about the surgery.
2. Assessing vital signs.
3. Auscultating lung and bowel sounds.
4. Inspecting the dressing.

1. *Correct. In the first hours following surgery*

of any type, priority should be paid to potential operative complications. Most clients are not ready to deal with the impact of the surgery at this time.

2. *No, this is NOT low priority! Assessing vital signs is a very important part of postoperative care.*
3. *No, this NOT low priority! Lung and bowel sounds are important assessments to identify potential postoperative problems.*
4. *No, this is NOT low priority! The presence of bleeding on the dressing could indicate hemorrhage. It is a very important assessment at this time.*

42. **The nurse is teaching a client about premenstrual syndrome (PMS). The nurse's teaching plan is guided by the knowledge that which intervention would have the least effect on the manifestations of PMS?**

1. Decreasing or eliminating caffeine from the diet.
2. Using stress reduction techniques.
3. Involvement with support groups.
4. Elimination of strenuous exercise programs.

1. *No, this is an effective intervention. It has been suggested that eliminating, or at least decreasing, caffeine intake will reduce the manifestations of PMS.*
2. *No, this is an effective intervention. Stress reduction techniques have been shown to promote wellbeing in the client with PMS.*
3. *No, this is an effective intervention. Support groups provide information regarding PMS that help them regain control of their lives.*
4. *Correct. Avoiding strenuous exercise is not indicated in PMS. In fact, establishing a regular exercise program such as fast walking, jogging or aerobics is strongly suggested as part of the plan of care.*

43. **An antepartum client complains of frequent leg cramps. Which nursing intervention is indicated at this time?**

1. Instruct the client to take calcium supplements.
2. Instruct the client to do specific leg exercises to decrease the incidence of the cramps.
3. Ask the client to write down her intake for two days.
4. Suggest that the client she drink more milk to prevent the leg cramps.

1. *Wrong. Leg cramps in pregnancy are related to an imbalance between calcium and phosphorus. This answer presumes that the client has insufficient calcium but, in fact, the leg cramps may be the result of too much calcium.*
2. *Incorrect. Leg exercises do not have any effect on the leg cramps, which are related to dietary im-*

balances.

3. **Correct! Before you can tell whether the leg cramps are the result of too much or too little calcium, the nurse must assess the dietary intake.**

4. *Wrong. This answer presumes the client has a deficiency of calcium in her diet. Leg cramps in pregnancy most often are related to an imbalance between calcium and phosphorus.*

44. A client comes to the prenatal clinic early in pregnancy. She tells the nurse that she has lost 60 pounds over the last year on a 1200 calorie balanced diet. She is concerned about weight gain in this pregnancy and wants to limit her gain to 10 pounds. What is the nurse's best reply?

1. "Now that you're pregnant, you'll have to go off your diet."
2. "You've done very well, however, sufficient weight gain is important to the developing fetus."
3. "You can keep your caloric intake low by eating primarily proteins, which are good for the developing fetus."
4. "As long as you eat properly in the first half of the pregnancy when most fetal development is occurring, you may decrease caloric intake in the later months."

1. *No, this response suggests that she may eat anything she wants now that she's pregnant.*

2. **Good choice. The antepartum client needs to be aware of the importance of balanced intake and progressive weight gain (25-35 pounds) throughout the pregnancy.**

3. *Incorrect. A balanced diet must include all of the food groups to provide adequate nutrition to the developing fetus.*

4. *Wrong. The largest part of fetal weight gain is accomplished in the last weeks of pregnancy. Maternal dieting at this time may result in a small for gestational age fetus.*

45. Following delivery, which of the following nursing actions should be done first to care for the newborn?

1. Stimulate the infant to cry.
2. Dry the infant off and cover the head.
3. Clear the respiratory tract.
4. Instill silver nitrate into the eyes.

1. *Wrong, one should never stimulate the infant to cry until the airway has been cleared! If the infant breathes prior to clearing the airway, there is a risk of aspirating fluid into the lungs.*

2. *Wrong. Drying the infant is a priority — but if the infant is unable to breathe, warmth is unimportant.*

3. **Correct. An open airway is the most impor-**

tant aspect of care for the newborn infant following delivery. A bulb syringe, DeLee mucous trap or manual suction are common methods to achieve this.

4. *No, prophylactic eye care can safely be delayed until the infant is admitted to the newborn nursery. This is not the priority action at this time.*

46. An antepartum client is scheduled to have a blood test to check for alpha-fetoprotein (AFP) at 15 weeks gestation. The nurse understands that this test screens most effectively for the possibility of:

1. Spinal defects in the fetus.
2. Chromosomal abnormalities in the fetus.
3. Inborn errors of metabolism in the fetus.
4. Maternal spinal cord defects.

1. **Excellent! When elevated levels of AFP are found in maternal blood, the fetus should be assessed through ultrasound examination for defects in the fetal spinal cord.**

2. *Wrong. There is some correlation between AFP levels and chromosomal abnormalities in the fetus, however, this blood test is most effective in screening for spinal defects. The way to diagnose chromosomal abnormalities in the fetus is by amniocentesis or chorionic villi sampling.*

3. *Incorrect. Most inborn errors of metabolism are diagnosed through neonatal testing, and in recent years there have been advances in prenatal diagnosis through amniocentesis. AFP testing cannot effectively screen for inborn errors of metabolism. Select another option.*

4. *Wrong. Elevated levels of AFP in maternal blood are related to defects in the fetal spinal cord, not the mother's.*

47. An antepartum client's blood work reveals: Rubella, negative; VDRL, negative; O positive; Coombs, negative. From these results, the nurse understands that which intervention is indicated at this time?

1. Discuss with the client the need for rubella vaccine after she delivers.
2. The client needs to receive penicillin immediately.
3. Blood work needs to be ordered for the father of the baby to check his Rh and type.
4. The client needs to know that she will have frequent blood work to check for an incompatibility of her blood with the fetus.

1. **Correct. Any time a mother's rubella titer is negative, she needs to be given a rubella vaccine immediately following delivery and to avoid pregnancy for at least three months after the vaccine.**

2. *Wrong. A negative VDRL means the client does not have syphilis. No antibiotic is indicated.*

3. *Incorrect. The fetus born to a mother with O type blood is at risk for an ABO incompatibility but, since there is no prenatal screening for this disorder, knowing the father's type is of no value.*

4. *Wrong. The negative Coombs means there are no antibodies present in the mother's blood that could affect the developing fetus. If the mother was Rh negative, a repeat Coombs would be done later in the pregnancy.*

48. **The nurse is monitoring the fetal heart rate of a laboring woman. The nurse's assessment is based on the knowledge that the normal baseline fetal heart rate is:**

1. 100-150 beats per minute.
2. 110-160 beats per minute.
3. 120-160 beats per minute.
4. 120-170 beats per minute.

1. *Wrong. This rate is too low.*
2. *Incorrect. The lower rate of 110 is too low.*
3. **Correct. Normal baseline is between 120-160 beats per minute.**
4. *Wrong. The upper rate of 170 is too high.*

49. **The nurse is teaching an antepartum client about counting fetal movements. Which statement by the client demonstrates to the nurse that the client understands this procedure?**

1. "I will count the times my fetus moves for a period of one hour at various times throughout a day."
2. "I will call my doctor if my baby's movements increase considerably at any time."
3. "I will count my baby's fetal movements after meals for 20 to 30 minutes."
4. "It is normal for the fetus to have sleep times, so if I do not feel fetal movement early in the morning it's okay."

1. *Wrong. Consistency is important in the timing of fetal movements. Research has proven that the fetus is most active after meals. If you count prior to eating one time and after eating another, there may be drastic differences.*
2. *Wrong. Increased fetal movement is a good prognostic sign.*
3. **Correct. Whenever possible, the antepartum client is encouraged to do fetal movement counts three times daily, preferably after meals.**
4. *Wrong. The fetus may move less while the mother is sleeping, but when the mother awakens she usually will feel fetal movements. Failure to feel fetal movement in the early morning upon arising could be a cause for concern. The mother needs to eat and or drink, and try again to count fetal movements.*

50. **A first time mother who is breast feeding tells the nurse she is concerned about whether her baby is receiving enough intake. Which is the best nursing assessment to use in evaluating the adequacy of hydration?**

1. How often the baby cries.
2. The number of wet diapers per day.
3. The baby's skin turgor.
4. The fit of the baby's clothes.

1. *Wrong. Babies cry for reasons other than hunger.*
2. **Good choice. The easiest and most reliable method to evaluate hydration is urinary output. Six to eight wet diapers per day is generally considered adequate.**
3. *Wrong. Loss of skin turgor will not occur in the early stages of dehydration, whereas decreased urination will.*
4. *Wrong. The fit of the newborn's clothes is not a good evaluation tool for hydration because there are too many variables (e.g., shrinking in dryer, different sizing).*

51. **In developing a plan to improve the self-image of an eight-year-old with asthma, the nurse should consider that:**

1. The client is not able to understand the causes or limitations of chronic illness.
2. The client's peers, parents, and teachers should be instructed in strategies for encouraging her.
3. Teaching the client self-care skills will increase her sense of control.
4. The client should be told about all potential long-term complications.

1. *Incorrect. This child is in third grade at school, where science is part of the curriculum. Cause and effect is understood if the terms used are appropriate. Make another choice.*
2. *This isn't the best choice. Her peers are also eight years old, and they are not necessarily supportive or encouraging. These are all external sources of approval, not a measure of self-esteem. Select again.*
3. **Very good! A sense of control will increase self-esteem. Teaching her about her medications and how to handle her asthma attacks will increase her self-esteem by increasing her sense of control over her illness.**
4. *Incorrect. School age children cannot comprehend long-term complications. This would not improve her self-esteem, either. Make another selection.*

52. **A 10-year-old is overweight. He has no dietary restrictions. The nurse is helping him make out his menu. Which diet**

would the nurse plan to encourage?

1. A glass of whole milk, hot dog on a roll with pickles, and a candy bar.
2. A glass of skim milk, baked fish sandwich on whole wheat roll with lettuce, and a medium apple.
3. A glass of diet lemonade, hamburger and roll, medium orange and mashed potatoes.
4. A salad plate of low fat cottage cheese, potato salad, and macaroni salad with a croissant and a glass of water.

1. *No, this diet is not well balanced and lacks vitamins and minerals. There is an excess of carbohydrates and fats in the candy and hot dog. Try again.*
2. **Correct! The menu includes selections from several food groups, has complex carbohydrates, and is low in fat, which should be encouraged during weight reduction.**
3. *No, this diet doesn't include an adequate source of calcium and has fairly high carbohydrates. Try again.*
4. *Incorrect. This may look OK at first, but there is too much fat in the ingredients of the salads and croissant. This choice also lacks fruit and has no green vegetable. Choose again.*

53. The mother of a two-year-old who is hospitalized asks how she should handle her son's temper tantrums. The nurse should advise the mother to:

1. Restrain the child physically.
2. Ignore the behavior.
3. Let the child know his temper tantrums are not acceptable.
4. Play a game with him, or rock him quietly.

1. *Incorrect. This may actually cause the behavior to intensify. Select an option that will diminish the behavior.*
2. **Good work! This is the recommended approach, since it does not reinforce the behavior. Ignoring a negative behavior is a basic concept in behavior modification.**
3. *No, this is not preferred. This behavior is due to lack of self-control, which is gradually being gained at this age. Select again.*
4. *This would reinforce the negative behavior, so it is incorrect. Choose another answer.*

54. The nurse knows that instructions for the mother of a school age girl with pediculosis have been successful when the mother states:

1. "My child must have a physician's note to return to school."
2. "I will treat family members who have lice."
3. "Before I put the shampoo on, I'll cut her hair."

4. "All toys must be thrown out if they can't be dry cleaned or washed."

1. *Incorrect. The school nurse will examine the child upon returning, to determine if the child is free of nits.*
2. **Very good! Only the members who actually have lice should be treated, because there are side effects with the treatment as with any medication.**
3. *No! Cutting her hair would be psychologically traumatic for the child. This is not done. Choose again.*
4. *Incorrect and unnecessary. Items that can't be dry cleaned or washed can be closed into a plastic bag for 10 to 14 days. The lice can't live without a host. Choose again.*

55. A five-month-old must undergo a spinal tap to rule out meningitis. The nurse who is planning to assist with the procedure should:

1. Have several other nurses to help hold the infant.
2. Position the child seated on the side of table.
3. Hold chin to chest and knees to abdomen.
4. Utilize a papoose board to restrain limbs.

1. *Wrong! Look at the age of the child. There isn't room for three people to hold onto this child. Pick another option.*
2. *Wrong! This might be an option for an adolescent or adult, but not an infant! Select again.*
3. **Yes, this is the correct position. For a five-month-old, one nurse should be adequate.**
4. *Wrong. This would be used for a procedure done on the anterior side of the body. Choose again.*

56. A hospitalized eight-year-old is losing a game of checkers. He stands up and says, "I quit." The nurse understands that this behavior probably is:

1. A personality change due to hospitalization.
2. Immaturity for his age.
3. A sign that this game is too hard for him.
4. Normal for his social development.

1. *No, this behavior is probably not a change. Select again.*
2. *Incorrect. Look for another reason for this behavior.*
3. *No, this is an age appropriate activity. Remember, play is the way children learn. Try again.*
4. **Yes, you got it right. Children will frequently "quit" at this age if they can not succeed, until they learn that the social interaction is more important than winning.**

57. The nurse knows that the observations most likely to be made on a child with celiac disease include:

1. Pale, small arms, large belly.
2. Periorbital edema and weight gain.
3. Retractions, flushing, increased respirations.
4. Diaphoresis and increased bowel sounds.

1. *Correct. These are the signs of a child who is malnourished. Since celiac disease interferes with absorption, this would be the clinical appearance.*
2. *Incorrect. These aren't the signs found in a child with malabsorption. Select again.*
3. *No, this sounds like a respiratory disease, not celiac. Try again.*
4. *These would be found in children experiencing diarrhea, but they are nonspecific for celiac disease. Pick another answer.*

58. The nurse would interpret which finding as an indication that an infant's dehydration has been corrected?

1. Weight gain of three ounces in 24 hours.
2. Specific gravity of 1.028.
3. Cool skin with tenting.
4. Frequent stooling.

1. *Yes, weight gain is the best indicator of rehydration in infants and small children.*
2. *Incorrect. This indicates dehydration. Select again.*
3. *Incorrect. Cool skin and tenting are signs of dehydration. The skin is cool and less elastic due to the decrease in circulating volume. Choose another response.*
4. *Incorrect. This answer doesn't tell you anything about hydration status, but you might suspect that if stooling continues, dehydration may worsen or at least will not improve. Try again.*

59. The nurse is evaluating the effectiveness of the teaching performed for the mother of a six-month-old who is teething. The nurse would consider the teaching to be successful if the mother:

1. Provides the infant with a hard rubber toy to bite.
2. Places aspirin against the erupting tooth.
3. Rubs a topical anesthetic on the sensitive area.
4. Places sherry and water mixture on gums at bedtime.

1. *Yes, this is correct! This is safe and at the same time will speed the tooth's erupting by providing a firm surface to help the tooth break through the skin.*
2. *No! This is unsafe, since the infant may aspirate the aspirin. Try again.*
3. *Definitely not! Topical anesthetics are not to be taken internally or used in the mouth. Only oral anesthetics can be used safely. Make another selection.*

4. *No! Although many parents will remember someone in the family using alcohol to reduce teething pain, this is never recommended for children. Select again.*

60. At nine months of age, an infant has been in the hospital four times for a total of 42 days. The nurse notices that the infant does not seem upset when her parents leave. The nurse would evaluate this behavior as:

1. An infant with an easy temperament.
2. A mature infant who is very secure.
3. A strong attachment to the nurses.
4. Experiencing detachment.

1. *Incorrect. Even children with an easy temperament would not normally feel comfortable with parents leaving them. Fear of abandonment is strong at this age. Try again.*
2. *No, there is no reason to believe this is a true statement. This child has had four interruptions in a sensitive period of development: the period where trust in the primary care giver needs to be developed. Choose again.*
3. *Incorrect. The infant must first develop a sense of trust with one individual (the primary care giver) before meaningful relationships can occur with others. Due to many separations, this child has not had the opportunity to develop that trust. Make another selection.*
4. *Yes, this is correct. The infant is exhibiting the third stage of separation anxiety, which is detachment. The characteristic superficial interaction with the environment might appear to be an acceptance by the child of being left by parents.*

61. The nurse explains a bone marrow aspiration to a seven-year-old. Which response would the nurse interpret as indicating that the child understood the teaching?

1. "I hope my headache won't be too bad."
2. "The doctor will put me to sleep for a little while."
3. "I'll have to lay on my belly while it's done."
4. "My doctor will push on my chest, but it won't hurt."

1. *Incorrect. Bone marrow aspiration will not effect the brain or its fluids. Perhaps you were thinking of a lumbar puncture. Select again.*
2. *No, this test is not normally done under anesthesia. Try again.*
3. *Yes, the position for children having a bone marrow aspiration is usually on the abdomen, since the specimen is obtained from the iliac crest.*

4. *Incorrect. This position is used in adults for obtaining a bone marrow aspiration. It can be frightening and, since the bones are softer in childhood, the sternum is not the preferred site. Choose another option.*

62. **In preparing a teaching plan for families about Reye's syndrome, the nurse knows that the most important part of the plan is:**

   1. Avoiding the use of aspirin with children; only acetaminophen is safe.
   2. Treating all streptococcal infections immediately.
   3. Keeping the fever down with cool baths.
   4. Calling the child's doctor if a sick child is recovering and then becomes ill again.

   1. *Incorrect. Although aspirin is unsafe to use in children with certain viral infections, aspirin is still a safe drug for children with other diseases. Make another choice.*
   2. *Wrong choice. This action is correct to avoid complications of strep, but strep is bacterial and is not implicated in Reye's syndrome.*
   3. *No, this does not treat or prevent Reye's syndrome. Select again.*
   4. **Yes, this is correct! If the child has been ill, is improving and then there is a return of manifestations of illness, this should always be reported to the doctor. Delay can be fatal.**

63. **The parents of a child with Hodgkin's lymphoma ask about their son's prognosis. The nurse's response should be based on the knowledge that Hodgkin's lymphoma:**

   1. Is frequently a fatal disease.
   2. Is associated with excellent survival rates.
   3. Is associated with remissions that are usually short, and then manifestations return.
   4. Is completely unpredictable.

   1. *No, this is incorrect. Select again, based on the prognosis of this disorder.*
   2. **Yes, this is correct. If diagnosed early, survival rates approach 95 percent.**
   3. *This response is incorrect; it does not describe the pattern that usually follows treatment of Hodgkin's. Try again.*
   4. *Not true. Although it is not possible to predict each individual's response in advance, we do have data based on a large number of clients with this disease. What is the experience with Hodgkin's?*

64. **A client is being treated for an intracranial tumor. A CAT scan with contrast dye was ordered by the physician to determine if the tumor is shrinking. The client asks the nurse what to expect during the procedure. The most appropriate response by the nurse is:**

   1. "Just try to relax and go to sleep."
   2. "It is important to remain still. You will be on your back on an x-ray table. Your head will be immobilized, and you will hear clicking sounds."
   3. "The contrast dye will make you sleepy and may make your skin itch."
   4. "Although the procedure may be uncomfortable, you have to do it because your physician ordered it."

   1. *This is an inappropriate response. The nurse needs to provide the client with relevant information about the procedure. Choose another option.*
   2. **Correct. This is an accurate explanation of what the client will experience during the procedure.**
   3. *This statement is untrue. The contrast dye may cause a flushed feeling, a salty taste, or nausea and vomiting. Choose another option.*
   4. *Incorrect. This is not an appropriate response. It uses the communication block of referring to an inappropriate person (the physician). The nurse needs to be empathetic toward the client and help to allay his fears by providing correct information about the procedure. The nurse should address the issue raised by the client. Choose another option.*

65. **When a contrast dye is used during a CAT scan, the nurse should observe the client for signs of an allergic reaction. Which finding would the nurse identify as indicating an allergic reaction to the dye?**

   1. Flushed feeling.
   2. Nausea and vomiting.
   3. Headache.
   4. Dyspnea and urticaria.

   1. *Incorrect. This is an expected side effect of the contrast dye, not an allergic reaction. Try again.*
   2. *Incorrect. This is an expected side effect of the contrast dye, not an allergic reaction. Try again.*
   3. *Incorrect. This is an expected side effect of the contrast dye, not an allergic reaction. Try again.*
   4. **Good work! These are manifestations of an allergic reaction to the contrast dye.**

66. **The nurse has prepared a client for an MRI of the lower back to rule out a herniated disc. The nurse is aware that MRI procedures are generally contraindicated for clients who have a fear of:**

   1. Closed spaces.
   2. Dark places.
   3. Immobilization.
   4. Needles.

1.   *Correct. This condition is known as claustro-phobia.*
2.   *Incorrect. There is a light source at both openings of the MRI machine.*
3.   *Incorrect. Fear of remaining still is usually not a factor for this procedure.*
4.   *Incorrect. Needles are not used for this procedure.*

67.   The Tensilon test, used to diagnose myasthenia gravis, is administered intravenously and usually lasts about 15-30 minutes. If the client has myasthenia gravis, following administration of edrophonium chloride (Tensilon) the nurse would expect that muscle strength should:

1.   Stay the same.
2.   Decrease immediately.
3.   Improve immediately.
4.   Develop fasciculations.

1.   *Incorrect. This does not occur if the client has myasthenia gravis.*
2.   *Incorrect. This does not occur if the client has myasthenia gravis.*
3.   *Correct. The degree of improvement depends on the muscle group being tested.*
4.   *Incorrect. This is a reaction demonstrated if the client does not have myasthenia gravis.*

68.   To determining how much fluid the client loses during hemodialysis, the nurse measures the client's:

1.   Abdominal girth.
2.   Blood pressure.
3.   Ankle and calf measurements.
4.   Body weight.

1.   *Incorrect. This is not an accurate indicator of a client's fluid status. Try again!*
2.   *Incorrect. This measurement has nothing to do with fluid losses, or gains, from dialysis. Try again!*
3.   *Incorrect. These measurements will not accurately reflect fluid changes during dialysis. Try again!*
4.   *Correct. This is the most accurate method used to compare fluid changes during dialysis.*

69.   In a client with Cushing's syndrome, which clinical manifestation(s) would the nurse expect to observe?

1.   Large extremities.
2.   Decreased body and facial hair.
3.   Moon face, truncal obesity, and hyperpigmentation.
4.   Muscle twitching, seizures.

1.   *Incorrect. Clients have thin extremities. Try again.*
2.   *Incorrect. There is an increase in body and facial hair. Try again.*
3.   *Correct. Additionally, there is a "buffalo*

hump," purple striae on the trunk, acne, and pendulous abdomen.*
4.   *Incorrect. These are not common manifestations in Cushing's syndrome. They would occur in a neurological disorder. Try again.*

70.   A client has returned from the operating room following repair of the ligaments in his left knee. Upon awakening, he complains of severe pain. The physician has ordered morphine sulfate for the control of pain. Which assessment should be made by the nurse before administering the drug?

1.   Radial pulse rate.
2.   Blood pressure.
3.   Respiratory rate.
4.   Pulse pressure.

1.   *Incorrect. This assessment is not required prior to administration of narcotic analgesics. The pulse should be monitored per routine orders, and significant bradycardia (below 60 beats per minute) should be reported to the physician.*
2.   *Incorrect. This assessment is not required prior to administration of narcotic analgesics. Blood pressure should be monitored per routine orders, and significant hypotension should be reported to the physician.*
3.   *Correct. Narcotic drugs depress the respiratory center in the brain and should not be administered if the respiratory rate is below 12 per minute.*
4.   *Incorrect. This is not a routine assessment before administering narcotic analgesics.*

71.   A client develops a fecal impaction. Before digital removal of the mass, what type of enema is usually given by the nurse to loosen the feces?

1.   Fleets.
2.   Oil retention.
3.   Soap suds.
4.   Tap water.

1.   *Incorrect. A Fleets enema, which is a hypertonic solution, is given to cleanse the bowel. It is usually given after digital removal of the impaction.*
2.   *Correct. Before digital removal of the fecal mass, an oil retention enema is often given to soften the stool. This makes the digital removal less painful for the client.*
3.   *No. A soap suds enema acts as an irritant to increase peristalsis and thus facilitate the removal of stool. The soap suds enema is usually given after the fecal impaction has been digitally removed in order to completely cleanse the bowel.*
4.   *Wrong. Tap water enemas were previously used to cleanse the bowel, but now are contraindicated because of the possibility of fluid and electrolyte*

imbalances. Tap water, which is hypotonic, can be drawn into the cells, causing a fluid overload (hypervolemic state).

72. **A nurse is caring for a client with a diagnosis of cancer of the colon. He is scheduled for a bowel resection in two days. Which order can the nurse expect to see included in his preoperative plan of care?**

1. NPO for three days prior to surgery.
2. Administration of cleansing enemas.
3. Administration of IV antibiotics as a bowel preparation.
4. Instructions on colostomy irrigations.

1. *Absolutely not! This action could put the client in serious jeopardy with fluid and electrolyte imbalances, especially dehydration and negative nitrogen balance.*
2. **Yes. Clients undergoing a bowel resection need a bowel prep to minimize bacterial growth in the colon and decrease the chance of postoperative wound infection. This prep usually includes administration of enemas to cleanse the bowel, as well as the oral administration of neomycin sulfate.**
3. *No, IV antibiotics are not typically used as part of the bowel prep to decrease bacterial growth in the colon and decrease the chance of a postoperative wound infection. Oral antibiotics such as neomycin sulfate are given.*
4. *Incorrect. This information should be given in the postoperative period prior to discharge, if even indicated at all.*

73. **A client just returned from the operating room, where he underwent a left-sided cardiac catheterization. One of the complications of this surgery can be an arterial embolus or thrombus in the affected limb. Which nursing action would be harmful in caring for this client?**

1. If ordered, administer a vasodilator to relieve painful constriction.
2. Administer an anticoagulant as ordered, and monitor for signs of bleeding.
3. Protect the affected limb from pressure, and maintain the limb at a level or slightly dependent position with respect to the heart.
4. Massage the limb to promote circulation.

1. *Wrong choice. This is an appropriate action that increases the blood flow in the limb, relieving the constriction.*
2. *Wrong choice. This is an appropriate action when ordered by the physician. It can prevent the development of emboli, which can be life-threatening.*
3. *Wrong choice. This is an appropriate action to protect the integrity of the limb.*
4. **Good work! You have identified the dangerous**

action. Massaging could result in dislodging a clot.

74. **A client was admitted to the neurological unit of the hospital because of exacerbation of her multiple sclerosis. Her family asks the nurse what will happen, and how to deal with the client's emotional changes. The nurse would demonstrate an understanding of the family's emotional needs by:**

1. Encouraging the family to look on the bright side.
2. Advising the family to overlook the client's mood swings, since she really doesn't mean to be angry or depressed.
3. Providing the family with medical journals describing the latest research on multiple sclerosis.
4. Spending time listening to the family, and encouraging them to ventilate their feelings.

1. *Incorrect. This response by the nurse uses a cliché and is not helpful or productive. This response does not properly address the family's feelings, fails to provide any information, and does nothing to promote a realistic and a positive outlook of the disease on the part of the family. The family members are the clients in this question, and the nurse's response must be therapeutic for them.*
2. *Incorrect. Overlooking the client's mood changes will not help the family to deal with them effectively. The client's emotional state has an effect on the family — and vice versa. The family members are the clients in this question, and the nurse's response must be therapeutic for them.*
3. *Incorrect. Technical material may confuse and intimidate the family. Instead, to address the family's need for information, the nurse may provide them with appropriate client education materials and refer them to the National Multiple Sclerosis Society.*

TEST-TAKING TIP: *When answering a communication question, be sure you have correctly identified the client — and remember that the priority is to address the client's feelings. Can you identify an option that uses a therapeutic communication tool?*

4. **Excellent! The family members are the clients in this question, and the nurse's response must be therapeutic for them. Spending time listening to the family conveys that they are worthy of the nurse's attention. It is important that the nurse recognize the family's needs and provide them an opportunity to express their concerns and feelings.**

75. **A female client with a history of severe multiple sclerosis has requested a living will and has asked the nurse to witness it. The appropriate response is:**

1. "I would be honored to witness the will."
2. "I think your physician should witness the will."
3. "It would be a conflict of interest for me to witness the will, since I do not believe in living wills."
4. "I am unable to witness the will because of my professional relationship with you. Is there someone else you know who could do so?"

1. *Incorrect. A nurse is not permitted to witness the living will of her/his client. Such a witness would be invalid because of the nurse's professional relationship with the client.*
2. *Incorrect. A physician is not permitted to witness the living will of his/her client. Such a witness would be invalid because of the physician's professional relationship with the client.*
3. *Incorrect. There is a conflict of interest here, but it is because of the nurse's professional relationship with the client, not the client's beliefs. A nurse is prohibited from witnessing the living will of his/her client, and such a witness would be invalid. Note that this response also uses the communication block of referring to an inappropriate issue: the nurse's beliefs are not important.*
4. **Correct. The nurse is prohibited from witnessing the living will because of his/her professional relationship with the client. Such a witness would be invalid.**

76. A client with chronic osteoarthritis complains of discomfort when performing exercises prescribed by the physical therapist. Which response by the nurse is most appropriate?

1. "The exercises will prevent pain."
2. "The exercises will prevent worsening of the disease."
3. "The exercises will help to maintain as near normal joint function as possible, as well as range of motion."
4. "The exercises will make you feel better."

1. *Wrong. This statement is not true, and the exercises themselves may cause some mild discomfort.*
2. *Incorrect. The exercises will not prevent worsening of the disease. There is no cure for osteoarthritis.*
3. **Correct. The exercises will help maintain joint function and range of motion if done on a regular basis. This response is therapeutic because it provides correct information.**
4. *Wrong choice. The exercises may help the client to feel better, but this is not the most appropriate response.*

77. A client is to undergo cholecystosonography, which is the preferred method for detecting gallstones. The nurse explains to the client that this diagnostic evaluation of the gallbladder involves:

1. X-ray of the abdomen.
2. Radioisotope imaging of the gallbladder.
3. Drinking an oral contrast medium.
4. Ultrasound imaging of the gallbladder and bile ducts.

1. *Incorrect. An abdominal x-ray is able to visualize only calcified gallstones. Choose again.*
2. *Incorrect. This test is called cholescintigraphy and is used in clients who are allergic to iodine-containing contrast agents.*
3. *Incorrect. This test can visualize gallstones, as well as the filling and emptying of the gallbladder.*
4. **Correct. This test can also differentiate hepatic disease from biliary obstruction.**

78. Acute renal failure usually follows direct injury to the kidneys or overwhelming physiologic stress such as burns, severe shock, or nephrotoxic drugs. Which manifestations would the nurse identify as inconsistent with a diagnosis of acute renal failure?

1. Generalized edema.
2. Anorexia, nausea, and vomiting.
3. Irritability, restlessness, and headache.
4. Polyuria.

1. *Incorrect. This is a common sign of acute renal failure.*
2. *Incorrect. These common manifestations of acute renal failure can progress to dehydration and electrolyte imbalance.*
3. *Incorrect. These manifestations of acute renal failure can progress to muscle twitching and convulsions.*
4. **Correct. Anuria, not polyuria, occurs in acute renal failure.**

79. A diabetic client with acute renal failure is receiving peritoneal dialysis, in addition to medication therapy. The nurse knows that a complication of peritoneal dialysis is:

1. Hypoglycemia.
2. Metabolic acidosis.
3. Infection.
4. Hyponatremia.

1. *Incorrect. HYPERglycemia, not HYPOglycemia, occurs in diabetic clients undergoing dialysis and those receiving hypertonic dialysates.*
2. *Incorrect. Metabolic alkalosis, not acidosis, can occur if the dialysis is prolonged. The dialysates contain 45 mEq/liter of sodium acetate or sodium lactate, both of which are metabolized to bicarbonate.*
3. **Correct. The danger of peritonitis requires sterile techniques, closed sterile instillation and drainage systems, and frequent cultures of**

peritoneal drainage.

4. *Incorrect. HYPERnatremia, not HYPOnatremia, can occur, especially if hypertonic dialysate is used and water is removed in excess of electrolytes.*

80. **In explaining the treatment of peptic ulcers, the nurse would emphasize the need to avoid which substances that can aggravate a peptic ulcer?**

1. Smoking, coffee and tea.
2. Antacids.
3. Sedatives.
4. Bland diet.

1. **Correct. These substances increase stomach acidity. Nurses should advise clients to limit their consumption.**
2. *Incorrect. These drugs are used to neutralize excess stomach acidity.*
3. *Incorrect. These drugs are used to decrease anxiety and restlessness, allowing physical and psychological relaxation.*
4. *Incorrect. Although not as rigidly prescribed as in the past, a bland diet does not aggravate a peptic ulcer.*

81. **The doctor prescribes tube feedings for an elderly client who is hospitalized. The nurse understands that tube feedings may be prescribed when:**

1. The client is unable to swallow foods by mouth.
2. The client prefers this feeding method, since it is easier.
3. The client refuses to eat solid foods in the hospital because they contain meat and dairy products.
4. The family requests this method because it is more efficient.

1. **Correct. This is a common intervention for clients who are unable to eat by mouth.**
2. *Incorrect. This is not a valid reason for prescribing of tube feedings. Oral feeding is preferred over tube feedings.*
3. *Incorrect. This is never a reason for prescription of tube feedings! A vegetarian diet and dairy-free diet can be provided for the client in the hospital after consultation with a dietitian.*
4. *Incorrect. This is not a valid reason for prescribing of tube feedings. Consultation with a dietitian is important to ensure that the nutritional requirements of the elderly client are met, in the hospital or at home.*

82. **The nurse understands that a guaiac test detects microscopic particles in the feces of:**

1. Bile.
2. Lipid.
3. Bacteria.
4. Blood.

1. *Incorrect. The test does not measure bile in the stool.*
2. *Incorrect. The test does not measure lipid in the stool.*
3. *Incorrect. The test does not measure bacteria in the stool.*
4. **Correct. This is a useful diagnostic screening test for colon cancer.**

83. **In planning preoperative care for a client, the nurse is aware that obtaining legal, informed consent to perform surgery is the responsibility of:**

1. The nurse.
2. The surgeon.
3. The client's family physician.
4. The client.

1. *Incorrect. The nurse's responsibility is to ensure that a signed informed consent is in the chart. The nurse may present a form for the client to sign, and the nurse may sign the form as a witness to the signature. However, this does not transfer legal liability for informed consent for medical care to the nurse.*
2. **Yes. To attain the right to operate, it is necessary for the surgeon to obtain a voluntary and informed consent from the client. Before the client signs the consent form, the surgeon should inform the client in clear and simple terms what a reasonable person would want to be told, including an explanation of what the surgery will entail, as well as the possible risks and complications of the surgical procedure.**
3. *No. The client's family physician does not have responsibility for obtaining the informed consent. The family physician's role is purely advisory in this situation.*
4. *Not possible. The client cannot give himself informed consent! He needs information from the expert in the clinical area.*

84. **In writing the plan of care for a client with an ileostomy, the nurse states the need to protect the skin around the ileostomy stoma. The nurse's rationale for this client is based on the fact that:**

1. Friction causes irritation.
2. Urine causes skin excoriation.
3. Intestinal juices are irritating to the skin.
4. Organisms present on the skin can cause infection in the stoma.

1. *Not correct. This would be the rationale for cleansing the peristomal area gently with soap and water so that the skin is not damaged by vigorous rubbing and scrubbing.*

2. *No. An ileostomy does not drain urine. That is done via an ileal conduit.*

3. **Correct. Drainage from an ileostomy contains enzymes and bile salts that are damaging to the skin. A protective skin barrier paste or liquid, which serves to prevent contact between the skin and the ileostomy drainage, is placed on the peristomal skin after cleansing and prior to the application of a collection device.**

4. *Wrong choice. Unless there is a break in the skin or mucous membrane (that is, the lining of the stoma), there should be no danger of skin organisms causing infection.*

85. **Which intervention would be most important for the nurse to include in the plan of care for a client with hepatitis B?**

    1. Bedrest with bathroom privileges.
    2. High calorie, high protein diet.
    3. Force fluids to 3,000 ml in 24 hours.
    4. Medicate for pain every three to four hours as needed.

    1. **Yes, this is very important. Bedrest is usually recommended until the manifestations of hepatitis have subsided. Bedrest will "rest" the liver and decrease energy demands.**

    2. *Wrong option. Adequate nutrition should be maintained, but proteins are restricted when the liver's ability to metabolize protein by-products is impaired, as demonstrated by manifestations. Because the client tends to be anorexic, small, high-calorie, moderate-protein meals are indicated rather than three normal meals.*

    3. *Incorrect. Clients with hepatitis B are anorexic and often experience nausea/vomiting. If emesis is a problem, the client is treated with intravenous therapy. It is not realistic to expect the client to drink 3,000 ml in 24 hours.*

    4. *Wrong. Clients with hepatitis B may be anorexic and experience dyspepsia, generalized aching, malaise, and weakness. Medications are avoided if at all possible, in order to "rest" the liver.*

86. **The nurse is caring for a male client, age 65, who has undergone a below-the-knee amputation because of persistent peripheral vascular disease (PVD). The orders are for wet to dry dressing changes b.i.d. The nurse knows that which dressing technique is the most appropriate?**

    1. Clean technique, using nonsterile gloves.
    2. Sterile technique, using sterile gloves.
    3. Sterile technique for the first week postoperatively, then clean technique.
    4. Mask, gown, and sterile gloves for all dressing changes.

    1. *Incorrect. This wound requires sterile technique while in the hospital.*

    2. **Correct. This is a sterile procedure.**

    3. *Incorrect. This is a sterile procedure while it is done in the hospital.*

    4. *Incorrect. Sterile procedure does not require a mask unless it is a central line dressing change. A gown is not required unless the nurse feels the wound has excessive drainage that may soil the nurse's uniform.*

87. **A young male client, age 11 years, sustained a broken tibia while playing football. The physician set the fracture in the operating room and applied a cast. The client returned to his room drowsy and complaining of mild pain. At this time, the nurse should:**

    1. *Use a hair dryer to hasten the drying of the cast.*
    2. *Keep the casted leg in a flat position.*
    3. *Observe for signs of circulatory impairment, infection, swelling, and hemorrhage.*
    4. *Teach the client to keep his leg in contact with the floor while sitting.*

    1. *No! The cast is left uncovered to promote drying. The heat from a hair dryer will prolong the drying process.*

    2. *No! The leg needs to be elevated on a pillow to reduce swelling.*

    3. **Correct. Any change in sensation, change in color or skin temperature, decrease in pedal pulse, odor from the cast, swelling, elevated body temperature, or bleeding from the cast, indicates a problem that needs to be addressed immediately.**

    4. *No! The casted leg needs to be elevated when sitting, to reduce swelling.*

88. **A client underwent a below-the-knee bilateral amputation of both lower extremities following a severe motor vehicle accident. On the first postoperative day, it is inappropriate for the nurse to:**

    1. Start range of motion exercises to both stumps.
    2. Encourage the client not to sit in any one position for prolonged periods of time.
    3. Elevate the stumps on a pillow.
    4. Apply compression bandages.

    1. **Good work, range of motion exercises would be inappropriate. Exercises are contraindicated for about 10 days postoperatively.**

    2. *Wrong choice. This is an appropriate instruction for the client with lower extremity amputation. Inactivity can cause hip flexion contractures.*

    3. *Wrong choice, this is appropriate. Elevation of the stumps will decrease swelling and pain.*

    4. *Wrong choice, this is appropriate. Compression is*

important in decreasing edema and in preparing for a prosthesis fitting.

89. **A male client has developed right-sided heart failure. The nurse is aware that right-sided heart failure results in an increase in:**

1. Central venous pressure (CVP).
2. Blood pressure (BP).
3. Pulse pressure.
4. Intraocular pressure.

1. ***Correct. Right-sided heart failure results in an increase in pressure in the right atrium, resulting in an increase in pressure in the vena cava and, consequently, in the CVP.***
2. *Incorrect. Although BP may be elevated in heart failure clients, this is not always the case.*
3. *Incorrect. Pulse pressure is the difference between the systolic and diastolic pressures. A normal pulse pressure is 40 to 50 mm Hg. A widening of the pulse pressure can occur with an increase intracranial pressure.*
4. *Incorrect. An increase in intraocular pressure occurs with glaucoma.*

90. **Which characteristic is inconsistent with a client diagnosed with varicose veins?**

1. Peripheral edema of the lower leg(s) that appears during the day, is aggravated by prolonged standing, and decreases or disappears during the night, when the client is sleeping.
2. Reddish discoloration of the lower legs.
3. Dryness and scaling over prominent varices.
4. Ulcerations, including long-standing varicose ulcers.

1. *Wrong choice. This is a normal characteristic with varicose veins.*
2. ***Correct. The nurse would not expect to see reddish discoloration of the lower legs. There is a brownish discoloration of the lower legs with varicose veins.***
3. *Wrong choice. This is a common characteristic with varicose veins.*
4. *Wrong choice. Ulcerations can occur with varicose veins and are often difficult to treat.*

91. **The nurse teaching a group of hypertensive clients about the prevention of arteriosclerosis is guided by the knowledge that a factor contributing to the development of arteriosclerosis is:**

1. Hypotension.
2. Elevated levels of high density lipoproteins (HDLs).
3. Cholesterol levels less than 200 mg.
4. Fat intake greater than 30% of daily calorie consumption.

1. *Incorrect. This is not a contributing factor in the development of arteriosclerosis.*
2. *Incorrect. Elevated HDLs have a protective effect on the development of arteriosclerosis.*
3. *Incorrect. Cholesterol levels less than 200 mg are a recommended goal because this helps to decrease the incidence of arteriosclerosis.*
4. ***Correct. Fat intake greater than 30% of daily calorie consumption is a contributing factor in the development of arteriosclerosis. Clients are advised to substitute polyunsaturated fat (vegetable fat) for saturated fats (animal origin).***

92. **The nurse would select which infection control precautions as appropriate in caring for an AIDS client?**

1. Strict isolation.
2. Respiratory isolation.
3. Contact isolation.
4. Universal blood and body fluid precautions.

1. *Incorrect. Strict isolation is instituted for clients with highly contagious infections spread by air and contact, such as chicken pox and diphtheria.*
2. *Incorrect. Respiratory isolation prevents transmission of infectious diseases over short distances through air droplets. It is appropriate for measles, mumps, pneumonia, and meningitis.*
3. *Incorrect. Contact isolation prevents transmission of highly transmissible infections spread by close or direct contact that do not warrant strict precautions. It is appropriate for impetigo, herpes simplex infections, and acute respiratory infections in infants and young children.*
4. ***Correct. Universal precautions prevent contact with pathogens transmitted by direct or indirect contact with infective blood or body fluids containing blood.***

93. **In assessing a client, the nurse would recognize which manifestations or findings as consistent with AIDS?**

1. Persistent fever, swollen glands, diarrhea, weight loss, and fatigue.
2. Elevated hemoglobin level, increased urinary glucose, elevated BUN.
3. Elevated BP, tachycardia, dyspnea, and edema.
4. Hypotension, dehydration, and pallor in the nail beds, conjunctivae, lips, and skin.

1. ***Correct. The manifestations of AIDS are vague and can be confused with other conditions such as mononucleosis or chronic fatigue syndrome.***
2. *Incorrect. These laboratory results are not indicative of active AIDS. Decreased hemoglobin can occur with anemia. Increased urinary glucose can*

occur in diabetes. An elevated BUN can occur in kidney disease. Try again.

3.   *Incorrect. These are manifestations of congestive heart failure. Try again.*

4.   *Incorrect. These manifestations may be indicative of shock. Try again.*

94.   **The nurse monitors a client who is taking digoxin (Lanoxin) for his heart condition. The nurse would interpret which manifestation as an indication that the client may be developing digitalis toxicity?**

1.   Polydipsia.
2.   Diplopia (double vision).
3.   Nausea and vomiting.
4.   Constipation.

1.   *Incorrect. This is not a sign of digoxin toxicity. Choose another option.*

2.   *Incorrect. This is not a sign of digoxin toxicity. Choose another option.*

3.   **Correct. These are early signs of digoxin toxicity.**

4.   *Incorrect. This is not a sign of digoxin toxicity.*

95.   **Before giving preoperative medication to a client going to surgery, the nurse must make sure that:**

1.   The client has an empty bladder.
2.   Vital signs are documented on the preoperative check list.
3.   Dentures are removed.
4.   The consent form has been signed.

1.   *Incorrect. This assessment is desirable, but not critical prior to administering the preoperative medication. If a client expresses the need to urinate after the preoperative medication has been given, then the urinal or bedpan would be used. Remember that, for safety reasons, the client cannot get out of bed after the preoperative medication has been given.*

2.   *No, this is important prior to the client's transport to the surgical suite, but it's not necessary that the data be documented prior to giving the preoperative medication. What would be important is the fact that the vital signs were TAKEN prior to the administration of the medication.*

3.   *Incorrect. The client may wish to keep the dentures in place until called to the operating room. It is not critical that they be removed at this time.*

4.   **Correct. The nurse must always check to see that a consent form has been signed before giving the preoperative medication. For legal purposes, the client cannot be under the influence of narcotics or sedatives when signing the consent form, or the client's "mental competence" could be challenged.**

96.   **A client with advanced cirrhosis is admitted with bleeding esophageal varices. A Sengstaken-Blakemore tube has been inserted. In planning care for this client, the nurse knows that the primary purpose of the Sengstaken-Blakemore tube is to:**

1.   Coagulate the bleeding varices.
2.   Prevent the aspiration of blood into the lungs.
3.   Apply direct pressure to the bleeding varices.
4.   Provide a means for removing blood from the stomach.

1.   *No, the Sengstaken-Blakemore tube does not have the capability to coagulate the bleeding varices.*

2.   *Wrong choice. Although the Sengstaken-Blakemore tube, when properly inflated, will prevent aspiration of blood into the lungs, this is not the primary purpose for the tube. The three openings in the tube are for specific purposes: gastric aspiration, inflation of the gastric balloon, and inflation of the esophageal balloon.*

3.   **Correct. The Sengstaken-Blakemore tube compresses the bleeding vessels by inflation of the esophageal balloon, which applies direct pressure to the site. This is the primary purpose of the Sengstaken-Blakemore tube.**

4.   *Incorrect. The Sengstaken-Blakemore tube does have an opening that can be used for aspirating gastric contents, but that is not the primary function of the tube.*

97.   **When planning care for the client receiving a narcotic antitussive, the nurse's main goal is to:**

1.   Deliver analgesia.
2.   Provide intervals of rest.
3.   Encourage productive coughing.
4.   Suppress the cough center.

1.   *The narcotic antitussives, codeine and hydrocodone bitartrate (Hycodan), do offer some analgesia. However, this is not the primary purpose of these medications. There are medications available that are more appropriate for providing analgesia.*

2.   **Very good! The main goal of administering an antitussive is to control chronic coughing and allow the client rest periods. Since a productive cough is beneficial to the body, the need for rest should be measured against the client's need for airway clearance.**

3.   *Productive coughs are encouraged through deep breathing and coughing exercises and encouraging fluids, as well as through judicious use of expectorants/mucolytics. An antitussive suppresses coughing.*

4.   *No, this is not really correct. A productive cough clears the airway of secretions and is beneficial to*

the body. It should not be the goal to suppress the cough center, but rather to provide intervals where the cough is suppressed enough to provide rest for the client. A goal takes into account why the intervention is performed, not merely how the intervention is performed.

98. The nurse is assessing a young child with asthma in order to determine the usefulness of a metered dose inhaler. Which factor would the nurse assess as discouraging the use of the inhaler.

1. The child's inability to follow directions.
2. The family's poor financial situation.
3. The size of the medication particles.
4. The severity of the child's disease.

1. *Good! In order to effectively use a metered dose inhaler, the child must be able to inhale as the medication is released. Children can use an inhaler as soon as they can follow these directions.*
2. *No, this would not discourage use. The relative costs of oral medications, metered dose inhalers, and nebulizers are the same. In fact, nebulizers may be more costly initially.*
3. *No, this would not discourage use. Medication particles are the smallest when delivered by metered dose inhaler. Because children's airways are narrower than adults' airways, a metered dose inhaler is the route of choice. The inhaler cannot be used, however, by children too young to understand how to use the inhaler.*
4. *When used properly, a metered dose inhaler can deliver a sufficient amount of medication to treat an asthma attack. The inhaler has the advantage of being more transportable and, therefore, more readily available. The severity of the illness, therefore, is a poor factor in determining effectiveness.*

99. A client received discharge instructions regarding side effects of his kanamycin sulfate (Kantrex) therapy. Which of the following statements by the client indicates to the nurse the need for further teaching?

1. "I know I should drink extra fluids while taking this medicine — at least two quarts a day."
2. "I'll call the doctor if I notice any ringing in my ears or a change in my hearing."
3. "I won't forget to call the doctor's office to make an appointment for lab work, to check on the medication's blood level."
4. "I won't worry about slight numbness or tingling in my legs because I know it's just a side effect I have to live with while I'm on this medicine."

1. *No, the client is correct in stating that he should drink extra fluids while taking aminoglycosides to prevent nephrotoxicity. You are looking for an INCORRECT statement. Choose another option.*
2. *No, the client would be correct in reporting any changes in hearing or tinnitus (monitoring for ototoxicity). You are looking for an INCORRECT statement. Choose another option.*
3. *No, the client correctly understands that it is important to monitor the serum kanamycin level while the client is taking this medicine. A peak level that is too high may be associated with an increased incidence of toxicity. The client understands the rationale for this lab work. You are looking for an INCORRECT statement. Choose another option.*
4. *Good evaluation! The client does not understand the importance of reporting these CNS manifestations, which can be early indications of neurotoxicity. Numbness, tingling, and muscle twitching should be reported immediately to the physician.*

100. A client is diagnosed with active tuberculosis and is started on a treatment regimen of isoniazid (INH) and ethambutol (Myambutol). Which of the following manifestations would the nurse identify as demanding the discontinuation of ethambutol?

1. Anorexia, nausea/vomiting.
2. Loss of color discrimination.
3. Edema of feet and hands.
4. Red-orange discoloration to all body fluids.

1. *Incorrect. These side effects are not common when a client is taking ethambutol, which is well absorbed from the GI tract in either the presence or absence of food. Try again.*
2. *Correct! The most commonly reported toxic reaction to normal therapeutic doses of ethambutol is indeed visual disturbance. Examples include changes of color vision (especially red and green) and loss of visual acuity. These signs are cause to terminate ethambutol use.*
3. *No, this side effect is not related to ethambutol therapy. Try again.*
4. *This is not related to ethambutol therapy. Recall that discoloration of body fluids is a side effect of rifampin (Rifadin) and is harmless. Make another selection.*

NOTES

NCLEX-PN

Test 7

NCLEX-PN TEST 7

1. A client has left her used insulin syringe on the bedside table. What is the best action by the nurse to help prevent spread of infection by way of the contaminated needle?

    1. Explain to the client that the syringe should be disposed of in the garbage can, to avoid a potential needle stick by someone providing care for the client.
    2. Cap the syringe and take it to the needle disposal container.
    3. Place the uncapped syringe in the needle disposal container.
    4. Have the nurse administer the injection, since the client is not responsible enough to follow through with the correct procedure.

2. An confused elderly client has wrist restraints for safety reasons. To provide for the client's safety, the nurse should give priority to which intervention?

    1. Checking the pulse, color, and temperature of extremities every shift and reporting these findings.
    2. Making sure the call light is within the client's reach.
    3. Notifying the client's family of the restraints and explaining the rationale for their use.
    4. Removing the restraints at night while the client is sleeping.

3. An elderly client is admitted to the hospital following a stroke. He has paralysis of the right side and is at risk of developing decubitus ulcers. In caring for this client, the nurse should:

    1. Move the client up in bed by sliding him.
    2. Roll the client to his side once a day.
    3. Change the client's position every two hours.
    4. Keep the client in a wheel chair during the morning and afternoon hours.

4. An elderly client has a draining pressure sore. The culture of the drainage reveals staphylococci. The most important nursing action is to:

    1. Reinforce the pressure dressing with a sterile towel before ambulating the client.
    2. Wear gown and gloves when changing the client's bed linen.
    3. Use sterile technique when changing the dressing on the pressure sore.
    4. Discourage the client's use of his personal effects until they have been sterilized.

5. A client complains that he is unable to rest because of the noise from his roommate's TV. The best action by the nurse is to:

    1. Have the client moved to a private room.
    2. Provide ear phones for the client who is watching television.
    3. Explain that the roommate is hard of hearing, so the television is louder than usual.
    4. Ask the roommate to shut off the television so the client can rest.

6. An elderly client is to receive a tub bath. In preparing the bath, which action by the nurse would be unsafe?

    1. Check the temperature of the tub room.
    2. Gather and take all of the necessary equipment to the tub room prior to the bath.
    3. Test the temperature of the bath water by having the client place his hand in the water.
    4. Place a mat or towel in the bottom of the tub.

7. While bathing a preschooler in a tub, which action by the nurse is inappropriate?

    1. Check the temperature of the water with a thermometer.
    2. Never leave the child unattended.
    3. Make sure the temperature in the room is warm.
    4. Allow the child to determine if the water temperature is comfortable by placing the child's feet in the water.

8. When making rounds, the nurse notices that a client who is receiving oxygen via nasal cannula has a pack of cigarettes at the bedside. The best nursing action is to:

    1. Remove the pack of cigarettes from the bedside.
    2. Remind the client not to smoke when oxygen is in use.
    3. Ask the client how he obtained the cigarettes.
    4. Review the rules of safety with the client's family.

9. The nurse is caring for an elderly client in a long-term care facility. When applying a hot water bottle to the client, it would be unsafe for the nurse to:

    1. Wrap the hot water bottle in a cloth before placing it next to the client's skin.
    2. Fill the hot water bottle with as much hot water as

it will hold.

3. Eliminate as much air as possible from the hot water bottle.

4. Check the temperature of the water with a thermometer.

10. The nurse is about to instruct parents of young children about poison control in the home. The nurse should:

1. Instruct the parents to induce vomiting with syrup of ipecac.

2. Instruct the parents to immediately bring the child to the emergency room.

3. Provide labels for the parent's telephone, with the Poison Control Center's telephone number, and give instructions to call that number after an accidental ingestion.

4. Notify social services to investigate the home situation for safety.

11. A adolescent client is to have a water system heating device ("K-Pad"), applied to a pulled muscle. The client tells the nurse that the device does not feel very warm. The most appropriate nursing action is to:

1. Tell the client that these heating devices never feel hot.

2. Check the temperature setting on the heating unit and feel the pad for warmth.

3. Call the appropriate repair department and have them fix the unit.

4. Turn the temperature up on the unit if it doesn't feel warm enough to the client.

12. During the resuscitation of a client, the physician orders the client to be defibrillated by receiving a controlled electrical shock. The nurse knows that it would be unsafe to:

1. Move away from the bed while the client is defibrillated.

2. Observe the other nurses to be sure they are not in contact with the client or the bed during defibrillation.

3. Hold the IV pole out of the way while the client is defibrillated.

4. Make sure the client's chest is dry, except where the electrode paste or pads are applied for placement of the defibrillator paddles.

13. Which statement would the nurse use to best describe the diagnosis and treatment of ovarian cancer?

1. Early detection has reduced the mortality rate in recent years.

2. Early diagnosis is very difficult, so prognosis remains poor.

3. Early detection is accomplished by routine vagi-

nal exam every three months.

4. Extensive radiation is highly successful in treating ovarian cancer.

14. The nurse is caring for an infant who is born small for gestational age (SGA) at 40 weeks gestation. The nurse's plan of care for this client should include:

1. Prevention of hyaline membrane disease.

2. Prevention of hyperglycemia.

3. Limitation of daily fluid intake due to small stomach capacity.

4. Careful suctioning of airways at delivery.

15. The nurse is caring for a three-day-old infant who is receiving phototherapy for an elevated bilirubin. Which nursing goal is least appropriate for the infant's care?

1. Protection of the eyes.

2. Prevention of fluid volume excess.

3. Maintenance of stable body temperature.

4. Promotion of mother-infant bonding.

16. The nurse is caring for an infant born to a mother who is addicted to crack cocaine. Which nursing action would be inappropriate?

1. Small frequent feedings.

2. Tight swaddling of infant.

3. Frequent stimulation.

4. Promoting mother-infant bonding.

17. A client's husband asks the nurse what he can do about his wife's rapid mood swings during her pregnancy. What is the best nursing response?

1. "They are the result of hormone imbalances. There is little you can do to help her."

2. "Try to ignore them. Paying attention to her as a result of these mood swings will only increase the problem."

3. "Talk to your wife about the mood swings and exhibit loving behaviors in spite of her mood."

4. "They are the result of hormone changes. You might suggest that she ask her doctor for medication to reduce their incidence."

18. An expectant father tells the nurse that he feels resentful of the added attention others are giving to his wife since the pregnancy was first announced several weeks ago. What is the most therapeutic nursing response to the father?

1. "It would be wise for you to speak to a therapist about these feelings."

2. "Has your wife sensed your anger towards her and the baby?"

3. "I'm sure that it's really hard to accept this, when it's your baby too."
4. "These feelings are very common to expectant fathers in early pregnancy."

19. **An antepartum client in her first trimester asks the nurse at the clinic if she may safely continue her aerobics program throughout her pregnancy. The appropriate nursing response is:**

    1. "Perhaps you should check with the doctor."
    2. "No problem. Go ahead and continue what you have been doing."
    3. "You may continue, but be careful not to go to the point of exhaustion."
    4. "It is probably wise to change to something less stressful during pregnancy."

20. **An obstetrical client tells the nurse that her last menstrual period began on July 8th. Based upon Naegle's rule, the nurse would calculate her baby's expected date of birth as:**

    1. April 15.
    2. April 1.
    3. October 15.
    4. October 1.

21. **Which finding would the nurse identify as a cause for concern in the antepartum client?**

    1. A +1 glucose in urine.
    2. WBC 15,000 mm³.
    3. Hematocrit 33%.
    4. Reactive VDRL.

22. **A client has a slight drop in blood pressure at her prenatal visits between 13 and 24 weeks gestation. The nurse understands that this is the result of:**

    1. Increased estrogen levels.
    2. Decreased circulating blood volume.
    3. Increased progesterone levels.
    4. Impending complications in the pregnancy.

23. **The nurse is caring for a client in labor. An epidural block is administered during the intrapartum period for pain relief. The nurse must be alert for the complication of:**

    1. Severe headaches.
    2. Hypotension.
    3. Nausea and vomiting.
    4. Pulmonary edema.

24. **A child is admitted with a possible diagnosis of Wilms' tumor (nephroblastoma). The nurse should obtain a**

sign to be placed over the child's bed, with which warning?

1. "Do not palpate abdomen."
2. "No blood work or BPs in arms."
3. "Isolation."
4. "No rectal temperatures."

25. **In assisting the doctor in examining a two-year-old who has otitis media, the nurse should have the child:**

    1. Lie down on the examining table while his throat and ears are examined, and then allow him to sit up for the rest of the exam.
    2. Lie down on the examining table, while the physician starts with examining the head and proceeds downward with the exam.
    3. Sit in his mother's lap while the heart and lungs are auscultated, and then examine the rest of his body, doing the throat and ears last.
    4. Allow him to sit in his mother's lap while his ears are examined with an otoscope, and then take his BP and vital signs.

26. **The father of a four-year-old son tells the nurse that his child believes there are "monsters and boogeymen" in his closet at bedtime. The nurse's best suggestion for dealing with this problem is:**

    1. Letting the child sleep with his parents.
    2. Keeping a night light on in the child's bedroom.
    3. Tell the child that these fears are not real.
    4. Staying with the child until he falls asleep.

27. **A three-year-old is brought to the clinic for evaluation because he is thin and his mother is concerned about his appetite. The best response the nurse can give his mom is:**

    1. "His appetite should be increasing, so he needs to be fed."
    2. "You should discourage food rituals."
    3. "His growth is slow, and so his appetite is too."
    4. "If this continues, he will need testing."

28. **The nurse is assessing a child for pediculosis capitis. Which sign is the most definitive indication of this condition?**

    1. Firmly attached white particles on the hair.
    2. Itching and scratching of the head.
    3. Patchy areas of hair loss.
    4. Areas of round, serous weeping patches.

29. **A 15-year-old was admitted with burns to his face and hands. Which observation would indicate to the nurse**

that he has achieved adaptation to his changed body image?

1. The client meets family and peers in the visiting room.
2. The client states that he'll see his friends when he gets home.
3. The client asks for pain medication each day before visiting hours.
4. The client tells everyone that he is on protective isolation.

30. **A toddler is in Bryant's traction. Which assessment by the nurse should be immediately reported to the RN?**

    1. Absent pedal pulse on unaffected leg.
    2. Buttocks off the bed.
    3. Ace wrap coming off affected leg.
    4. Child sleeping in supine position.

31. **The nurse determines that the mother of an eight-year-old with impetigo has demonstrated understanding of instructions when she states that she will treat the affected areas by:**

    1. Washing with half peroxide and half normal saline.
    2. Treating with Silvadene cream (silver sulfadiazine).
    3. Applying antibiotic ointment and leaving open.
    4. Covering with occlusive dressing after rinsing with water.

32. **The nurse's teaching about the side effects of DPT vaccine would be considered effective if the mother states:**

    1. "I will call if the baby has a high-pitched cry."
    2. "It is important to give aspirin as soon as we get home."
    3. "I'll expect her to be awake later than usual tonight."
    4. "Some tremors are expected after this first DPT shot."

33. **After taking a course in child maltreatment, the LPN is asked to describe her role in regard to child abuse. The nurse best describes the role of the LPN in possible child abuse cases as:**

    1. To allow the charge nurse to decide if the case is to be reported.
    2. To report only observed cases of abuse to the state hotline.
    3. To report any suspected abuse case.
    4. Applying only while on duty as an LPN.

34. **The nurse is planning care for an adolescent with men-**

ingitis. Which nursing intervention would be inappropriate?

1. Measuring head circumference every shift.
2. Keep lights dimly lit.
3. Maintain Semi-Fowler's position.
4. Measure I & O.

35. **To meet the nutritional needs of a child with an extensive first and second degree burn, the nurse plans to:**

    1. Perform dressing changes at least one hour before or after meals.
    2. Administer oral pain medication one-half hour before each meal.
    3. Feed low fat, low carbohydrate, high protein meals.
    4. Allow the child to eat at his own pace, providing privacy.

36. **An 18-month-old is admitted for lead poisoning. A specific gravity is ordered. The nurse anticipates that preparation most likely includes:**

    1. Obtaining a catheter.
    2. Applying a pediatric urine collector.
    3. Obtaining a syringe to extract urine.
    4. Catching the urine during mid-stream.

37. **A client questions why his physician wants to test every stool specimen. The nurse explains that the purpose of the guaiac test is to detect the presence of:**

    1. Fat.
    2. Parasites.
    3. Microorganisms.
    4. Blood.

38. **The nurse caring for an AIDS client accidentally pierces her hand with a needle used to give the client his pain medication. The priority nursing action is to:**

    1. Report the incident to the charge nurse.
    2. Cover the wound with a sterile gauze dressing and report the incident to employee health.
    3. Complete an incident report.
    4. "Bleed" the site and rinse under water, apply an antibiotic ointment, and cover the area with a dry dressing.

39. **A young client has been admitted to the acute diseases unit. She has recently been diagnosed with AIDS. When the nurse enters her room, the nurse finds the client is crying. What is the most appropriate response demonstrated by the nurse?**

    1. Ignore the crying and proceed to take the client's vital signs.

2. Acknowledge her feelings and offer to help.
3. Consult with the charge nurse immediately.
4. Notify her physician and suggest an antidepressant medication.

40. **In providing postoperative care to a client who has just received a permanent pacemaker, which nursing action is inappropriate?**

    1. Have the client perform active range of motion exercises on the affected shoulder to prevent development of a "frozen" shoulder.
    2. Prevent infection by using sterile dressings over the operative site.
    3. Monitor the cardiac rhythm to verify correct functioning of the pacemaker.
    4. Provide psychological support by allowing the client to express his feelings about having a pacemaker.

41. **A client has been diagnosed with iron deficiency anemia. To supplement his iron medication, which foods would the nurse recommend as good sources of iron?**

    1. Red meat, eggs, and green leafy vegetables.
    2. White bread, and yellow vegetables.
    3. Citrus fruit and dairy products.
    4. Fish, pasta, and cereals.

42. **In caring for a client with AIDS, the nurse understands that a factor that puts the client at risk for the development of potentially fatal secondary infections is:**

    1. Intact skin integrity.
    2. Exposure to someone with a respiratory infection.
    3. Diet high in protein and vitamin C.
    4. WBC count of count of 4,100 to 10,900 per microliter.

43. **Which exposure would place the nurse at greatest risk for contracting AIDS?**

    1. Vaginal secretions and semen.
    2. Blood.
    3. Cerebrospinal fluid.
    4. Sputum.

44. **A client is admitted to the hospital with a high fever, chills, and dehydration. Of the following laboratory tests ordered by the physician, the nurse should avoid using which test to screen for infection:**

    1. WBC count.
    2. Erythrocyte sedimentation rate.
    3. Blood glucose.
    4. Cultures of wound, sputum, urine and blood.

45. **The nurse understands that one factor that places a client at risk for the development of infection is:**

1. Positive nitrogen balance.
2. Physiological stress.
3. Middle-age adulthood.
4. Intact immune system.

46. **A client is at risk for tuberculosis because of a recent diagnosis in his immediate family. The nurse understands that the most accurate tuberculin test method currently available is:**

    1. Mono-Vacc tests.
    2. Aplitest.
    3. Tine test.
    4. Mantoux test.

47. **Because a client has multiple sclerosis (MS), the nurse's plan of care should include teaching to avoid:**

    1. Laxatives.
    2. Cool baths.
    3. Exercise.
    4. Caffeine.

48. **A female client is scheduled for magnetic resonance imaging (MRI). Prior to the study, the nurse should explain to the client that:**

    1. She must fast from midnight the night before the test.
    2. The study will take about 15 minutes.
    3. She will be asleep during the study.
    4. She must remove all metal-containing objects from her body.

49. **A client is diagnosed with a C-6 complete spinal cord transection following a motor vehicle accident. Which intervention should receive highest priority in the nursing plan of care?**

    1. Turning the client every two hours to prevent pressure sores.
    2. Elevating the head of the bed to 30 degrees to decrease intracranial pressure.
    3. Monitoring respiratory status every hour to detect changes in breathing patterns.
    4. Forcing fluids to prevent dehydration.

50. **A client with a history of bleeding esophageal varices is concerned about preventing further episodes of bleeding. What caution should the nurse give to the client?**

    1. Include high fiber and roughage in your diet.
    2. Avoid drinking hot liquids.
    3. Restrict activities and exercise in warm weather.
    4. Avoid bearing down when having a bowel movement.

51. A client is scheduled for a sigmoidoscopy. The nurse should advise the client that, during the procedure, he will be placed in which position?

    1. Supine.
    2. Prone.
    3. Left lateral.
    4. Semi-Fowler's.

52. In performing ileostomy care, the nurse measures the circumference of the collection device opening so that it is at least how much larger than the stoma circumference?

    1. 1/8 inch.
    2. 1/4 inch.
    3. 1/2 inch.
    4. 3/4 inch.

53. A trauma client, admitted through the Emergency Room, has a urinary catheter inserted to monitor kidney function and assess for early signs of shock. The nurse would report which urinary output measurements as suggestive of cardiac failure or hypovolemia?

    1. 20 ml/hour.
    2. 35 ml/hour.
    3. 40 ml/hour.
    4. 50 ml/hour.

54. A postoperative client should be assessed frequently for manifestations of hemorrhage, which can lead to hypovolemic shock. In hypovolemic shock, which assessment would most likely be made by the nurse?

    1. Rising blood pressure.
    2. Hyperthermia.
    3. Bradycardia.
    4. Tachypnea.

55. The nurse should assess an immobilized client for manifestations of a fecal impaction, the most definitive of which is:

    1. The absence of bowel sounds.
    2. Diarrhea stools with abdominal cramping.
    3. A rigid board-like abdomen.
    4. Constipation with liquid fecal seepage.

56. A postoperative client is developing manifestations of a paralytic ileus following abdominal surgery. Which assessment can the nurse expect to make?

    1. Abdominal cramping, diarrhea.
    2. Vomiting, chest pain.
    3. Abdominal distention, hypoactive bowel sounds.
    4. Rigid, board-like abdomen, elevated temperature.

57. A postoperative client has an infected surgical incision. The area is red and swollen with a small amount of thick, yellow drainage. The correct term for the nurse to use in describing this drainage is:

    1. Purulent.
    2. Sanguineous.
    3. Serous.
    4. Serosanguineous.

58. In assessing postoperative clients for manifestations of early hypovolemic shock, the nurse notes that an initial observation would most likely be:

    1. Thirst.
    2. Warm, flushed skin.
    3. Irritability.
    4. Bradycardia.

59. A client is diagnosed with acute pyelonephritis. The nursing plan of care should include teaching the client to:

    1. Drink 4,000 ml of fluid per day.
    2. Maintain complete bedrest until manifestations decrease.
    3. Complete the entire cycle of antibiotic therapy.
    4. Do daily weights with notification of the physician if any fluctuation occurs.

60. The physician has ordered a urine specimen to be sent to the lab for analysis of specific gravity. How should the nurse collect the specimen?

    1. Clean-catch midstream urine.
    2. Catheterized urine specimen.
    3. Random urine sample.
    4. 24-hour urine collection.

61. A client is admitted with a cerebrovascular accident (CVA). A goal of care is to reduce intracranial pressure. Which of the following interventions should be included in the nurse's plan of care?

    1. Administer sedative medications at regular intervals.
    2. Cough and deep breathe every two hours.
    3. Elevate head of bed 30 degrees.
    4. Limit fluid intake to 500 ml in 24 hours.

62. A client, admitted with a tentative diagnosis of cholecystitis, is scheduled for an oral cholecystogram (gallbladder series) in the morning. Which question asked by the nurse is critical prior to this test?

    1. "What is your height and weight?"
    2. "What is your age and occupation?"
    3. "Have you ever had this test performed before?"
    4. "Are you allergic to any seafood?"

63. Which postoperative intervention by the nurse should receive the highest priority for a client who had a cholecystectomy this morning?

    1. Coughing and deep breathing.
    2. Dangling and ambulation.
    3. Use of anti-embolic stockings.
    4. Irrigation of the nasogastric tube.

64. A postoperative client's knee dressing becomes completely saturated with blood one hour after returning to the clinical unit. Initially, the nurse should:

    1. Reinforce the knee dressing.
    2. Apply a tourniquet around the closest artery.
    3. Apply direct pressure to the knee.
    4. Apply ice to the knee.

65. Following spinal cord injury at or above T-6, the nurse should watch the client closely for signs of autonomic dysreflexia. The nurse is aware that this potentially dangerous response could be triggered by:

    1. Elevated blood pressure.
    2. Severe headache.
    3. Distended bladder.
    4. Edema of the spinal cord.

66. A client who had surgery 24 hours ago is experiencing dyspnea and tachycardia, and has developed a fever. The nurse suspects atelectasis. If this complication is present, the nurse's auscultation of the client's lung sounds would reveal:

    1. Diminished breath sounds.
    2. Rhonchi.
    3. A pleural friction rub.
    4. Absent breath sounds.

67. When doing a physical assessment on a client with early common bile duct obstruction, the nurse would expect to see which clinical manifestation?

    1. Dark yellow urine.
    2. Ascites.
    3. Clay-colored feces.
    4. Petechiae.

68. A client with a fractured right hip is taken to surgery for an open reduction and internal fixation. A gravity suction device is placed in the surgical wound. The nurse understands that the purpose of this device is to:

    1. Prevent the development of a wound infection.
    2. Monitor the amount of bleeding from the surgical site.

    3. Prevent fluid from accumulating in the wound.
    4. Eliminate the need for wound irrigations.

69. A client has just returned to the clinical unit following a myelogram. Which of the following manifestations manifested by the client should the nurse report immediately to the charge nurse?

    1. Leg cramps.
    2. Pain at the needle insertion site.
    3. Oral temperature reading of 99.8° F.
    4. Neck pain and stiffness.

70. A truck driver is diagnosed with thrombophlebitis and is started on anticoagulant therapy. During the time the client is on anticoagulants, the nurse should advise the client:

    1. Not to drive his truck.
    2. To use an electric razor.
    3. To carry the antidote with him at all times.
    4. To stay in bed.

71. A client is diagnosed with a urinary tract infection and is placed on ciprofloxacin (Cipro) 500 mg P. O. every 12 hours. Which of the following instructions should the nurse include in the teaching plan for this client?

    1. Drink extra fluids (one to two quarts) each day while taking Cipro.
    2. If the medicine causes an upset stomach, take an antacid at the same time.
    3. Cipro may cause photosensitivity. Wear protective clothing when out in the sun.
    4. Please report any blurred vision or ringing in the ears to your physician immediately.

72. In caring for a client taking isoniazid (INH), the nurse knows that which diagnostic study is done frequently to monitor for toxic effects?

    1. AST, ALT.
    2. WBC count.
    3. Bone marrow aspirations.
    4. Creatinine & BUN.

73. A client has returned after major surgery and is complaining of pain. The physician ordered morphine sulfate to control her pain. Before administering the medication, the nurse would first:

    1. Discuss the side effects with the client.
    2. Take the client's vital signs.
    3. Provide mouth care.
    4. Have the client turn, cough and deep breathe.

74. A two-year-old admitted with seizures is receiving phenytoin (Dilantin) in oral suspension form. What should the nurse do before administering each dose?

    1. Be sure the client has not eaten within the hour.
    2. Shake the container vigorously.
    3. Perform mouth care.
    4. Warm the solution before administering.

75. A 66-year-old client is receiving hemodialysis via left arteriovenous fistula (AVF) for management of chronic renal disease. The nurse should instruct the client to:

    1. Check the access hourly for patency.
    2. Maintain skin integrity through frequent cleansing and application of lotion over the site.
    3. Avoid tight clothing around the access site.
    4. Sleep on his left side to maintain patency of the access site.

76. The nurse is instructing the client regarding good food sources for potassium. Which menu choice by the client indicates to the nurse that the client has understood the instruction?

    1. Baked chicken, boiled potato, pudding.
    2. Boiled chicken, rice, cranberry juice.
    3. Broiled meat, baked potato, citrus fruit salad.
    4. Beef stew, bread and butter, Jell-O.

77. A client is in the hospital and he is dying. He is very weak, tired, and short of breath. The nursing plan of care for the client and his family should emphasize:

    1. Limiting visiting hours to help conserve his energy.
    2. Having the client do as much as he can for himself to increase his self-esteem and independence.
    3. Encouraging the family to spend as much time as possible with him and do whatever they feel comfortable with in caring for him.
    4. Planning to perform as much of his care as possible at one time, so he can rest for long intervals.

78. A client is taking acetaminophen (Tylenol) for muscular aches and pains. She reports to the nurse that she is lonely and has been drinking heavily in the evenings. The nurse should advise the client that:

    1. Alcohol and Tylenol may result in a diuretic effect, depleting fluid volume and electrolytes.
    2. Sodium and fluid retention may result from this combination.
    3. Alcoholic beverages should be avoided because they increase the risk of liver toxicity when taken with Tylenol.
    4. This combination has an increased potential for causing palpitations.

79. A client diagnosed with schizophrenia says to the nurse, "They lied about me and are trying to poison my food." The therapeutic nursing response is:

    1. "You are mistaken. Nobody has told lies about you or tried to poison you."
    2. "You're having very frightening thoughts."
    3. "Tell me more about your concerns about being poisoned."
    4. "Tell me who would do such things to you?"

80. The nurse enters an anorexic client's room and finds her doing vigorous push-ups on the floor. What is the most therapeutic nursing action?

    1. Remind her that if her weight decreases she will lose a privilege.
    2. Leave the room and permit her to exercise in private.
    3. Ask her to stop doing the push-ups and suggest she pursue a less strenuous activity.
    4. Wait for her to finish exercising and ask her why she feels the need to exercise.

81. The nurse is caring for a bulimic client. The best initial nursing intervention to help the client deal more effectively with her bulimic behavior is:

    1. Establishing a behavioral contract to control these urges.
    2. Keeping a journal of eating behavior and feelings experienced before, during, and after eating.
    3. Supervising the client's behavior at all times.
    4. Eating only when other persons are present.

82. A 20-year-old college student is brought to the emergency room by the campus police. She was raped while walking to the parking lot after one of her classes. What action by the nurse is most therapeutic initially?

    1. Ask questions to get the client to talk about the attack.
    2. Treat the client's physical wounds.
    3. Explain to the client that she is now in a safe place.
    4. Have a calm and accepting attitude.

83. One morning the nurse asks an elderly client if she had any visitors the day before. She responds that several members of her church choir had been to see her. The nurse knows that only her daughter had visited the day before. The nurse understands that a fabrication that is told to mask memory loss is an example of:

    1. Delusion.
    2. Illusion.
    3. Confabulation.
    4. Dissociation.

84. **Which statement by the nurse indicates the best understanding of the principles of reality orientation?**

    1. "Good morning, Mr. Jones. Did you sleep well? It's time to get dressed."
    2. "Good morning. This is your second day in Shady Pines and I am your nurse for the day."
    3. "Do you remember who I am? We met yesterday when you were admitted."
    4. "Good morning, how are you today? I am your nurse for the day. My name is Mrs. Smith."

85. **The nurse caring for clients in a long-term care facility understands that remotivation therapy is used to:**

    1. Stimulate and encourage social participation.
    2. Reorient clients with cognitive problems.
    3. Encourage clients to share memories of past experiences and events.
    4. Resolve emotional problems.

86. **The nurse is planning orientation to the unit for a new client who is severely depressed. Which nursing approach is best initially?**

    1. Introduce the client to other clients on the unit and staff members.
    2. Tour the unit and introduce her to everyone they meet on the way.
    3. Explain the unit policies and answer any questions she may have.
    4. Accompany the client to her room and stay with her while she unpacks, offering only minimal information.

87. **In planning activities for a depressed client during his early stages of hospitalization, which nursing plan is best?**

    1. Provide one activity a day, to avoid fatigue.
    2. Let the client choose an activity that is appealing.
    3. Provide a structured daily program of activities for the client.
    4. Wait until the client's mood improves and he indicates an interest in productive activity.

88. **The nurse learns that an elderly client's sleeping problems began six months ago, when his physician diagnosed prostatic cancer. Prior to that time, he had enjoyed good physical health. The nurse also knows that his wife of 50 years died one year ago. One day the client tells the nurse, "I'd be better off dead because I am totally worthless." The nurse's most therapeutic response is:**

    1. "I have seen some very valuable things about you."
    2. You feel worthless now because you are so de-

pressed. You will feel differently when you depression begins to improve."
    3. "You really have a great deal to live for."
    4. "You have been feeling very sad and alone for some time now."

89. **An elderly client is able to walk with a cane and enjoys ambulating in the hall. Since he has memory problems, he has great difficulty remembering which room is his. What nursing action would best alleviate this problem?**

    1. Assign him a room close to the nursing station so staff members will be available to help him.
    2. Assign him to a room with a roommate who can watch out for him.
    3. Do not allow him to leave his room unaccompanied.
    4. Put his picture and his name written in large letters on the door to his room.

90. **A client who has just been diagnosed with cancer tells the nurse that he would rather be dead than go through the treatment for cancer. The most appropriate nursing response is:**

    1. "What is it about the cancer treatment that concerns you?"
    2. "If you don't receive the treatment, you will get your wish."
    3. "Why don't you talk to your doctor about your feelings?"
    4. "That wouldn't be fair to your family, would it?"

91. **A client is admitted to the hospital. He has been on bed rest at home and has been incontinent of urine. His wife has been caring for him, and there is a strong odor of urine. The wife state that she is sorry and embarrassed about the unpleasant smell. Which response by the nurse is therapeutic?**

    1. "It must be difficult to care for someone who is confined to bed. How have you been able to manage?"
    2. "Don't worry about it. He will get a bath, and that will take care of the odor."
    3. "A lot of clients that are cared for at home have the same problem."
    4. "When was the last time that he had a bath?"

92. **The client tells the nurse that he does not know how he is ever going to stay on the low cholesterol diet that his doctor ordered after his heart attack. The best response by the nurse is:**

    1. "If you don't follow the diet, you will probably have another heart attack, which could kill you."
    2. "What is it about the low cholesterol diet that seems to be a problem for you?"
    3. "I've been on that same diet for the last five years,

and I'm sure you will learn how to change your eating habits after a while."

4. "I will have the dietitian talk to you before you are discharged. She's the expert, and she can be really helpful."

93. An elderly client with Alzheimer's disease is admitted to the hospital. His daughter says to the nurse, "I really feel guilty about leaving my father, but I need to go home." The most helpful response by the nurse to the daughter is:

1. "Your father is well cared for here."
2. "Your worried feelings are normal."
3. "When you are getting ready to leave, tell me. I will sit with your father."
4. "Can I call another family member to stay with him?"

94. A client is diagnosed with active tuberculosis. He and his family have many questions for the nurse. They ask, "How did this happen? What can we do to prevent this? What will happen next?" Which is the most helpful response by the nurse?

l. "The tuberculosis was probably contracted from someone else with TB."
2. "You need not be concerned. TB is very curable."
3. "Tuberculosis can be treated at home with medications."
4. "You seem very worried about the TB. What concerns you most?"

95. During a client's postoperative recovery from an ileostomy, the nurse begins teaching her stoma care, when the nurse notices that the client will not look at her ostomy. The client states, "I'd rather be dead than have to live with this all my life." Which is the most therapeutic nursing response?

l. "I can't imagine what you must be feeling like; it must be awful."
2. "I'll call your physician and see if he will order something to help you to relax."
3. "There's no reason to feel like that. Things will get better."
4. "You appear upset. Would you like to talk?"

96. Which is the best nursing action to maintain maximum privacy for the client during a medical procedure?

1. Closing the door of the client's room.
2. Pulling the curtains around the client's bed.
3. Asking family members to leave the room.
4. Using sterile drapes to cover the client.

97. A client is to have a rectal temperature taken. A glass thermometer is available at the client's bedside. The mercury bulb on the insertion end of the thermometer is long and slender. The safest action by the nurse is to:

1. Obtain a thermometer with a short, blunt insertion end.
2. Take the client's temperature with the available thermometer, and report any elevations.
3. Carefully insert the long end of the thermometer after lubricating that end.
4. Put gloves on before using the thermometer available at the client's bedside.

98. While working the night shift, the nurse notices a mouse running down the hallway of the clinical unit. The correct nursing action is to:

1. Place rat poison in the vicinity where the mouse was seen.
2. Set some mouse traps to catch the mouse, and then dispose of it in a plastic bag labeled as contaminated.
3. Notify the supervisor of the problem.
4. Call the environmental health department of the hospital, and report the incident.

99. A vest restraint is placed on a confused elderly client who is at high risk for falling. Which nursing action is inappropriate?

1. Provide an opportunity for the client to use the bedpan, toilet, or other toilet facilities at regular intervals.
2. Assess the respiratory status of the client frequently.
3. Utilizing help from other nurses, approach the client and apply the vest as quickly as possible, in order to avoid any resistance from the client.
4. Change the client's position at least every two hours.

100. A vest restraint is placed on a confused elderly client who is at high risk for falling. He is partially paralyzed and is at risk for developing pressure sores. How should the nurse handle the linen when changing this client's bed?

1. When removing the linen from the bed, hold it close to the body to avoid dropping it.
2. After removing the linen from the bed, place it on the floor until finished making the bed.
3. When removing the linen from the bed, hold it away from the uniform.
4. Shake the clean linen to unfold it, before making the bed.

NCLEX-PN

Test 7

Questions with Rationales

NCLEX-PN TEST 7 WITH RATIONALES

1. **A client has left her used insulin syringe on the bedside table. What is the best action by the nurse to help prevent spread of infection by way of the contaminated needle?**

   1. Explain to the client that the syringe should be disposed of in the garbage can, to avoid a potential needle stick by someone providing care for the client.
   2. Cap the syringe and take it to the needle disposal container.
   3. Place the uncapped syringe in the needle disposal container.
   4. Have the nurse administer the injection, since the client is not responsible enough to follow through with the correct procedure.

   1. *This is not correct. The syringe should not be disposed of in the garbage can because the employees that take care of the trash can incur a needle stick while handling the trash. Furthermore, needles should NOT be recapped, since there is a potential risk of sticking oneself during this action. Try again to find the correct action that protects everyone from potential needle sticks.*
   2. *Wrong! Needles should not be recapped because there is a potential risk of sticking oneself during this action.*
   3. **Best choice! Special containers are available for syringe and needle disposal. These containers should be utilized. Remember that needles should not be recapped, however, because there is a potential risk of sticking oneself during this action.**
   4. *This is not appropriate. The client should be reminded or taught about the potential injuries and infections that can result from a needle stick. The client should continue to administer the insulin, with closer supervision by the nurse concerning disposal of the needle and syringe.*

2. **An confused elderly client has wrist restraints for safety reasons. To provide for the client's safety, the nurse should give priority to which intervention?**

   1. Checking the pulse, color, and temperature of extremities every shift and reporting these findings.
   2. Making sure the call light is within the client's reach.
   3. Notifying the client's family of the restraints and explaining the rationale for their use.
   4. Removing the restraints at night while the client is sleeping.

   1. *Wrong! This will not be adequate to protect the client from permanent injury, since the client is at risk of decreased circulation. The extremities should be assessed at least every two hours. Try again.*
   2. **Great job! Even though the client is confused, the call light must be available to allow the client to communicate his or her needs. This option is the best choice because it is the only action that provides for the client's immediate safety.**
   3. *The family should be informed, however, there is another option that is more necessary for the client's immediate safety.*
   4. *No. If the client requires restraints because of confusion, the restraints should not be removed at night. This action is incorrect.*

3. **An elderly client is admitted to the hospital following a stroke. He has paralysis of the right side and is at risk of developing decubitus ulcers. In caring for this client, the nurse should:**

   1. Move the client up in bed by sliding him.
   2. Roll the client to his side once a day.
   3. Change the client's position every two hours.
   4. Keep the client in a wheel chair during the morning and afternoon hours.

   1. *No. Sliding the client causes friction between the sheets and the client, resulting in possible damage to his skin, and possible infection.*
   2. *No. The client must be turned at least every two hours!*
   3. **Good work! Changing the client's position every two hours helps prevent bed sores.**
   4. *No, this is an incorrect action. Keeping the client in a wheel chair most of the day can cause pressure sores due to lack of circulation to the areas of skin that are in constant contact with the wheelchair.*

4. **An elderly client has a draining pressure sore. The culture of the drainage reveals staphylococci. The most important nursing action is to:**

   1. Reinforce the pressure dressing with a sterile towel before ambulating the client.
   2. Wear gown and gloves when changing the client's bed linen.
   3. Use sterile technique when changing the dress-

ing on the pressure sore.

4. Discourage the client's use of his personal effects until they have been sterilized.

1. No. Reinforcing the dressing will not prevent the spread of the pathogens.

2. Right! The nurse should always wear a gown and gloves when changing the client's bed linen. This is to prevent the spread of pathogens, which may attach to the nurse's clothing during the bed change, then when the nurse goes to another client's room, there is no threat of contaminating that client with this client's pathogens.

> **TEST-TAKING TIP:** This question is a prioritizing question. Since no physiological need is identified, the priority is safety. The nurse will provide the safest environment by this action.

3. Sterile technique will help prevent secondary pathogens from infecting the wound, but it will not prevent the spread of the pathogens. This is not the best option.

4. Sterilizing the client's linen and personal effects will not prevent the spread of the pathogens.

5. A client complains that he is unable to rest because of the noise from his roommate's TV. The best action by the nurse is to:

1. Have the client moved to a private room.
2. Provide ear phones for the client who is watching television.
3. Explain that the roommate is hard of hearing, so the television is louder than usual.
4. Ask the roommate to shut off the television so the client can rest.

1. Moving the client to a private room would eliminate the noisy television. The client, however, would need input to determine if his insurance will cover the cost of a private room, and if not, whether he is willing to pay the difference. This is not the best action by the nurse at this time.

2. Yes, great thinking! Providing ear phones provides both clients with a solution to the problem.

3. Wrong! Explaining the action of the roommate indicates to the client that his concerns are not important since nothing is being done to decrease the noise. This action also fails to promote rest for the client.

4. Wrong! Telling the roommate to turn off the television interferes with his right to watch television.

6. An elderly client is to receive a tub bath. In preparing the bath, which action by the nurse would be unsafe?

1. Check the temperature of the tub room.

2. Gather and take all of the necessary equipment to the tub room prior to the bath.
3. Test the temperature of the bath water by having the client place his hand in the water.
4. Place a mat or towel in the bottom of the tub.

1. This is a safe action. The tub room should not be too cold or too hot because the client may either become chilled or too warm. The question, however, asked you to identify an UNSAFE action.

2. This is a safe action. All of the supplies should be available before taking the client to the tub room. The question, however, asks you to identify an UNSAFE action.

3. Excellent choice! This action is incorrect, and the question asked you to select an option that is UNSAFE. The elderly client's sensitivity to hot and cold decreases as part of the aging process. The client is, therefore, at risk for becoming chilled or incurring a burn if his decreased sensory ability is depended upon to check the bath temperature. The client also is at risk for burns because an elderly client's skin is often thin and fragile.

4. This is a safe nursing action. A mat or towel will help prevent a slip or fall by the client getting into or out of the tub. The question, however, asks you to identify an UNSAFE action.

7. While bathing a preschooler in a tub, which action by the nurse is inappropriate?

1. Check the temperature of the water with a thermometer.
2. Never leave the child unattended.
3. Make sure the temperature in the room is warm.
4. Allow the child to determine if the water temperature is comfortable by placing the child's feet in the water.

1. Wrong choice! This action is appropriate. Water temperature should be between 100° and 105° F, since the small child's skin is easily burned at higher temperatures. You are looking for an INAPPROPRIATE action.

2. Wrong choice! A small child may be able to turn the water faucet on and may turn on the hot water and receive burn injuries. There also is a danger of drowning when a small child is left unattended. You are looking for an INAPPROPRIATE action.

3. Wrong choice! The temperature of the room should be warm, to avoid chilling the child. You are looking for an INAPPROPRIATE action.

4. Good work, you have identified the incorrect action! If the water is too hot, the child may sustain burned feet. Instead, the nurse should use a thermometer to ensure that the temperature is in the correct range of between 100° and 105° F.

8. When making rounds, the nurse notices that a client who is receiving oxygen via nasal cannula has a pack of cigarettes at the bedside. The best nursing action is to:

1. Remove the pack of cigarettes from the bedside.
2. Remind the client not to smoke when oxygen is in use.
3. Ask the client how he obtained the cigarettes.
4. Review the rules of safety with the client's family.

1. Correct. It may appear restrictive, however, this is the correct procedure, because the presence of the cigarettes creates a hazard for all the clients in the room and in the vicinity.
2. Close, but this is incorrect! This action also is appropriate, but it is not sufficient to provide for the safety of the clients in the room. Try again.
3. Wrong. This would be appropriate if possession of the cigarettes were prohibited, however, this action alone will not provide for the safety of the clients in the room. Try again.
4. Wrong. This action is appropriate, but it is not sufficient to provide for the safety of the clients in the room.

9. The nurse is caring for an elderly client in a long-term care facility. When applying a hot water bottle to the client, it would be unsafe for the nurse to:

1. Wrap the hot water bottle in a cloth before placing it next to the client's skin.
2. Fill the hot water bottle with as much hot water as it will hold.
3. Eliminate as much air as possible from the hot water bottle.
4. Check the temperature of the water with a thermometer.

1. Incorrect, this is safe! The cover provides comfort and prevents burns, because the cloth acts as an insulator. This question is asking you to select an action that is UNSAFE.
2. You are right, this action is unsafe. The bag should be filled only two-thirds full, to keep the bag easy to mold.
3. Eliminating excess air is important, since air is a poor conductor of heat. The question, however, asks you to identify an UNSAFE action.
4. The temperature of the water should be close to 115^0 F, to avoid burning the client. Checking the temperature of the water is a correct nursing action. The question, however, asks you to select an action that is UNSAFE.

10. The nurse is about to instruct parents of young children about poison control in the home. The nurse should:

1. Instruct the parents to induce vomiting with syrup of ipecac.
2. Instruct the parents to immediately bring the child to the emergency room.
3. Provide labels for the parent's telephone, with the Poison Control Center's telephone number, and give instructions to call that number after an accidental ingestion.
4. Notify social services to investigate the home situation for safety.

1. No! In some poisons, such as lye or petroleum products, vomiting is contraindicated! Identification of the poison is most important before treatment can be initiated.
2. No! Immediate measures usually can be instituted by the parents to lessen the severity of the poisoning by preventing or slowing absorption. Depending on the location of the hospital, time may be a factor in the outcome of the situation.
3. Congratulations! The phone number for the Poison Control Center can place the parents in contact with an immediate source of information for initial emergency measures that can be implemented to help decrease the severity of the poisoning prior to transportation to the emergency room.
4. Wrong! Accidental poisoning often occurs because of a lack of knowledge on the part of the parents. A social service consult is not necessary unless a pattern of practices indicates an unsafe environment for the children.

11. A adolescent client is to have a water system heating device ("K-Pad"), applied to a pulled muscle. The client tells the nurse that the device does not feel very warm. The most appropriate nursing action is to:

1. Tell the client that these heating devices never feel hot.
2. Check the temperature setting on the heating unit and feel the pad for warmth.
3. Call the appropriate repair department and have them fix the unit.
4. Turn the temperature up on the unit if it doesn't feel warm enough to the client.

1. Wrong. Although these heating units do feel warm and not hot, the unit may not be at a therapeutic temperature, and should be assessed to see if it is working properly.
2. Correct! The nurse should check that the device is set to the temperature recommended by the manufacturer. The nurse should also assess whether the pad feels warm.
3. Incorrect! The unit may not be malfunctioning. It should be assessed by the nurse before any other action is taken. If the unit is malfunctioning, it

should be replaced with another unit, and the malfunctioning unit should be sent to the repair department.

4. *Incorrect! The temperature should not be set above the recommended setting, to avoid causing a burn to the client.*

12. **During the resuscitation of a client, the physician orders the client to be defibrillated by receiving a controlled electrical shock. The nurse knows that it would be unsafe to:**

1. Move away from the bed while the client is defibrillated.
2. Observe the other nurses to be sure they are not in contact with the client or the bed during defibrillation.
3. Hold the IV pole out of the way while the client is defibrillated.
4. Make sure the client's chest is dry, except where the electrode paste or pads are applied for placement of the defibrillator paddles.

1. *This is a safe action, and, therefore, not the correct answer to this question. Touching the bed or the client may result in the nurse receiving an electrical shock, since the electricity the client receives can be conducted to anything with which the client is in contact.*
2. *This is a safe action, and, therefore, not the correct answer to this question. You should observe for other nurses who may be so involved in performing a particular task, such as starting an intravenous line, that the physician's order may not be heard. Observing their actions and alerting them may protect them from an electrical injury.*
3. ***This action is unsafe, so this is the correct answer in this question with a false response stem. The IV pole may conduct electricity by way of the IV fluid that the client is receiving. Touching the pole could result in an electrical shock to the nurse.***
4. *This is a safe action, and, therefore, not the correct answer to this question. Moisture is an excellent conductor of electricity. During defibrillation, the electricity will follow the path of least resistance, including any moisture on the chest, which could result in burns to the chest area where the moisture is present.*

13. **Which statement would the nurse use to best describe the diagnosis and treatment of ovarian cancer?**

1. Early detection has reduced the mortality rate in recent years.
2. Early diagnosis is very difficult, so prognosis remains poor.
3. Early detection is accomplished by routine vaginal exam every three months.

4. Extensive radiation is highly successful in treating ovarian cancer.

1. *Wrong. Early detection of ovarian cancer is very difficult. Most often, by the time the diagnosis is made, the cancer has spread.*
2. ***Correct. There is no test found to be useful for early detection of ovarian cancer. Once diagnosis is made, prognosis is poor, even with aggressive treatment.***
3. *No, early detection may be accomplished frequent vaginal abdominal ultrasound examinations in the client at high risk. Vaginal exam is not enough.*
4. *Wrong. Radiation has not been found to be effective in the treatment of ovarian cancer.*

14. **The nurse is caring for an infant who is born small for gestational age (SGA) at 40 weeks gestation. The nurse's plan of care for this client should include:**

1. Prevention of hyaline membrane disease.
2. Prevention of hyperglycemia.
3. Limitation of daily fluid intake due to small stomach capacity.
4. Careful suctioning of airways at delivery.

1. *Wrong. Hyaline membrane disease is most commonly seen in premature infants, not infants born at term.*
2. *Incorrect. SGA babies are at high risk for hypoglycemia, not hyperglycemia.*
3. *Wrong. The SGA baby needs more frequent feedings to assure adequate caloric intake to promote weight gain and prevent hypoglycemia.*
4. ***Correct. When a fetus is SGA, there usually has been intrauterine hypoxia with resulting meconium amniotic fluid. Careful suctioning of airways at delivery is needed to prevent meconium aspiration.***

15. **The nurse is caring for a three-day-old infant who is receiving phototherapy for an elevated bilirubin. Which nursing goal is least appropriate for the infant's care?**

1. Protection of the eyes.
2. Prevention of fluid volume excess.
3. Maintenance of stable body temperature.
4. Promotion of mother-infant bonding.

1. *Wrong choice, this goal is appropriate. The effects of the high intensity lights on the baby's retinas are unknown. The eyes should be covered to provide protection from damage. Look for a goal that is NOT appropriate for this client.*
2. ***Correct. This goal is NOT appropriate because this infant is not at risk for fluid volume excess. On the contrary, phototherapy may cause liquid stool and increased water loss. Additional feedings are needed to prevent a***

fluid volume deficit.

3.   *Wrong choice, this goal is appropriate. The infant receiving phototherapy is at risk for hyperthermia due to the high intensity lights. Careful assessment is needed to monitor for alterations in body temperature. Look for a goal that is NOT appropriate for this client.*

4.   *Wrong choice, this goal is appropriate. This is a very important part of the care of an infant receiving phototherapy. Mothers are often reluctant to hold and touch their infants while they are under the lights and they should be encouraged to do so. Look for a goal that is NOT appropriate for this client.*

16.   **The nurse is caring for an infant born to a mother who is addicted to crack cocaine. Which nursing action would be inappropriate?**

1.   Small frequent feedings.
2.   Tight swaddling of infant.
3.   Frequent stimulation.
4.   Promoting mother-infant bonding.

1.   *Wrong choice, this action is appropriate. The drug addicted infant often has an uncoordinated suck and swallow predisposing to aspiration. Small frequent feedings provide adequate caloric intake and reduce the risk of aspiration. Look for the action that is NOT appropriate for this client.*

2.   *Wrong choice, this action is appropriate. Tight swaddling of the infant discourages hyperactivity and provides comfort in the newborn. Look for the action that is NOT appropriate for this client.*

3.   **Good work, this action is not appropriate. This infant needs a quiet, calm, dim environment with minimal stimulation, to promote rest and reduce stress.**

4.   *Wrong choice, this action is appropriate. Mother-infant bonding is an important part of this baby's care. The mother's drug use, as well as the baby's hyperactive behavior often interfere with establishment of the mother-infant relationship.*

17.   **A client's husband asks the nurse what he can do about his wife's rapid mood swings during her pregnancy. What is the best nursing response?**

1.   "They are the result of hormone imbalances. There is little you can do to help her."
2.   "Try to ignore them. Paying attention to her as a result of these mood swings will only increase the problem."
3.   "Talk to your wife about the mood swings and exhibit loving behaviors in spite of her mood."
4.   "They are the result of hormone changes. You might suggest that she ask her doctor for medication to reduce their incidence."

1.   *Wrong. The mood swings are the result of hormone imbalances, but there is much the partner can do to provide support during these difficult psychological times.*

2.   *Incorrect. Ignoring the mood swings can be perceived as unloving and uncaring by the partner, which will only make the problems worse.*

3.   **Correct. This is often a very difficult thing to do, but open communication between partners will promote understanding. Exhibiting loving behaviors promotes a feeling of well-being in the woman.**

4.   *Wrong. Medication is not indicated in this situation, even though the mood swings are the result of hormone imbalances.*

18.   **An expectant father tells the nurse that he feels resentful of the added attention others are giving to his wife since the pregnancy was first announced several weeks ago. What is the most therapeutic nursing response to the father?**

1.   "It would be wise for you to speak to a therapist about these feelings."
2.   "Has your wife sensed your anger towards her and the baby?"
3.   "I'm sure that it's really hard to accept this, when it's your baby too."
4.   "These feelings are very common to expectant fathers in early pregnancy."

1.   *Wrong! This response suggests that these feelings need to be studied further when, in actuality, they are common to expectant fathers in early pregnancy.*

2.   *Incorrect. This response suggests that this anger could be a cause for concern, when it is a very common response to early pregnancy by the father.*

3.   *Wrong! This response appears empathetic, but it suggests that the father has every right to be resentful. This response will probably accelerate the negative feelings and is not therapeutic for the father.*

4.   **Good choice. This father needs to be reassured that these feelings are very normal to the expectant father. Reassure him that when the pregnancy becomes obvious he will feel more involved in the pregnancy. This therapeutic response addresses the client's feelings by providing information.**

19.   **An antepartum client in her first trimester asks the nurse at the clinic if she may safely continue her aerobics program throughout her pregnancy. The appropriate nursing response is:**

1.   "Perhaps you should check with the doctor."
2.   "No problem. Go ahead and continue what you

have been doing."

3. "You may continue, but be careful not to go to the point of exhaustion."
4. "It is probably wise to change to something less stressful during pregnancy."

1. *Wrong. A practical nurse working with an antepartum client should be able to advise the client on such things as exercise.*
2. *This option is a good distractor! This answer carries no caution about overdoing. As the client advances in pregnancy, she may not be able to tolerate the regime she is used to doing.*
3. **Good choice. The client may continue, but she should be cautioned not to overdo to the point of exhaustion.**
4. *Wrong. If the client is used to an aerobics program, she may continue as long as she uses moderation.*

20. **An obstetrical client tells the nurse that her last menstrual period began on July 8th. Based upon Naegle's rule, the nurse would calculate her baby's expected date of birth as:**

1. April 15.
2. April 1.
3. October 15.
4. October 1.

1. **Good work! The expected date of birth is predicted by counting back three months from the first day of the last menstrual period and adding seven days.**
2. *Wrong. You counted back three months but you subtracted seven days instead of adding them.*
3. *Incorrect. To get this answer you counted ahead three months and added seven days. Try to find the option that uses the correct formula.*
4. *Wrong. This calculation reflects counting ahead three months and subtracting seven days. Try to find the option that uses the correct formula.*

21. **Which finding would the nurse identify as a cause for concern in the antepartum client?**

1. A +1 glucose in urine.
2. WBC 15,000 mm³.
3. Hematocrit 33%.
4. Reactive VDRL.

1. *Incorrect. Because of the increase glomerular filtration rate, glycosuria is commonly seen in the antepartum client. It is not a cause for concern unless it is consistently present at each prenatal visit or the client has other manifestations related to diabetes.*
2. *Wrong. For some unknown reason the leukocyte*

count of the antepartum woman is often elevated above the norm of 5,000 to 12,000 mm³. It is not uncommon to see WBC's in laboring women at 25,000 mm³ with no pathology.
3. *Wrong. During pregnancy there is an increase in blood volume, composed mainly of plasma. Hematocrit measures the percentage of red blood cells in a volume of blood, which normally drops during pregnancy. This is referred to as physiologic anemia of pregnancy and is not a cause for concern unless the hematocrit drops below 30%.*
4. **Correct. The VDRL test is a diagnostic tool for syphilis. A reactive test usually means the client has syphilis and should be treated with antibiotics.**

22. **A client has a slight drop in blood pressure at her prenatal visits between 13 and 24 weeks gestation. The nurse understands that this is the result of:**

1. Increased estrogen levels.
2. Decreased circulating blood volume.
3. Increased progesterone levels.
4. Impending complications in the pregnancy.

1. *No, estrogen levels do not have any effect on maternal blood pressure.*
2. *Incorrect. Blood volume actually increases in pregnancy, thus predisposing the client to fluid volume excess and a rise in blood pressure.*
3. **Very good! Progesterone levels are significantly increased throughout pregnancy. Since progesterone results in relaxation in smooth muscle, the blood vessels experience vasodilation, with a corresponding drop in blood pressure. As the circulatory system adjusts to the high progesterone levels, the vasodilation resolves and the blood pressure returns to early pregnancy values.**
4. *No, this drop in blood pressure is an expected clinical finding in the antepartum client.*

23. **The nurse is caring for a client in labor. An epidural block is administered during the intrapartum period for pain relief. The nurse must be alert for the complication of:**

1. Severe headaches.
2. Hypotension.
3. Nausea and vomiting.
4. Pulmonary edema.

1. *Wrong. Headaches are associated with spinal anesthesia but are not a complication of epidural anesthesia.*
2. **Right! A very common complication of epidural anesthesia is hypotension. This is generally prevented through rapid intravenous fluid administration.**

3. No, nausea and vomiting are not seen in clients as a result of epidural anesthesia.

4. Wrong. Pulmonary edema is not seen in clients who receive epidural anesthesia. If the client had a condition that put her at risk for pulmonary edema, care would have to be taken in intravenous fluid administration.

24. **A child is admitted with a possible diagnosis of Wilms' tumor (nephroblastoma). The nurse should obtain a sign to be placed over the child's bed, with which warning?**

   1. "Do not palpate abdomen."
   2. "No blood work or Bps in arms."
   3. "Isolation."
   4. "No rectal temperatures."

   1. **Correct. This tumor is encapsulated, and palpation may cause it to rupture, which would allow "seeding" of the tumor into the pelvic cavity.**
   2. Incorrect. There is no particular reason to avoid the use of the arms. Look back at the diagnosis, before you select another option.
   3. Incorrect. You missed part of the information in the stem, which states this is a "possible" diagnosis. In cancer treatment, isolation is required during periods of immunosuppression during chemotherapy, but it is not required before the treatment is begun. Select again.
   4. No, rectal temps would be all right. Rectal temps are contraindicated when there is a high risk of bleeding, or interruption of the rectal mucosa. Make another choice.

25. **In assisting the doctor in examining a two-year-old who has otitis media, the nurse should have the child:**

   1. Lie down on the examining table while his throat and ears are examined, and then allow him to sit up for the rest of the exam.
   2. Lie down on the examining table, while the physician starts with examining the head and proceeds downward with the exam.
   3. Sit in his mother's lap while the heart and lungs are auscultated, and then examine the rest of his body, doing the throat and ears last.
   4. Allow him to sit in his mother's lap while his ears are examined with an otoscope, and then take his BP and vital signs.

   1. No, this approach is likely to have the child crying and upset. Select another approach to the physical exam.
   2. Incorrect. In young children it is not recommended to start at the head and work down. This method is recommended for school age and above. Try an-

other answer.

3. **Very good. This is the correct sequence, leaving the most invasive procedures until last.**

4. No, this may result in inaccurate vital signs, or great difficulty in even obtaining them. Following the exam of the ears, the child is likely to be upset and crying. Select again.

26. **The father of a four-year-old son tells the nurse that his child believes there are "monsters and boogeymen" in his closet at bedtime. The nurse's best suggestion for dealing with this problem is:**

   1. Letting the child sleep with his parents.
   2. Keeping a night light on in the child's bedroom.
   3. Tell the child that these fears are not real.
   4. Staying with the child until he falls asleep.

   1. Incorrect. This is apt to develop a habit that will interfere with the parents' need for privacy and the child's ability to settle himself for sleep. Select again.
   2. **Yes, this is right! After the parent reassures the child, the light helps the child "see" for himself that there is nothing hiding in the shadows.**
   3. Incorrect. Although the "monsters and boogeymen" are not, the fears are real! This is not the best suggestion for the child of age four, who has difficulty distinguishing between real and make-believe. Choose again.
   4. Not recommended, since this encourages procrastination going to sleep. This easily becomes a habit that is difficult to break. Make another choice.

27. **A three-year-old is brought to the clinic for evaluation because he is thin and his mother is concerned about his appetite. The best response the nurse can give his mom is:**

   1. "His appetite should be increasing, so he needs to be fed."
   2. "You should discourage food rituals."
   3. "His growth is slow, and so his appetite is too."
   4. "If this continues, he will need testing."

   1. No! Three-year-olds do not like being fed. They want to do it themselves. Choose again.
   2. Food fads and rituals are a normal part of the developing toddler. Ignoring them is recommended, rather than drawing attention to them. Make another selection.
   3. **Good work! The term for this is "physiologic anorexia." The child's appetite decreases in response to the plateau of growth at this age.**
   4. No, this is incorrect information. Think about the norms for this age child and then choose another answer.

28. The nurse is assessing a child for pediculosis capitis. Which sign is the most definitive indication of this condition?

    1. Firmly attached white particles on the hair.
    2. Itching and scratching of the head.
    3. Patchy areas of hair loss.
    4. Areas of round, serous weeping patches.

    1. *Right! That's what the nits look like. Unlike dandruff, they are attached at the base of the hair shaft.*
    2. *Wrong choice. Although scratching may be a manifestation, there may be many other causes of itching. This is not a definitive manifestation of pediculosis. Try another answer.*
    3. *Wrong choice. Hair loss is not a manifestation that would be definitive of pediculosis. Choose again.*
    4. *Incorrect. This may be a sign of other disease, and it should be reported to the RN. Select again.*

29. A 15-year-old was admitted with burns to his face and hands. Which observation would indicate to the nurse that he has achieved adaptation to his changed body image?

    1. The client meets family and peers in the visiting room.
    2. The client states that he'll see his friends when he gets home.
    3. The client asks for pain medication each day before visiting hours.
    4. The client tells everyone that he is on protective isolation.

    1. *Terrific! This best demonstrates a positive self-image. He is seeing both family and peers in a public setting.*
    2. *No, this would indicate that he does not feel comfortable with his peer group. Since they are very important to him as an adolescent, acceptance of his disfigurement has not been achieved. Choose again.*
    3. *Incorrect. This would indicate the desire to escape the interaction at some level. It does not indicate acceptance of his disfigurement. Make another selection.*
    4. *Incorrect. On the contrary, this response is an attempt to escape from interpersonal contact, which indicates that acceptance of his disfigurement has not been achieved. Pick another answer.*

30. A toddler is in Bryant's traction. Which assessment by the nurse should be immediately reported to the RN?

    1. Absent pedal pulse on unaffected leg.
    2. Buttocks off the bed.
    3. Ace wrap coming off affected leg.
    4. Child sleeping in supine position.

    1. *Correct. You remembered that the child in Bryant's traction has both legs wrapped and elevated by the weights. Absent pulses should always be reported.*
    2. *No, this is expected with Bryant's traction. This indicates correct alignment. Select again.*
    3. *No, this does not need to be reported to the RN. This should be rewrapped, as with any skin traction. Try again.*
    4. *No, this is expected. Since both legs are in traction, side-lying or prone positioning is not possible. Select another answer.*

31. The nurse determines that the mother of an eight-year-old with impetigo has demonstrated understanding of instructions when she states that she will treat the affected areas by:

    1. Washing with half peroxide and half normal saline.
    2. Treating with Silvadene cream (silver sulfadiazine).
    3. Applying antibiotic ointment and leaving open.
    4. Covering with occlusive dressing after rinsing with water.

    1. *Incorrect. This is not the treatment for impetigo, which is a bacterial infection. Choose again.*
    2. *Incorrect. Silvadene cream is used to treat burns, not impetigo, which is a bacterial infection. Pick another option.*
    3. *Correct. The crust is removed gently, and then antibiotic ointment is used to treat the infection, which is left open to the air.*
    4. *Incorrect. Occlusive dressing is not used, and there is nothing in this option that will treat the pathophysiology of impetigo. Choose again.*

32. The nurse's teaching about the side effects of DPT vaccine would be considered effective if the mother states:

    1. "I will call if the baby has a high-pitched cry."
    2. "It is important to give aspirin as soon as we get home."
    3. "I'll expect her to be awake later than usual tonight."
    4. "Some tremors are expected after this first DPT shot."

    1. *Correct. This data could indicate increased intracranial pressure, which is the most serious side effect of DPT vaccines and could put the child at risk for seizures.*
    2. *Wrong! Although some physicians recommend medicating the child for the fever and discomfort normally associated with immunizations, acetaminophen, not aspirin, is the drug of choice.*
    3. *Lethargy or malaise is most common, not increased activity. Try again.*
    4. *Wrong! This is a sign of meningeal irritation and*

seizure activity. This is not an expected outcome, and the mother should be taught to call the pediatrician if this occurs. Choose again.

33. **After taking a course in child maltreatment, the LPN is asked to describe her role in regard to child abuse. The nurse best describes the role of the LPN in possible child abuse cases as:**

    1. To allow the charge nurse to decide if the case is to be reported.
    2. To report only observed cases of abuse to the state hotline.
    3. To report any suspected abuse case.
    4. Applying only while on duty as an LPN.

    1. *Incorrect. The LPN is also a mandated reporter, and may be considered legally responsible if reporting is not done. Select again.*
    2. *No, you do not have to "see" abuse to have indications that an abusive situation exists. There are parent, child, and environmental indicators that are covered in child abuse education. Try again.*
    3. **Yes, this is absolutely right. This is the definition of a mandated reporter. You are not responsible for investigating or proving the abuse. You are responsible for recognition of indicators, and reporting.**
    4. *Incorrect! The LPN is a mandated reporter, and this law applies to all situations that may encountered by the LPN. Choose again.*

34. **The nurse is planning care for an adolescent with meningitis. Which nursing intervention would be inappropriate?**

    1. Measuring head circumference every shift.
    2. Keep lights dimly lit.
    3. Maintain Semi-Fowler's position.
    4. Measure I & O.

    1. **Good work, you identified the inappropriate nursing intervention. The head circumference of an adolescent can't increase, since the fontanels are closed. All other responses are helpful in either monitoring or decreasing intracranial pressure.**
    2. *Wrong choice, this action is important! Dimming the lights reduces the sensory stimuli. You are looking for an INAPPROPRIATE action. Select again.*
    3. *Wrong choice, this action is important. Semi-Fowler's position will reduce edema to the brain. You are looking for an INAPPROPRIATE action. Make another choice.*
    4. *Wrong choice, this should be done to monitor the fluids. Fluid overload could increase cerebral pressure. You are looking for an INAPPROPRIATE action. Make another choice.*

35. **To meet the nutritional needs of a child with an extensive first and second degree burn, the nurse plans to:**

    1. Perform dressing changes at least one hour before or after meals.
    2. Administer oral pain medication one-half hour before each meal.
    3. Feed low fat, low carbohydrate, high protein meals.
    4. Allow the child to eat at his own pace, providing privacy.

    1. **Yes, that's right. Dressing changes are painful, so they should not be done close to the time of feeding, since appetite and digestion may be negatively affected.**
    2. *Incorrect. If medication is needed, one-half hour before a meal would not produce pain relief in time for the meal. Choose another response.*
    3. *Incorrect. In fact, the child who has a burn needs a high carbohydrate diet, with adequate fat and high protein for healing. Select another answer.*
    4. *Incorrect. Children who are in pain, which the second degree burn would indicate, will probably not do well feeding themselves alone. They need feeding and socializing during meals. Try another option.*

36. **An 18-month-old is admitted for lead poisoning. A specific gravity is ordered. The nurse anticipates that preparation most likely includes:**

    1. Obtaining a catheter.
    2. Applying a pediatric urine collector.
    3. Obtaining a syringe to extract urine.
    4. Catching the urine during mid-stream.

    1. *No, the normal means of obtaining a specific gravity is not an invasive procedure. Specific gravity may be tested on the same child repeatedly during a hospitalization. Choose again.*
    2. *Incorrect. This method is used to obtain a routine urine in a child who is not toilet trained, but it is not necessary for a specific gravity alone. Select again.*
    3. **Yes, you're right. It's that simple! Peel back the liner of the child's diaper (with gloves on, of course), and pinch out some of the absorbent material. Put this into the syringe and express a drop onto the refractometer.**
    4. *No, nothing this difficult required. A specific gravity does not need to be free of bacterial contamination. Try again.*

37. **A client questions why his physician wants to test every stool specimen. The nurse explains that the purpose of the guaiac test is to detect the presence of:**

    1. Fat.
    2. Parasites.

3. Microorganisms.
4. Blood.

1. *No. A fecal fat collection is a 72-hour collection of stool for analysis.*
2. *Incorrect. Stool for parasites is usually collected from three different specimens, and sent immediately to the lab for analysis.*
3. *Wrong. Stool for culture is a single collection, sent to the lab for analysis in a sterile container to decrease the risk of outside contamination.*
4. **Yes! Guaiac tests are done to detect "occult" blood, invisible to the naked eye because of its minute quantity. False positive results may occur if the client has eaten red meat or poultry before the test. Medications such as iron, aspirin, steroids, and Vitamin C may also cause false positive results. Clients are instructed to restrict these products for three days prior to the test.**

38. The nurse caring for an AIDS client accidentally pierces her hand with a needle used to give the client his pain medication. The priority nursing action is to:

1. Report the incident to the charge nurse.
2. Cover the wound with a sterile gauze dressing and report the incident to employee health.
3. Complete an incident report.
4. "Bleed" the site and rinse under water, apply an antibiotic ointment, and cover the area with a dry dressing.

1. *Wrong choice, this would be the second action taken by the nurse, not the first. What should the nurse do first?*
2. *Incorrect. This wound requires more than a sterile dry dressing.*
3. *Wrong choice, an incident report is indicated, but it is not the first action by the nurse. What should the nurse do first?*
4. **Correct. The initial action is to bleed the area to rid the wound of any pathogens. Then an antibiotic ointment should be applied and the area protected with a dry dressing.**

39. A young client has been admitted to the acute diseases unit. She has recently been diagnosed with AIDS. When the nurse enters her room, the nurse finds the client is crying. What is the most appropriate response demonstrated by the nurse?

1. Ignore the crying and proceed to take the client's vital signs.
2. Acknowledge her feelings and offer to help.
3. Consult with the charge nurse immediately.
4. Notify her physician and suggest an antidepressant medication.

1. *No! This is disrespectful of the client's feelings and demonstrates a lack of caring by the nurse. The nurse should never ignore the client.*
2. **Correct. This demonstrates acceptance of the client by the nurse. Acknowledging the client's feelings is the therapeutic communication tool of empathy. Offering to help is the therapeutic communication tool of offering self. This response is therapeutic by the client.**
3. *Incorrect. This is not indicated at this time. The nurse should address the client's feelings.*
4. *Incorrect. This is not the appropriate response. The nurse must address the client's feelings and try to help her deal with them.*

TEST-TAKING TIP: This is a communication question, so look for a response that uses a therapeutic communication tool.

40. In providing postoperative care to a client who has just received a permanent pacemaker, which nursing action is inappropriate?

1. Have the client perform active range of motion exercises on the affected shoulder to prevent development of a "frozen" shoulder.
2. Prevent infection by using sterile dressings over the operative site.
3. Monitor the cardiac rhythm to verify correct functioning of the pacemaker.
4. Provide psychological support by allowing the client to express his feelings about having a pacemaker.

1. **Good work! Active range of motion exercises are not indicated in the immediate postoperative period. Therapeutic exercises are appropriate only after healing has occurred.**
2. *No, this is appropriate. Sterile dressings are indicated postoperatively. You are looking for an INAPPROPRIATE action.*
3. *No, this is appropriate. The cardiac rhythm must be monitored to determine any irregularity. You are looking for an INAPPROPRIATE action.*
4. *No, this is appropriate. The client must be encouraged to express his feelings in a supportive atmosphere. You are looking for an INAPPROPRIATE action.*

41. A client has been diagnosed with iron deficiency anemia. To supplement his iron medication, which foods would the nurse recommend as good sources of iron?

1. Red meat, eggs, and green leafy vegetables.
2. White bread, and yellow vegetables.
3. Citrus fruit and dairy products.
4. Fish, pasta, and cereals.

1. *Correct. These foods are high in iron. Red meat should be lean, and eggs should be restricted to three per week because of their high cholesterol content.*

2. *Incorrect. Whole grain bread is preferred because it has a higher iron content than white refined bread. Yellow vegetables, while not high in iron, are good sources of vitamin A.*

3. *Incorrect. Citrus fruits are a good source of vitamin C, and dairy products contain high amounts of calcium. You are looking for good sources of iron.*

4. *Incorrect. None of these is high in iron. Fish is a good source of a complete protein. Pasta contains B complex vitamins. Cereals are a source of carbohydrates. However, both pasta and cereals may be fortified with iron, so advise the client to read the nutritional labels.*

42. **In caring for a client with AIDS, the nurse understands that a factor that puts the client at risk for the development of potentially fatal secondary infections is:**

1. Intact skin integrity.
2. Exposure to someone with a respiratory infection.
3. Diet high in protein and vitamin C.
4. WBC count of count of 4,100 to 10,900 per microliter.

1. *Incorrect. This does not put the client at risk. Intact skin is the body's first defense against infection.*

2. **Correct. The AIDS client has an impaired immune system and should not associate with persons who have respiratory infections.**

3. *Incorrect, this would not put the client at risk. Protein and vitamin C are needed to maintain an intact immune system.*

4. *Incorrect, this does not put the client at risk. This is a normal WBC range.*

43. **Which exposure would place the nurse at greatest risk for contracting AIDS?**

1. Vaginal secretions and semen.
2. Blood.
3. Cerebrospinal fluid.
4. Sputum.

1. *Incorrect. These secretions must contain blood to be contaminating.*

2. **Correct. Blood contains the AIDS virus. Universal precautions must always be used when dealing with blood from any source.**

3. *Incorrect. These secretions must contain blood to be contaminating.*

4. *Incorrect. These secretions must contain blood to be contaminating.*

44. **A client is admitted to the hospital with a high fever, chills, and dehydration. Of the following laboratory tests ordered by the physician, the nurse should avoid using which test to screen for infection:**

1. WBC count.
2. Erythrocyte sedimentation rate.
3. Blood glucose.
4. Cultures of wound, sputum, urine and blood.

1. *Incorrect, this is a common test to screen for infection. Normal values are 5000-10,000/mm^3. Which test is NOT used to screen for infection?*

2. *Incorrect, this test result will be elevated in the presence of anti-inflammatory process. Normal values are up to 15 mm/hr for men and 20 mm/hr for women. Which test is NOT used to screen for infection?*

3. **Correct. This test is used to screen for diabetes mellitus, not for infection. Normal values are 80-120 mm/dl.**

4. *Incorrect, these tests will show the presence of infectious microorganism growth. Which test is NOT used to screen for infection?*

45. **The nurse understands that one factor that places a client at risk for the development of infection is:**

1. Positive nitrogen balance.
2. Physiological stress.
3. Middle-age adulthood.
4. Intact immune system.

1. *Incorrect. A negative nitrogen balance predisposes a client to develop an infection. This may be seen in the AIDS or cancer client, for example.*

2. **Correct. Continued physiological stress results in an elevation of cortisone levels, which results in decreased resistance to infection.**

3. *Incorrect. The very young and the very old are susceptible to infection because of their compromised immune systems. Middle age is not typically a time of increased risk.*

4. *Incorrect. This is the body's strongest protector against invading pathogens.*

46. **A client is at risk for tuberculosis because of a recent diagnosis in his immediate family. The nurse understands that the most accurate tuberculin test method currently available is:**

1. Mono-Vacc tests.
2. Aplitest.
3. Tine test.
4. Mantoux test.

1. *Incorrect. This is a multipuncture test that is impregnated with PPD or OT. A positive test requires a Mantoux test for confirmation.*
2. *Incorrect. This is a multipuncture test that is impregnated with PPD or OT. A positive test requires a Mantoux test for confirmation.*
3. *Incorrect. This is a multipuncture test that is impregnated with PPD or OT. A positive test requires a Mantoux test for confirmation.*
4. ***Correct. This test employs a single-needle intradermal injection of PPD (purified protein derivative), permitting precise measurement of dosage. The multipuncture tests employ intradermal injections using tines impregnated with OT (old tuberculin) or PPD. Multipuncture tests are generally used for screening because they require less skill and are more rapidly administered than the Mantoux test.***

47. Because a client has multiple sclerosis (MS), the nurse's plan of care should include teaching to avoid:

1. Laxatives.
2. Cool baths.
3. Exercise.
4. Caffeine.

1. ***Correct. Laxatives and enemas should be avoided. A high-fiber diet, bulk formers, and stool softeners are useful for maintaining stool consistency.***
2. *No, cool baths are not harmful to this client. The client should not be exposed to excessive heat or hot baths, as this can cause the weakness associated with MS to become much worse. Cool baths would be appropriate.*
3. *No, exercise is not harmful for this client. In fact, the MS client's daily routine should include physical exercise balanced by rest periods to prevent fatigue.*
4. *No, caffeine is not contraindicated for clients with MS. There is no known correlation between caffeine and MS manifestations at this time.*

48. A female client is scheduled for magnetic resonance imaging (MRI). Prior to the study, the nurse should explain to the client that:

1. She must fast from midnight the night before the test.
2. The study will take about 15 minutes.
3. She will be asleep during the study.
4. She must remove all metal-containing objects from her body.

1. *Incorrect. The MRI can visualize soft tissue without the use of contrast media or ionizing radiation. No dietary restrictions are needed.*

2. *No, the MRI takes 30 minutes for a body region and approximately 60 minutes for a total body scan. The body part to be imaged is moved inside a large machine. Some clients do become claustrophobic and are unable to tolerate the confinement of MRI.*
3. *Not true. The client must remain still during the study, but she does not have to be sedated.*
4. ***Correct! In the MRI, an electromagnet is used to detect radio frequency pulses produced by alignment of hydrogen protons in the magnetic field. Therefore, it cannot be used in the presence of metal. All jewelry must be removed prior to this test. Clients who are not candidates for MRI include those with any metal inside the body (aneurysm clips, orthopedic hardware, artificial heart valves, intrauterine devices, pacemakers, etc.).***

49. A client is diagnosed with a C-6 complete spinal cord transection following a motor vehicle accident. Which intervention should receive highest priority in the nursing plan of care?

1. Turning the client every two hours to prevent pressure sores.
2. Elevating the head of the bed to 30 degrees to decrease intracranial pressure.
3. Monitoring respiratory status every hour to detect changes in breathing patterns.
4. Forcing fluids to prevent dehydration.

1. *Not the best choice. This intervention is important, along with maintenance of proper body alignment and passive range of motion exercises to extremities, but it does not have the highest priority.*
2. *No! The client will be placed in some form of skeletal traction to reduce the fracture dislocation and maintain alignment of the cervical spine. Elevating the head of the bed will not be possible, as the client will be placed on a Stryker or other turning frame. Spinal cord injuries cause edema of the spinal cord, not the brain. Concerns about increasing intracranial pressure are not the priority.*
3. ***Exactly! The muscles contributing to respirations are the abdominals, intercostals, and the diaphragm. Ventilation is affected when these muscles are paralyzed, decreasing chest excursion. In high cervical cord injury, acute respiratory failure is the leading cause of death.***
4. *No, definitely not! IV fluids may be indicated in the immediate post-trauma phase, but not forcing fluids. This client may be kept slightly dehydrated to help decrease edema of the spinal cord. High-dose steroids may also be administered to counteract cord edema.*

50. A client with a history of bleeding esophageal varices is concerned about preventing further episodes of bleeding. What caution should the nurse give to the client?

    1. Include high fiber and roughage in your diet.
    2. Avoid drinking hot liquids.
    3. Restrict activities and exercise in warm weather.
    4. Avoid bearing down when having a bowel movement.

    1. *No, absolutely not! Esophageal varices can often bleed after irritation of the dilated vessels by poorly chewed foods or irritating fluids. Foods that are high in fiber and roughage can also mechanically irritate the varices, causing them to bleed.*
    2. *No, not necessary. There is no indication that drinking hot liquids will cause varices to bleed.*
    3. *No, not necessary. There is no connection between exercise in warm weather and bleeding esophageal varices. Look for an option that may increase portal pressure.*
    4. ***Yes! The client should avoid all straining maneuvers that increase intra-abdominal or intrathoracic pressure: straining, coughing, sneezing, bending over, etc.***

51. A client is scheduled for a sigmoidoscopy. The nurse should advise the client that, during the procedure, he will be placed in which position?

    1. Supine.
    2. Prone.
    3. Left lateral.
    4. Semi-Fowler's.

    1. *Incorrect. This position would not allow for proper insertion of the sigmoidoscope and could cause bowel perforation.*
    2. *No. This position is not used because it does not provide the client with adequate lung aeration during the procedure and does not allow for proper insertion of the sigmoidoscope, following the natural curvature of the bowel.*
    3. ***Good choice. The left lateral, or Sim's position, is the preferred position, just as for enema administration. It provides the most comfort for the client and allows the scope to be inserted along the natural curvature of the sigmoid colon.***
    4. *Absolutely not! This position is never used for colonoscopic examinations. It offers no visibility of the rectal opening and is dangerous for the client with the possible complication of bowel perforation.*

52. In performing ileostomy care, the nurse measures the circumference of the collection device opening so that it is at least how much larger than the stoma circumference?

    1. 1/8 inch.
    2. 1/4 inch.
    3. 1/2 inch.
    4. 3/4 inch.

    1. ***Correct. The 1/8 inch edge around the stoma opening means that as little skin as possible is exposed to the irritating drainage from the ileostomy.***
    2. *No, this is not the correct amount of peristomal skin to be exposed to the irritating effects of the ileostomy drainage.*
    3. *Incorrect. The amount of skin to be exposed to the irritating effects of the ileostomy drainage is less than this.*
    4. *Wrong choice. This amount of skin exposed to the ileostomy drainage will lead to peristomal skin irritation.*

53. A trauma client, admitted through the Emergency Room, has a urinary catheter inserted to monitor kidney function and assess for early signs of shock. The nurse would report which urinary output measurements as suggestive of cardiac failure or hypovolemia?

    1. 20 ml/hour.
    2. 35 ml/hour.
    3. 40 ml/hour.
    4. 50 ml/hour.

    1. ***Correct. Normal urine flow is 50 ml/hour. A urinary output of 30 ml/hour or less is suggestive of cardiac failure or inadequate volume replacement.***
    2. *Incorrect. This output would be within safe parameters, but the client should be monitored closely to watch for further changes.*
    3. *Incorrect. This urinary output amount is within safe limits. The client will need continued monitoring to evaluate further changes in urinary output.*
    4. *Incorrect. Normal urine flow is 50 ml/hour. This output would suggest normal kidney function.*

54. A postoperative client should be assessed frequently for manifestations of hemorrhage, which can lead to hypovolemic shock. In hypovolemic shock, which assessment would most likely be made by the nurse?

    1. Rising blood pressure.
    2. Hyperthermia.
    3. Bradycardia.

4. Tachypnea.

1. *Incorrect. As the client's blood volume decreases, the cardiac output decreases, causing a decrease in arterial and venous blood pressure. Try again.*
2. *Incorrect. One of the clinical manifestations of hypovolemic shock due to hemorrhage is a falling body temperature, not hyperthermia. Try again.*
3. *Incorrect. In the case of hemorrhage, the pulse rises (tachycardia) as the body attempts to compensate for decreased cardiac output and falling blood pressure, which result in tissue hypoxia. Try again.*
4. **Yes! In hypovolemic shock, the respirations are rapid and deep, often of the gasping type spoken of as "air hunger." As shock worsens, the respirations become increasingly shallow and rapid. Tachypnea is the body's attempt to provide more oxygen to the cells.**

55. **The nurse should assess an immobilized client for manifestations of a fecal impaction, the most definitive of which is:**

    1. The absence of bowel sounds.
    2. Diarrhea stools with abdominal cramping.
    3. A rigid board-like abdomen.
    4. Constipation with liquid fecal seepage.

    1. *No. Absence of bowel sounds is seen in a paralytic ileus when peristalsis has stopped. That is not the problem with a fecal impaction.*
    2. *Incorrect. Diarrhea stools with abdominal cramping are often caused by gastroenteritis. Although both manifestations may be present in the case of a fecal impaction, they are not the most definitive assessments that can be made.*
    3. *Wrong choice. A rigid, board-like abdomen is seen in peritonitis, an inflammation of the peritoneum. As the affected area of the abdomen becomes extremely tender, the muscles become rigid, giving the board-like appearance to the abdomen.*
    4. **Yes, these are the classic manifestations of a fecal impaction. Other manifestations of a fecal impaction include painful defecation, a feeling of fullness in the rectum, abdominal distention, and sometimes cramps and watery stools. Very often, liquid fecal material may bypass the hardened mass.**

56. **A postoperative client is developing manifestations of a paralytic ileus following abdominal surgery. Which assessment can the nurse expect to make?**

    1. Abdominal cramping, diarrhea.
    2. Vomiting, chest pain.
    3. Abdominal distention, hypoactive bowel sounds.
    4. Rigid, board-like abdomen, elevated temperature.

1. *No. Diarrhea is a result of hyperperistalsis. A client with a paralytic ileus would not have a hyperactive bowel.*
2. *Incorrect. Chest pain would be present with cardiac or lung pathology. Nausea/vomiting may be seen in clients with an ileus, however, it is associated with abdominal pain and tenderness.*
3. **Correct assessment! Paralytic ileus quickly leads to distention of the intestinal tract and abdominal cavity. Other objective signs include hypoactive or absent bowel sounds and no passage of feces or gas rectally.**
4. *Wrong choice. The manifestations of a rigid, boardlike abdomen and elevated temperature are indicative of peritonitis, an inflammation of the peritoneum usually caused by a bacterial infection.*

57. **A postoperative client has an infected surgical incision. The area is red and swollen with a small amount of thick, yellow drainage. The correct term for the nurse to use in describing this drainage is:**

    1. Purulent.
    2. Sanguineous.
    3. Serous.
    4. Serosanguineous.

    1. **Correct. Purulent drainage is commonly known as pus, the thick yellow secretion from an infected wound that is composed of bacteria, necrotic tissue, and white blood cells.**
    2. *No. Sanguineous refers to "blood" and would designate bleeding from a surgical incision.*
    3. *Incorrect. Serous drainage, typically seen on the original surgical dressing, is clear to light yellow in color with a thin consistency. This drainage is serum, the clear liquid portion of blood that does not contain fibrinogen or blood cells.*
    4. *Wrong. Serosanguineous drainage contains both serum and blood. It is pink to cherry red in color and does not indicate an infectious process.*

58. **In assessing postoperative clients for manifestations of early hypovolemic shock, the nurse notes that an initial observation would most likely be:**

    1. Thirst.
    2. Warm, flushed skin.
    3. Irritability.
    4. Bradycardia.

    1. *Incorrect. Thirst is not an early sign of hypovolemic shock. True thirst is caused by fluid volume deficits, but it comes after other diagnostic manifestations.*
    2. *Incorrect. Warm, flushed skin is seen in early septic shock, which is usually caused by gram-negative bacteria. It is not an early sign of hypovolemic shock.*
    3. **Good work! Early in hypovolemic shock, hy-**

peractivity of the sympathetic nervous system with increased secretion of epinephrine usually causes the client to feel anxious, nervous, and irritable.

4. *Incorrect. Bradycardia is not seen in shock conditions. The pulse is rapid and becomes weaker, thready and irregular as shock progresses.*

59. **A client is diagnosed with acute pyelonephritis. The nursing plan of care should include teaching the client to:**

1. Drink 4,000 ml of fluid per day.
2. Maintain complete bedrest until manifestations decrease.
3. Complete the entire cycle of antibiotic therapy.
4. Do daily weights with notification of the physician if any fluctuation occurs.

1. *Wrong. This amount of fluid intake is unrealistic to expect of a client. Force fluids means 2,000-3,000 ml in 24 hours.*
2. *No! The client should NOT be placed on complete bedrest. Commode or bathroom privileges will help prevent complications of bedrest such as constipation and urinary stasis.*
3. **Yes! It is very important that the client take the full prescription of antibiotic therapy to decrease the chance of regrowth of the causative organism.**
4. *Incorrect. This action is not indicated for acute pyelonephritis. Intake and output should be monitored and fluids encouraged. NOTE: Even if a client is on daily weights in the hospital, after discharge he is instructed to weigh himself one to two times per week and report significant gain or loss. This will help to prevent needless worry over day to day fluctuations in weight.*

60. **The physician has ordered a urine specimen to be sent to the lab for analysis of specific gravity. How should the nurse collect the specimen?**

1. Clean-catch midstream urine.
2. Catheterized urine specimen.
3. Random urine sample.
4. 24-hour urine collection.

1. *Not necessary. A clean-catch midstream urine would be collected if the physician is looking for a causative organism for a urinary tract infection. Specific gravity measurements do not detect bacteria.*
2. *No, it is not necessary to have a catheterized specimen to measure specific gravity of urine. A catheterized specimen is ordered the least frequently because of the chance of introducing bacteria into the urinary system.*

3. *Yes! Only a random sample is needed to test for specific gravity of urine, which measures the concentration of the urine. A fresh morning specimen is preferred, but the urine can be collected at any time; at least 10 ml should be obtained.*
4. *No, 24-hour urine collections are not necessary when testing for specific gravity, which can give a clue as to the body's hydration status.*

61. **A client is admitted with a cerebrovascular accident (CVA). A goal of care is to reduce intracranial pressure. Which of the following interventions should be included in the nurse's plan of care?**

1. Administer sedative medications at regular intervals.
2. Cough and deep breathe every two hours.
3. Elevate head of bed 30 degrees.
4. Limit fluid intake to 500 ml in 24 hours.

1. *No! Sedative medications are contraindicated because they may mask signs of increased intracranial pressure, particularly changes in level of consciousness.*
2. *No! Coughing is to be avoided since it increases intracranial pressure. Deep breathing would be appropriate.*
3. **Correct. The head of the bed is elevated 15 to 30 degrees to promote venous drainage from the head. The head and neck must be kept in the midline so that venous drainage into the body is not restricted.**
4. *No! This amount of fluid intake could predispose the client to dehydration and would not be appropriate. Although fluid intake is restricted somewhat, this amount is too drastic and could cause other problems for the client.*

62. **A client, admitted with a tentative diagnosis of cholecystitis, is scheduled for an oral cholecystogram (gallbladder series) in the morning. Which question asked by the nurse is critical prior to this test?**

1. "What is your height and weight?"
2. "What is your age and occupation?"
3. "Have you ever had this test performed before?"
4. "Are you allergic to any seafood?"

1. *No, this question is not critical prior to the gallbladder series. It would be part of the admission assessment data obtained earlier.*
2. *No, this information would have no bearing on the test or the client's safety during the procedure.*
3. *No, this is not a critical question. Although this question is an important part of the teaching done prior to the test, it is not as important as another question posed above.*

4. *Correct. The client is asked about allergies to iodine or seafood because an iodide-containing contrast medium is given orally on the evening prior to the exam. This contrast medium is excreted by the liver and concentrated in the gallbladder. The normal gallbladder fills with this radiopaque substance. If gallstones are present, they appear as shadows on the radiograph.*

63. Which postoperative intervention by the nurse should receive the highest priority for a client who had a cholecystectomy this morning?

    1. Coughing and deep breathing.
    2. Dangling and ambulation.
    3. Use of anti-embolic stockings.
    4. Irrigation of the nasogastric tube.

    1. *Absolutely! This client is especially prone to pulmonary complications, as are all clients with upper abdominal incisions. Thus, he should be taught to take deep breaths and cough every hour to expand the lungs fully and remove secretions. These actions will help to prevent atelectasis or pneumonia.*
    2. *No, this is not the highest priority in the first 24 hours after upper abdominal surgery — although these actions will help to prevent many postoperative complications, especially thrombophlebitis. Look for an option that is more important in the first postoperative day.*
    3. *Sorry, this is not the priority. Anti-embolic stockings are helpful in preventing thrombophlebitis, but this is not the major concern after gallbladder surgery.*
    4. *Wrong choice. Patency of the nasogastric tube is important to prevent gastric distention and nausea/vomiting, but it's not the priority concern after high abdominal surgery.*

64. A postoperative client's knee dressing becomes completely saturated with blood one hour after returning to the clinical unit. Initially, the nurse should:

    1. Reinforce the knee dressing.
    2. Apply a tourniquet around the closest artery.
    3. Apply direct pressure to the knee.
    4. Apply ice to the knee.

    1. *No, this would not be effective. This action is more for cosmetic purposes and does not reflect the seriousness of the client's condition. Something must be done to stop or slow the bleeding.*
    2. *No, this is not appropriate at this time. This action is somewhat drastic and should only be used as a last resort when the hemorrhage cannot be controlled by any other method.*

3. *Correct! Almost all bleeding can be stopped by direct pressure, except when a major artery has been severed. The charge nurse should then be notified, so that appropriate action can be taken by the surgeon. The client usually has to return to surgery for ligation of the bleeder(s).*
4. *No, this is inappropriate in this situation — even though ice is a vasoconstrictor and will help decrease edema and hematoma formation. Reread the options and try again.*

65. Following spinal cord injury at or above T-6, the nurse should watch the client closely for signs of autonomic dysreflexia. The nurse is aware that this potentially dangerous response could be triggered by:

    1. Elevated blood pressure.
    2. Severe headache.
    3. Distended bladder.
    4. Edema of the spinal cord.

    1. *Incorrect. A rapid rise in blood pressure, severe hypertension, is the most serious response seen in autonomic dysreflexia, due to vasoconstriction of the arterioles. It is not a triggering factor, but a result.*
    2. *Incorrect. A severe headache is one of the results of autonomic dysreflexia. It is not a causative agent.*
    3. *Excellent! There are many kinds of stimulation that can precipitate autonomic dysreflexia. Most are related to the bladder, bowel, and skin of the client: for example, catheter changes, a distended bladder or bowel, enemas, and sudden position changes.*
    4. *Incorrect. Edema of the spinal cord is a natural result of a spinal cord injury, not a causative factor of autonomic dysreflexia.*

66. A client who had surgery 24 hours ago is experiencing dyspnea and tachycardia, and has developed a fever. The nurse suspects atelectasis. If this complication is present, the nurse's auscultation of the client's lung sounds would reveal:

    1. Diminished breath sounds.
    2. Rhonchi.
    3. A pleural friction rub.
    4. Absent breath sounds.

    1. *Correct. Assessment of atelectasis (collapse of lung tissue) would include increased pulse and temperature, and decreased breath sounds or fine crackles on auscultation.*
    2. *No. Rhonchi are coarse, low-pitched, sonorous rattling sounds caused by secretions in the larger air passages. They are heard in clients with bronchitis,*

pulmonary edema, and resolving pneumonia.

3. *Incorrect. A pleural friction rub, which is a grating or scratchy sound similar to creaking shoe leather, occurs when irritated visceral and parietal pleura rub against each other, as in pleurisy.*

4. *Wrong. Lung sounds would be absent in the case of a pneumothorax, which is the presence of air or gas within the pleural cavity.*

67. **When doing a physical assessment on a client with early common bile duct obstruction, the nurse would expect to see which clinical manifestation?**

1. Dark yellow urine.
2. Ascites.
3. Clay-colored feces.
4. Petechiae.

1. *Incorrect. Dark yellow urine is a normal manifestation for clients with concentrated urine, possibly due to low fluid intake or dehydration. It is not symptomatic of a common bile duct obstruction.*

2. *No, ascites is a complication of liver failure caused by portal hypertension. This accumulation of fluid in the abdominal cavity is not an early manifestation of common bile duct obstruction.*

3. ***Correct. Clay-colored feces indicates that bile has been obstructed from entering the intestinal tract, causing the absence of urobilin (which gives the characteristic brown color to feces).***

4. *Wrong choice. Petechiae, small pinhead hemorrhages, are typically associated with bleeding disorders, not with bile duct obstruction.*

68. **A client with a fractured right hip is taken to surgery for an open reduction and internal fixation. A gravity suction device is placed in the surgical wound. The nurse understands that the purpose of this device is to:**

1. Prevent the development of a wound infection.
2. Monitor the amount of bleeding from the surgical site.
3. Prevent fluid from accumulating in the wound.
4. Eliminate the need for wound irrigations.

1. *Incorrect. Although the removal of blood and fluid from the operative site decreases the chance of infection developing in the area, the suction device will not prevent a wound infection.*

2. *Incorrect. It is possible to measure the amount of drainage that collects in the suction device, but this is not the primary purpose of this piece of equipment. Other factors would help in monitoring the amount of bleeding at the surgical site, such as the saturation of the dressing and observance of hematoma formation at the incision site.*

3. ***Correct. Fluid and blood accumulating at the surgical site are generally drained with a portable gravity suction device. This prevents accumulation of fluid, which could contribute to discomfort and could provide a site for infection. Drainage of 200 to 500 ml in the first 24 hours is expected. By 48 hours postoperatively, the total drainage in eight hours usually decreases to 30 ml or less.***

4. *Not correct. A wound irrigation is indicated when there is an infection in the surgical incision. A gravity suction device would not be used as a substitute for wound irrigation.*

69. **A client has just returned to the clinical unit following a myelogram. Which of the following manifestations manifested by the client should the nurse report immediately to the charge nurse?**

1. Leg cramps.
2. Pain at the needle insertion site.
3. Oral temperature reading of 99.8° F.
4. Neck pain and stiffness.

1. *No, leg cramps (muscle spasms) may occur when the legs are immobile for an extended period of time, but they are not life-threatening. Look for an option that may be serious and would require immediate intervention.*

2. *Incorrect. Discomfort at the needle insertion site (usually between L-3 and L-4, or L-4 and L-5) can be controlled with a mild analgesic such as acetaminophen.*

3. *Wrong. An oral temperature of 99.8° F is not a significant elevation and would not need to be reported immediately to the charge nurse.*

4. ***Very good! Nuchal rigidity (pain and stiffness in the neck) is a sign of meningeal irritation. Meningitis can be caused by the accidental introduction of infectious agents into the spinal canal during lumbar puncture. The most outstanding manifestation of meningitis is a severe and persistent headache that is greatly aggravated by shaking the head. Other manifestations include exaggerated deep tendon reflexes, irritability, and photophobia.***

70. **A truck driver is diagnosed with thrombophlebitis and is started on anticoagulant therapy. During the time the client is on anticoagulants, the nurse should advise the client:**

1. Not to drive his truck.
2. To use an electric razor.
3. To carry the antidote with him at all times.
4. To stay in bed.

1. *No, the client will be allowed to drive his truck when he leaves the hospital. He will be on oral anticoagulants and will need to be taught ways to increase his circulation. He will also need to have an ID that states he is on anticoagulants, in case of an accident.*

2. ***Excellent! He is less likely to cut himself with an electric razor.***

3. *No, clients do not need to carry the antidote with them, but they should have an ID card or bracelet in case of an emergency.*

4. *No, staying in bed the whole time he is on anti-coagulants would lead to many complications of immobility, including thrombophlebitis.*

71. **A client is diagnosed with a urinary tract infection and is placed on ciprofloxacin (Cipro) 500 mg P. O. every 12 hours. Which of the following instructions should the nurse include in the teaching plan for this client?**

    1. Drink extra fluids (one to two quarts) each day while taking Cipro.
    2. If the medicine causes an upset stomach, take an antacid at the same time.
    3. Cipro may cause photosensitivity. Wear protective clothing when out in the sun.
    4. Please report any blurred vision or ringing in the ears to your physician immediately.

    1. ***Correct! Drinking extra fluids will reduce the risk of crystalluria. Cipro is excreted primarily via the kidneys.***

    2. *No, the Cipro is best absorbed on an empty stomach with a full glass of water. If an antacid needs to be taken, instruct the client to take it at least two hours after administering the Cipro. Choose again!*

    3. *No, the Cipro can cause photophobia—eye sensitivity to light—not skin photosensitivity. Make another selection.*

    4. *Incorrect. Tinnitus, a sign of ototoxicity, is not a side effect of quinolone therapy. This is a major concern with aminoglycosides and salicylates. Try again!*

72. **In caring for a client taking isoniazid (INH), the nurse knows that which diagnostic study is done frequently to monitor for toxic effects?**

    1. AST, ALT.
    2. WBC count.
    3. Bone marrow aspirations.
    4. Creatinine & BUN.

    1. ***Correct!! AST (SGOT) and ALT (SGPT) are studies of liver function. These liver enzymes are monitored to detect the effects of INH that might be toxic to the liver. They should be***

monitored before drug therapy is started and at least monthly during the course of therapy.

2. *Wrong. The WBC would not be monitored separately to assess for complications from INH therapy. Select another option.*

3. *Incorrect. Although aplastic anemia can result from INH therapy, it is not common. A complete blood count would be a more effective screening tool than invasive (and painful) bone marrow aspirations. Try again.*

4. *INH is not considered to be a nephrotoxic agent; therefore, kidney function studies would not be indicated. Try again.*

73. **A client has returned after major surgery and is complaining of pain. The physician ordered morphine sulfate to control her pain. Before administering the medication, the nurse would first:**

    1. Discuss the side effects with the client.
    2. Take the client's vital signs.
    3. Provide mouth care.
    4. Have the client turn, cough and deep breathe.

    1. *No, this is not the first nursing action. Clients do need to be informed of possible side effects, but the nurse should save any teaching until the client is more alert. Make another selection.*

    2. ***Correct! Vital signs should be taken before administering morphine to provide a baseline for measuring respiratory depression, which can occur afterwards.***

    3. *This is not the first nursing action. Mouth care will be needed postoperatively but it is not needed prior to morphine administration.*

    4. *Wrong. The client will be better able to cooperate when she has less pain, after the medication is administered. Make another choice.*

74. **A two-year-old admitted with seizures is receiving phenytoin (Dilantin) in oral suspension form. What should the nurse do before administering each dose?**

    1. Be sure the client has not eaten within the hour.
    2. Shake the container vigorously.
    3. Perform mouth care.
    4. Warm the solution before administering.

    1. *No! Phenytoin should be given with meals to decrease gastric problems.*

    2. ***Correct! It is important for the nurse to shake the container, as clients can be under-medicated if the medication is not evenly distributed.***

    3. *Wrong choice. Although mouth and dental care are needed, and clients do need to consult their dentist, mouth care is not needed before each dose. Read all the options and try again.*

    4. *This action is not necessary. The diluent for oral*

suspension of the drug will hasten dissolution if warmed. Try again.

75. **A 66-year-old client is receiving hemodialysis via left arteriovenous fistula (AVF) for management of chronic renal disease. The nurse should instruct the client to:**

    1. Check the access hourly for patency.
    2. Maintain skin integrity through frequent cleansing and application of lotion over the site.
    3. Avoid tight clothing around the access site.
    4. Sleep on his left side to maintain patency of the access site.

    1. *Wrong. It is only necessary to check the access site two times daily for the "buzz" that indicates adequate blood flow. Hourly checks are unnecessary.*
    2. *Wrong. The use of creams or lotions are to be avoided over the access site to prevent infection.*
    3. ***Good work! Tight clothing may decrease the blood flow and cause clotting.***
    4. *Wrong. Sleeping on the side of the access may cause impairment of blood flow and clotting to occur.*

76. **The nurse is instructing the client regarding good food sources for potassium. Which menu choice by the client indicates to the nurse that the client has understood the instruction?**

    1. Baked chicken, boiled potato, pudding.
    2. Boiled chicken, rice, cranberry juice.
    3. Broiled meat, baked potato, citrus fruit salad.
    4. Beef stew, bread and butter, Jell-O.

    1. *Wrong choice! Chicken and potato are both good sources of potassium, but since the potato is boiled it has lost significant amounts of potassium. Milk products contain some potassium but are not considered a good source.*
    2. *Wrong choice! Chicken is a good source of potassium, but since it is boiled it has lost significant amounts of potassium. Rice and cranberry juice contain only small amounts of potassium.*
    3. ***Very good! Broiled meat, baked potato and citrus fruit salad are all good sources of potassium and the cooking methods have not depleted this nutrient.***
    4. *Wrong choice! Beef is a good source of potassium, but bread, butter and Jell-O are not.*

77. **A client is in the hospital and he is dying. He is very weak, tired, and short of breath. The nursing plan of care for the client and his family should emphasize:**

    1. Limiting visiting hours to help conserve his energy.
    2. Having the client do as much as he can for himself to increase his self-esteem and independence.
    3. Encouraging the family to spend as much time as possible with him and do whatever they feel com-

fortable with in caring for him.

    4. Planning to perform as much of his care as possible at one time, so he can rest for long intervals.

    1. *Wrong! The question tells you that the client is dying. Limiting visiting hours serves no purpose and denies the client, family and friends valuable time together.*
    2. *Wrong! The client is weak and short of breath. Self-care activities will increase oxygen needs and cause more physiological distress for the client.*
    3. ***Correct choice! This plan provides support systems for the client and allows the family to spend as much time as possible with the client before his death, which is important when working through the grieving process.***
    4. *Wrong! This will further exhaust the client and increase oxygen consumption. A better approach is to provide frequent rest periods. Try again.*

78. **A client is taking acetaminophen (Tylenol) for muscular aches and pains. She reports to the nurse that she is lonely and has been drinking heavily in the evenings. The nurse should advise the client that:**

    1. Alcohol and Tylenol may result in a diuretic effect, depleting fluid volume and electrolytes.
    2. Sodium and fluid retention may result from this combination.
    3. Alcoholic beverages should be avoided because they increase the risk of liver toxicity when taken with Tylenol.
    4. This combination has an increased potential for causing palpitations.

    1. *This is incorrect. A diuretic effect occurs when alcohol is taken with ibuprofen, not Tylenol. Make another selection.*
    2. *Wrong. Sodium and fluid retention occurs when NSAIDs are given with steroids. Make another choice.*
    3. ***Good! Liver toxicity is likely to occur, as alcohol potentiates the hepatic effects of Tylenol.***
    4. *This is incorrect. Alcohol and Tylenol taken together will cause hepatic changes, not cardiac changes.*

79. **A client diagnosed with schizophrenia says to the nurse, "They lied about me and are trying to poison my food." The therapeutic nursing response is:**

    1. "You are mistaken. Nobody has told lies about you or tried to poison you."
    2. "You're having very frightening thoughts."
    3. "Tell me more about your concerns about being poisoned."
    4. "Tell me who would do such things to you?"

    1. *This is not correct. This statement, if made by the nurse, is directly confronting her delusion, which*

could make the client feel more angry and misunderstood. There is a better option.

2. **Correct. Instead of responding literally to the client's statement, the nurse is responding to the feelings that the client was attempting to communicate. By so doing, the nurse is shifting the focus from the beliefs, which are not real, to the client's fear, which is real.**

3. *This is not correct. This statement is supporting the content of the delusion, so it is not a therapeutic response. Look again at the other options.*

4. *Incorrect, because this statement is supporting the client's delusional thinking.*

80. **The nurse enters an anorexic client's room and finds her doing vigorous push-ups on the floor. What is the most therapeutic nursing action?**

1. Remind her that if her weight decreases she will lose a privilege.
2. Leave the room and permit her to exercise in private.
3. Ask her to stop doing the push-ups and suggest she pursue a less strenuous activity.
4. Wait for her to finish exercising and ask her why she feels the need to exercise.

1. *This is not correct. Vigorous physical exercise is a compulsive behavior in anorexic clients, and the threat of losing privileges will not deter the client from this activity.*

2. *This is not correct. Active intervention is required to prevent the client from continuing to lose weight.*

3. **Correct. Maslow's theory dictates that physiological needs receive priority. This response by the nurse identifies a physiological need. Active intervention is required to prevent the client from continuing to lose weight. The goal of treatment is to promote weight gain through behavior modification. The nurse should actively intervene to interrupt undesirable behaviors, such as vigorous exercise.**

4. *This is not correct. Active intervention on the part of the nurse is needed to prevent further weight loss by burning calories. Discussing feelings indicates that the nurse does not understand the compulsive nature of some of the client's behaviors.*

81. **The nurse is caring for a bulimic client. The best initial nursing intervention to help the client deal more effectively with her bulimic behavior is:**

1. Establishing a behavioral contract to control these urges.
2. Keeping a journal of eating behavior and feelings experienced before, during, and after eating.
3. Supervising the client's behavior at all times.

4. Eating only when other persons are present.

1. *This is not the best option. Behavioral contracts are often used to help bulimic clients, but they are not the best initial intervention.*

2. **Correct. The use of journals to record the types and amounts of food eaten as well as the feelings that occur when eating will help the client become more aware of the relationship between her feelings and eating behavior. Also, initially it may be easier for the bulimic client to write about her feelings than to talk about them.**

3. *Constant supervision of the client's behavior will not assist the client to develop better insight into her eating behavior.*

4. *This action will not assist the client to develop better insight into her eating behavior. Look for an option that indicates a better understanding of problems confronting the bulimic client.*

82. **A 20-year-old college student is brought to the emergency room by the campus police. She was raped while walking to the parking lot after one of her classes. What action by the nurse is most therapeutic initially?**

1. Ask questions to get the client to talk about the attack.
2. Treat the client's physical wounds.
3. Explain to the client that she is now in a safe place.
4. Have a calm and accepting attitude.

1. *One principle of crisis intervention is to encourage discussion of what happened. However, there is another nursing intervention that will promote this intervention and that is more important initially. Read the other options and choose again.*

2. *Rape victims often experience the treatment of the wounds as a continuation of the invasive trauma of the rape. Unless the wounds are life-threatening, there is a more important priority for the nurse.*

3. *The client needs to feel safe, but there is a better option that would provide even greater reassurance for the client.*

4. **Correct. A calm and accepting attitude on the part of the nurse will establish an atmosphere of safety and security for the rape survivor, and is necessary for establishing a therapeutic relationship with the client.**

83. **One morning the nurse asks an elderly client if she had any visitors the day before. She responds that several members of her church choir had been to see her. The nurse knows that only her daughter had visited the day before. The nurse understands that a fabrication that is told to mask memory loss is an example of:**

1. Delusion.
2. Illusion.
3. Confabulation.
4. Dissociation.

1. This is not correct. A delusion is a false, fixed belief. Delusional thinking is most often associated with schizophrenia and other psychotic disorders.

2. This is not correct. An illusion is a sensory misperception and not a thinking problem.

3. Correct. Confabulation is making up responses that may be inaccurate but sound appropriate. It is done to avoid embarrassment about memory loss.

4. This is not correct. Dissociation is the defense mechanism of separating aspects of memory or emotions from the rest of one's conscious awareness or identity.

84. **Which statement by the nurse indicates the best understanding of the principles of reality orientation?**

    1. "Good morning, Mr. Jones. Did you sleep well? It's time to get dressed."
    2. "Good morning. This is your second day in Shady Pines and I am your nurse for the day."
    3. "Do you remember who I am? We met yesterday when you were admitted."
    4. "Good morning, how are you today? I am your nurse for the day. My name is Mrs. Smith."

    1. This is not correct because it does not actually orient the client to anything other than his name. Also, the nurse should wait for the client to answer her initial question before telling him it is time to get dressed. Short statements, made one at a time, should be used with persons who have memory and other cognitive deficits.

    2. Correct. This statement orients to client to time of day, place, and the nurse's identity. It also is a clear statement that does not contain any irrelevant information that could be confusing to the client.

    3. This is not correct. The client with memory deficits will probably not recognize the nurse or remember meeting her the previous day. The question does not orient the client to time or place, and even fails to identify the nurse.

    4. This greeting does not orient the client to place. There is a better option.

85. **The nurse caring for clients in a long-term care facility understands that remotivation therapy is used to:**

    1. Stimulate and encourage social participation.
    2. Reorient clients with cognitive problems.
    3. Encourage clients to share memories of past experiences and events.

4. Resolve emotional problems.

*1. **Correct. The goals of remotivation therapy are to stimulate and encourage social participation using structured group approaches.***

2. This is not correct. This option describes reality orientation programs.

3. This is not correct. This option describes reminiscence therapy.

4. This is not correct. Psychotherapy, either individual or group, is used to assist clients to resolve emotional and psychological difficulties. This is not the rationale for remotivation therapy.

86. **The nurse is planning orientation to the unit for a new client who is severely depressed. Which nursing approach is best initially?**

    1. Introduce the client to other clients on the unit and staff members.
    2. Tour the unit and introduce her to everyone they meet on the way.
    3. Explain the unit policies and answer any questions she may have.
    4. Accompany the client to her room and stay with her while she unpacks, offering only minimal information.

    1. This is not correct, because this approach would be overwhelming for the client at this time.

    > **TEST-TAKING TIP:** This option says essentially the same thing as Option 2 — so both must be wrong!

    2. This approach would be overwhelming for the client at this time.

    > **TEST-TAKING TIP:** This option says essentially the same thing as Option 1 — so both must be wrong!

    3. This is not the best approach initially because severely depressed persons are easily confused. Can you identify an approach that uses another communication tool that is more suitable for the nurse to use in establishing a therapeutic relationship with the client?

    4. Correct. Severely depressed persons have problems with concentration and easily become confused. A nursing approach that focuses on giving simple information, slowly and directly, is best. This initial approach also uses the communication tool of offering self. The presence of the nurse conveys to the client that she is worthy of the nurse's attention, and will help the client adjust to her new surroundings.

87. In planning activities for a depressed client during his early stages of hospitalization, which nursing plan is best?

    1. Provide one activity a day, to avoid fatigue.
    2. Let the client choose an activity that is appealing.
    3. Provide a structured daily program of activities for the client.
    4. Wait until the client's mood improves and he indicates an interest in productive activity.

    1. *Providing only one activity a day will reinforce the client's feelings of inadequacy and withdrawal. This is not the correct option.*
    2. *Wrong. The depressed person has great difficulty making decisions.*
    3. ***Correct. A regular schedule provides structure for the depressed client, who has difficulty making decisions and providing structure for himself. Good work!***
    4. *This is not a recommended approach because inactivity reinforces a depressed mood by preventing satisfaction and social recognition.*

88. The nurse learns that an elderly client's sleeping problems began six months ago, when his physician diagnosed prostatic cancer. Prior to that time, he had enjoyed good physical health. The nurse also knows that his wife of 50 years died one year ago. One day the client tells the nurse, "I'd be better off dead because I am totally worthless." The nurse's most therapeutic response is:

    1. "I have seen some very valuable things about you."
    2. You feel worthless now because you are so depressed. You will feel differently when you depression begins to improve."
    3. "You really have a great deal to live for."
    4. "You have been feeling very sad and alone for some time now."

    1. *This may look like a positive and encouraging statement, but it is not therapeutic for the client because it does not address his feelings. The nurse should accept the client's perceptions without agreeing with his conclusions.*
    2. *This response does address the client's feelings of worthlessness, but in an incorrect manner. This client has suffered some serious losses, and the nurse should accept the client's feelings and help the client to explore them. Instead, this response blocks communication by using false reassurance, because the nurse does not know how the client will feel in the future.*
    3. *This response is not therapeutic. It uses cliché and false reassurance. From the client's point of view, this statement is simply not true. The nurse should accept the client's feelings and encourage him to explore them.*
    4. ***Correct. Depressed persons have great difficulty expressing their feelings. This response by the nurse uses the communication tool of empathy and is a good way to begin to help him become more aware and accepting of his feelings.***

89. An elderly client is able to walk with a cane and enjoys ambulating in the hall. Since he has memory problems, he has great difficulty remembering which room is his. What nursing action would best alleviate this problem?

    1. Assign him a room close to the nursing station so staff members will be available to help him.
    2. Assign him to a room with a roommate who can watch out for him.
    3. Do not allow him to leave his room unaccompanied.
    4. Put his picture and his name written in large letters on the door to his room.

    1. *This is not correct. This action is not feasible in most settings, and even if it were, would only serve to make him more dependent on the nursing staff. This is a better option.*
    2. *This is not correct. The nursing staff is responsible for assuring the client's safety, not the roommate. This action it would also foster increasing dependency and loss of a sense of control. There is a better option.*
    3. *This is not correct! It is unnecessarily restrictive and would foster increasing dependency. The client "is able to walk with a cane and enjoys ambulating." The client should be assisted to maintain his level of independence. There is a better option.*
    4. ***Correct. This is an orienting device that would allow the client to locate his room independently. This will assist the client to maintain his level of independence. This option is therapeutic for the client.***

90. A client who has just been diagnosed with cancer tells the nurse that he would rather be dead than go through the treatment for cancer. The most appropriate nursing response is:

    1. "What is it about the cancer treatment that concerns you?"
    2. "If you don't receive the treatment, you will get your wish."
    3. "Why don't you talk to your doctor about your feelings?"
    4. "That wouldn't be fair to your family, would it?"

    1. ***Excellent! This response is therapeutic because it focuses on the client's feelings and concerns.***

This response encourages the client to further express his feelings about cancer treatments. The nurse may also be able to clarify any misinformation that the client may have concerning the treatments.

2. *This response is inappropriate and unprofessional. It fails to respect the client's feelings and does not address the client's immediate concerns. This response blocks further communication, instead of encouraging the client to express his feelings concerning the treatments. The nurse must always be in a therapeutic role! Make another choice.*

3. *With this response, the nurse avoids the discussion with the communication block of "putting the client's concern on hold." This response is not appropriate, because it tells the client that the nurse does not want to hear about the client's feelings. The nurse must always be in a therapeutic role. Make another choice.*

4. *This response uses the communication block of "referring to an inappropriate person." By addressing the needs of the family instead of the needs of the client, the nurse indicates that the needs of the family are more important. This statement also expresses disapproval by the nurse, which is not therapeutic. The nurse must always be in a therapeutic role. Make another choice.*

91. **A client is admitted to the hospital. He has been on bed rest at home and has been incontinent of urine. His wife has been caring for him, and there is a strong odor of urine. The wife state that she is sorry and embarrassed about the unpleasant smell. Which response by the nurse is therapeutic?**

1. "It must be difficult to care for someone who is confined to bed. How have you been able to manage?"
2. "Don't worry about it. He will get a bath, and that will take care of the odor."
3. "A lot of clients that are cared for at home have the same problem."
4. "When was the last time that he had a bath?"

1. *Excellent! The wife is the client in this question. The nurse's response must be therapeutic for the client. This response addresses the feelings of the client by using the communication tool of showing empathy. It also facilitates therapeutic communication because it is nonjudgmental and encourages the client to express her feelings.*

2. *Telling the client not to worry blocks communication by devaluing her feelings and her concern about the odor. This is a communication question, and the nurse's response must be therapeutic for the client. Look for a response by the nurse that addresses the feelings of the client and uses a therapeutic communication tool. Try again.*

3. *This response implies that caregivers in the home are not able to keep the client odor free. It is a judgmental statement that is not therapeutic. Look for a response by the nurse that addresses the feelings of the client and uses a therapeutic communication tool. Try again.*

4. *Asking about the last bath implies to the client that the odor of urine indicates that her husband has not been bathed for some time. This is a communication question, and the nurse's response must be therapeutic for the client. Who is the client in this question? Look for a response by the nurse that addresses the feelings of the client and uses a therapeutic communication tool. Try again.*

92. **The client tells the nurse that he does not know how he is ever going to stay on the low cholesterol diet that his doctor ordered after his heart attack. The best response by the nurse is:**

1. "If you don't follow the diet, you will probably have another heart attack, which could kill you."
2. "What is it about the low cholesterol diet that seems to be a problem for you?"
3. "I've been on that same diet for the last five years, and I'm sure you will learn how to change your eating habits after a while."
4. "I will have the dietitian talk to you before you are discharged. She's the expert, and she can be really helpful."

1. *Wrong choice. A low cholesterol diet decreases the amount of fat in the diet. High fat content in the diet causes plaque to be deposited in the blood vessels, which results in narrowed blood vessels that can cause a heart attack. Telling the client that he may die if he doesn't follow this diet, however, is perceived as a threat and blocks therapeutic communication. Make another choice.*

2. **Excellent! This response uses the therapeutic communication tool of clarification. It lets the client know that his concerns are important to the nurse, and encourages him to tell the nurse more about his concerns. When you cannot identify a therapeutic response focusing on the client's feelings, look for a response that addresses the client's concerns and uses a therapeutic communication tool.**

3. *The fact that the nurse has personal experience with this diet may be beneficial when teaching the client about the diet. As a response to the client's comment in the case scenario, however, this response is not therapeutic. It blocks communication by focusing on an inappropriate person — the nurse — instead of on the client's feelings and concerns. The nurse must always be in a therapeutic role. Try again.*

4. *This response blocks communication by putting*

the client's concern on hold. The nurse should address the client's concern and should obtain more information from the client about the problem before deciding to ask the dietitian to talk with the client.

93. **An elderly client with Alzheimer's disease is admitted to the hospital. His daughter says to the nurse, "I really feel guilty about leaving my father, but I need to go home." The most helpful response by the nurse to the daughter is:**

    1. "Your father is well cared for here."
    2. "Your worried feelings are normal."
    3. "When you are getting ready to leave, tell me. I will sit with your father."
    4. "Can I call another family member to stay with him?"

    1. *This may sound good, but it is not correct. This response blocks therapeutic communication by using cliché and false reassurance. Remember, the client in this test question is the daughter! The nurse's response should address the feelings and concerns that she has shared with the nurse.*
    2. *Wrong choice! This is an example of the communication block of cliché and false reassurance. Also, this response incorrectly identifies the client's feelings as "worry," and it does not address the client's concern about leaving her father.*
    3. **Good choice! In this response the nurse offers to help the daughter by sitting with the father. The nurse is using the therapeutic communication tool of offering self.**
    4. *Wrong! By suggesting getting someone else to sit with the father, the nurse makes the daughter feel all the more guilty about leaving.*

94. **A client is diagnosed with active tuberculosis. He and his family have many questions for the nurse. They ask, "How did this happen? What can we do to prevent this? What will happen next?" Which is the most helpful response by the nurse?**

    1. "The tuberculosis was probably contracted from someone else with TB."
    2. "You need not be concerned. TB is very curable."
    3. "Tuberculosis can be treated at home with medications."
    4. "You seem very worried about the TB. What concerns you most?"

    1. *This answers only one of the questions that were asked, and it may not be the true cause of the illness.*
    2. *Incorrect. This response devalues the clients' feelings and uses false reassurance, since TB can be difficult to treat. This response does not answer their*

questions or allay their fears, and it is not therapeutic.

    3. *Incorrect. This response only addresses only one of the clients' questions and does not encourage further communication. Read all the options before selecting the best one!*
    4. **Good choice! This response invites the family to ask questions and obtain answers to everything that concerns them, while focusing on the "here and now."**

95. **During a client's postoperative recovery from an ileostomy, the nurse begins teaching her stoma care, when the nurse notices that the client will not look at her ostomy. The client states, "I'd rather be dead than have to live with this all my life." Which is the most therapeutic nursing response?**

    1. "I can't imagine what you must be feeling like; it must be awful."
    2. "I'll call your physician and see if he will order something to help you to relax."
    3. "There's no reason to feel like that. Things will get better."
    4. "You appear upset. Would you like to talk?"

    1. *No! Expressing excessive approval can be as harmful to nurse/client relationship as stating disapproval.*
    2. *No, this ignores the clients statement and changes the subject, which conveys a lack of empathy.*
    3. *No, this offers false reassurance to the client, which blocks therapeutic communication.*
    4. **Good choice. This response uses the communication tool of empathy to convey to the client a caring attitude. The nurse, in offering to listen, is also offering self. This will be therapeutic for the client.**

96. **Which is the best nursing action to maintain maximum privacy for the client during a medical procedure?**

    1. Closing the door of the client's room.
    2. Pulling the curtains around the client's bed.
    3. Asking family members to leave the room.
    4. Using sterile drapes to cover the client.

    1. *This action may be appropriate and will help maintain a secure environment, but it is not the best action to maintain privacy for the client. If someone opens the door or enters the room, the client's privacy may be violated.*
    2. **Very good. This is the best action for providing maximum privacy for the client. In each of the other options, the client's privacy will not be protected if someone enters the room.**
    3. *This is appropriate but it is not the best action to maintain privacy for the client. After family members leave, someone else may enter the room.*

4. *This may be an appropriate action, but it is not the best action to maintain privacy for the client. During a procedure, the body part that is involved will be exposed to provide access for the nurse or physician. The client's privacy will not be protected if someone enters the room.*

97. **A client is to have a rectal temperature taken. A glass thermometer is available at the client's bedside. The mercury bulb on the insertion end of the thermometer is long and slender. The safest action by the nurse is to:**

    1. Obtain a thermometer with a short, blunt insertion end.
    2. Take the client's temperature with the available thermometer, and report any elevations.
    3. Carefully insert the long end of the thermometer after lubricating that end.
    4. Put gloves on before using the thermometer available at the client's bedside.

    1. *Yes, great job! The thermometer that is available is an axillary or oral thermometer. It has the long mercury bulb in order to provide more surface area contact with the tissues under the tongue or in the axilla. Because the bulb end is long and narrow, it has a greater potential for breaking, and could injure or puncture rectal tissue easily. Using this thermometer to obtain a rectal temperature is not safe.*
    2. *The available thermometer is not safe to use to obtain a rectal temperature. The long, thin bulb has the potential for breaking and/or puncturing the rectal tissues.*
    3. *Wrong! A rectal thermometer should be lubricated prior to use, for ease of insertion. However, the available thermometer is an oral or axillary thermometer, which is not safe to use in obtaining a rectal temperature because it has the potential for causing injury to the rectal tissues.*
    4. *Wrong! Gloves should be worn when the possibility of coming in contact with body fluids exists. However, the thermometer available at the bedside is an oral thermometer, which should not be used to obtain a rectal temperature because of the potential for injuring rectal tissues.*

98. **While working the night shift, the nurse notices a mouse running down the hallway of the clinical unit. The correct nursing action is to:**

    1. Place rat poison in the vicinity where the mouse was seen.
    2. Set some mouse traps to catch the mouse, and then dispose of it in a plastic bag labeled as contaminated.

    3. Notify the supervisor of the problem.
    4. Call the environmental health department of the hospital, and report the incident.

    1. *Wrong! Poison should not be placed in an area that clients, staff and visitors utilize, because of the risk of accidental exposure or poisoning.*
    2. *It is not the nurse's responsibility to catch mice. To prevent infection, however, the problem should be reported to the department responsible for rodent control.*
    3. *The supervisor is not responsible for rodent control. If the nurse has a problem getting the department that is responsible for environmental health to take care of the mouse, then the supervisor may be needed to intervene on behalf of the nurse.*
    4. *Yes! The department that is responsible for environmental health deals with pest and rodent control and should be notified of this problem.*

99. **A vest restraint is placed on a confused elderly client who is at high risk for falling. Which nursing action is inappropriate?**

    1. Provide an opportunity for the client to use the bedpan, toilet, or other toilet facilities at regular intervals.
    2. Assess the respiratory status of the client frequently.
    3. Utilizing help from other nurses, approach the client and apply the vest as quickly as possible, in order to avoid any resistance from the client.
    4. Change the client's position at least every two hours.

    1. *Placing a vest restraint on a client results in a the client's being dependent on the nurse for many basic needs. This client cannot get a bed pan or go to the bathroom without assistance. This is a true statement, but it is not the correct answer because the question asks you to select an option that is incorrect.*
    2. *A vest restraint can interfere with respiratory effort if the restraint is too tight, therefore, frequent assessment is necessary. This question asks for an inappropriate action, however, so this is not the correct answer.*
    3. *This is the correct answer because the question asks you to identify the inappropriate action. Applying a restraint can be threatening to an agitated or confused client. The client should be approached slowly and calmly, utilizing only as much help as is deemed necessary to ensure the safety of the client and the nurse.*

4. *In order to avoid complications that may develop as a result of immobility, the client should have a position change at least every two hours. However, this question asks you to identify an incorrect action, so this is not the correct option.*

100. **A vest restraint is placed on a confused elderly client who is at high risk for falling. He is partially paralyzed and is at risk for developing pressure sores. How should the nurse handle the linen when changing this client's bed?**

    1. When removing the linen from the bed, hold it close to the body to avoid dropping it.
    2. After removing the linen from the bed, place it on the floor until finished making the bed.
    3. When removing the linen from the bed, hold it away from the uniform.
    4. Shake the clean linen to unfold it, before making the bed.

    1. *No. The linen will contaminate the nurse's uniform and should be placed in the dirty linen bag immediately.*
    2. *No. The linen should be placed in the dirty linen bag immediately.*
    3. ***This choice is correct, because the linen is considered "dirty" and should be held away from the uniform to avoid contaminating it.***
    4. *Sorry, try again. Shaking linen spreads bacteria and other harmful organisms.*

NCLEX-PN

Test 8

NCLEX-PN TEST 8

1. A client has advanced cancer of the lung with metastasis. His wife says to the nurse, "I know my husband is in severe pain. I wish I could do something to make him feel better." Which of the following responses by the nurse would be most helpful to the wife?

   1. "It must be very difficult for you to see your husband suffering."
   2. "I wish there was more that I could do to relieve his pain, too."
   3. "I'm sure he will begin to feel better after his next pain medication."
   4. "Your husband tries hard not to show the pain when you are with him."

2. A 17-year-old client had an appendectomy. When the nurse offers meperidine (Demerol) for postoperative pain, the client says, "No, I don't want to get hooked." Which is the most appropriate nursing response?

   1. "You are right. Why take a chance?"
   2. "Tell me what you mean by getting hooked."
   3. "You will not get addicted for the short amount of time that you will be in the hospital."
   4. "The Demerol will make you more comfortable, not make you an addict."

3. A 29-year-old diabetic is admitted to the hospital for dialysis because of poor renal function. He says to the nurse, "I don't even know why I'm doing this. There is no cure." Which of the following is the most appropriate nursing response?

   1. "There is always a chance that through research a cure will be found."
   2. "Dialysis will help you live longer."
   3. "You shouldn't complain! You are fortunate to be in this good a shape, considering the type of diabetes you have."
   4. "It sounds as though you have given up on life."

4. A couple is in the hospital because of a fetal death at 37 weeks gestation. The husband is trying to comfort the wife, who is crying. The husband says to the nurse, "We wanted this baby so much." Which of the following is an appropriate response by the nurse?

   1. "You are both young and you can have other children."
   2. "It is God's will, and it must be accepted."
   3. "It must be very difficult for you both. I will be available if you need anything."

   4. "I think you should call your minister. He can help comfort you."

5. A chronic alcoholic has been hospitalized following a drinking binge. The nurse enters the room and finds the client shouting in a terrified voice, "Get those ants out of my room!" At this time, which of the following responses by nurse would be most appropriate?

   1. "Tell me more about the ants that you see in your room."
   2. "I'm sure that the ants you see will not harm you."
   3. "I don't see any ants, but you seem very frightened."
   4. "I do not see anything. This is part of your illness."

6. A 69-year-old client is admitted to the hospital. She brings all of her medicines, including a bottle with no label. She says this is her cough medicine, which she put in a small bottle so it would fit in her purse. At this time, the best nursing action is to:

   1. Pour the liquid down the drain, since it has no label.
   2. Instruct the client concerning safety issues related to this practice, and suggest that she have the pharmacy put the medication in smaller containers that will fit in her purse.
   3. Send the bottle home with a family member.
   4. Tell the client that this is a dangerous practice, which could result in the death of one of her small grandchildren.

7. A postoperative client has an electronic blood pressure machine automatically measuring her blood pressure every 15 minutes. The blood pressure machine is reading the client's blood pressure at more frequent intervals, and the readings are not similar. The nurse checks the machine settings and observes additional readings, but the problem continues. At this time, the nurse should:

   1. Record only those blood pressures that are needed for the 15-minute intervals.
   2. Disconnect the machine and measure the blood pressure with a sphygmomanometer and stethoscope.
   3. Turn on the machine every 15 minutes to obtain the client's blood pressure.
   4. Measure the blood pressure manually and compare readings obtained by the machine with readings obtained manually.

8. A client in an extended care facility is in the dining room, having dinner with the other clients. The client

has stopped eating, is grasping his throat with his hands, and cannot talk. The first and most effective action by the nurse is to:

1. Call a code and obtain assistance, before taking further action.
2. Perform the Heimlich Maneuver.
3. Place the client on the floor and begin mouth-to-mouth resuscitation.
4. Slap the client on the back several times.

9. The nurse discovers a fire in the hospital. Which of the following nursing actions would be unsafe?

1. Sound the nearest fire alarm.
2. Move clients who are in the immediate area of the fire.
3. Turn off any oxygen or electrical equipment.
4. Open the doors and windows to let the smoke out.

10. A client who gave birth two days ago, is in the bathroom after taking a shower. The nurse hears a loud thud and when she opens the bathroom door, she sees the client on the floor and a hair dryer in the sink with the basin full of water. The first nursing action is to:

1. Assess the client to determine if she is breathing.
2. Assess the client for a heart rate.
3. Unplug the hair dryer, while taking care not to touch the client or any water or wet surface.
4. Perform a neurological assessment.

11. A young client is paralyzed from the waist down. He has a TV, radio, video tape player, stereo, and video game unit, which are all turned on most of the day. The nurse notices that there are not enough electrical outlets, and that extension cords with multiple outlets are in use to accommodate this equipment. The best nursing action is to:

1. Have the client's family take some of the equipment home.
2. Unplug as much of the client's equipment as necessary, after informing the client that an overloaded circuit can cause an electrical fire, and, therefore, the extension cords are not allowed.
3. Tell the client that only single-outlet cords can be used, and that you will check often to see if he wants to use anything not currently connected.
4. Call the maintenance department and have more wall outlets installed in the client's room.

12. A client is admitted to a long-term care facility. She requires total care. In providing mouth care to the client, the nurse should:

1. Place the client on her back with a pillow under her head.
2. Use her thumb and index finger to keep the client's mouth open.
3. Use a stiff toothbrush to clean the client's teeth.
4. Place the client on her side before starting mouth care.

13. While caring for a client, the nurse notices that the call light cord is frayed. The nurse should:

1. Tell the client not to use the call light until it is fixed.
2. Remove the call light, and report the problem to the supervising nurse immediately.
3. Tape up the cord until the maintenance people can fix it, so the client will have a call light.
4. Tell the client to call out if he needs help, and to use the call light only in an emergency.

14. An elderly client is scheduled for surgery tomorrow. As the nurse enters the client's room, she notices that flames are coming out of the waste basket. The nurse would demonstrate an understanding of safety priorities by first:

1. Placing the folded blanket from the client's bed over the entire opening of the waste basket.
2. Finding the nearest fire extinguisher to put the fire out.
3. Telling the client that he is not supposed to be smoking.
4. Pulling the nearest fire alarm.

15. A client spills hot coffee on himself during breakfast. The first action by the nurse is to:

1. Remove the clothing from the burn area and apply cold water to the area.
2. Call the physician.
3. Make out an incident report.
4. Cover the area with sterile towels.

16. An elderly client has an IV with an infusion pump. While examining the infusion pump, the nurse notices a slight tingling in her hand as the plug is checked. What is the next nursing action?

1. Shut the pump off immediately.
2. Inform the repair department to immediately shut off the pump.
3. Recheck the equipment in one hour.
4. Use a different electrical outlet site.

17. While caring for an infant you notice that one of the infant's stuffed animals in the crib has eyes that can easily be pulled off. The appropriate nursing action is to:

1. Take the toy out of the crib.
2. Remove the eyes from the stuffed animal and return it to the crib.
3. When the mother comes to visit, show her the eyes and explain that the infant could pull them off and choke on them.
4. Send the toy home with the mother.

18. **A client is to have an electrical heating device applied to his lower back area. The plug on the heating device has three prongs, and the electrical wall outlet available only has two-pronged openings. The client's radio is plugged into a three-pronged outlet. The best action by the nurse at this time is:**

    1. Unplug the client's radio, which is plugged into a three-pronged outlet, and use that outlet for the heating device.
    2. Obtain an extension cord with a three-pronged outlet on it.
    3. Use a 2-pronged adapter to plug into the wall outlet, then plug the heating device into the adapter.
    4. Call central supply to see if you can get a heating device with a two-pronged plug on it.

19. **The nurse is assisting an elderly client to eat. The client suddenly coughs a few times, then appears to be attempting to cough, making a whistling sound as he inhales. When using the Heimlich Maneuver on a conscious client, which of the following nursing actions is most effective?**

    1. Ask the client what he is choking on.
    2. Place your arms around the client and position your fist in the abdomen, between the bottom of the breast bone and the navel.
    3. Slap the client on the back until the object is expelled or until the client becomes unconscious.
    4. Stand in front of the person.

20. **A client is ordered to have a hypothermic or cooling blanket applied because of a very high body temperature. When caring for this client, which of the following is an inappropriate nursing action?**

    1. Check the client's body temperature frequently.
    2. Place a layer of cloth, such as a bath blanket, between the client and the cooling blanket if the cooling blanket does not have a protective covering.
    3. Keep the cooling blanket in place until the client's body temperature is a couple of degrees below the desired level recommended by the physician.
    4. Remove the cooling blanket when the client's body temperature is a couple of degrees above the desired level recommended by the physician.

21. **In a long-term care facility, the nurse finds an elderly client on the floor. After having the client examined by the physician, the most important nursing action is to:**

    1. Call the family and ask them to stay with the client.
    2. Provide for the safety and protection of the client.
    3. Apply wrist and leg restraints to prevent the client from falling from the bed.
    4. Obtain an order for medication to sedate the client.

22. **A client is confused and confined to bed. He has attempted to crawl over the side rails. The safe nursing action is to:**

    1. Apply restraints to the client immediately.
    2. Stay with the client and notify the supervising nurse.
    3. Remind the client to stay in bed.
    4. Tell the client to stay in bed, or else the nursing staff will have to restrain him.

23. **The nurse is caring for a client who is on a moderate sodium diet for her pregnancy induced hypertension. Which of the following lunch selections by the client would signify an understanding of the diet?**

    1. Grilled cheese sandwich and tomato soup.
    2. Bologna sandwich and dill pickles.
    3. Chinese vegetables with soy sauce.
    4. Chicken salad sandwich with tossed salad.

24. **Which observation by the nurse would warrant further teaching to prevent infection in the postpartum client?**

    1. Wiping the perineum from back to front.
    2. Large amounts of fluid intake.
    3. Use of tap water for peri-care.
    4. Frequent use of sitz bath.

25. **A client has mild preeclampsia. The nurse anticipates that which of these measures is likely to be included in her plan of care?**

    1. Bedrest.
    2. One gram sodium diet.
    3. Administration of magnesium sulfate.
    4. Hospitalization for close observation.

26. **The nurse is caring for a client admitted to the labor unit with premature rupture of membranes (PROM) at 30 weeks gestation. Which of the following nursing interventions should receive priority in the client's care?**

    1. Frequent assessment for vaginal bleeding.
    2. Assessment of blood pressure every two hours.
    3. Careful assessment for signs of infection.

4. Continuous fetal heart rate monitoring.

27. **An infant's respiratory rate is irregular, 52 breaths per minute with several periods of apnea lasting five to 10 seconds. The infant's color is pink with acrocyanosis. What nursing measures are indicated at this time?**

    1. Notify the RN immediately.
    2. Place the infant in a warmer environment.
    3. Continue to routinely monitor the infant.
    4. Assess the infant's blood sugar.

28. **A client is experiencing morning sickness early in her pregnancy. She asks the nurse in the prenatal clinic what she can do to alleviate the problem. The nurse should recommend which of the following diets to reduce nausea and vomiting?**

    1. Low residue diet.
    2. Fat free diet.
    3. Dry diet in a.m.
    4. Low carbohydrate diet.

29. **Which of the following would the nurse teach the antepartum client to report to her health care provider immediately?**

    1. White vaginal discharge.
    2. Urinary frequency.
    3. Unable to get wedding ring off.
    4. Nausea and vomiting.

30. **The client is seen at prenatal clinic in the first trimester. She tells the nurse that she is upset because, although she and her husband planned this pregnancy, she has been having many ambivalent feelings about the upcoming change in her life. The best response by the nurse is:**

    1. "Have you spoken to your husband about these feelings?"
    2. "I would like you to see a counselor to discuss these feelings further."
    3. "These feelings are quite common in women early in pregnancy."
    4. "Don't worry, these feelings will go away."

31. **Which of the following manifestations should the nurse anticipate in a baby born to a heroin-addicted mother?**

    1. Exaggerated reflexes.
    2. Poor muscle tone.
    3. Respiratory rate below 30 per minute.
    4. Extended periods of sleep.

32. **How would the nurse assess an antepartum client for the presence of quickening?**

    1. Complete a vaginal exam.
    2. Ask the mother if she has felt the baby move.
    3. Request an ultrasound exam.
    4. Provide a contraction stress test.

33. **The nurse knows that which of the following can be used to positively confirm a pregnancy?**

    1. A positive pregnancy test.
    2. Chadwick's sign.
    3. Fetal movement felt by the midwife.
    4. Braxton-Hicks contractions.

34. **Which technique would be best when the nurse wants a four-year-old to take deep breaths following an abdominal operation?**

    1. "I will give you a star each time you take a deep breath."
    2. "You can go to the playroom when you finish doing your deep breathing."
    3. "I'll leave your blow bottle here on your table, so that you can use it in a few minutes."
    4. "Let's play a game of blowing cotton balls across your table."

35. **A 16-year-old male is to receive an intramuscular injection. To gain cooperation with this procedure, the nurse's first intervention is to:**

    1. Tell him what he will feel.
    2. Explain the purpose of the medication.
    3. Offer him a choice of injection sites.
    4. Describe the steps in the procedure.

36. **While the nurse is caring for a seven-month-old female infant, she aspirates a small toy. She begins to cough and becomes cyanotic, and then no sound is made. At this time, which nursing action would be most appropriate?**

    1. Perform a chest thrust.
    2. Turn the client prone and administer back blows.
    3. Stimulate further coughing.
    4. Perform a modified Heimlich maneuver with one hand.

37. **While working in a pediatric unit, the nurse encounters all ages of children. The nurse knows that a child's social interactions with peers are very important. During which periods of a child's life is this need greatest?**

    1. Preschool and school age.
    2. Toddler and preschool.
    3. School age and adolescent.
    4. Late adolescence and early adulthood.

38. **The nurse knows that it is characteristic of the development of a 30-month-old child to:**

1. Tell tall tales.
2. Have a command vocabulary of about 10 words.
3. Weigh double his birth weight.
4. Have achieved complete primary dentition.

39. The nurse knows that the most likely observable manifestation of impetigo is:

    1. Raised reddened areas.
    2. Blisters with scattered pustules.
    3. Crusted lesions with serous drainage.
    4. Severe itching with sand-like rash.

40. The nurse is doing postoperative teaching for a three-month-old recovering from an umbilical hernia repair. Before discharge, the mother demonstrates understanding by stating she will:

    1. Maintain positioning in semi-Fowler's after meals.
    2. Limit activities for four weeks.
    3. Expect bulging of the incision with coughing or crying.
    4. Keep the infant's diaper away from the incision.

41. The nurse has completed preoperative teaching on a child scheduled for surgery to treat Hirschsprung's disease. The father expresses understanding when he says:

    1. "I'm glad my child will have normal BMS now."
    2. "Now the diarrhea will finally stop."
    3. "The operation will straighten out the kink in the intestine."
    4. "The ostomy is only temporary."

42. The nurse knows that the best way to determine the parent's ability to care for their child who has had an ostomy is to:

    1. Make sure both parents can explain the procedure.
    2. Allow the parents to ask questions while the nurse is performing the procedure.
    3. Supervise the parents while they are doing the procedure.
    4. Have the ostomy nurse do teaching before discharge.

43. In developing a plan for perioperative teaching for an adolescent, the nurse should be guided by the knowledge that:

    1. He may act as if he knows much more than he actually does.
    2. He will only be interested in reassurance that things will go well.
    3. The major part of the teaching should be delayed until after the surgery.

4. His parents should be the major focus of the teaching.

44. A 15-year-old client has had an appendectomy. As the nurse prepares to give discharge instructions, the best approach is:

    1. Instruct both parents.
    2. Explain to the client and one parent.
    3. Explain to only one parent.
    4. Any family member may be instructed.

45. The nurse would best describe the most important aspect of planning the discipline of a hospitalized toddler as:

    1. Consistency in enforcing the rules.
    2. Delaying punishment for wrong doing until parents are present.
    3. Eliminating discipline while the child is ill.
    4. Giving several warnings before actually disciplining.

46. To relieve thirst immediately after a tonsillectomy, the best fluid for the nurse to offer a child would be:

    1. Anything the child likes.
    2. Ice cream.
    3. Orange Popsicle.
    4. Grapefruit juice.

47. A client is to undergo various diagnostic tests and procedures for evaluation of neurologic function. When the client asks the nurse which test uses a gas as a contrast medium, the nurse responds that the test is the:

    1. Pneumoencephalogram.
    2. Echoencephalogram.
    3. Brain scan.
    4. Electroencephalogram.

48. In preparing a client for a bone marrow aspiration, which of these actions by the nurse should receive highest priority?

    1. Explaining the procedure to the client.
    2. Shaving the site to be used for the aspiration.
    3. Premedicating the client with a mild sedative.
    4. Obtaining a set of vital signs immediately prior to the procedure.

49. Which intervention should be included in the nurse's plan of care for a client who has returned from surgery for a below-the-knee amputation?

1. Elevate the stump on a pillow for 24 hours.
2. Keep suture removal set at bedside.
3. Elevate head of bed 60 degrees at all times.
4. Irrigate nasogastric tube every four hours.

50. **While caring for a client in the oliguric phase of acute renal failure, the nurse's plan of care should include:**

    1. Maintaining reverse isolation to prevent infection.
    2. Increasing the client's protein intake to prevent muscle wasting.
    3. Encouraging fluid intake to prevent dehydration.
    4. Meticulous skin care to prevent skin breakdown.

51. **A client returns from surgery with two Penrose drains in place. In anticipation of frequent dressing changes, what should the nurse use to most effectively reduce skin irritation around the incision area?**

    1. Montgomery straps.
    2. Silicone spray.
    3. Hypoallergenic tape.
    4. Large, bulky absorbent pads.

52. **A post-mastectomy client returns to the surgical unit with a closed-wound gravity suction device (Hemovac) in place. Which action by the nurse would ensure proper operation of the device?**

    1. Irrigate the tubing with sterile normal saline once each shift.
    2. Empty the device when it's full.
    3. Keep the tubing above the level of the surgical incision.
    4. Recollapse the device whenever it's one-half to two-thirds full of air.

53. **An 18-year-old client admitted with ulcerative colitis is being treated with sulfasalazine (Azulfidine). The nurse explains to the client that the major action of Azulfidine is to:**

    1. Suppress inflammation of the bowel wall.
    2. Reduce peristaltic activity.
    3. Neutralize gastrointestinal tract acidity.
    4. Prevent a secondary infection.

54. **A client is admitted with open-angle glaucoma. He is started on a treatment regimen of timolol (Timoptic) and pilocarpine (Pilocar) eye drops. The nurse understands that these drugs will be administered:**

    1. Until the client's intraocular pressure returns to normal.
    2. For three to six months or until manifestations subside.

3. On a regular schedule for the rest of the client's life.
4. For approximately 10 days, followed by a gradual tapering to discontinuance.

55. **In assessing a client with Addison's disease, the nurse recognizes that a classic, characteristic sign associated with Addison's disease is:**

    1. Hirsutism.
    2. Intention tremors.
    3. Skin discoloration.
    4. Petechiae.

56. **A client is diagnosed with Cushing's disease. The nurse recognizes that the signs and manifestations of Cushing's disease are primarily related to what endocrine dysfunction?**

    1. Adrenal hyperfunction.
    2. Thyroid hyperfunction.
    3. Pituitary hypofunction.
    4. Parathyroid hypofunction.

57. **A client with acquired immunodeficiency syndrome (AIDS) is taking zidovudine (Retrovir) 200 mg every six hours. Which side effect should the nurse anticipate with the use of this drug?**

    1. Nausea.
    2. Fever.
    3. Hypotension.
    4. Lethargy.

58. **A client is admitted with burns to his upper chest and arms. The burns are wet and shiny with large blisters. The nurse understands that these burns would be classified as:**

    1. Superficial.
    2. Partial-thickness.
    3. Full-thickness.
    4. Fourth degree.

59. **Which burn client would be at greatest risk for developing respiratory problems secondary to burns and would require a priority respiratory assessment by the nurse?**

    1. A client with singed nasal hair.
    2. A client burned on the lower chest while lighting a charcoal fire outside.
    3. A client with a history of smoking, burned on the abdomen and upper thigh areas.
    4. A client with blackened soot around his face and neck.

60. **Which intervention should be included in the nursing plan of care for a client who has just been admitted with a myocardial infarction?**

   1. Complete bedrest.
   2. Limit fluid intake to 1500 cc in 24 hours.
   3. Ambulate in hallway four times a day.
   4. Monitor oxygen via nasal cannula.

61. **In planning to teach a client who has the human immunodeficiency virus (HIV), the nurse should remember to alert the client that the virus can be transmitted:**

   1. As soon as the client develops manifestations.
   2. To anyone having contact with the client's blood.
   3. Via the respiratory route, like tuberculosis.
   4. Only during the active phase of the virus, but not while it is inactive.

62. **What should be the nurse's priority goal of care for a client admitted with multiple myeloma?**

   1. Prevention of decubitus ulcers.
   2. Adequate nutritional intake.
   3. Relief from pain.
   4. Maintenance of a patent airway.

63. **Six hours into the collection of a 24-hour urine specimen, one voided specimen is accidentally discarded by the client. The nurse should:**

   1. Continue the collection, noting the loss on the lab slip.
   2. Notify the nurse in charge.
   3. Discard the previously collected urine and start the collection again.
   4. Notify the lab so that the collection can be reduced to six hours.

64. **If a nurse takes the following actions to prepare a client for an electroencephalogram (EEG), which one should be questioned?**

   1. The client is given a mild sedative the evening prior to the procedure.
   2. The client's intake of coffee and alcohol is restricted 48 hours prior to the procedure.
   3. The client is told that the procedure is painless.
   4. The nurse washes and dries the client's hair prior to the procedure.

65. **A client complains of a throbbing headache after a lumbar puncture. Which action by the nurse would be most appropriate at this time?**

   1. Darken the client's room and close the door.
   2. Keep the client flat in bed for six to eight hours after the procedure.

   3. Encourage the client to limit fluid intake for eight hours after the procedure.
   4. Report the headache to the charge nurse.

66. **During cardiopulmonary resuscitation (CPR), the nurse should assess the adult's pulse by feeling the:**

   1. Carotid pulse in the neck.
   2. Brachial pulse in the arm.
   3. Femoral pulse in the groin.
   4. Radial pulse in the wrist.

67. **Which sign/symptom is least likely to be observed by the nurse in a client who is admitted with a myocardial infarction?**

   1. Cyanosis.
   2. Nausea.
   3. Chest pressure.
   4. Acute indigestion.

68. **The nurse can expect that a client diagnosed with AIDS related complex (ARC) would have which manifestation?**

   1. No manifestations.
   2. Evidence of opportunistic infection.
   3. Fatigue and weight loss.
   4. Inactive human immunodeficiency virus.

69. **The nurse understands that the primary purpose of the water seal in a chest tube drainage system is to:**

   1. Prevent the return of air to the chest cavity.
   2. Monitor the amount of drainage from the chest cavity.
   3. Serve as a suction control for the drainage system.
   4. Prevent the return of fluid to the chest cavity.

70. **A client has just returned from surgery following a radical neck dissection with placement of a tracheostomy tube. Which assessment by the nurse should receive highest priority during the first 24 hours postoperatively?**

   1. Lung sounds and respiratory rate.
   2. Patency of the tracheostomy airway.
   3. Surgical dressing site.
   4. Pulse and blood pressure.

71. **In the initiation of cardiopulmonary resuscitation (CPR), which assessment should be made by the nurse PRIOR to beginning chest compressions?**

   1. Absence of respirations.
   2. Dilated pupils.
   3. Absence of pulse.
   4. Unresponsiveness.

72. Which is the first nursing action when preparing to do tracheostomy care?

    1. Open all sterile supplies and solutions.
    2. Hyperoxygenate the client with 100% oxygen.
    3. Apply sterile gloves.
    4. Wash hands thoroughly.

73. A client is admitted with thrombophlebitis. Which intervention can the nurse anticipate will be included in the plan of care?

    1. Bedrest for 10-14 days.
    2. Application of warm, moist heat.
    3. Restriction of oral fluids.
    4. Administration of vasodilating medications.

74. When caring for a client in the phase immediately following a myocardial infarction, the priority goal for the nurse is to:

    1. Decrease the client's anxiety.
    2. Prevent constipation.
    3. Relieve the client's pain.
    4. Restore fluid and electrolyte balance.

75. A client is seen in the health clinic and is diagnosed with conjunctivitis of the right eye. An antibiotic ophthalmic ointment has been ordered. Which instruction would be appropriate for the nurse to give to this client?

    1. Use a sterile glove and applicator to apply the antibiotic ointment.
    2. When washing your face, wash the infected eye first.
    3. Other family members may share your washcloth as long as you rinse it out first.
    4. Apply the ointment in a thin line, beginning at the inner corner and proceeding outward.

76. The nurse is preparing a client for an arthroscopic examination of her left knee. She asks the nurse about her level of activity following the procedure. Which response by the nurse is appropriate?

    1. "You will be on bedrest for 24 hours."
    2. "You will have to use crutches with no weight bearing on the left leg for several days."
    3. "You will probably be allowed to walk after the procedure."
    4. "You can return to all your normal activities immediately."

77. A client with chronic renal failure is undergoing peritoneal dialysis. Which nursing measure will help most to promote outflow drainage of the dialyzing solution?

    1. Push the peritoneal catheter in approximately one inch further.
    2. Elevate the height of the dialysate bag.
    3. Apply manual pressure to the client's lower abdomen.
    4. Turn the client from side to side.

78. Which manifestations can the nurse expect to see in a client admitted with emphysema?

    1. Dyspnea, bradycardia.
    2. Barrel chest, shallow respirations.
    3. Cyanosis, productive cough.
    4. Asymmetrical chest, dry cough.

79. A client has a positive Mantoux test following a screening for tuberculosis. The nurse interprets this to mean that the client:

    1. Has active tuberculosis.
    2. Was infectious at one time, but now has inactive tuberculosis.
    3. Will require further evaluation.
    4. Has never been exposed to the tubercle bacillus.

80. To get the best ferrous sulfate absorption, the nurse should give this drug with:

    1. Milk.
    2. Water.
    3. Orange juice.
    4. Meals.

81. The nurse knows codeine is used cautiously in clients with chronic obstructive pulmonary disease because:

    1. Coughs are not associated with COPD.
    2. There is a high abuse potential.
    3. Increased secretions may be produced.
    4. Interaction with beta agonists may be fatal.

82. The nurse would assess which of the following as an early manifestation of a complication of medication with hydrocodone bitartrate (Dihydrocodeine Bitartrate)?

    1. Tachycardia.
    2. Slowed respirations.
    3. Change in level of consciousness.
    4. Fixed pupils.

83. The nurse understands that, for most clients with a cough that interferes with recovery, guaifenesin (Robitussin) is the medication of choice because:

    1. The respiratory system is not depressed.
    2. There is an added analgesic effect.
    3. It is considered more effective than a narcotic.
    4. Guaifenesin is available without a prescription.

84. **A client is diagnosed with hypertension and is treated with clonidine (Catapres) in the transdermal form. What statement by the client indicates to the nurse a need for further teaching about her drug therapy?**

   1. "I have trimmed the patch to make it fit better under my blouse."
   2. "I am reapplying the patch every seven days."
   3. "I understand that I can shower as usual."
   4. "I will notify my doctor if I get a rash."

85. **A client takes ibuprofen (Motrin) for her arthritis. To reduce esophageal irritation, the nurse should advise the client to take the medication:**

   1. Not with meals or any food.
   2. With a full glass of water and remain upright for 15-30 minutes afterwards.
   3. Before meals with a snack.
   4. After meals; then lie down for an hour.

86. **A client is a truck driver who sits for hours in his truck while driving. He has a swollen and inflamed right calf and is diagnosed with thrombophlebitis. He is hospitalized immediately and is started on a continuous heparin infusion and placed on bed rest. He asks the nurse how long it will take for the heparin to dissolve his clot. What is the best response by the nurse?**

   1. "It usually takes two to three days for heparin to work."
   2. "I'm not sure. You will need to ask your doctor."
   3. "Heparin begins to work immediately, but it does not actually dissolve clots. It prevents new clots from forming, and the present one from getting bigger."
   4. "Heparin thins the blood quickly."

87. **A client will go home on warfarin (Coumadin). It is important for the nurse to instruct the client to:**

   1. Carry an ID card with him at all times.
   2. Take only aspirin for headaches.
   3. Eat lots of foods high in vitamin K, like broccoli, liver, and spinach.
   4. Avoid any exercise.

88. **A client has been receiving moxalactam (Moxam) 800 mg IV for septicemia. He is now ready for discharge. Which discharge instructions would be most appropriate for the nurse to give?**

   1. Do not drink any alcohol for at least three days after discharge.
   2. Report any shortness of breath to your physician immediately.
   3. Be sure to continue taking the Moxam (P.O.) until

the entire prescription is gone.
   4. Drink extra fluids for at least one week to help prevent kidney damage from the IV Moxam.

89. **The nursing staff decide to develop a behavioral program to help a young anorexic client gain weight. Which of the following nursing interventions is inappropriate for this client?**

   1. Provide positive reinforcement for each pound that she gains.
   2. Permit her to spend some quiet time in her room after each meal.
   3. Allow her to select her meals from the same daily menu offered to all clients.
   4. Refrain from commenting about her eating during meal times.

90. **In caring for the elderly, the nurse is guided by Erikson's observation that the elderly need to resolve conflicts between:**

   1. Ego integrity and despair.
   2. Intimacy and isolation.
   3. Generativity and stagnation.
   4. Identity and isolation.

91. **An 82-year-old widow is admitted to the hospital for hip replacement surgery. She appears alert and cooperative, although in great pain. While doing an assessment, the nurse learns she is disoriented to time and believes she is in a hotel. The nurse identifies acute confusion as a nursing problem. The nurse understands that which of the following would least influence the client's confusion:**

   1. Her age.
   2. Relocation to the hospital.
   3. Her physical pain.
   4. Bed confinement.

92. **The nurse has been caring for an elderly client who was admitted for hip replacement and is disoriented to time and place. The nurse requests to be assigned to stay with the client when she returns to the unit after her surgery. The rationale for this request is:**

   1. The elderly client requires close postoperative supervision because of her unpredictable preoperative behavior.
   2. The elderly client will most likely be agitated when she regains consciousness after surgery.
   3. The many stresses associated with surgery could lead to further cognitive impairment in this elderly client.
   4. Elderly clients are particularly vulnerable to the development of postoperative complications.

93. A client taking lithium is discharged from the hospital after being taught to recognize the manifestations of lithium toxicity. The nurse knows learning has occurred when the client states that she will call the psychiatrist if she experiences:

    1. Vomiting and diarrhea.
    2. Fine hand tremor.
    3. Polyuria.
    4. Drowsiness and lethargy.

94. A nursing goal for abusive parents is for them to learn more effective parenting skills. Which of the following support groups would be an appropriate referral by the nurse to further this goal?

    1. Parents Without Partners.
    2. Al-Anon.
    3. Parents Anonymous.
    4. Recovery, Inc.

95. In developing a nursing care plan for an abused wife, which of the following is inappropriate?

    1. Mutual goal setting.
    2. Assisting the client to mobilize her available support system.
    3. Providing information about available resources, such as the local women's shelter, child care services, and legal counseling.
    4. Notifying the appropriate authorities.

96. The nursing care plan for the antisocial client should stress:

    1. Setting clear rules and expectations for the client's behavior on the unit, with the consequences for any violations clearly spelled out.
    2. Ignoring the client's past antisocial acts and focusing on current here-and-now issues.
    3. Supervising the client's behavior closely, to prevent any acting-out or destructive behavior while hospitalized.
    4. Helping the client to identify feelings and gain insight into what motivates his behavior.

97. The nurse is caring for an elderly client who will soon be discharged to a long-term care facility. What nursing action is most important for promoting her continued recovery?

    1. Reviewing the client's nursing care plan with the client's daughter.
    2. Discussing the client's nursing care needs with her physician.
    3. Telephoning the charge nurse at the long-term care facility to explain the client's nursing care needs.
    4. Sending a written summary of the nursing care plan for the client to the long-term care facility.

98. The nurse working with elderly clients knows that organic mental disorders:

    1. Are the most prevalent type of psychiatric problem in this age group.
    2. Are almost always chronic.
    3. Need careful evaluation as they may be caused by a medical problem that could be treated effectively.
    4. Can be controlled with supportive and behavioral approaches, but eventually will lead to further deterioration and death.

99. The nurse working with elderly clients should remember that dementia in the elderly:

    1. Is easy to distinguish from depression.
    2. May coexist with depression.
    3. Is not affected by medications.
    4. Cannot be concealed by the client.

100. A woman is admitted to the psychiatric unit with a diagnosis of depression. Her husband reported that she has been despondent since their youngest child left for college two months before. The client states, "Do not bother with me because I am totally worthless." Which of the following is the most helpful response by the nurse to the client?

    1. "I have seen many valuable things about you."
    2. "You feel worthless now because you are so depressed. You will feel differently when you begin to recover."
    3. "You have been feeling very sad and alone for some time now."
    4. "You really have a great deal to live for."

NCLEX-PN

Test 8
Questions with Rationales

NCLEX-PN TEST 8 WITH RATIONALES

1. A client has advanced cancer of the lung with metastasis. His wife says to the nurse, "I know my husband is in severe pain. I wish I could do something to make him feel better." Which of the following responses by the nurse would be most helpful to the wife?

    1. "It must be very difficult for you to see your husband suffering."
    2. "I wish there was more that I could do to relieve his pain, too."
    3. "I'm sure he will begin to feel better after his next pain medication."
    4. "Your husband tries hard not to show the pain when you are with him."

    1. *This answer is correct. The wife is the client in this question. The nurse is responding to her feelings. Her response is therapeutic and illustrates the communication tool of empathy. Good choice!*
    2. *Wrong! This option focuses on the nurse rather than the client and is not therapeutic.*
    3. *This choice illustrates the non-therapeutic communication block of false reassurance. This is not the answer.*
    4. *The client in this question is the wife. The response in this option is incorrect because it focuses on the husband. It might also cause the wife to feel guilty and is non-therapeutic. Look for a response that addresses the wife's feelings and uses a therapeutic communication tool.*

2. A 17-year-old client had an appendectomy. When the nurse offers meperidine (Demerol) for postoperative pain, the client says, "No, I don't want to get hooked." Which is the most appropriate nursing response?

    1. "You are right. Why take a chance?"
    2. "Tell me what you mean by getting hooked."
    3. "You will not get addicted for the short amount of time that you will be in the hospital."
    4. "The Demerol will make you more comfortable, not make you an addict."

    1. *Wrong. The client appears to have made an incorrect assumption concerning risks of the medication. This response is not therapeutic because it does not properly address the client's concern about addiction or the issue of the client's physical discomfort. It also blocks communication by using a cliché ("Why take a chance?").*
    2. *Excellent choice! This response enhances*

therapeutic communication by asking for clarification. The nurse is addressing the client's concern and asking for important information about the client's knowledge and feelings.

3. *Sorry, try again! This statement uses false reassurance and devalues the client's feelings. The nurse should communicate therapeutically by trying to learn more about the client's knowledge and feelings.*
4. *Wrong. The first part of this response gives the client correct information and addresses the issue of the client's pain. However, the nurse should first ask for clarification of the client's concerns about "getting hooked."*

3. A 29-year-old diabetic is admitted to the hospital for dialysis because of poor renal function. He says to the nurse, "I don't even know why I'm doing this. There is no cure." Which of the following is the most appropriate nursing response?

    1. "There is always a chance that through research a cure will be found."
    2. "Dialysis will help you live longer."
    3. "You shouldn't complain! You are fortunate to be in this good a shape, considering the type of diabetes you have."
    4. "It sounds as though you have given up on life."

    1. *Wrong! This statement is an example of cliché and false reassurance. The client has expressed his feelings to the nurse. Instead of helping the client deal with his feelings, the nurse focuses on the possibility of a future cure.*
    2. *This statement is true, but it does not address the client's feelings. The client has just expressed his feelings to the nurse. To be therapeutic, the nurse's response should focus on the client's feelings.*
    3. *No. This statement expresses the nurse's disapproval of the client's feelings, and devalues his concerns about the future. This response blocks communication and is not appropriate in the nurse-client relationship.*
    4. *Great work! The nurse is using the communication tool of restatement to encourage the expression of feelings, which is therapeutic for the client. The nurse must maintain a nonjudgmental attitude so that the client will feel free to express his feelings. Note that Option 3 blocks communication by expressing the nurse's disapproval of the client's feelings.*

4.   A couple is in the hospital because of a fetal death at 37 weeks gestation. The husband is trying to comfort the wife, who is crying. The husband says to the nurse, "We wanted this baby so much." Which of the following is an appropriate response by the nurse?

1.   "You are both young and you can have other children."
2.   "It is God's will, and it must be accepted."
3.   "It must be very difficult for you both. I will be available if you need anything."
4.   "I think you should call your minister. He can help comfort you."

1.   *This statement may be true, but the nurse cannot know what will happen in the future. This response does not acknowledge the feelings of the clients and blocks communication. This is an example of cliché and false assurance.*
2.   *This is a cliché that expresses the nurse's beliefs and values. It is not empathetic and does not recognize the clients' feelings. This is a communication block.*
3.   ***Correct! This statement acknowledges the clients' feelings. The nurse is showing empathy, and is also offering self by offering to assist them.***
4.   *Wrong! This statement implies that the minister is needed for comforting and that the nurse is not available discuss the clients' feelings. This response is also giving advice to the client.*

5.   A chronic alcoholic has been hospitalized following a drinking binge. The nurse enters the room and finds the client shouting in a terrified voice, "Get those ants out of my room!" At this time, which of the following responses by nurse would be most appropriate?

1.   "Tell me more about the ants that you see in your room."
2.   "I'm sure that the ants you see will not harm you."
3.   "I don't see any ants, but you seem very frightened."
4.   "I do not see anything. This is part of your illness."

1.   *This option is an inappropriate response because it reinforces the client's hallucination.*
2.   *This option is an inappropriate response because it reinforces the client's hallucination.*
3.   ***Very good! This response presents reality ("I don't see any ants"). Also, this response illustrates the therapeutic communication tool of showing empathy. By saying, "You seem frightened," the nurse acknowledges the client's feelings.***

TEST-TAKING TIP: *If you did not know the answer to this question, the test-taking strategy of looking for similar words in the stem and one of the options would be effective here. The words "frightened" and "terrified" are similar.*

4.   *Wrong! In this option the nurse attempts to present reality ("I do not see anything"). The statement, however, is not as specific as it should be ("I don't see any ants"). Also, the response is not empathetic. To be therapeutic, the nurse should acknowledge the client's feelings.*

6.   A 69-year-old client is admitted to the hospital. She brings all of her medicines, including a bottle with no label. She says this is her cough medicine, which she put in a small bottle so it would fit in her purse. At this time, the best nursing action is to:

1.   Pour the liquid down the drain, since it has no label.
2.   Instruct the client concerning safety issues related to this practice, and suggest that she have the pharmacy put the medication in smaller containers that will fit in her purse.
3.   Send the bottle home with a family member.
4.   Tell the client that this is a dangerous practice, which could result in the death of one of her small grandchildren.

1.   *No! Although placing medication in an unlabelled container is not a safe practice, the medication belongs to the client and may be expensive. The nurse should not dispose of it without the client's consent. The client should be informed of the hazard and told of safer alternatives.*
2.   ***Yes, best choice! Instructing the client regarding safety issues and discussing alternatives allows the client to participate in health care decisions, which results in a higher rate of compliance.***
3.   *The bottle can be sent home with a family member; however, this is a safety issue that should be discussed with the client. In addition, sending the bottle home with a family member will not resolve the problem of medication in an unlabelled bottle. This is not the best option.*
4.   *No. Using fear as an approach is not appropriate, and this response by the nurse is not therapeutic. In addition, labeling the bottle will not prevent small children from ingesting the contents if given access to the medication. All medications must be kept out of the reach of children.*

7.   A postoperative client has an electronic blood pressure machine automatically measuring her blood pressure every 15 minutes. The blood pressure machine is reading the client's blood pressure at more frequent intervals, and the readings are not similar. The nurse checks

the machine settings and observes additional readings, but the problem continues. At this time, the nurse should:

1. Record only those blood pressures that are needed for the 15-minute intervals.
2. Disconnect the machine and measure the blood pressure with a sphygmomanometer and stethoscope.
3. Turn on the machine every 15 minutes to obtain the client's blood pressure.
4. Measure the blood pressure manually and compare readings obtained by the machine with readings obtained manually.

1. *This is incorrect. Although blood pressure readings are being obtained, the fact that the machine is taking the blood pressure more frequently and the measurements obtained are not similar suggests that the machine is malfunctioning and is in need of repair.*
2. ***Very good. If there is a question concerning the reliability of the monitoring equipment, a manual check should be made, so that a client does not receive medical treatment because of an erroneous measurement.***
3. *No. Since the measurements and the operation of the machine appear to be questionable, the machine should be taken out of service and repaired.*
4. *Although this option appears to provide a means of checking the machine, the fact that it is not operating correctly suggests that it should not be used until it has been checked by a biomedical technician.*

8. **A client in an extended care facility is in the dining room, having dinner with the other clients. The client has stopped eating, is grasping his throat with his hands, and cannot talk. The first and most effective action by the nurse is to:**

1. Call a code and obtain assistance, before taking further action.
2. Perform the Heimlich Maneuver.
3. Place the client on the floor and begin mouth-to-mouth resuscitation.
4. Slap the client on the back several times.

1. *It is not necessary to call a code at this time. Also, choking requires immediate intervention. Waiting for help places the client at further risk.*
2. ***Excellent choice! The Heimlich Maneuver is the most effective method to clear an obstructed airway of a choking person.***
3. *No! This action is inappropriate and might cause further danger to the client. Mouth-to-mouth resuscitation is indicated after the airway has been cleared, for a client who has ceased breathing. Mouth-to-mouth resuscitation performed on a chok-*

ing client could lodge the food even further into the airway.
4. *Wrong, try again. The client is choking. Slapping a person on the back is not the best intervention for choking.*

9. **The nurse discovers a fire in the hospital. Which of the following nursing actions would be unsafe?**

1. Sound the nearest fire alarm.
2. Move clients who are in the immediate area of the fire.
3. Turn off any oxygen or electrical equipment.
4. Open the doors and windows to let the smoke out.

1. *This is a safe action in case of fire. This question has a negative response stem and requires an answer that is NOT correct. Try again.*
2. *This is a safe action in case of fire. The stem of this question asks for an option that is NOT safe.*
3. *This is a safe action in case of fire. This question has a false response stem and asks for an option that is NOT safe.*
4. ***Good work, you have identified the unsafe action. Opening doors and windows makes the fire worse by providing more oxygen. Doors and windows should be shut.***

10. **A client who gave birth two days ago, is in the bathroom after taking a shower. The nurse hears a loud thud and when she opens the bathroom door, she sees the client on the floor and a hair dryer in the sink with the basin full of water. The first nursing action is to:**

1. Assess the client to determine if she is breathing.
2. Assess the client for a heart rate.
3. Unplug the hair dryer, while taking care not to touch the client or any water or wet surface.
4. Perform a neurological assessment.

1. *While this is important and should be done, it is not the first action, since the safety of the nurse may also be at stake in this situation.*
2. *Assessing the heart rate is not the first nursing action during an emergency. The safety of the nurse may also be at stake during this situation.*
3. ***Good! The hair dryer in a basin of water appears to be the cause of this client's problem. The dryer still poses a serious electrical hazard and should be carefully unplugged, so that the nurse does not also become injured.***
4. *While this is an appropriate measure, the safety of the nurse may be at stake in this situation. This option is not the first action to initiate.*

11. **A young client is paralyzed from the waist down. He has a TV, radio, video tape player, stereo, and video**

game unit, which are all turned on most of the day. The nurse notices that there are not enough electrical outlets, and that extension cords with multiple outlets are in use to accommodate this equipment. The best nursing action is to:

1. Have the client's family take some of the equipment home.
2. Unplug as much of the client's equipment as necessary, after informing the client that an overloaded circuit can cause an electrical fire, and, therefore, the extension cords are not allowed.
3. Tell the client that only single-outlet cords can be used, and that you will check often to see if he wants to use anything not currently connected.
4. Call the maintenance department and have more wall outlets installed in the client's room.

1. *The client should not be deprived of activities that he finds entertaining. This option does not solve the problem at hand, either, since an electrical fire could occur while waiting for the family to take the equipment home.*
2. *This action would provide for the client's safety, but it does not provide any alternatives for consideration of the client. See if you can identify a better option.*
3. ***Good choice. This option allows the client the continued use of his electrical devices, and provides for the client's immediate safety by decreasing the possibility of an electrical fire.***
4. *Revamping the physical structure of a building is an administrative decision. Adding electrical outlets is expensive, and may not comply with fire or electrical codes. Also, this option does not solve the problem at hand, since an electrical fire could occur while waiting for the electrical work to be done.*

12. **A client is admitted to a long-term care facility. She requires total care. In providing mouth care to the client, the nurse should:**

1. Place the client on her back with a pillow under her head.
2. Use her thumb and index finger to keep the client's mouth open.
3. Use a stiff toothbrush to clean the client's teeth.
4. Place the client on her side before starting mouth care.

1. *No! Placing the client on her back during mouth care could result in aspiration of fluid into the lungs.*
2. *No. A padded tongue blade—not a thumb or an index finger—should be used to keep the client's mouth open.*
3. *No. A soft toothbrush should be used, not a stiff one.*

4. ***This is correct, because placing the client on her side encourages fluids to run out of her mouth.***

13. **While caring for a client, the nurse notices that the call light cord is frayed. The nurse should:**

1. Tell the client not to use the call light until it is fixed.
2. Remove the call light, and report the problem to the supervising nurse immediately.
3. Tape up the cord until the maintenance people can fix it, so the client will have a call light.
4. Tell the client to call out if he needs help, and to use the call light only in an emergency.

1. *This will not protect the client from potential electrical burns or shocks. A frayed cord is an electrical hazard.*
2. ***Correct. Removal of a frayed cord is the only way to protect the client from potential electrical burns. The supervising nurse will make arrangements for another call light or system for the client.***
3. *This is not a proper repair, and it will not protect the client from potential electrical burns or shocks. A frayed cord is an electrical hazard.*
4. *This will not protect the client from potential electrical burns or shocks. A frayed cord is an electrical hazard.*

14. **An elderly client is scheduled for surgery tomorrow. As the nurse enters the client's room, she notices that flames are coming out of the waste basket. The nurse would demonstrate an understanding of safety priorities by first:**

1. Placing the folded blanket from the client's bed over the entire opening of the waste basket.
2. Finding the nearest fire extinguisher to put the fire out.
3. Telling the client that he is not supposed to be smoking.
4. Pulling the nearest fire alarm.

1. ***Excellent! Placing the blanket over the waste basket will eliminate the source of oxygen, which is an element needed for a fire to burn. This is the fastest method in this scenario for putting out a small fire.***
2. *While an extinguisher will put out this small fire, it is not the best first action in this situation. While you are getting the extinguisher, the fire will increase.*
3. *This is not an appropriate first action during this emergency situation. Providing for the immediate safety of the client is most important.*

> **TEST-TAKING TIP:** The case scenario in this question does not tell you that the client has been smoking, and it is incorrect to assume this. Do not "read into" the question!

4. An attempt should be made to quickly extinguish a small fire at the time it is found, since it can become out of control within ten minutes. The fire alarm should be pulled as soon as initial measures to extinguish the fire have been implemented.

15.   **A client spills hot coffee on himself during breakfast. The first action by the nurse is to:**

1.   Remove the clothing from the burn area and apply cold water to the area.
2.   Call the physician.
3.   Make out an incident report.
4.   Cover the area with sterile towels.

1.   *Correct! Removing the "hot" clothing and applying cold water helps to stop the burning process.*
2.   *The physician should be notified, but after emergency first aid measures have been initiated.*
3.   *An incident report should be completed for any client who receives an injury while in a health care facility, but not until after steps have been taken to help the client.*
4.   *The area should be kept as clean as possible to prevent infection, but this is not the first action in the care of a burn.*

16.   **An elderly client has an IV with an infusion pump. While examining the infusion pump, the nurse notices a slight tingling in her hand as the plug is checked. What is the next nursing action?**

1.   Shut the pump off immediately.
2.   Inform the repair department to immediately shut off the pump.
3.   Recheck the equipment in one hour.
4.   Use a different electrical outlet site.

1.   *No! The question is trying to determine if you know what to do to prevent an electrical injury to the client and yourself. The pump should be turned off, but since the nurse has already felt tingling when she touched the plug, she should not shut the pump off herself! Look for a safer option.*
2.   *Correct. The repair department should be notified to immediately shut off the pump to protect the client and nurse from risk of electrical injury.*
3.   *No! The pump must be shut off to protect the client from the risk of electrical injury. Leaving the equipment operating and rechecking it in an hour increases risk for the client.*

4.   *No! This is an incorrect action that increases the risk of electrical injury for the client. Switching the electrical outlet will not ensure the client's safety. The pump must be shut off to protect the client from the risk of electrical injury.*

17.   **While caring for an infant you notice that one of the infant's stuffed animals in the crib has eyes that can easily be pulled off. The appropriate nursing action is to:**

1.   Take the toy out of the crib.
2.   Remove the eyes from the stuffed animal and return it to the crib.
3.   When the mother comes to visit, show her the eyes and explain that the infant could pull them off and choke on them.
4.   Send the toy home with the mother.

1.   *Best choice! The stuffed animal has the potential for causing the infant to choke. This is a safety issue, and steps should be taken to prevent an accident from occurring.*
2.   *Wrong! Since the case scenario indicates that the stuffed toy belongs to the infant and not the hospital, the nurse should not remove the eyes unless she discusses it with the mother first.*
3.   *No. Waiting for the mother to visit before providing for the infant's safety is not appropriate. The situation should be discussed with the mother, but this is not the best initial action. The immediate safety of the infant needs to be addressed.*
4.   *No. The toy can be sent home with the mother, especially if it has sentimental value and can be kept intact until the child is old enough that it is no longer a safety issue. However, the immediate safety of the infant needs to be addressed.*

18.   **A client is to have an electrical heating device applied to his lower back area. The plug on the heating device has three prongs, and the electrical wall outlet available only has two-pronged openings. The client's radio is plugged into a three-pronged outlet. The best action by the nurse at this time is:**

1.   Unplug the client's radio, which is plugged into a three-pronged outlet, and use that outlet for the heating device.
2.   Obtain an extension cord with a three-pronged outlet on it.
3.   Use a 2-pronged adapter to plug into the wall outlet, then plug the heating device into the adapter.
4.   Call central supply to see if you can get a heating device with a two-pronged plug on it.

1.   *This is correct. The third prong on the heating device when plugged into a grounded outlet is the ground, which prevents the client from*

receiving an electrical injury if the heating device malfunctions and causes a short in the circuit. The grounded electrical outlet provides a pathway for any stray electrical current.

2. *This action is unsafe. Extension cords should be avoided because of the potential for fire. In this case scenario, the client would not be protected from an electrical injury since there is no ground on the wall outlet or the extension cord. The ground prong on the heating device is not in contact with any pathway for stray electricity, which places the client at risk for electrical injury if the heating device shorts out.*

3. *This action is unsafe. Plug adapters or "cheater plugs" should never be used, since they eliminate the pathway for stray electricity, placing the client at risk for an electrical injury if the heating device shorts out.*

4. *This action is unsafe. Only grounded equipment should be used for any client. A two-pronged plug does not provide a ground to protect the client from an electrical injury.*

19. **The nurse is assisting an elderly client to eat. The client suddenly coughs a few times, then appears to be attempting to cough, making a whistling sound as he inhales. When using the Heimlich Maneuver on a conscious client, which of the following nursing actions is most effective?**

   1. Ask the client what he is choking on.
   2. Place your arms around the client and position your fist in the abdomen, between the bottom of the breast bone and the navel.
   3. Slap the client on the back until the object is expelled or until the client becomes unconscious.
   4. Stand in front of the person.

   1. *This is not appropriate because the client requires immediate assistance to dislodge the object that is obstructing the airway. It does not matter what the client is choking on, and the client will be unable to speak if he is choking.*
   2. **This is the correct placement for the fist in the Heimlich maneuver: above the navel and below the end of the sternum or breast bone. This is the necessary emergency action by the nurse.**
   3. *It is not helpful to slap someone who is choking. The client requires immediate assistance to dislodge the object that is obstructing the airway.*
   4. *This choice is the same as doing nothing at all. The client requires immediate assistance to dislodge the object that is obstructing the airway.*

20. **A client is ordered to have a hypothermic or cooling blanket applied because of a very high body tempera-**

ture. When caring for this client, which of the following is an inappropriate nursing action?

   1. Check the client's body temperature frequently.
   2. Place a layer of cloth, such as a bath blanket, between the client and the cooling blanket if the cooling blanket does not have a protective covering.
   3. Keep the cooling blanket in place until the client's body temperature is a couple of degrees below the desired level recommended by the physician.
   4. Remove the cooling blanket when the client's body temperature is a couple of degrees above the desired level recommended by the physician.

   1. *This action is appropriate. The client's temperature needs to be checked frequently in order to determine the body's response to the therapy and to prevent hypothermia. Look for something the nurse should NOT do.*
   2. *This action is appropriate. The client's skin should never come in direct contact with any method used for cooling purposes since tissue damage can occur. Look for something the nurse should NOT do.*
   3. **Good work, this action would be inappropriate. The client's body temperature will continue to cool after the blanket is removed. The client will become too cold if the blanket is not taken off until the temperature is below the desired level.**
   4. *This action is appropriate. The cooling blanket should be removed when the client's temperature is a couple of degrees higher than the desired level indicated by the physician, since the body will continue to cool after the blanket is removed. Look for something the nurse should NOT do.*

21. **In a long-term care facility, the nurse finds an elderly client on the floor. After having the client examined by the physician, the most important nursing action is to:**

   1. Call the family and ask them to stay with the client.
   2. Provide for the safety and protection of the client.
   3. Apply wrist and leg restraints to prevent the client from falling from the bed.
   4. Obtain an order for medication to sedate the client.

   1. *Wrong choice! Having a member of the family stay with the client may be a possibility if it can be arranged. This provides for the client's safety and allows some mobility for the client while in bed. However, this is not the best option.*
   2. **Excellent! This option in effect includes providing all appropriate interventions that address the safety needs of the client.**

TEST-TAKING TIP: *This is the global response option. It is a more comprehensive statement about providing for the client's safety. When you cannot identify the correct answer using your nursing knowledge alone, try to identify an option that is more global.*

3. *No! Application of a vest restraint may be appropriate to ensure the safety of the client, but leg and wrist restraint would be inappropriate because they do not allow for the client's mobility and are likely to cause agitation. This is not the least restrictive option for providing for this client's safety and therefore cannot be the first nursing action in this case scenario.*

4. *No! Sedating a client often makes the client more confused and more likely to behave inappropriately. Try to identify another measure that would be more appropriate for this client.*

22. **A client is confused and confined to bed. He has attempted to crawl over the side rails. The safe nursing action is to:**

    1. Apply restraints to the client immediately.
    2. Stay with the client and notify the supervising nurse.
    3. Remind the client to stay in bed.
    4. Tell the client to stay in bed, or else the nursing staff will have to restrain him.

    1. *This is incorrect. Applying restraints unnecessarily can be considered false imprisonment.*

    2. **Good work! This client is at risk for falling. Staying with the client protects him from harm. The supervising nurse can then notify the physician and request orders.**

    3. *This action will not provide for the client's safety because the client is confused. Try again.*

    4. *This is incorrect, because restraints should never be used as a punishment. Restraints are to be used only when necessary, to protect the client from harm.*

23. **The nurse is caring for a client who is on a moderate sodium diet for her pregnancy induced hypertension. Which of the following lunch selections by the client would signify an understanding of the diet?**

    1. Grilled cheese sandwich and tomato soup.
    2. Bologna sandwich and dill pickles.
    3. Chinese vegetables with soy sauce.
    4. Chicken salad sandwich with tossed salad.

    1. *Wrong. Most processed and canned foods are high in sodium. The cheese in the sandwich and the soup are high in sodium.*

    2. *Incorrect. Most cold cuts are high in sodium, and the dill pickles are very high.*

    3. *No, the Chinese vegetables are safe, but the soy sauce is very high in sodium.*

4. **Good choice. Chicken salad and tossed salad are both low in sodium.**

24. **Which observation by the nurse would warrant further teaching to prevent infection in the postpartum client?**

    1. Wiping the perineum from back to front.
    2. Large amounts of fluid intake.
    3. Use of tap water for peri-care.
    4. Frequent use of sitz bath.

    1. **Correct reasoning, this observed action is incorrect. All clients should be taught that correct perineal cleaning should always be done from front to back.**

    2. *No, this behavior by the client is helpful. Intake of large amounts of fluid reduces the chances of UTIs in postpartum women. This question has a false response stem, so you are looking for an INCORRECT behavior.*

    3. *No, this behavior by the client is correct. Clients are taught to use warm tap water for peri-care after each voiding and BM. This question has a false response stem, so you are looking for an INCORRECT behavior.*

    4. *No, this behavior by the client is correct. Frequent use of the sitz bath promotes circulation to the perineal area and promotes healing. This question has a false response stem, so you are looking for an INCORRECT behavior.*

25. **A client has mild preeclampsia. The nurse anticipates that which of these measures is likely to be included in her plan of care?**

    1. Bedrest.
    2. One gram sodium diet.
    3. Administration of magnesium sulfate.
    4. Hospitalization for close observation.

    1. **Correct. Mild preeclampsia is most commonly treated with bedrest. The client may or may not be hospitalized, depending on her ability to rest at home.**

    2. *Wrong. Restriction of sodium in the diet of a client with preeclampsia is not indicated. The client is usually put on a moderate sodium diet, not to exceed six grams per day.*

    3. *No, magnesium is not indicated unless the client has manifestations of severe preeclampsia.*

    4. *No, the client with mild preeclampsia may or may not be hospitalized. If she is hospitalized, she is usually admitted to the antepartum unit with routine assessments, every four to eight hours. Close monitoring would be indicated for the client with severe preeclampsia, for which 1:1 nursing care is common.*

26. The nurse is caring for a client admitted to the labor unit with premature rupture of membranes (PROM) at 30 weeks gestation. Which of the following nursing interventions should receive priority in the client's care?

    1. Frequent assessment for vaginal bleeding.
    2. Assessment of blood pressure every two hours.
    3. Careful assessment for signs of infection.
    4. Continuous fetal heart rate monitoring.

    1. *Wrong. There is no reason to suspect that PROM will increase the risk of vaginal bleeding.*
    2. *No, PROM has no effect on the maternal blood pressure.*
    3. ***Good choice. Whenever a woman's membranes rupture early, there is an increased risk for maternal and/or fetal sepsis.***
    4. *No, the fetal heart rate will be assessed routinely throughout the day, but continuous monitoring is not indicated.*

27. An infant's respiratory rate is irregular, 52 breaths per minute with several periods of apnea lasting five to 10 seconds. The infant's color is pink with acrocyanosis. What nursing measures are indicated at this time?

    1. Notify the RN immediately.
    2. Place the infant in a warmer environment.
    3. Continue to routinely monitor the infant.
    4. Assess the infant's blood sugar.

    1. *Wrong. This statement describes a normal pattern for a newborn infant. No action is indicated at this time.*
    2. *No, this infant is not exhibiting any signs of hypothermia.*
    3. ***Correct. This baby is exhibiting a normal respiratory rate and rhythm. No additional measures are needed at this time.***
    4. *No, this infant has no evidence of hypoglycemia such as jitteriness or poor suck.*

28. A client is experiencing morning sickness early in her pregnancy. She asks the nurse in the prenatal clinic what she can do to alleviate the problem. The nurse should recommend which of the following diets to reduce nausea and vomiting?

    1. Low residue diet.
    2. Fat free diet.
    3. Dry diet in a.m.
    4. Low carbohydrate diet.

    1. *No, the amount of residue in a diet does not affect nausea and vomiting related to pregnancy.*
    2. *Incorrect. Clients are taught to avoid greasy foods, but elimination of all fat from the diet could adversely affect the mother's health as well as the*

development of the fetus.
    3. ***Good choice. Eating dry crackers or toast in the morning before rising will reduce the risk of nausea in pregnancy.***
    4. *No. On the contrary, some researchers believe that low carbohydrate levels predispose the pregnant woman to nausea. Eating frequent small meals throughout the day that are high in protein and complex carbohydrates seems to decrease the incidence of nausea.*

29. Which of the following would the nurse teach the antepartum client to report to her health care provider immediately?

    1. White vaginal discharge.
    2. Urinary frequency.
    3. Unable to get wedding ring off.
    4. Nausea and vomiting.

    1. *Incorrect. The high levels of estrogen present throughout pregnancy often result in thick, white vaginal discharge. This is a good opportunity to teach the client about daily bathing and avoiding douching during pregnancy.*
    2. *Wrong. Urinary frequency is a common complaint in the first trimester, resulting from pressure of the enlarging uterus on the bladder.*
    3. ***Correct. Edema of the hands and face is found in the client with preeclampsia. The client who is unable to get her rings off is experiencing increased fluid retention and should be assessed for the presence of preeclampsia.***
    4. *Wrong. Nausea and vomiting are common in the first trimester and only need to be reported to the health care provider when the client is unable to ingest an adequate caloric intake.*

30. The client is seen at prenatal clinic in the first trimester. She tells the nurse that she is upset because, although she and her husband planned this pregnancy, she has been having many ambivalent feelings about the upcoming change in her life. The best response by the nurse is:

    1. "Have you spoken to your husband about these feelings?"
    2. "I would like you to see a counselor to discuss these feelings further."
    3. "These feelings are quite common in women early in pregnancy."
    4. "Don't worry, these feelings will go away."

    1. *No, this option is a good distractor. Communication between partners is important, but relating these feelings to her husband may worry him unnecessarily about these feelings, which are normal in early pregnancy. This response is not therapeutic for the client because it anticipates a yes/no*

reply from the client and refers to an inappropriate person. The response should address the client's feelings and concerns about the pregnancy.

2. *This response incorrectly indicates that the client's feelings are a cause for concern. The feelings are normal in early pregnancy.*

3. **Correct. The statement is true and reassures the client that many antepartum women experience similar feelings in early pregnancy. This response uses the therapeutic communication tool of providing information in addressing the client's concerns and feelings.**

4. *Wrong. This response devalues the client's feelings and fails to provide important information about them. The client has expressed concern about the feelings and needs to be reassured that they are normal in early pregnancy.*

31. Which of the following manifestations should the nurse anticipate in a baby born to a heroin-addicted mother?

1. Exaggerated reflexes.
2. Poor muscle tone.
3. Respiratory rate below 30 per minute.
4. Extended periods of sleep.

1. **Good work! The drug addicted newborn usually exhibits signs of hyperactivity within the central nervous system. Exaggerated reflexes is indicative of CNS irritability.**

2. *Incorrect. In fact, drug addicted babies usually have increased muscle tone.*

3. *Incorrect. The addicted baby often experiences respiratory distress that is manifested by rapid respirations, greater than 60 per minute.*

4. *No. Extended periods of sleep is a sign of CNS depression, not hyperactivity. This would not be anticipated in a drug addicted baby.*

32. How would the nurse assess an antepartum client for the presence of quickening?

1. Complete a vaginal exam.
2. Ask the mother if she has felt the baby move.
3. Request an ultrasound exam.
4. Provide a contraction stress test.

1. *No, a vaginal exam will not reveal if the mother has felt the fetus moving.*

2. **Good choice. The mother's first awareness of fetal movement, called quickening, generally occurs in the fourth or fifth month of pregnancy.**

3. *This is a possible answer, but it is not the best choice. Ultrasound exam will verify the presence or absence of fetal movement but it is expensive and it cannot confirm whether fetal movement has been detected by the mother.*

4. *No, this is not correct. A contraction stress test involves evaluating fetal response to artificially stimulated uterine contractions in an antepartum client.*

33. The nurse knows that which of the following can be used to positively confirm a pregnancy?

1. A positive pregnancy test.
2. Chadwick's sign.
3. Fetal movement felt by the midwife.
4. Braxton-Hicks contractions.

1. *No, this test is not definitive, because there are several other conditions that can cause a positive pregnancy test. These include menopause, choriocarcinoma and hydatidiform mole.*

2. *Incorrect. Chadwick's sign is a bluish discoloration in the cervix, vagina and vulva associated with pregnancy. After the first pregnancy, this discoloration may remain, making it of little value in subsequent pregnancies.*

3. **Correct! When fetal movement is felt by an experienced examiner, it is considered positive proof of pregnancy. Remember, the examiner must be experienced — so the mother's report of fetal movement is not positive proof of pregnancy.**

4. *Sorry. Braxton-Hicks contractions, which are painless tightenings of the uterus, can also result from hematomas or soft myomas in the uterus.*

34. Which technique would be best when the nurse wants a four-year-old to take deep breaths following an abdominal operation?

1. "I will give you a star each time you take a deep breath."
2. "You can go to the playroom when you finish doing your deep breathing."
3. "I'll leave your blow bottle here on your table, so that you can use it in a few minutes."
4. "Let's play a game of blowing cotton balls across your table."

1. *Not the best answer. This is going to be painful, and the child may not respond to this positive reinforcement, which occurs after the pain. Select another answer.*

2. *No, there is a better choice. This answer suggests a reward to be given after doing a painful procedure.*

3. *Incorrect. This probably will not be successful. Since the deep breathing will be uncomfortable, it is unlikely the child will perform it without coaching. Select again.*

4. **Yes, this is the best answer. By engaging the child in a form of play, the nurse may effectively distract him from the discomfort associ-**

ated with deep breathing following abdominal surgery.

35. **A 16-year-old male is to receive an intramuscular injection. To gain cooperation with this procedure, the nurse's first intervention is to:**

1. Tell him what he will feel.
2. Explain the purpose of the medication.
3. Offer him a choice of injection sites.
4. Describe the steps in the procedure.

1. Incorrect. Try to think about what is said when you go into an adolescent's room. Do you start off saying it's going to hurt? Try again.

2. Correct. After identifying the client, you state the purpose of the medication. An adolescent is capable of understanding and cooperating based on this information.

3. This choice may be offered, but it is not the first intervention, especially with an adolescent. Try again.

4. Incorrect. This is unnecessary and may increase anxiety. Many adults don't want to know all the details. Select another answer.

36. **While the nurse is caring for a seven-month-old female infant, she aspirates a small toy. She begins to cough and becomes cyanotic, and then no sound is made. At this time, which nursing action would be most appropriate?**

1. Perform a chest thrust.
2. Turn the client prone and administer back blows.
3. Stimulate further coughing.
4. Perform a modified Heimlich maneuver with one hand.

1. Incorrect. This is not the first step of when a coughing infant is identified. Select again.

2. Yes, this is the recommendation of the American Red Cross and American Heart Association for the treatment of choking in an infant.

3. No! The case scenario indicates that the coughing is ineffective, since no sound is heard. Effective action needs to be taken immediately. Choose again.

4. No, this is not the age-appropriate recommendation of the American Red Cross and American Heart Association for the treatment of choking in an infant. Try this one again.

37. **While working in a pediatric unit, the nurse encounters all ages of children. The nurse knows that a child's social interactions with peers are very important. During which periods of a child's life is this need greatest?**

1. Preschool and school age.
2. Toddler and preschool.
3. School age and adolescent.
4. Late adolescence and early adulthood.

1. No, this is incorrect. Think about the type of interactions a child has at each age. Select again.

2. Incorrect. The toddler's world is still the family. Make another choice.

3. Yes, this is correct. School age children begin to extend beyond the nuclear family, while adolescents need peers to help them develop their identity and independence.

4. Incorrect. Note that young adulthood is beyond childhood. This is a clue that this option is not the best choice. Choose again.

38. **The nurse knows that it is characteristic of the development of a 30-month-old child to:**

1. Tell tall tales.
2. Have a command vocabulary of about 10 words.
3. Weigh double his birth weight.
4. Have achieved complete primary dentition.

1. No, this is true of children of about four years old. Try again.

2. Incorrect. Language is much more developed at this age; the child's vocabulary consists of approximately 300 words.

3. Incorrect. This important developmental milestone should be attained by six months. Select again.

4. Terrific! This was a tough one. The 20 primary teeth should be erupted by approximately 30 months.

39. **The nurse knows that the most likely observable manifestation of impetigo is:**

1. Raised reddened areas.
2. Blisters with scattered pustules.
3. Crusted lesions with serous drainage.
4. Severe itching with sand-like rash.

1. No, this is not a sign of impetigo. Select again.

2. No, there are no blisters or pustules in impetigo. Try again.

3. Excellent! You have correctly identified a description of the lesions of impetigo.

4. No, this is not the sign of impetigo. This actually describes Fifth's disease. Choose again.

40. **The nurse is doing postoperative teaching for a three-month-old recovering from an umbilical hernia repair. Before discharge, the mother demonstrates understanding by stating she will:**

1. Maintain positioning in Semi-Fowler's after meals.
2. Limit activities for four weeks.
3. Expect bulging of the incision with coughing or crying.
4. Keep the infant's diaper away from the incision.

1. *No, this is not necessary and will not improve the postoperative surgical outcome. Make another selection.*
2. *No, you have probably forgotten the age of this child! You need to keep this in mind with all pediatric questions. Select again.*
3. *Incorrect. After surgery there should be no bulging when intra-abdominal pressure is increased. This would mean that the repair has been unsuccessful. Try another option.*
4. **Yes, this is correct. To prevent infection, the mother should be able to verbalize and demonstrate proper folding of the diaper to protect the surgical incision from contamination.**

41. **The nurse has completed preoperative teaching on a child scheduled for surgery to treat Hirschsprung's disease. The father expresses understanding when he says:**

1. "I'm glad my child will have normal BMS now."
2. "Now the diarrhea will finally stop."
3. "The operation will straighten out the kink in the intestine."
4. "The ostomy is only temporary."

1. *This statement indicates an erroneous expectation that the surgery will correct Hirschsprung's disease. The child will probably have three surgeries over a one-and-a-half to two-year period of time before normal bowel function is obtained. Select again.*
2. *Incorrect. Diarrhea is not a manifestation of this disease, so it would not be expected that this would be resolved by surgery. Try another option.*
3. *This statement refers inaccurately to the pathophysiology of this disease. Hirschsprung's is an area of the intestine without nerve innervation. Select again.*
4. **Yes, this statement by the client's father is correct. The initial surgery to treat Hirschsprung's is an ostomy, which relieves the obstructed area and allows the bowel distal to the ostomy to rest.**

42. **The nurse knows that the best way to determine the parent's ability to care for their child who has had an ostomy is to:**

1. Make sure both parents can explain the procedure.
2. Allow the parents to ask questions while the nurse

is performing the procedure.
3. Supervise the parents while they are doing the procedure.
4. Have the ostomy nurse do teaching before discharge.

1. *Incorrect. Did you read all the options before choosing the best one? This isn't the best way to know that the parents will be prepared at home. Try again.*
2. *No, this is not a method of evaluating knowledge. Reread your choices and select again.*
3. **Terrific! Always observe when possible, to see what the client and/or family can do. This is the real test of skill acquisition. This is how your clinical instructor evaluates your ability in a particular skill.**
4. *Incorrect. The ostomy nurse's seeing the client/ family does not indicate competency. Look again for an answer that will provide objective data for you.*

43. **In developing a plan for perioperative teaching for an adolescent, the nurse should be guided by the knowledge that:**

1. He may act as if he knows much more than he actually does.
2. He will only be interested in reassurance that things will go well.
3. The major part of the teaching should be delayed until after the surgery.
4. His parents should be the major focus of the teaching.

1. **Yes, of course! Adolescents may have a difficult time asking questions or being open to explanations. This is part of their struggle for independence.**
2. *Wrong. Adolescents are capable of abstract thought and realize that there are risks. Select again.*
3. *Incorrect. The content of perioperative teaching for an adolescent should be similar to that of an adult, since they have the ability to understand the concept of time as well as abstract reasoning.*
4. *Wrong. In adolescence, health professionals should switch the direction of teaching to the client. This does not mean that parents are excluded, but that they are no longer the focus, as they were in earlier periods. Make another choice.*

44. **A 15-year-old client has had an appendectomy. As the nurse prepares to give discharge instructions, the best approach is:**

1. Instruct both parents.
2. Explain to the client and one parent.
3. Explain to only one parent.
4. Any family member may be instructed.

1. *Not the best choice. Look at the age of the client, then try again.*
2. **Absolutely! When the client is an adolescent, the nurse needs to teach him too, or compliance will probably not be achieved.**
3. *No, this is not optimal. Look at the age of the client! Select again.*
4. *Incorrect. You are missing an important element in the question.*

45. **The nurse would best describe the most important aspect of planning the discipline of a hospitalized toddler as:**

1. Consistency in enforcing the rules.
2. Delaying punishment for wrong doing until parents are present.
3. Eliminating discipline while the child is ill.
4. Giving several warnings before actually disciplining.

1. **Correct. Although this may be a hard sell to parents who have guilty feelings about the hospitalization. Parents need to be reminded that discipline communicates love to children.**
2. *This is inappropriate. Rules should be maintained, even in the parents' absence. Select again.*
3. *This is inappropriate. Although some parents feel that this is appropriate. Choose again.*
4. *This is inappropriate because it encourages testing on the child's part to determine the limits. It could actually be dangerous, depending on the behavior. Choose again.*

46. **To relieve thirst immediately after a tonsillectomy, the best fluid for the nurse to offer a child would be:**

1. Anything the child likes.
2. Ice cream.
3. Orange Popsicle.
4. Grapefruit juice.

1. *Incorrect. In the immediate postoperative period, several types of fluids are contraindicated. Select again.*
2. *Wrong. Dairy products are contraindicated, since they may increase the viscosity of the mucous. Select again.*
3. **Correct. This is the best choice because it is a clear fluid and the cold temperature will decrease swelling and pain in the operative area.**
4. *Wrong. Citrus juices are acidic and will cause irritation to the incision site and increase pain. Select another choice.*

47. **A client is to undergo various diagnostic tests and procedures for evaluation of neurologic function. When the client asks the nurse which test uses a gas as a** contrast medium, the nurse responds that the test is the:

1. Pneumoencephalogram.
2. Echoencephalogram.
3. Brain scan.
4. Electroencephalogram.

1. **Correct. A pneumoencephalogram involves the instillation of air or a gas into the ventricular and subarachnoid system through a lumbar puncture. The CSF is partially replaced by the gas, and x-rays are taken. The air or gas serves as a contrast medium because air is less dense than fluid to x-rays.**
2. *Incorrect. An echoencephalogram is the recording of sound waves reflected by the brain structures in response to ultrasound signals. There is no contrast medium used.*
3. *Incorrect. A brain scan involves the use of a radio-isotope that is absorbed easily by abnormal tissue, such as a tumor. After the isotope is injected, the client waits one to three hours for absorption. A scintillation scanner is then used to image the brain.*
4. *No. An electroencephalogram (EEG) is a diagnostic test that evaluates the electrical activity of the brain. Electrodes are applied on the scalp surface and a reading is taken on graph paper. There is no contrast medium used.*

48. **In preparing a client for a bone marrow aspiration, which of these actions by the nurse should receive highest priority?**

1. Explaining the procedure to the client.
2. Shaving the site to be used for the aspiration.
3. Premedicating the client with a mild sedative.
4. Obtaining a set of vital signs immediately prior to the procedure.

1. **Yes, absolutely! As part of the hospitalized client's Bill of Rights, a client has the right to information about every procedure, including any risks or possible complications.**
2. *No, shaving the site is usually not necessary. Bone marrow aspirations are done either over the sternum or the iliac crest. It is now known that shaving can increase the chance of infection due to skin abrasions or irritations.*
3. *Incorrect. Bone marrow aspirations are done using a local injection of an anesthetic agent such as Novocain into the aspiration site. Premedication with a mild sedative is not indicated.*
4. *Not necessary. The procedure is invasive, but should have little impact upon the cardiovascular system of the client. Vital signs can be obtained per hospital policy.*

49. Which intervention should be included in the nurse's plan of care for a client who has returned from surgery for a below-the-knee amputation?

1. Elevate the stump on a pillow for 24 hours.
2. Keep suture removal set at bedside.
3. Elevate head of bed 60 degrees at all times.
4. Irrigate nasogastric tube every four hours.

1. *Correct choice. The stump is elevated for 24 to 48 hours to decrease edema, but no longer than 48 hours because of the danger of hip contractures, which would block rehabilitation efforts to achieve ambulation.*
2. *Not necessary. A large tourniquet should be kept at the bedside in case of hemorrhage. Fresh bleeding onto the stump dressing should be reported immediately.*
3. *No! The head of the bed should be elevated for meals and then lowered to a semi-Fowler's position. If the head of the bed is elevated 60 degrees at all times, the position predisposes the client to hip flexion contractures.*
4. *Incorrect. A nasogastric tube would not be indicated for a client with an amputation. Nasogastric tubes are generally indicated after surgery on the gastrointestinal tract or surgery in the abdominal region when the bowel has to be handled.*

50. While caring for a client in the oliguric phase of acute renal failure, the nurse's plan of care should include:

1. Maintaining reverse isolation to prevent infection.
2. Increasing the client's protein intake to prevent muscle wasting.
3. Encouraging fluid intake to prevent dehydration.
4. Meticulous skin care to prevent skin breakdown.

1. *Not necessary. The client in acute renal failure is not immunocompromised and does not require any form of isolation.*
2. *No, this would not be indicated during the oliguric phase of acute renal failure. Remember that the client's urine output is greatly decreased during this time.*
3. *No! Remember that the client is in the oliguric phase of renal failure, resulting in a decreased urine output. Encouraging fluids would only add to the client's problems of fluid retention.*
4. *Correct. The poor systemic nutrition and edema that go along with renal failure may cause skin breakdown. Meticulous skin care, frequent turning, and special pressure-relieving mattresses are very important.*

51. A client returns from surgery with two Penrose drains in place. In anticipation of frequent dressing changes, what

should the nurse use to most effectively reduce skin irritation around the incision area?

1. Montgomery straps.
2. Silicone spray.
3. Hypoallergenic tape.
4. Large, bulky absorbent pads.

1. *Correct. Montgomery straps are adhesive strips applied to the skin on either side of the surgical wound. The strips have holes for the use of gauze to "tie" the dressing secure. When the dressing needs changing, the ties are released, the dressing changed, and the ties then secured again without removing the adhesive strips. This taping technique will decrease irritation to the skin around the wound edges.*
2. *Incorrect choice. Silicone spray is appropriate, but its purpose is not to reduce skin irritation. Silicone spray is used OVER the adhesive to hold the dressing in place. The silicone waterproofs the dressing so that the client can bathe. It also isolates the area from contamination.*
3. *Incorrect choice. Hypoallergenic tape is used when a client is sensitive to adhesive material, but it still has to be removed with each dressing change. This could increase the risk of skin irritation.*
4. *Wrong. Large, bulky absorbent pads would certainly absorb more wound drainage, but would not prevent skin irritation around the incisional area.*

52. A post-mastectomy client returns to the surgical unit with a closed-wound gravity suction device (HemoVac) in place. Which action by the nurse would ensure proper operation of the device?

1. Irrigate the tubing with sterile normal saline once each shift.
2. Empty the device when it's full.
3. Keep the tubing above the level of the surgical incision.
4. Recollapse the device whenever it's one-half to two-thirds full of air.

1. *No! The Hemovac has a drainage catheter connected to a spring-loaded drum. It is not possible to irrigate the tubing. Patency is accomplished through another option.*
2. *No! The device should be emptied when it STARTS to fill, to prevent the weight of the collected drainage from pulling on the insertion site. There is no suction if the collecting device is full of drainage.*
3. *No! This action would defeat the purpose of a portable gravity suction device. The tubing should always be below the level of the incision to enhance drainage.*
4. *Yes, you understand the functioning of the*

Hemovac! The Hemovac, which has a drainage catheter connected to a spring-loaded drum, must be collapsed periodically to create the desired suction, which pulls fluid into the collection area of the device. As drainage or air accumulates, it is emptied and the Hemovac recompressed.

53. An 18-year-old client admitted with ulcerative colitis is being treated with sulfasalazine (Azulfidine). The nurse explains to the client that the major action of Azulfidine is to:

   1. Suppress inflammation of the bowel wall.
   2. Reduce peristaltic activity.
   3. Neutralize gastrointestinal tract acidity.
   4. Prevent a secondary infection.

   1. Correct. Azulfidine, an antibiotic, exhibits some antibacterial activity but it also serves as an anti-inflammatory agent to decrease irritation within the colon.
   2. Incorrect. Azulfidine will not reduce peristaltic activity. In fact, some of the common side effects of the drug are nausea, vomiting, and diarrhea.
   3. Incorrect. Azulfidine does not act to reduce GI tract acidity. This would be the action of an antacid.
   4. Incorrect. Azulfidine, although classified as an antibiotic, is not used to prevent a secondary infection. Recall that the client with ulcerative colitis already has an infection and treatment is aimed at correcting this problem first.

54. A client is admitted with open-angle glaucoma. He is started on a treatment regimen of timolol (Timoptic) and pilocarpine (Pilocar) eye drops. The nurse understands that these drugs will be administered:

   1. Until the client's intraocular pressure returns to normal.
   2. For three to six months or until manifestations subside.
   3. On a regular schedule for the rest of the client's life.
   4. For approximately 10 days, followed by a gradual tapering to discontinuance.

   1. Incorrect. This would not be a safe practice. The client's intraocular pressure is being controlled only by the medications. This practice would result in worsening of the client's condition after the medications were discontinued.
   2. Incorrect. This practice would result in worsening of the client's condition after the medications were discontinued. The client's intraocular pressure is being controlled only by the medications.
   3. Correct. Drugs prescribed for glaucoma are intended to enhance aqueous outflow or decrease

its production, or both. The client must continue the eye drops on an uninterrupted basis for life. These medications are not a cure, but they can control the disease and prevent further vision loss.
   4. Incorrect. The client's intraocular pressure is being controlled only by the medications. This practice would result in worsening of the client's condition after the medications were discontinued.

55. In assessing a client with Addison's disease, the nurse recognizes that a classic, characteristic sign associated with Addison's disease is:

   1. Hirsutism.
   2. Intention tremors.
   3. Skin discoloration.
   4. Petechiae.

   1. Incorrect. Hirsutism (increased facial and body hair) is seen in Cushing's disease, which is a hypersecretion of the adrenal gland hormones, especially glucocorticoids and mineralocorticoids. Addison's disease is hyposecretion of the adrenals and results in loss of body hair.
   2. Incorrect. Intention tremors are seen in multiple sclerosis, a neuromuscular disorder that affects primarily the central nervous system.
   3. Yes. An insufficient supply of cortisol signals the pituitary to secrete more ACTH, which results in increased dark pigmentation (bronzing) of the skin.
   4. Wrong choice. Petechiae (small intradermal or submucosal bleeds) are seen in Cushing's disease, which is a hypersecretion of the hormones from the adrenal glands.

56. A client is diagnosed with Cushing's disease. The nurse recognizes that the manifestations of Cushing's disease are primarily related to what endocrine dysfunction?

   1. Adrenal hyperfunction.
   2. Thyroid hyperfunction.
   3. Pituitary hypofunction.
   4. Parathyroid hypofunction.

   1. Correct! Cushing's disease, a hypersecretion problem, can be caused by an adrenal tumor, excessive secretion of corticotropin (ACTH) by the pituitary, or ectopic production of ACTH by tumors outside the pituitary, most commonly lung and thyroid cancers.
   2. Wrong. Cushing's disease is not a disorder of the thyroid gland. This would be known as Grave's disease.
   3. Incorrect. Pituitary hypofunction would affect the

adrenal glands (remember the release of ACTH from the pituitary), and would result in manifestations seen in Addison's disease, not Cushing's disease.

4. *Wrong. Cushing's disease is not a disorder of the parathyroid glands.*

57. A client with acquired immunodeficiency syndrome (AIDS) is taking zidovudine (Retrovir) 200 mg every six hours. Which side effect should the nurse anticipate with the use of this drug?

1. Nausea.
2. Fever.
3. Hypotension.
4. Lethargy.

1. ***Correct! Side effects of Retrovir include nausea, headache, muscular pain, sleeplessness, anemia, and granulocytopenia.***
2. *No, fever is not a side effect of Retrovir therapy. However, the client's CBC, BUN, and serum creatinine levels do need to be checked periodically because of the drug's cytotoxicity and nephrotoxicity.*
3. *Incorrect. Blood pressure is not affected by Retrovir therapy.*
4. *Wrong choice. Lethargy is typically a manifestation of AIDS—not Retrovir therapy.*

58. A client is admitted with burns to his upper chest and arms. The burns are wet and shiny with large blisters. The nurse understands that these burns would be classified as:

1. Superficial.
2. Partial-thickness.
3. Full-thickness.
4. Fourth degree.

1. *Incorrect. Superficial burns, known as first-degree, appear as dry, red skin without blisters.*
2. ***Correct. A partial-thickness burn, known as second-degree, appears as a mottled color with wet, shiny skin, with or without blisters.***
3. *Incorrect. Full-thickness burns, known as third-degree, appear as whitish and leathery with dry skin.*
4. *Incorrect. Fourth-degree burns, which include muscle and bone, appear as dead white with charred skin.*

59. Which burn client would be at greatest risk for developing respiratory problems secondary to burns and would require a priority respiratory assessment by the nurse?

1. A client with singed nasal hair.
2. A client burned on the lower chest while lighting a charcoal fire outside.
3. A client with a history of smoking, burned on the abdomen and upper thigh areas.
4. A client with blackened soot around his face and neck.

1. ***Good choice! Clients should be watched closely for signs of developing respiratory problems if they have burns of the face and neck, singed nasal hair, darkened membranes in the nose and mouth, or a history of having been burned in an enclosed space.***
2. *No. This client would not be at greatest risk because the burn did not occur around the face and/or neck.*
3. *Incorrect. Even though this client has a history of smoking, his burns are low enough on the body to avoid interference with respirations and a patent airway.*
4. *No. Although the presence of soot around the face and neck should be cause for further assessment, it does not prove the presence of a BURN to that area, which would put the client at high risk for a respiratory problem.*

60. Which intervention should be included in the nursing plan of care for a client who has just been admitted with a myocardial infarction?

1. Complete bedrest.
2. Limit fluid intake to 1500 cc in 24 hours.
3. Ambulate in hallway four times a day.
4. Monitor oxygen via nasal cannula.

1. *Wrong. The client is typically placed on bedrest with commode privileges in order to decrease the chances of the client performing the Valsalva maneuver when getting on and off the bedpan.*
2. *Not necessary. Although the client will be on intake and output, there is no need to limit fluid intake. Clients are always assessed for signs of heart failure, but there is no indication of this problem in the situation provided.*
3. *Incorrect action. Remember that the client was just admitted with a myocardial infarction. Walking is certainly an important part of the cardiac rehabilitation program, but it is not indicated at this time.*
4. ***Yes! Oxygen administration should be included, along with the administration of analgesia (usually morphine) to assure maximum relief of pain. Inhalation of oxygen even in low doses raises the circulating level of oxygen and reduces pain associated with low levels of circulating oxygen.***

61. In planning to teach a client who has the human immunodeficiency virus (HIV), the nurse should remember to alert the client that the virus can be transmitted:

   1. As soon as the client develops manifestations.
   2. To anyone having contact with the client's blood.
   3. Via the respiratory route, like tuberculosis.
   4. Only during the active phase of the virus, but not while it is inactive.

   1. *Incorrect. HIV can be transmitted BEFORE the client develops manifestations of an opportunistic infection or is diagnosed with AIDS. Because the client is asymptomatic and is not aware that he/she has the virus, the virus is usually transmitted during this time.*
   2. ***Correct. The concentration of the virus is highest in blood, and has been isolated in several body fluids, including sputum, saliva, cerebrospinal fluid, urine, and semen. Clients with HIV are cautioned to practice safe sex and to avoid donating blood or sharing needles with others.***
   3. *Incorrect. HIV has not been found to be transmitted via the respiratory route, although the virus has been isolated in sputum. It is not a disease of airborne transmission, like tuberculosis. Evidence has indicated that HIV is transmitted only through intimate sexual contact, parenteral exposure to infected blood or blood products, and perinatal transmission from mother to neonate.*
   4. *Incorrect! The HIV can be transmitted at any time— there is no such thing as an active or inactive phase of transmission of this disease.*

62. What should be the nurse's priority goal of care for a client admitted with multiple myeloma?

   1. Prevention of decubitus ulcers.
   2. Adequate nutritional intake.
   3. Relief from pain.
   4. Maintenance of a patent airway.

   1. *This is not a priority goal of care. Multiple myeloma is a malignant disease of plasma cells that infiltrate bone, lymph nodes, liver, spleen, and kidneys. It does not decrease skin integrity. The client should remain as active as possible to decrease the chance of hypercalcemia. Try again.*
   2. *Incorrect. Clients with multiple myeloma do not have gastrointestinal tract manifestations. However, good hydration is essential to prevent renal damage from precipitation of protein in the renal tubules. Try again.*
   3. ***Yes! Clients with multiple myeloma may be unable to perform activities of daily living because of constant bone pain. Remember that multiple myeloma results in bone marrow infiltration by malignant plasma cells. Bone frac-***

tures are common, especially in the vertebrae or ribs.
   4. *No, there is no reason to be concerned that the client's airway would be affected. Multiple myeloma is a malignant disease affecting primarily the bone marrow. Try again.*

63. Six hours into the collection of a 24-hour urine specimen, one voided specimen is accidentally discarded by the client. The nurse should:

   1. Continue the collection, noting the loss on the lab slip.
   2. Notify the nurse in charge.
   3. Discard the previously collected urine and start the collection again.
   4. Notify the lab so that the collection can be reduced to six hours.

   1. *Incorrect. This action would give false results because the values would be based on less than a 24-hour collection of ALL voided urine.*
   2. *Not necessary. There is an action that the nurse can take independently prior to notifying the nurse in charge.*
   3. ***Yes, this is the correct action by the nurse. If a specimen is lost or contaminated in any way during the 24-hour collection, the process must begin again. ALL urine voided in 24 hours must be collected or the test results will not be valid. Remember that lab values are being monitored based on the average elimination of those elements in a 24-hour time period.***
   4. *Not appropriate. 24-hour collections are designed to be just that: no less and no more. Lost specimens mean delays and time lost in the analysis of the urine. Try again.*

64. If a nurse takes the following actions to prepare a client for an electroencephalogram (EEG), which one should be questioned?

   1. The client is given a mild sedative the evening prior to the procedure.
   2. The client's intake of coffee and alcohol is restricted 48 hours prior to the procedure.
   3. The client is told that the procedure is painless.
   4. The nurse washes and dries the client's hair prior to the procedure.

   1. ***Good work, you have identified the inappropriate nursing action! Tranquilizers and stimulants should be withheld for 24 to 48 hours before an EEG because these medications can alter the EEG wave patterns or mask the abnormal wave patterns of a seizure disorder.***

2. No, this action is correct and should not be questioned. Stimulants and tranquilizers should be withheld because they can alter EEG wave patterns or mask abnormal wave patterns.

3. No, this is a correct action. Electrodes are arranged on the scalp to record the electrical activity in various regions of the head. The procedure takes 45 to 60 minutes or longer if a sleep EEG is performed, and does not cause an electric shock.

4. No, this is a correct action. The hair should be clean and dry prior to the test. Remember that electrodes are going to be placed on the scalp.

65.   A client complains of a throbbing headache after a lumbar puncture. Which action by the nurse would be most appropriate at this time?

1. Darken the client's room and close the door.
2. Keep the client flat in bed for six to eight hours after the procedure.
3. Encourage the client to limit fluid intake for eight hours after the procedure.
4. Report the headache to the charge nurse.

1. No, this action would not be the most appropriate as it doesn't address the cause of the headache. Although this action is helpful for any client in pain, there is another option that is more therapeutic in this case.

2. **Yes! The headache following a lumbar puncture is probably due to continuing cerebrospinal fluid (CSF) leakage through the opening in the dura made by the needle. The headache is usually relieved when the client lies down. Increasing fluids to 2,000-3,000 ml in 24 hours is also helpful in replacing fluid and CSF quickly, unless contraindicated.**

3. No! Just the opposite should be done. Fluid intake should be encouraged to replace the cerebrospinal fluid that was removed during the test. This will help decrease the likelihood of post-spinal headaches.

4. Wrong action at this time. There are independent nursing actions that you can take to decrease the severity of post-spinal headaches, an uncomfortable but not life-threatening side effect of a lumbar puncture.

66.   During cardiopulmonary resuscitation (CPR), the nurse should assess the adult's pulse by feeling the:

1. Carotid pulse in the neck.
2. Brachial pulse in the arm.
3. Femoral pulse in the groin.
4. Radial pulse in the wrist.

1. **Correct. The carotid area is the pulse of choice because of its closeness to the heart and the**

ease with which it can be assessed after establishing an airway and giving the rescue breaths.

2. No, this not correct in an adult — but it is the correct pulse site to assess in the infant when performing CPR.

3. Incorrect. The femoral site is not preferred because of its distance from the heart and difficulty in palpating quickly during the pulse check, which occurs after four cycles of 15 compressions and two breaths, and every few minutes thereafter.

4. Incorrect. The radial pulse is one of the most distant from the heart and is not as reliable as another site that is closer to the heart.

67.   Which manifestation is least likely to be observed by the nurse in a client who is admitted with a myocardial infarction?

1. Cyanosis.
2. Nausea.
3. Chest pressure.
4. Acute indigestion.

1. **Yes! A client having a myocardial infarction typically exhibits pallor and cold, clammy skin (diaphoresis), not cyanosis.**

2. No, this is often a manifestation evident in a client who has had a myocardial infarction. Vomiting may also be present. Look for an option that is NOT usually seen.

3. Incorrect. Clients having a myocardial infarction typically present with continuous chest pain or a feeling of intense pressure, usually over the lower sternal region and the upper abdomen. In some cases, the pain may radiate to the jaw and neck. You are asked to choose an option NOT commonly seen.

4. Wrong. Clients with a myocardial infarction often deny the severity of their condition, referring to the pain or pressure as a "bad case of indigestion." Look for an option that would NOT commonly be seen.

68.   The nurse can expect that a client diagnosed with AIDS related complex (ARC) would have which manifestation?

1. No manifestations.
2. Evidence of opportunistic infection.
3. Fatigue and weight loss.
4. Inactive human immunodeficiency virus.

1. Wrong choice. Clients with ARC do have manifestations of AIDS, along with evidence of immunodeficiency.

2. No. The presence of an opportunistic infection in a client who is HIV positive would mean that the client has AIDS, not ARC.

3. **Correct! Clients with ARC have two or more mani-**

festations of AIDS and at least two laboratory test results that indicate a state of immunodeficiency.

4. *Incorrect. Clients with ARC do have the virus in its active phase. Choose a more appropriate option.*

69. **The nurse understands that the primary purpose of the water seal in a chest tube drainage system is to:**

    1. Prevent the return of air to the chest cavity.
    2. Monitor the amount of drainage from the chest cavity.
    3. Serve as a suction control for the drainage system.
    4. Prevent the return of fluid to the chest cavity.

    1. *True. The primary purpose of the water seal is to prevent air from returning to the chest cavity. The water seal allows air and fluid to escape from the chest, but basically serves as a one-way exit system, preventing collapse of the lung from the accumulation of air and/or fluid.*
    2. *Incorrect. In a one-bottle system, the water seal bottle does serve as a collection unit for the chest drainage, but this is not its primary purpose.*
    3. *No, the water seal bottle can never serve as a suction control bottle. In a two-bottle system, the suction control bottle acts as a trap to control and decrease the amount of suction within the chest tube. Otherwise, the suction might be too forceful and damage the pleural membrane.*
    4. *Incorrect! The water seal does act as a one-way valve, but not for the purpose of preventing fluid from entering the chest cavity once it has been removed.*

70. **A client has just returned from surgery following a radical neck dissection with placement of a tracheostomy tube. Which assessment by the nurse should receive highest priority during the first 24 hours postoperatively?**

    1. Lung sounds and respiratory rate.
    2. Patency of the tracheostomy airway.
    3. Surgical dressing site.
    4. Pulse and blood pressure.

    1. *Incorrect. Although respiratory rate and lung sounds are important assessments for every postoperative client, they are not the priority for a client with a new tracheostomy.*
    2. *Yes! You remembered the basic principle that an open airway is essential for life. Since the client's airway may become obstructed by swelling or bleeding at the surgical site, this assessment is most critical and has the highest priority.*

3. *No, inspection of the dressing site to monitor for hemorrhage is important, but not as critical as another assessment that is a priority for a tracheostomy client.*
4. *Incorrect. Vital signs are important assessments for every postoperative client, but they are not as critical as another option given. What is the highest priority for every client?*

71. **In the initiation of cardiopulmonary resuscitation (CPR), which assessment should be made by the nurse PRIOR to beginning chest compressions?**

    1. Absence of respirations.
    2. Dilated pupils.
    3. Absence of pulse.
    4. Unresponsiveness.

    1. *Incorrect. The nurse would assess for absence of respirations prior to beginning mouth-to-mouth resuscitation.*
    2. *No. Dilated pupils (failure of the pupils to react to light) will eventually occur as the brain is deprived of its oxygen supply, but this is a late sign and is not assessed in the early initiation of CPR.*
    3. *Correct. Prior to beginning chest compressions, it is essential that the nurse assess for the absence of a pulse. The carotid site is assessed for five to 10 seconds. If no pulse is felt, then chest compressions are begun. Doing chest compressions on a client who has a pulse can lead to cardiac arrhythmias and death.*
    4. *No, establishing unresponsiveness is the first step in CPR. It is done prior to establishing an airway or beginning ventilations. Only after two breaths are given does the nurse do a further assessment. Remember the ABC's of CPR!*

72. **Which is the first nursing action when preparing to do tracheostomy care?**

    1. Open all sterile supplies and solutions.
    2. Hyperoxygenate the client with 100% oxygen.
    3. Apply sterile gloves.
    4. Wash hands thoroughly.

    1. *Incorrect. This action will be necessary in performing tracheostomy care, but it is not the first action.*
    2. *Incorrect. This action would be necessary prior to suctioning a client's tracheostomy. It is not needed prior to tracheostomy care.*
    3. *This would not be the first action in preparing to do tracheostomy care. Sterile procedure is necessary, but there is another option that should be performed first.*
    4. *Correct. A basic principle of medical and surgical asepsis is thorough hand washing be-*

fore contact with clients or equipment. This reduces the risk of transmission of microbes from other areas of the hospital to either the client or to equipment used with that client.

73. **A client is admitted with thrombophlebitis. Which intervention can the nurse anticipate will be included in the plan of care?**

    1. Bedrest for 10-14 days.
    2. Application of warm, moist heat.
    3. Restriction of oral fluids.
    4. Administration of vasodilating medications.

    1. *No, bedrest is usually ordered for five to seven days. A longer period of bedrest could predispose the client to other complications, such as pneumonia, constipation, and pressure ulcers.*
    2. **Correct. Warm, moist heat is used for its ability to decrease inflammation and edema, relieve muscle spasms, and promote comfort.**
    3. *Incorrect. Fluids would most likely be encouraged to prevent dehydration, which can contribute to concentration of the blood, further increasing venous stasis and clot formation.*
    4. *No, anticoagulant drugs such as heparin and warfarin (Coumadin) are used to prevent further clot formation. Vasodilating drugs would have no effect upon the existing thrombus.*

74. **When caring for a client in the phase immediately following a myocardial infarction, the priority goal for the nurse is to:**

    1. Decrease the client's anxiety.
    2. Prevent constipation.
    3. Relieve the client's pain.
    4. Restore fluid and electrolyte balance.

    1. *Incorrect choice. Although decreasing the client's anxiety is important, it is not the priority action in the immediate phase following a myocardial infarction. Try again.*
    2. *No. This action would certainly be important AFTER the immediate phase (defined as the first 24-48 hours). Straining at stool (Valsalva maneuver) will cause a transient drop in arterial blood pressure, along with decreased cardiac output. This may result in cardiac arrhythmias, the leading cause of death in clients following a myocardial infarction. Try again.*
    3. **Yes, this is the priority goal in the immediate phase following a myocardial infarction. Decreasing the client's chest pain will also decrease the oxygen consumption of the myocardium. The drug of choice is morphine sulfate, given intravenously. In addition to relieving the client's chest pain, morphine causes vasodilation of the vascular smooth muscle,**

helping to reduce myocardial workload. Try again.
    4. *Wrong choice. This is not the priority goal in the immediate post-myocardial infarction phase. The major concern is for adequate tissue perfusion. Try again.*

75. **A client is seen in the health clinic and is diagnosed with conjunctivitis of the right eye. An antibiotic ophthalmic ointment has been ordered. Which instruction would be appropriate for the nurse to give to this client?**

    1. Use a sterile glove and applicator to apply the antibiotic ointment.
    2. When washing your face, wash the infected eye first.
    3. Other family members may share your washcloth as long as you rinse it out first.
    4. Apply the ointment in a thin line, beginning at the inner corner and proceeding outward.

    1. *Not necessary. Ophthalmic ointments are applied directly from the tube, using clean technique. The tube should not be allowed to touch the eye and should be recapped as soon as the ointment has been applied.*
    2. *No! Remember the basic principle of asepsis: clean to dirty. The client should be taught to wash the unaffected eye first, then wash the infected eye. This prevents cross-contamination.*
    3. *No, not true! This would not be good aseptic practice. Conjunctivitis is highly contagious. The washcloth used by the client should NOT be used by any other family member.*
    4. **Correct. This is the proper procedure for applying ophthalmic ointment. Always proceed from the inner to the outer eye corner, to prevent the medication from entering the lacrimal duct and thus the general circulation.**

76. **The nurse is preparing a client for an arthroscopic examination of her left knee. She asks the nurse about her level of activity following the procedure. Which response by the nurse is appropriate?**

    1. "You will be on bedrest for 24 hours."
    2. "You will have to use crutches with no weight bearing on the left leg for several days."
    3. "You will probably be allowed to walk after the procedure."
    4. "You can return to all your normal activities immediately."

    1. *Incorrect. When a client has recovered from any sedation, she will be allowed to walk but should not overuse or strain the joint for a few days.*
    2. *Incorrect. The client may do partial weight bearing*

as soon as she has recovered from any sedation. Crutches and/or a knee immobilizer are often indicated if a biopsy or surgery was performed.

3. **Correct. The client will be allowed to walk but should not overuse or strain the joint. Crutches and/or a knee immobilizer are often ordered by the physician to increase the client's comfort and safety.**

4. *Not true. The client will need to prevent strain on the operative site for several days, and even weeks if surgery was performed.*

77. **A client with chronic renal failure is undergoing peritoneal dialysis. Which nursing measure will help most to promote outflow drainage of the dialyzing solution?**

1. Push the peritoneal catheter in approximately one inch further.
2. Elevate the height of the dialysate bag.
3. Apply manual pressure to the client's lower abdomen.
4. Turn the client from side to side.

1. *No! Pushing in the peritoneal catheter is contraindicated because it introduces bacteria into the peritoneal cavity.*

2. *No! The question asks how to promote OUTFLOW. Raising the height of the dialysate bag will only increase the rate of the inflow.*

3. *No! This technique is not recommended as it may cause displacement of the catheter and/or damage to the peritoneal lining as pressure is applied to the lower abdomen and to the catheter.*

4. **Excellent! Sometimes the peritoneal catheter is buried in the omentum, which will slow or stop the outflow drainage. If the fluid is not draining properly, move the client from side to side to facilitate removal of peritoneal drainage.**

78. **Which manifestations can the nurse expect to see in a client admitted with emphysema?**

1. Dyspnea, bradycardia.
2. Barrel chest, shallow respirations.
3. Cyanosis, productive cough.
4. Asymmetrical chest, dry cough.

1. *Wrong. Although dyspnea is seen in clients with emphysema, bradycardia is not. The heart rate will increase as the heart tries to compensate for less oxygen to the tissues.*

2. **Correct assessment! Clients with emphysema lose lung elasticity, the diaphragm becomes permanently flattened by overdistention of the lungs, the muscles of the rib cage become rigid, and the ribs flare outward. This produces the "barrel chest" typical of emphysema clients. Res-**

pirations are also shallow because of decreased lung elasticity.

3. *Incorrect. Clients with emphysema have skin that is pink in color, due to retained carbon dioxide (hypercapnia). Emphysema clients have only a small amount of mucous, unlike the client with bronchitis.*

4. *No, clients with emphysema would not have an asymmetrical (unequal) chest. The chest wall, although altered in shape, is not unequal. Remember that an asymmetrical chest occurs when two or more ribs are fractured, leading to unequal movement of the chest wall on inspiration and expiration. A dry cough may be present, but it is not a characteristic sign.*

79. **A client has a positive Mantoux test following a screening for tuberculosis. The nurse interprets this to mean that the client:**

1. Has active tuberculosis.
2. Was infectious at one time, but now has inactive tuberculosis.
3. Will require further evaluation.
4. Has never been exposed to the tubercle bacillus.

1. *No, a positive Mantoux is not diagnostic for active tuberculosis. Remember, the Mantoux is a screening test.*

2. *Incorrect. A positive Mantoux indicates that the body tissues are sensitive to tuberculin, but it does not mean that the client has had the disease.*

3. **Correct! A positive Mantoux indicates that the person has been infected with the tubercle bacillus (has been exposed) and further evaluation through sputum cultures and chest x-rays is needed.**

4. *Not true. A Mantoux is a screening test for tuberculosis and will detect tissue sensitivity to the tubercle bacillus.*

80. **To get the best ferrous sulfate absorption, the nurse should give this drug with:**

1. Milk.
2. Water.
3. Orange juice.
4. Meals.

1. *No! Milk or dairy products cause a decrease in iron absorption.*

2. *No, try again. Water does not facilitate absorption.*

3. **Correct. Vitamin C will potentiate the absorption of iron.**

4. *No, this is not correct. Iron is highly protein bound, so meals, especially of eggs, beans, or cereals will inhibit absorption. When iron is taken with food, absorption may be decreased by 1/3 to 1/2.*

81. **The nurse knows codeine is used cautiously in clients with chronic obstructive pulmonary disease because:**

    1. Coughs are not associated with COPD.
    2. There is a high abuse potential.
    3. Increased secretions may be produced.
    4. Interaction with beta agonists may be fatal.

    1. *Coughing is not a cardinal sign of COPD, as it is in tuberculosis, however, some clients do experience chronic coughing. Since COPD is characterized by in effective airway clearance, a productive cough should be encouraged.*
    2. ***You're right! In any chronic disease where there will be long-term medication, a high abuse potential is a danger to the client.***
    3. *Antitussives suppress the cough and may result in the pooling of secretions, but they do not produce increased secretions.*
    4. *With codeine, one is primarily concerned about interactions with medications that cause sedation. Beta agonists do not produce sedation.*

82. **The nurse would assess which of the following as an early manifestation of a complication of medication with hydrocodone bitartrate (Dihydrocodeine Bitartrate)?**

    1. Tachycardia.
    2. Slowed respirations.
    3. Change in level of consciousness.
    4. Fixed pupils.

    1. *Wrong. Tachycardia would be of concern if the nurse were detecting complications of beta agonists, xanthins, or anticholinergics. Tachycardia, however, is not an initial sign of complications of hydrocodone, which is a narcotic.*
    2. ***Very good! One of the dangers of a narcotic, such as hydrocodone, is depressed respirations, which manifests initially as slowed respirations. A baseline assessment with frequent monitoring is recommended.***
    3. *No, this is not an early manifestation. If narcotic sedation is severe enough, central nervous system sedation will be evident. The nurse should be alert for earlier signs, however.*
    4. *No, this is not an early manifestation. While it is true that overuse of a narcotic will eventually produce fixed pupils, this is an extremely late sign. The alert nurse will pick up earlier signs long before the client reaches this point.*

83. **The nurse understands that, for most clients with a cough that interferes with recovery, guaifenesin (Robitussin) is the medication of choice because:**

    1. The respiratory system is not depressed.
    2. There is an added analgesic effect.

    3. It is considered more effective than a narcotic.
    4. Guaifenesin is available without a prescription.

    1. ***You are absolutely right. Guaifenesin is a non-narcotic antitussive. The narcotic antitussives depress the respiratory system, leading to further complications.***
    2. *No, this is not true. Actually, the analgesic effect is caused by the narcotic antitussives, not the non-narcotic antitussives.*
    3. *No, this is not true. Non-narcotic guaifenesin and the narcotic antitussives are considered equally effective.*
    4. *This option is a true statement, but it is not the answer. The fact that a medication is available over-the-counter is not necessarily a benefit. It may be more convenient for the client, but the client has less consistent, if any monitoring or client teaching.*

84. **A client is diagnosed with hypertension and is treated with clonidine (Catapres) in the transdermal form. What statement by the client indicates to the nurse a need for further teaching about her drug therapy?**

    1. "I have trimmed the patch to make it fit better under my blouse."
    2. "I am reapplying the patch every seven days."
    3. "I understand that I can shower as usual."
    4. "I will notify my doctor if I get a rash."

    1. ***Yes, this statement by the client indicates a need for further instruction. If the patch is trimmed, part of the medication will be removed, thus reducing the dose.***
    2. *No, this action by the client would be correct. The client is following the proper routine for Catapres patches by reapplying the patch every seven days.*
    3. *No misunderstanding here! The client is correct in understanding that she can shower or bathe as usual.*
    4. *No misunderstanding here! A rash may indicate hypersensitivity, and the client is quite right to report one. Remember this question asked for an option that indicated that the client did NOT understand the teaching.*

85. **A client takes ibuprofen (Motrin) for her arthritis. To reduce esophageal irritation, the nurse should advise the client to take the medication:**

    1. Not with meals or any food.
    2. With a full glass of water and remain upright for 15-30 minutes afterwards.
    3. Before meals with a snack.
    4. After meals, then lie down for an hour.

    1. *This is incorrect. Ibuprofen can be taken with a meal to prevent gastric irritation. Try again.*

2. *Good! To reduce the serious risk of esophageal irritation caused by tablets lodging against the esophageal lining, the client should take the medication with water and remain upright.*

3. *This is not the best option. Taking ibuprofen with food helps reduce esophageal irritation, but there is an even better method. Try again.*

4. *This is incorrect. Lying down may cause gastric reflux into the esophagus. Make another selection.*

86. A client is a truck driver who sits for hours in his truck while driving. He has a swollen and inflamed right calf and is diagnosed with thrombophlebitis. He is hospitalized immediately and is started on a continuous heparin infusion and placed on bed rest. He asks the nurse how long it will take for the heparin to dissolve his clot. What is the best response by the nurse?

1. "It usually takes two to three days for heparin to work."
2. "I'm not sure. You will need to ask your doctor."
3. "Heparin begins to work immediately, but it does not actually dissolve clots. It prevents new clots from forming, and the present one from getting bigger."
4. "Heparin thins the blood quickly."

1. *This response is inaccurate. Heparin starts to work immediately. Warfarin (Coumadin) takes two to three days to begin working.*

2. *No, this response is not appropriate. The nurse can answer this question!*

3. ***This is the correct response to the client's question. The option correctly describes the action of heparin.***

4. *No. Many times we hear of heparin thinning the blood, but this is not really its function.*

87. A client will go home on warfarin (Coumadin). It is important for the nurse to instruct the client to:

1. Carry an ID card with him at all times.
2. Take only aspirin for headaches.
3. Eat lots of foods high in vitamin K, like broccoli, liver, and spinach.
4. Avoid any exercise.

1. ***Correct. The client must be able to alert anyone to his anticoagulant use in case of an emergency.***

2. *No! Aspirin and the NSAIDs will prolong clotting times and potentiate the effects of Coumadin.*

3. *Wrong. Broccoli, liver, and spinach contain high amounts of Vitamin K, which may decrease the effects of Coumadin.*

4. *No! Avoiding any exercise will lead to venous stasis and thrombophlebitis. This would not be a wise thing to do.*

88. A client has been receiving moxalactam (Moxam) 800 mg IV for septicemia. He is now ready for discharge. Which discharge instructions would be most appropriate for the nurse to give?

1. Do not drink any alcohol for at least three days after discharge.
2. Report any shortness of breath to your physician immediately.
3. Be sure to continue taking the Moxam (P.O.) until the entire prescription is gone.
4. Drink extra fluids for at least one week to help prevent kidney damage from the IV Moxam.

1. ***Good job! You remembered that alcohol may cause a disulfiram-like reaction when taken with certain cephalosporins: Cefobid, Mandol, Cefotan, and Moxam. Manifestations include stomach pain, nausea/vomiting, headaches, hypotension, flushing of the face, and tachycardia. Clients are to avoid alcohol-containing beverages, medications and OTC medications containing alcohol during administration of these medications and for three days after the medicine is discontinued.***

2. *Incorrect choice. Although dyspnea is significant, this manifestation, often associated with bronchospasm secondary to anaphylaxis, would most likely occur during the first administration of this drug—not after discharge. Try again.*

3. *No. You need to review the fact that Moxam is not absorbed from the GI tract and must be given parenterally (IV, IM only). Make another selection.*

4. *Not the best choice. Although cephalosporins are excreted via the kidneys and should be used cautiously in clients with renal impairment, there is no indication for the client to drink extra fluids for one week after the medication is discontinued.*

89. The nursing staff decide to develop a behavioral program to help a young anorexic client gain weight. Which of the following nursing interventions is inappropriate for this client?

1. Provide positive reinforcement for each pound that she gains.
2. Permit her to spend some quiet time in her room after each meal.
3. Allow her to select her meals from the same daily menu offered to all clients.
4. Refrain from commenting about her eating during meal times.

1. *This is appropriate. Privileges are used to reinforce weight gain. This question asks you to identify an INAPPROPRIATE intervention.*

2. **Very good! Clients are monitored for ninety minutes after eating to ensure that they do not go to the bathroom and purge the food they have just ingested. Since this is an inappropriate intervention, it is the correct response to this question.**

3. *An important focus of treatment is to develop independence in eating behavior. Selecting food from a menu is one way for the client to develop more of a sense of her own autonomy. This intervention is appropriate! The question asked you to identify the option that is INAPPROPRIATE.*

4. *This is an appropriate intervention. Meal time conversation should focus on the client as a person and not on her eating behaviors. This approach is often a change from family patterns, which may have focused on urging her to eat and reinforced her eating difficulties by rewarding them with attention. This question asks you to identify the option that is NOT appropriate.*

90. **In caring for the elderly, the nurse is guided by Erikson's observation that the elderly need to resolve conflicts between:**

    1. Ego integrity and despair.
    2. Intimacy and isolation.
    3. Generativity and stagnation.
    4. Identity and isolation.

    1. **Correct. Integrity requires the acceptance of one's life, the ability to give up fantasies and goals that could not be achieved, making peace with oneself, and taking responsibility for how one's life has turned out. Failure to reach this level of self-acceptance may result in despair, contempt for others, and fear of death.**
    2. *This is not correct. Intimacy versus isolation is the psychosocial crisis associated with adulthood.*
    3. *This is not correct. Generativity versus stagnation is the psychosocial crisis associated with middle age.*
    4. *This is not correct. Identity versus isolation is the psychosocial crisis associated with adolescence.*

91. **An 82-year-old widow is admitted to the hospital for hip replacement surgery. She appears alert and cooperative, although in great pain. While doing an assessment, the nurse learns she is disoriented to time and believes she is in a hotel. The nurse identifies acute confusion as a nursing problem. The nurse understands that which of the following would least influence the client's confusion:**

1. Her age.
2. Relocation to the hospital.
3. Her physical pain.
4. Bed confinement.

1. **Correct. Although acute confusion commonly occurs in persons over the age of 80, this condition is caused by physical and psychological problems that occur in advanced old age, not by age itself. Acute confusion can be successfully resolved by diagnosing and treating the underlying problem(s).**
2. *Relocation to a new environment, particularly when the move is sudden or unplanned, can result in a period of acute confusion for an elderly person. You are looking for an option that is NOT a likely cause of this client's confusion. Try again.*
3. *Pain or discomfort from unmet physical needs is often the cause of acute confusion in persons of any age, including the elderly. You are looking for an option that is NOT a likely cause of this client's confusion. Try again.*
4. *Bed confinement, especially in a horizontal position, is often associated with acute confusion because the individual does not have access to the full range of visual cues needed to maintain good orientation. You are looking for an option that is NOT a likely cause of this client's confusion. Try again.*

92. **The nurse has been caring for an elderly client who was admitted for hip replacement and is disoriented to time and place. The nurse requests to be assigned to stay with the client when she returns to the unit after her surgery. The rationale for this request is:**

1. The elderly client requires close postoperative supervision because of her unpredictable preoperative behavior.
2. The elderly client will most likely be agitated when she regains consciousness after surgery.
3. The many stresses associated with surgery could lead to further cognitive impairment in this elderly client.
4. Elderly clients are particularly vulnerable to the development of postoperative complications.

1. *This is not correct. The client had disorientation to time and place preoperatively, but she was not described as unpredictable. Do not read into the question!*
2. *This is not the best option. The client exhibited disorientation to time and place preoperatively, but she was not described as agitated. This client is at risk for many problems, including agitation, postoperatively. Read the other options and try to identify a better nursing rationale.*
3. **Correct. The many stresses, both physiological and psychological, associated with surgery,**

place this client at risk for further cognitive impairment postoperatively. Her postoperative behavior requires ongoing nursing assessment and intervention. This can be best provided by a nurse in constant attendance. The continuity of care with the nurse who attended the client before surgery may also help the client in maintaining orientation.

4. *This is a true statement, but it does not specifically address the issues and risk factors in this question. Read the other options again, and try to identify a better option.*

93. **A client taking lithium is discharged from the hospital after being taught to recognize the manifestations of lithium toxicity. The nurse knows learning has occurred when the client states that she will call the psychiatrist if she experiences:**

    1. Vomiting and diarrhea.
    2. Fine hand tremor.
    3. Polyuria.
    4. Drowsiness and lethargy.

    1. **Correct. Vomiting and diarrhea are beginning signs of lithium toxicity. The client should omit the next dose of lithium and contact the physician to obtain further instructions.**
    2. *Fine hand tremor is a common side effect reported by about half of the clients on lithium. It is not a sign of impending toxicity.*
    3. *Polyuria is a common side effect reported by about 60% of the clients on lithium. It is not a sign of impending toxicity.*
    4. *Drowsiness and lethargy are common side effects of lithium and are not signs of impending toxicity.*

94. **A nursing goal for abusive parents is for them to learn more effective parenting skills. Which of the following support groups would be an appropriate referral by the nurse to further this goal?**

    1. Parents Without Partners.
    2. Al-Anon.
    3. Parents Anonymous.
    4. Recovery, Inc.

    1. *This is not correct. Parents Without Partners is designed to meet the needs of single parents. It provides educational and socialization experiences for its members and their children.*
    2. *This is not correct. Al-Anon is a support group for families who have been affected by the compulsive drinking of a family member or friend.*
    3. **Correct. Parents Anonymous is a support group for parents who have been abusive and would like to learn more effective ways of rais-**

ing their children.

4. *This is not correct. Recovery, Inc. is a support group to prevent relapses in former psychiatric clients.*

95. **In developing a nursing care plan for an abused wife, which of the following is inappropriate?**

    1. Mutual goal setting.
    2. Assisting the client to mobilize her available support system.
    3. Providing information about available resources, such as the local women's shelter, child care services, and legal counseling.
    4. Notifying the appropriate authorities.

    1. *This is an appropriate element of the nursing care plan. The nurse must assist the client to set her own goals, and refrain from imposing her own views because the client might not be ready to accept them. The client needs time and ongoing support to deal with the abusive situation. The question asks you to identify the INAPPROPRIATE option.*
    2. *The nurse should help the abused spouse to identify a support system and an action plan that she can mobilize when she is ready to do so. The question asks you to identify the INAPPROPRIATE option.*
    3. *The nurse should inform the client of community resources and services that are available to her. The question asks you to identify the INAPPROPRIATE option.*
    4. **You have identified the inappropriate action by the nurse! Unless the client is a minor, the nurse cannot notify the authorities without the client's permission. Instead, the nurse should help the client develop a greater sense of empowerment by informing her that physical abuse is illegal and there are legal options open to her.**

96. **The nursing care plan for the antisocial client should stress:**

    1. Setting clear rules and expectations for the client's behavior on the unit, with the consequences for any violations clearly spelled out.
    2. Ignoring the client's past antisocial acts and focusing on current here-and-now issues.
    3. Supervising the client's behavior closely, to prevent any acting-out or destructive behavior while hospitalized.
    4. Helping the client to identify feelings and gain insight into what motivates his behavior.

    1. **Correct. The most therapeutic environment for this client is one where reality therapy is practiced. Rules and expectations should be**

clearly stated, along with the penalties for any behavioral violations. This is the best approach for assisting the client to develop more adaptive behavior.

2. *This is not correct. The client should be encouraged to discuss events leading up to his hospitalization, to help break the pattern of denying responsibility for his own actions.*

3. *This is not correct. The staff should take measures to discourage acting-out or other destructive behaviors, but such behavior cannot be prevented by closely supervising the client. There is a better option.*

4. *Reality therapy, a form of behavioral therapy, is more effective for clients with antisocial behaviors than is insight-oriented treatment. This cannot be the correct option.*

97. **The nurse is caring for an elderly client who will soon be discharged to a long-term care facility. What nursing action is most important for promoting her continued recovery?**

   1. Reviewing the client's nursing care plan with the client's daughter.
   2. Discussing the client's nursing care needs with her physician.
   3. Telephoning the charge nurse at the long-term care facility to explain the client's nursing care needs.
   4. Sending a written summary of the nursing care plan for the client to the long-term care facility.

   1. *This is not the most important action. The family should know about the client's needs for care, but there is a better way to promote continuity of care.*

   2. *This is not the best action, even for clients who will continue to use the same physician. Select the option that would better promote the continuity of her nursing care.*

   3. *This is a possibility, but it is not the priority action in promoting continuity of care.*

   4. **Correct. A written summary of the nursing care plan for the client is the best way of conveying the client's nursing care needs to the nurses who will actually work with her in the long-term care facility.**

98. **The nurse working with elderly clients knows that organic mental disorders:**

   1. Are the most prevalent type of psychiatric problem in this age group.
   2. Are almost always chronic.
   3. Need careful evaluation as they may be caused by a medical problem that could be treated effectively.
   4. Can be controlled with supportive and behavioral approaches, but eventually will lead to further deterioration and death.

1. *This is not a true statement. About 4% of persons over the age of 65 suffer from a dementia, with this percentage increasing with age to about 20% of those over the age of 80. Depression is a psychiatric problem that is much more common in elderly persons, with an estimated 15% to 20% of older adults affected at any point in time.*

2. *This is not a true statement because many of the organic mental disorders are acute and reversible.*

3. **Correct. Cognitive changes, such as memory problems, disorientation, and confusion, require careful evaluation to determine whether a physiological or medical condition is responsible. The client's cognitive state will return to normal when the underlying cause is identified and effectively treated.**

4. *This statement is only partially true. Chronic and irreversible organic mental disorders, such as Alzheimer's disease and AIDS dementia complex, are called dementias. However, there are some dementias that can be reversed when treated, such as the dementia caused by hypothyroidism. Delirium, a third type of organic mental disorder, has a rapid onset and is reversible.*

99. **The nurse working with elderly clients should remember that dementia in the elderly:**

   1. Is easy to distinguish from depression.
   2. May coexist with depression.
   3. Is not affected by medications.
   4. Cannot be concealed by the client.

   1. *This is not a true statement. Many times the manifestations of depression in an elderly client are mistaken for those of dementia. Manifestations found in both conditions include apathy, memory loss, and disorientation. A thorough assessment is needed to identify the appropriate disorder and treatment.*

   2. **Correct. Persons with dementia, especially in the early stages of the disorder, may suffer a depression when the individual becomes aware of his or her memory loss and other cognitive problems. Treatment of the depression will improve the client's cognitive functioning, but will not return it to a pre-dementia level.**

   3. *This is not a true statement. Certain medications, such as sedatives and hypnotics, affect alertness and other cognitive functioning, and can make the manifestations of a dementia worse.*

   4. *This is not a true statement. Denial is a common defense mechanism used by a client with dementia to deal with the anxiety of the memory loss and other manifestations of dementia.*

100. A woman is admitted to the psychiatric unit with a diagnosis of depression. Her husband reported that she
has been despondent since their youngest child left for
college two months before. The client states, "Do not
bother with me because I am totally worthless." Which
of the following is the most helpful response by the
nurse to the client?

    1.   "I have seen many valuable things about you."
    2.   "You feel worthless now because you are so de-
         pressed. You will feel differently when you begin
         to recover."
    3.   "You have been feeling very sad and alone for
         some time now."
    4.   "You really have a great deal to live for."

    1.   *This statement may appear to be an attempt to
         raise self-esteem, but clients with low self-esteem
         do not benefit from feedback they do not perceive
         to be justified. This statement contradicts the
         client's statement to the nurse and does not pro-
         mote therapeutic communication. Look for an op-
         tion that addresses the client's feelings and uses a
         therapeutic communication tool.*
    2.   *The first part of this statement is a possibility be-
         cause it is teaching the client about the manifesta-
         tions of her depression. However, the second part
         uses the communication block of false reassur-
         ance. The nurse cannot assure the client that she
         will feel better when she recovers. Look for an
         option that addresses the client's feelings and uses
         a therapeutic communication tool.*
    3.   **Correct. This response reflects the client's feel-
         ings in a non-judgmental way that indicates
         the nurse is willing to listen and accept what
         she is expressing. This will help the client feel
         more comfortable expressing feelings to the
         nurse.**
    4.   *This response would block further comments by
         the client because the nurse, in an effort to help, is
         really belittling the client's perceptions. Look for
         an option that addresses the client's feelings and
         uses a therapeutic communication tool.*

NCLEX-PN

Test 9

NCLEX-PN TEST 9

1. **In a hospital pediatric unit, which action by the nurse is best for preventing accidental poisoning to a toddler?**

   1. Place cleaning supplies on a counter out of reach of the toddler.
   2. Do not allow any plant life on the pediatric unit.
   3. Place cleaning supplies in a locked cabinet.
   4. Place all toddlers in specific rooms where they are supervised frequently.

2. **The nurse, walking by a client's room, notices that the top sheet on the client's bed is on fire and the client is in the bed. What is the first action by the nurse?**

   1. Get a fire extinguisher and spray the entire bed, including the client, who is at risk for burns.
   2. Grab a towel and beat the flames out by hitting the burning sheet.
   3. Take the blanket at the foot of the bed, place the blanket over the burning sheets to smother the flames, and smooth the blanket to remove any pockets of oxygen.
   4. Use the nearest fire hose to extinguish the flames.

3. **When an infant is choking and turning blue, but still is conscious, the best action by the nurse is to:**

   1. Turn the child on his back and attempt mouth-to-mouth ventilation.
   2. Support the child in a prone position with the head down and give four back blows.
   3. Perform the Heimlich Maneuver.
   4. Call an ambulance.

4. **A heavy object is blocking a doorway and must be moved. What should the nurse do when lifting it?**

   1. Hold the object away from the body.
   2. Bend from the waist to lift the heavy object from the floor.
   3. Maintain good alignment of the body.
   4. Always try to lift the object first, to determine if a co-worker should be asked to help.

5. **An elderly client is to receive a bath. In preparing the bath, the nurse would avoid which unsafe action?**

   1. Check the temperature of the tub room.
   2. Gather and take all of the necessary equipment to the tub room prior to the bath.
   3. Test the temperature of the bath water by having the client place his hand in the water.
   4. Place a mat or towel in the bottom of the tub.

6. **In transferring a client with a newly applied leg cast from a wheelchair to a bed, which is the first nursing action?**

   1. Have the client help move himself or herself.
   2. Use a transfer belt or client mover.
   3. Lock the wheels on the wheelchair and the bed.
   4. Have several people available to help.

7. **The nurse notices a crack in an electrical outlet. The IV pump that is plugged into the outlet appears to be working without any problems. Which is the best nursing action?**

   1. Use another outlet, then call the maintenance department to have the outlet changed.
   2. Since the pump is working, no action is necessary.
   3. Test the outlet by moving the plug a bit in the outlet, and observing if this affects the pump.
   4. Since the outlet works, continue to use it until maintenance can replace it.

8. **A client is receiving oxygen following a heart attack. The nurse notices, upon entering the client's room, that his wife is smoking a cigarette. Which of the following actions by the nurse would be inappropriate?**

   1. Explain to the wife that smoking in a room with oxygen could cause a fire and is not permitted.
   2. Tell the wife that a smoking lounge is available, and that smoking in a room with oxygen could cause an explosion.
   3. Obtain a "No Smoking" sign and place it on the client's door.
   4. Provide an ashtray for the wife to extinguish the cigarette.

9. **The nurse caring for a client who is unconscious would place the unconscious client in which position?**

   1. Semi-Fowler's.
   2. Trendelenburg.
   3. Prone.
   4. Supine.

10. **A client is to receive eye drops. Which of the following nursing actions best prevents injury to the eye during administration?**

1. Apply gentle pressure over the opening to the na-solacrimal duct.
2. Hold the tip of the container above the conjunctival sac.
3. Instruct the client to look upward.
4. Deposit the drops into the conjunctival sac.

11. **The nurse is caring for a client who is scheduled for surgery. When the transporter arrives to take the client to the operating room, the client is sitting in a chair. To achieve the client's safe transfer onto the stretcher, the best nursing approach is to:**

    1. Assist the client to get back into bed, and then move her across to the stretcher with the help of a drawsheet.
    2. Have the client use the chair to step up onto the stretcher.
    3. Assist the client to climb up onto the stretcher.
    4. Together with the transporter, lift the client from the chair onto the stretcher, keeping a wide stance and a straight back.

12. **When caring for a client using a cane, which nursing action best provides for the client's safety?**

    1. Schedule physical therapy visits to strengthen muscle mass.
    2. Remind the client to place the cane on the strong side.
    3. Remove the rubber tips to enhance ambulation.
    4. Place the cane safely in the closet at nap and bedtime.

13. **An elderly client is admitted with a broken right arm and contusions to the left wrist following an automobile accident. The nurse is preparing to feed the client. Which of the following nursing actions is least effective in preventing aspiration?**

    1. Offer small bites of food.
    2. Order pureed foods.
    3. Have the client use her dentures while eating.
    4. Allow enough time for the client to chew the food well before offering more.

14. **While mixing a solution of bleach and water to be used as a disinfectant spray, the nurse discovers that there is more solution than will fit in the spray bottle. Which of the following actions by the nurse is unsafe?**

    1. Pour the excess solution into an empty container, label the container as to contents, and place it in the cleaning supply closet.
    2. Discard the excess solution.
    3. Use the excess solution for the immediate cleaning job, then discard what is left.

4. Pour the excess into another cleaning solution container that has only a small amount of an ammonia solution left in the bottom.

15. **During an electrical storm the lights go out for a few seconds. Some of the lights come back on, but the ventilator is not working. What is the first nursing action?**

    1. Remove the client from the ventilator and ventilate with a bag and mask.
    2. Quickly check the electrical outlets to determine if the ventilator is plugged into an emergency power outlet.
    3. Call a code.
    4. Ventilate the client with oxygen using a positive pressure bag attached to the endotracheal tube, until full power is restored.

16. **A client is admitted to the hospital with a compound fracture. While making the client's bed, the nurse finds a capsule of medication in the sheets. The nurse knows that it would be inappropriate to:**

    1. Administer the medication to the client.
    2. Notify the physician of the missed dose.
    3. Determine what medication the capsule contains.
    4. Document the incident in the nurse's notes.

17. **The nurse is teaching an antepartum client about the physiology of pregnancy. Which of the following statements by the client indicates to the nurse an understanding of the functions of amniotic fluid during pregnancy?**

    1. "My baby receives nourishment from the amniotic fluid he drinks."
    2. "My baby is able to get rid of unwanted waste by urinating the amniotic fluid he swallowed."
    3. "The amniotic fluid helps to regulate my baby's body temperature."
    4. "The amount of fluid around my baby doesn't really matter."

18. **In caring for an antepartum client, the nurse knows that the onset of labor is confirmed by:**

    1. Rupture of membranes.
    2. Fetal engagement.
    3. Progressive cervical changes.
    4. Blood-tinged vaginal discharge.

19. **Which statement made by a nursing mother would indicate to the nurse that the client has a good understanding of breast feeding?**

    1. "I need to add 500 calories to my pregnancy diet

to meet my own nutritional needs as well as my baby's needs."

2. "I must drink milk every day in order to assure good quality breast milk."
3. "Fluid intake is very important to adequate breast milk production."
4. "I should avoid nursing my baby more often than every four hours, or the baby will get used to it."

20. **An antepartum client is HIV positive, which has been confirmed by a repeat test. Which of the following will the nurse include in her antepartum/postpartum course?**

1. She will need regular blood testing to evaluate her HIV status.
2. She should abstain from sexual intercourse to reduce the risk of transmission of the virus to her partner.
3. She and her infant will need to be isolated following delivery.
4. Counseling sessions should be offered to the client.

21. **A client is admitted to the labor unit in early labor. Once the admission process is completed, the nurse knows that this time is best used for:**

1. Teaching baby care to the parents.
2. Quiet time for the parents together.
3. Teaching the parents the stages of labor.
4. Teaching the mother relaxation techniques.

22. **You are caring for a postpartum client with cardiac disease. Which nursing intervention would be inappropriate in her plan of care?**

1. Frequent assessment of maternal vital signs.
2. Encourage increased fluid intake to promote good kidney function.
3. Gradual, progressive increase in activity.
4. Semi-Fowler's position when in bed.

23. **A client calls the antepartum clinic at eight weeks gestation and tells the nurse that her nephew, whom she sees almost daily, has rubella. The client's antepartum record indicates that she is rubella negative. What information should the nurse give to the mother at this time?**

1. Reassure her that she is immune to rubella.
2. Tell her that rubella is only a concern if it is present at the time of delivery.
3. Teach her that there is no problem unless she herself actually contacts rubella.
4. Provide information regarding termination of pregnancy.

24. **A client calls the antepartum clinic and tells the nurse that she became very dizzy while lying in bed that morn-**

ing, but that the feeling went away when she turned to awaken her husband. At this time the nurse would:

1. Instruct the client to come to clinic so that a thorough assessment of her vital signs and blood levels can be completed.
2. Instruct the client about vena caval syndrome and measures she can take to prevent it.
3. Ask the client if she has any family history of diabetes in her family, as this could be a manifestation of hyperglycemia.
4. Ask the client if she has ingested any drugs not prescribed by her physician.

25. **A client reports urinary frequency at eight weeks gestation. She asks the nurse how long this will last. The correct nursing response is:**

1. "It's impossible to predict, as urinary frequency differs from client to client."
2. "Urinary frequency usually lessens by the end of the first trimester."
3. "Urinary frequency usually persists throughout the pregnancy."
4. "Most clients report that urinary frequency disappears by 20 weeks gestation."

26. **How many vessels would the nurse expect to see in the newborn infant's umbilical cord?**

1. Two arteries, one vein.
2. One artery, one vein.
3. Two veins, one artery.
4. Two arteries, two veins.

27. **The nurse understands that the diagnosis of pregnancy is based in part on testing maternal blood or urine to determine the presence of:**

1. Progesterone.
2. Estrogen.
3. Human Placental Lactogen.
4. Human Chorionic Gonadotropin.

28. **The first priority of the nurse caring preoperatively for a child scheduled for repair of pyloric stenosis is:**

1. Prevention of infection.
2. Prevention of aspiration.
3. Provision of age appropriate activities.
4. Treatment of anorexia.

29. **Acetaminophen (Tylenol) is ordered for a nine-year-old child with a temperature of 102° F. The nurse preparing to administer the medication to the client realizes that he looks very thin for his age. What action would the nurse take first?**

1. Give him one-half the ordered dose.
2. Give the prescribed dose.
3. Measure his weight and calculate the dosage range.
4. Call the doctor and question the dosage.

30. **At what age would the nurse expect that the anterior fontanel would be closed?**

    1. Three weeks.
    2. Three months.
    3. Eighteen months.
    4. Four years.

31. **When working with three-year-olds, the nurse expects to observe which speech patterns?**

    1. Speech that is not understood by strangers.
    2. Sentences average four to five words.
    3. Only direct commands are understood.
    4. Practices speech by talking constantly.

32. **The mother of a four-year-old says that she is worried about her son's fine motor development. The nurse expects the child to be able to:**

    1. Tie shoelaces.
    2. Copy a square and circle.
    3. Draw a stick man with seven to nine parts.
    4. Print name without errors.

33. **The nurse knows that a successful myringotomy will result in:**

    1. Ear drainage with less pain.
    2. Bloody drainage.
    3. Ear pulling and irritability.
    4. Fever and purulent drainage.

34. **The nurse is to explain to the parents that a barium enema is to be given to a child with intussusception. If the parents understand the diagnosis, they should be able to explain that intussusception is:**

    1. A piece of bowel that is telescoped like a sleeve over itself.
    2. A narrow area that is very tight.
    3. An interruption where bowel isn't connected.
    4. An area that is bulging, ready to burst.

35. **Genetic testing has revealed that a client is a carrier of hemophilia A, but her husband is free of the disease. The nurse determines that understanding of the disease has been achieved if the wife states:**

    1. "There's a 50/50 chance that each of our female children will inherit the disease."
    2. "There's a 50/50 chance each male child will in-

herit the disease."
3. "All our male children will inherit the disease."
4. "All our female children will be carriers.

36. **A newborn has a cleft palate. The nurse understands the best plan for feeding is to have the mother:**

    1. Come to the nursery to feed the baby.
    2. Observe while the baby is fed in the nursery.
    3. Go with the father to feed the baby the best they can, in private.
    4. Feed her in her room while the nurse remains with her.

37. **A child is returning from a T & A. In addition to a thermometer and BP cuff, which equipment is most important for the nurse to gather?**

    1. Hot water bottle.
    2. Flashlight.
    3. A mouth rinse.
    4. Pain medication.

38. **The nurse is planning to reinforce the doctor's preoperative teaching. The child is seven years old and is scheduled for repair of aganglionic megacolon (Hirschsprung's disease). The best nursing approach is to:**

    1. Explain the procedure to the child by pointing to the child's abdomen.
    2. Discuss the procedure only with the child's parents.
    3. Present an age-appropriate explanation of the procedure to the child.
    4. Demonstrate the procedure to the child using a drawing or doll.

39. **After a six-month-old has had his cleft lip repaired, in order to comfort him the nurse should:**

    1. Offer a pacifier.
    2. Place him in the nurses' station.
    3. Rock him with his favorite blanket.
    4. Wrap him snugly and place him on his abdomen.

40. **The most important element of nursing care for a child in sickle cell crisis is:**

    1. Increased fluids.
    2. Blood administration.
    3. Genetic counseling.
    4. Physical therapy.

41. **The nurse is observing the chest tube drainage system of a client who had a thoracotomy yesterday. There is continuous bubbling noted in the suction control bottle.**

What should be the nurse's response to this observation?

1. Encourage the client to cough and deep breathe.
2. Check the suction control outlet on the wall for air leaks.
3. Notify the charge nurse of this observation.
4. Continue to monitor the client's respiratory status.

42. **In preparing a client for Buck's traction, the nurse knows that the primary purpose of Buck's traction is to:**

    1. Provide temporary immobilization, support and comfort prior to definitive treatment.
    2. Maintain skeletal immobilization.
    3. Prevent contractures.
    4. Alleviate pain.

43. **The nurse is caring for a client who has been fitted with a below-the-knee prosthesis. The nurse understands that the purpose of a prosthesis in clients with an amputation is to:**

    1. Promote an increase in muscle mass.
    2. Prevent phantom limb pain.
    3. Prevent damage to the stump.
    4. Provide weight bearing and assist in ambulation.

44. **A client recently diagnosed with grand mal epilepsy following a head injury is treated with phenytoin (Dilantin) to control her seizures. Which action by the client indicates to the nurse that there has been a lack of effective client teaching?**

    1. Carries a medical alert tag at all times.
    2. Identifies an aura.
    3. Takes medication even when seizure free.
    4. Uses alcohol in moderation.

45. **A client is scheduled for a gastroscopy. His wife is with him and will wait for him to return from the procedure. Which nursing measure must be included in his immediate post-gastroscopy plan of care?**

    1. Connect the nasogastric tube to gravity drainage.
    2. Keep him flat in bed for at least two hours.
    3. Have him cough and deep breathe every two hours.
    4. Instruct his wife not to give him ice chips.

46. **A client diagnosed as having diabetes mellitus has been stabilized with insulin injections daily. The nurse should include which information when planning discharge teaching for this client?**

    1. Increase insulin dose prior to unusual exercise.
    2. Acetone in the urine indicates a need for less insulin.

3. Always keep insulin vials refrigerated.
4. Systematically rotate insulin injection sites.

47. **In addition to routine postoperative care, immediate plans by the nurse for a laryngectomy client will focus on the need for:**

    1. Adequate fluid and electrolyte balance.
    2. Prevention of hemorrhage.
    3. Pain control.
    4. Patent airway.

48. **A client is being discharged after insertion of a permanent pacemaker for complete heart block. Which instruction, if given to him by the nurse, could endanger his physical safety?**

    1. Wear loose fitting clothing around the area of the pacemaker.
    2. Take your radial pulse for a full minute once each week.
    3. You may participate in any sport that doesn't involve physical contact.
    4. Avoid exposure to metal detectors at airport security check points.

49. **Universal precautions requires that a nurse wear which protective equipment when performing a nasogastric tube irrigation on a client with acquired immunodeficiency syndrome (AIDS)?**

    1. Sterile gloves.
    2. Goggles and nonsterile gloves.
    3. Nonsterile gown, sterile gloves.
    4. Nonsterile gloves.

50. **What is the nurse's primary concern when caring for a client who has acquired immunodeficiency syndrome (AIDS)?**

    1. Prevention of infection.
    2. Relief from pain.
    3. Restoration of fluid and electrolyte balance.
    4. Provision of psychological support to client and significant others.

51. **A client was in an automobile accident. The initial assessment revealed fractures of the left femur and pelvis and a large contusion on the head. Which assessment would best help the nurse determine the client's neurological status?**

    1. Pupillary responses.
    2. Verbal responses.
    3. Limb movements.
    4. Level of consciousness.

52. In preparing a client to be discharged, the nurse teaches him to position himself for postural drainage. To achieve success in this teaching program, which information about the client is most important?

    1. The type of bed the client will be using at home for the procedure.
    2. The amount of time required for the client to change positions.
    3. The client's goal concerning his ability to be self-sufficient.
    4. The client's ability to move about without assistance from others.

53. A client had a myocardial infarction. The nurse visits him at home one week following his discharge. He is taking chlorothiazide (Diuril) 500 mg daily and digoxin (Lanoxin) 0.25 mg daily. The nurse should give priority to assessing the client's knowledge of:

    1. Sources of potassium.
    2. Sources of sodium.
    3. Activity restrictions.
    4. Signs of a heart attack.

54. A client has been diagnosed with paralytic ileus. Auscultation of the client's abdomen by the nurse reveals the bowel sounds to be:

    1. Absent.
    2. Decreased.
    3. Hyperactive.
    4. Normal.

55. The physician orders a urine test. The nurse understands that specific gravity of urine is used to determine the amount of:

    1. Proteins in the urine.
    2. Uric acid crystals in the urine.
    3. Solutes in the urine.
    4. Epithelial cells in the urine.

56. The nurse has been assigned to care for a recently diagnosed IDDM client who is resistant to learning self-injection of insulin. The client insists that the nurse administer all the injections. What is the appropriate nursing response in dealing with the client's resistance?

    1. "You won't be able to go home unless you learn to give yourself the insulin injection."
    2. "I will have to tell your doctor that you refuse to give yourself the insulin injections. I'm sure she will be angry with you."
    3. "Don't worry about it. Your daughter can come over to your house every morning to give you the insulin injections."

    4. "It is important that you learn to give yourself the insulin injections. What can I do to help you overcome your fear of giving the injections?"

57. At 8:45 p.m., a client tells the nurse that he is feeling short of breath and requests that the nurse assist him in changing position. In addition to repositioning the client, the nurse should give highest priority to which nursing action?

    1. Put the client on 15 minute checks.
    2. Call the charge nurse to report the shortness of breath.
    3. Observe the rate, depth, and character of the client's respirations.
    4. Give a back rub to help the client to relax.

58. A client is admitted to the hospital with a head injury and is unconscious. The nurse would place this client in which position?

    1. Supine, to promote adequate blood volume to the cerebral vessels.
    2. Side lying, to prevent aspiration of secretions into the lungs.
    3. Semi-Fowler's, to help alleviate edema of the cerebral tissues.
    4. Modified Trendelenburg, to decrease the risk of shock.

59. A client will receive her first dose of heparin today for treatment of thrombophlebitis. While the client is receiving heparin, which of the following medications should the nurse have available?

    1. Warfarin (Coumadin).
    2. Protamine sulfate.
    3. Vitamin K.
    4. Dicumarol.

60. During cardiopulmonary resuscitation (CPR), the preferred method that the nurse should use for opening the airway is:

    1. Turning the head and opening the mouth.
    2. Performing a finger sweep of the mouth.
    3. Using the jaw thrust and head tilt method.
    4. Tilting the head and lifting the chin.

61. When a nurse performs cardiopulmonary resuscitation (CPR) on an adult victim, the ratio of chest compressions to lung inflations is:

    1. Five compressions to one ventilation.
    2. Ten compressions to one ventilation.
    3. Ten compressions to two ventilations.
    4. Fifteen compressions to two ventilations.

62. Four days after admission for a myocardial infarction, a client becomes short of breath and complains of pain in his chest. What is the nurse's priority action?

    1. Give the client a sublingual nitroglycerin tablet.
    2. Report this information to the nurse in charge.
    3. Assess the client's lung sounds.
    4. Place the client in modified Trendelenburg position.

63. A client is transferred to the recovery room after a colon resection for adenocarcinoma. The client develops internal abdominal bleeding postoperatively. Which finding would be reported by the nurse as an early sign of postoperative bleeding?

    1. Tachycardia.
    2. Oliguria.
    3. Hyperthermia.
    4. Bradypnea.

64. The nurse is admitting a client who is suspected of having diabetes mellitus. Which characteristics would the nurse expect to observe?

    1. Shallow, labored respirations.
    2. Increased blood pressure associated with slight periorbital edema.
    3. Periods of altered pulse rate.
    4. Increased urinary output.

65. To monitor a client for the most common complication arising from the administration of total parenteral nutrition, the nurse should:

    1. Weigh the client at the same time each day using the same scale.
    2. Keep accurate records of total intake and total output.
    3. Determine the increase or decrease in body weight each day.
    4. Take the client's temperature at least every four hours.

66. Ileostomy and colostomy are two types of fecal diversion. In explaining the differences between an ileostomy and a colostomy, the nurse would state that the stool of the ileostomy is:

    1. More liquid.
    2. Hard and brown in color.
    3. Firm and formed
    4. Similar in consistency to that from a colostomy.

67. The nurse is to insert a Levin nasogastric tube. The nurse understands that an inappropriate use of the NG tube is:

    1. Maintaining NPO status.
    2. Decompression.
    3. Lavage.
    4. Gavage.

68. A client has been recently diagnosed with cirrhosis of the liver. Which nursing measure is inappropriate for this client?

    1. Administer supplemental vitamins to compensate for the liver's inability to store vitamins A, B complex, D, and K.
    2. Administer tube feedings if the client's condition necessitates it.
    3. Encourage use of sodium to correct electrolyte imbalances.
    4. Begin planning discharge teaching about the impact of cirrhosis on the client's ability to tolerate common over-the-counter medications.

69. A 22-year-old sustained a fracture of the tibia and fibula while playing football. A long leg cast has been applied, and the client is admitted to the orthopedic unit. In providing nursing care for the client, which of the following is a vital consideration?

    1. Elevation of the leg in the cast on a pillow will minimize edema.
    2. Healing of a fractured bone requires an extended period of time.
    3. A long period of immobility may lead to atrophy of the muscle.
    4. Analgesics may be needed for pain associated with the fracture.

70. In providing care to a client with COPD, what is the primary nursing consideration?

    1. To not overtire the client.
    2. To plan adequate rest periods.
    3. To give only low flow oxygen.
    4. To allow the client to move at his own pace.

71. A 38-year-old is admitted to the hospital for a severe episode of gastrointestinal bleeding secondary to a peptic ulcer. He is scheduled for an upper GI series. In preparing the client for this diagnostic procedure, which explanation by the nurse is accurate?

    1. "An upper GI series will take five or six hours to complete. Since you will be waiting much of this time, you should take something to read with you."
    2. "This is a series of x-rays in which the entire GI tract is delineated. A liquid suspension of barium sulfate taken orally is the contrast medium."
    3. "You should not eat or drink anything after midnight on the evening before the test. Following the

first x-rays, full liquids are allowed."

4. "A laxative is administered the day before the test. On the morning of the test, you will be given soap suds enemas are given until the returns are clear."

72. **A client with atelectasis of the left lower lung is to receive intermittent positive pressure breathing (IPPB) four times a day. It would be appropriate for the nurse to instruct the client that:**

1. The treatment will last 45 minutes to an hour each time.
2. The client should take short, quick breaths during the treatment to get the maximum benefit from the medication.
3. The medication used in the treatment may cause nausea, so the physician has prescribed an antiemetic to be given beforehand.
4. The client should notice an increase in productive coughing during and after the treatment. This means that the medication is working.

73. **A client with a chest tube drainage system is being transported to the x-ray department for a chest film. Which action by the nurse indicates proper knowledge of caring for the chest drainage system?**

1. The nurse keeps the drainage system below the level of the client's chest at all times.
2. The nurse pins the excess tubing to the client's gown to prevent pulling at the entry site.
3. The nurse clamps the chest tube prior to transferring the client to the wheelchair.
4. The nurse attaches the drainage system to portable suction while the client is transferred to the x-ray department.

74. **A client has been given instructions about taking enteric-coated erythromycin (E-Mycin). Which statement by the client indicates the need for further teaching?**

1. "I can take these pills with my meals."
2. "The medicine has been coated so that it dissolves in my intestine, not my stomach."
3. "It's okay to crush a tablet as long as I make sure it dissolves completely in water before swallowing it."
4. "It's important that I finish the entire prescription, even if I don't feel sick anymore."

75. **Which of the following statements by a client would indicate to the nurse that the client has an accurate understanding of oral cloxacillin (Tegopen) administration?**

1. "I'll take the medicine with milk or an antacid so that my stomach won't get upset."

2. "I'll take the Tegopen with a large glass of fruit juice so that I get extra Vitamin C for wound healing."
3. "I'll take the medicine either one hour before or two hours after meals so that it will work better."
4. "I'll take the Tegopen at the same time as my blood pressure and heart pills so that I don't forget to take it."

76. **The nurse is caring for a client with a myocardial infarction who is taking chlorothiazide (Diuril) and digoxin (Lanoxin). Which diet is indicated?**

1. Diet low in sodium and saturated fats, high in potassium.
2. Diet low in unsaturated fats, sodium and potassium.
3. Diet high in potassium, Vitamin C and protein.
4. Diet low in sodium and saturated and unsaturated fats.

77. **A client is to be medicated with narcotics for four to five days after surgery. What precautions should the nurse take?**

1. Provide bed rest for the first two to three days.
2. Put the client's water and cigarettes close to her bed, within her reach.
3. Encourage the client to call for help to ambulate.
4. Suggest that the client limit the use of her medications, as addiction may result.

78. **A client is pregnant and has iron deficiency anemia. The physician orders an injection of iron dextran (Imferon) IM. How should the nurse plan to administer the injection?**

1. Use a size 23-25 gauge needle and administer in the deltoid muscle.
2. Use a size 20 or 22 gauge needle and administer deep in the thigh.
3. Select a 19-20 gauge needle and use the Z-track method to administer.
4. Select an 18 gauge needle and give deep in the buttocks.

79. **The nurse observes that, in the first few days of hospitalization, an 18-month-old client sits quietly sucking her thumb in the corner of her crib. When the nurse approaches the crib, the client shyly turns her head away from the nurse. The nurse understands that the toddler's behavior:**

1. Indicates a pathological reaction to being hospitalized.
2. Indicates that the relationship between parents and child should be assessed.
3. Demonstrates an anxiety reaction to the stress of

hospitalization.

4. Is an example of negative behavior and a beginning attempt at autonomy.

80. An eight-year-old client with a diagnosis of acute rheumatic fever is admitted to the hospital. Which age-appropriate activity would the nurse recommend for this client?

1. Playing computer games in the game room.
2. Visiting with several school friends.
3. Completing school assignments.
4. Listening to favorite cassette tapes.

81. Before she is discharged from the hospital, the client and her husband attend a client education class on the topic of depression and learn to recognize behaviors that could indicate a recurrence of depression. The nurse knows which of the following is inconsistent with signs of depression?

1. Psychomotor retardation.
2. Grandiosity.
3. Self-devaluation.
4. Insomnia.

82. A client with blastomycosis is being treated with amphotericin B (Fungizone). Which of the following statements by the client indicates to the nurse an accurate understanding of amphotericin B?

1. "The nurse told me that the drug is destroyed by light, so I'll be getting the medicine on the 11:00 p.m. to 7:00 a.m. shift."
2. "It sure would be nice if they used my Hickman catheter for administration of this medicine, but I guess the medicine is too irritating to the material in the catheter."
3. "I'm glad that I'll only have to take this medicine for 10 days because of the numerous side effects."
4. "I'll be given some Tylenol before the medicine is given to help decrease the fever that I'll probably get when the medicine is being given."

83. A nurse observes a client on the psychiatric unit muttering to herself and standing near a window. The client states, "The voices are telling me to jump. They say test the glass and then jump through." Which is the best nursing response to this statement?

1. "Where are these voices coming from? Do you recognize them as belonging to anyone that you know?"
2. "I think you are hallucinating. The only voices in this room are yours and mine."
3. "Tell the voices that you are not going to listen to them."
4. "You say you are hearing voices that make you feel like jumping through the window. I understand the voices are frightening to you, but I want you to know that I do not hear any voices."

84. A woman is crying continuously after the death of her husband. The son is distressed over his mother's crying and reports to the nurse that she has said that she wants to die. He asks the nurse to help "calm her down." The nurse's best response to the son's request is:

1. "All right, I'll talk with her and see if I can comfort her."
2. "If you just sit quietly with her, I'm sure she will calm down when she gets these feelings out."
3. "It's hard to see her so upset, but she needs to let these feelings out. We can both stay with her for a while."
4. "This seems to bother you more than it does her."

85. A women is distressed over the death of her husband. The son remarks to the nurse, "My father has been dead for six months now. I think my mother needs to get on with her life." What is the most helpful response by the nurse to the son?

1. "A death is usually a crisis for the whole family. How has your father's death affected you?"
2. "I agree. How can you help her find more pleasure in her life?"
3. "I think it would be helpful if you could give her more support."
4. "Perhaps she needs more time. Grieving often takes a year or more to complete."

86. A client with Type I insulin dependent diabetes mellitus (IDDM) usually walks two miles each day after breakfast. She is planning to participate in a Walk-a-Thon, in which she may walk as much as six miles. Which of the following responses by the nurse would be best in preparing the client for the Walk-a-Thon?

1. "Participating in a Walk-a-Thon is much too strenuous for you."
2. "Ask your doctor to increase your insulin dose the day of the Walk-a-Thon."
3. "Test your blood glucose immediately following the Walk-a-Thon."
4. "Eat some additional carbohydrates before you begin the Walk-a-Thon."

87. A newly diagnosed adult diabetic is doing a return demonstration of the proper technique for insulin injection. He draws up the correct dose of insulin using the proper technique, but when he is ready to inject the needle, he hesitates and says, "I'm not sure I can do this." Which response by the nurse would be best initially?

1. "I'll show you again how to inject the needle."
2. "I'll inject the needle for you this time."

3. "You're doing fine so far. Give it a try."
4. "Why are you so nervous? Do you need help?"

88. **Soon after being admitted to a rehabilitation unit, a chronic alcoholic says to the nurse, "I don't really need to be here. My wife and family make me drink. My wife spends all my money. My kid just had an accident with his car that will cost me a fortune in repairs." The therapeutic nursing response is:**

   1. "Tell me more about how your wife is spending all your money."
   2. "Could you tell me more about why your child's car accident cost you money?"
   3. "It sounds like you are having a great deal of financial difficulty."
   4. "Tell me more about your feelings about being here in the hospital."

89. **A 25-year-old client was admitted to the hospital with a diagnosis of diabetes mellitus. She tells the nurse that she is very concerned about being placed on a calorie-controlled diet, since she has been losing weight even though she has been eating more food. The best response by the nurse is:**

   1. "You won't have to worry about weight loss once your sugar is regulated."
   2. "The doctor will order enough food for you."
   3. "You have been losing weight because your body is not producing insulin, which is needed to use the calories you eat. When you start receiving insulin, a calorie-controlled diet will be recommended to help maintain your weight."
   4. "You probably needed to lose some weight to decrease your need for insulin."

90. **A confused, elderly client has wet herself and is standing in the hospital corridor in a puddle of urine. She looks ashamed and says to the nurse, "I want to go outside for a walk now." At this time, what is the most appropriate response by the nurse?**

   1. "Before we go for a walk, perhaps we can make a list that will help you make your bathroom trips easier."
   2. "Right now, let me wipe up the urine on the floor, and let's get a change of clothing for you. I am sure that this problem is upsetting for you."
   3. "This has been a problem for you. Let's see if we can find a solution together."
   4. "Wetting yourself is very upsetting. Yes, let's take a walk."

91. **A 78-year-old client is admitted to the hospital for an exploratory laparotomy. The client's daughter says to the nurse, "I wish I could stay with my father, but I need to go home to see how my children are doing. I really hate to leave my father alone at this time." The most helpful response by the nurse to the daughter is:**

   1. "Your father needs opportunities to be independent. This will help him become self-sufficient."
   2. "Your father is capable of taking care of himself. Try to allow him more independence."
   3. "Stress is not good for your father at this time. Perhaps you could call your children."
   4. "You are feeling concern for both your dad and your children. Let me know when you are leaving, and I'll stay with him."

92. **A 20-day-old infant is recovering from surgery for pyloric stenosis. The client's mother asked the nurse, "Now that my son has had this surgery, is it likely that pyloric stenosis will cause trouble later?" An appropriate nursing response to the mother would be:**

   1. "Why don't you talk to the doctor about your uncertainties regarding your son's future?"
   2. "He might develop obstructive manifestations later. If so, take him immediately to an emergency room."
   3. "He will not have manifestations again in childhood, but may have digestive difficulties in his adult life."
   4. "Recurrence of the obstruction or repetition of the surgical procedure would be unlikely."

93. **A chronic alcoholic has been hospitalized following a drinking binge. During a lengthy conversation with the nurse about his long history of alcoholism, the client becomes tense and uncomfortable. Which of the following is the initial response by the nurse?**

   1. "What did I say to make you feel so uncomfortable?"
   2. "Drinking for a long time can make anyone feel uncomfortable."
   3. "At what point did you begin to feel uncomfortable?"
   4. "Talking about your drinking will help you to recover."

94. **A 62-year-old female has been diagnosed with breast cancer. She has become quiet and thoughtful and says to the nurse, "What do you think people will say about me when I'm gone?" Which response by the nurse is the most helpful to the client?**

   1. "You will be remembered as a very nice person."
   2. "Do you feel that people will be talking about you after your death?"
   3. "At this time, a positive attitude can influence your recovery."

4. "The thought of your breast cancer must seem hopeless."

95. A woman is admitted to the ICU on a ventilator after attempting suicide. As the husband is talking with the nurse, he begins to cry. He says, "It's all my fault. I should have been home more often to keep an eye on her." Which response to the husband by the nurse would be most helpful initially?

1. "You seem to regret not being there for your wife. How can you feel that way when you have to earn a living?"
2. "At this time you need your privacy. I will return later, and we can talk then."
3. "This is an important issue that you need to bring up at your family therapy session."
4. "It must have been hard to be away when your wife was so sick."

96. A client is admitted to the psychiatric unit with a diagnosis of acute depression. After being hospitalized for a few weeks, the client says to the nurse, "I'm a terrible person, and I should be dead." Which response by the nurse would be appropriate initially?

1. "That is why you are here. We are trying to help you with your bad feelings."
2. "Feeling that way must be awful. What makes you feel so terrible?"
3. "Feeling like a terrible person is part of your illness. As you get better, those feelings will lessen."
4. "You are not terrible. You are not a bad person."

97. The nurse observes a depressed client in the day room. The client is shivering. Which response by the nurse would be most helpful to this client?

1. "Come with me to your room, and we will get a sweater for you."
2. "Why do you sit here without a sweater when you are cold?"
3. "What color sweater do you want me to get from your room for you?"
4. "When you are in the day room, you should dress so that you are not cold."

98. After a depressed client is discharged, her husband stops attending family counseling sessions. The husband states, "I do not have time for all that talking." Which response to the husband by the nurse would be most appropriate?

1. "Because your wife's condition is improving, you will be less involved in family therapy."
2. "You should continue attending the counseling sessions until the therapist tells you to stop."
3. "It must be difficult for you to talk about these family problems."
4. "Continuing counseling is necessary if your wife is to continue making progress."

99. A client was admitted to the psychiatric unit with a diagnosis of manic-depression. At 3:00 a.m., the client ran to the nurses' station, demanding to see her therapist immediately. Which response by the nurse would be best initially?

1. "Calm down, go back to your room, and I'll try to get in touch with your therapist right away."
2. "Regulations state that I can't call the therapist in the middle of the night, except in an emergency."
3. "You must be very upset about something to want to see your therapist in the middle of the night."
4. "You are being unreasonable and I will not call your therapist at 3:00 in the morning."

100. A client who has a broken leg is to be discharged from the hospital after crutch training by physical therapy. His friend, who recently recovered from a similar injury, brings in a pair of crutches for him. What is the best nursing action?

1. Since the friend knows how to use crutches, cancel the physical therapy order and allow the client to go home with his friend.
2. Inform the client that crutches are custom fitted for each client, and that he cannot use his friend's crutches.
3. Have the client try the crutches to see if they are the right size.
4. Send the crutches to physical therapy with the client for evaluation by that department.

NOTES

NCLEX-PN

Test 9
Questions with Rationales

NCLEX-PN TEST 9 WITH RATIONALES

1. **In a hospital pediatric unit, which action by the nurse is best for preventing accidental poisoning to a toddler?**

   1. Place cleaning supplies on a counter out of reach of the toddler.
   2. Do not allow any plant life on the pediatric unit.
   3. Place cleaning supplies in a locked cabinet.
   4. Place all toddlers in specific rooms where they are supervised frequently.

   1. Wrong. A toddler is able to climb and can obtain many things that are "out of reach." Placing cleaning supplies on a high counter does not ensure the safety of the toddler.
   2. Wrong. Some plants are poisonous and should be recognized by the pediatric staff. Many are not poisonous and should not be banned or sent home from a client's room unless there is a safety issue.
   3. Good! Cleaning supplies should be locked up to provide for the safety of toddlers. They are very inquisitive and are able to open many doors without difficulty. If the door is locked, the toddler can't open the door.
   4. Wrong. Toddlers need constant supervision — not just frequent — in order to promote a safe environment.

2. **The nurse, walking by a client's room, notices that the top sheet on the client's bed is on fire and the client is in the bed. What is the first action by the nurse?**

   1. Get a fire extinguisher and spray the entire bed, including the client, who is at risk for burns.
   2. Grab a towel and beat the flames out by hitting the burning sheet.
   3. Take the blanket at the foot of the bed, place the blanket over the burning sheets to smother the flames, and smooth the blanket to remove any pockets of oxygen.
   4. Use the nearest fire hose to extinguish the flames.

   1. Wrong. The best action is to put the fire out as fast as possible. Obtaining the fire extinguisher takes time and allows the fire to worsen during that time. Some fire extinguisher chemicals should not come in contact with skin, so spraying the client may cause further injury.
   2. Wrong. Waving an object causes a fire to burn better by creating a fanning of the flames.
   3. Great choice! The blanket will smother the flames by eliminating the source of oxygen. This is the fastest action for putting out this fire.

   4. Wrong, try again! A fire hose has high pressure behind the water and is very difficult for one person to hold under control. In addition, the force of the water could push the client out of the bed and onto the floor, causing further injury.

3. **When an infant is choking and turning blue, but still is conscious, the best action by the nurse is to:**

   1. Turn the child on his back and attempt mouth-to-mouth ventilation.
   2. Support the child in a prone position with the head down and give four back blows.
   3. Perform the Heimlich Maneuver.
   4. Call an ambulance.

   1. This is not helpful in this case scenario. Mouth-to-mouth ventilation is done for a choking infant after he becomes unconscious, in an attempt to deliver some air around the obstruction. This infant is still conscious.
   2. Right! In the conscious infant that is choking, four back blows are the first action to attempt to dislodge the object. If this fails, then four chest thrusts are delivered. The infant's mouth is visually examined for the object. If the object is seen, it is removed. If it is not seen, then the sequence of four back blows, four chest thrusts and visual examination of the mouth is repeated until the object is dislodged or the infant becomes unconscious.
   3. This is not an appropriate first action for an infant who is choking. The Heimlich Maneuver involves administering abdominal thrusts, which can injure the liver or spleen of an infant, therefore chest thrusts are only used if necessary after back blows have been delivered.
   4. Wrong. Emergency measures should be initiated first. If the infant does not respond immediately to emergency measures, then an ambulance or rescue unit should be contacted.

4. **A heavy object is blocking a doorway and must be moved. What should the nurse do when lifting it?**

   1. Hold the object away from the body.
   2. Bend from the waist to lift the heavy object from the floor.
   3. Maintain good alignment of the body.
   4. Always try to lift the object first, to determine if a co-worker should be asked to help.

1. *This is incorrect. The heavy object should be carried close to the body, which provides the base of support.*
2. *Wrong. Instead of bending from the waist, the nurse should squat to lift heavy objects.*
3. **This is correct. Good body alignment during lifting prevents injury.**
4. *This is not correct. The nurse should get help if an object appears to be too heavy to lift safely.*

5. **An elderly client is to receive a bath. In preparing the bath, the nurse would avoid which unsafe action?**

   1. Check the temperature of the tub room.
   2. Gather and take all of the necessary equipment to the tub room prior to the bath.
   3. Test the temperature of the bath water by having the client place his hand in the water.
   4. Place a mat or towel in the bottom of the tub.

   1. *The tub room should not be too cold or too hot, since the client may become chilled or too warm. This safe action is not the correct answer because the question is asking you to choose an UNSAFE action.*
   2. *All of the supplies should be available before taking the client to the tub room. This safe action is not the correct answer because the question is asking you to choose an UNSAFE action.*
   3. **Good! This action is unsafe. Sensitivity to hot and cold decreases as part of the aging process. There is a potential for the client to become chilled or to incur a burn if he determines the bath temperature. Also, the skin of an elderly client is often thin and fragile, which puts them at a high risk for burns.**
   4. *A mat or towel will help prevent a slip or fall as the client gets into or out of the tub. This safe action is not the correct answer because the question is asking you to choose an UNSAFE action.*

6. **In transferring a client with a newly applied leg cast from a wheelchair to a bed, which is the first nursing action?**

   1. Have the client help move himself or herself.
   2. Use a transfer belt or client mover.
   3. Lock the wheels on the wheelchair and the bed.
   4. Have several people available to help.

   1. *The client should participate in the transfer if possible. However, this is not the first action.*
   2. *Using a transfer belt or client mover may be appropriate, but it is not the first action.*
   3. **Very good! Before anything is done to transfer a client, the first action is to lock the wheels on all equipment so that the equipment will not move. If this is not done, the client may fall and be injured. The client's safety is at**

risk if the wheels are not locked.
   4. *It may be necessary to have other staff available to help. However, this is not the first action.*

7. **The nurse notices a crack in an electrical outlet. The IV pump that is plugged into the outlet appears to be working without any problems. Which is the best nursing action?**

   1. Use another outlet, then call the maintenance department to have the outlet changed.
   2. Since the pump is working, no action is necessary.
   3. Test the outlet by moving the plug a bit in the outlet, and observing if this affects the pump.
   4. Since the outlet works, continue to use it until maintenance can replace it.

   1. **This is the correct choice! A cracked electrical outlet should never be used and should be replaced, since it has the potential to start an electrical fire or to cause an electrical shock to any person who attempts to insert a plug.**
   2. *No, this is unsafe. Although the electrical outlet is presently working, it could quit working or cause a short and start an electrical fire.*
   3. *No, this is unsafe. Moving the plug in the outlet may cause the outlet to become further damaged and cause an electrical shock or electrical fire.*
   4. *No, this is unsafe. A broken electrical outlet should never be used because of the potential for an electrical fire or short.*

8. **A client is receiving oxygen following a heart attack. The nurse notices, upon entering the client's room, that his wife is smoking a cigarette. Which of the following actions by the nurse would be inappropriate?**

   1. Explain to the wife that smoking in a room with oxygen could cause a fire and is not permitted.
   2. Tell the wife that a smoking lounge is available, and that smoking in a room with oxygen could cause an explosion.
   3. Obtain a "No Smoking" sign and place it on the client's door.
   4. Provide an ashtray for the wife to extinguish the cigarette.

   1. *This option is appropriate. Oxygen supports combustion, which means it burns readily in the presence of a spark or flame. You are looking for an INAPPROPRIATE action.*
   2. **Correct choice! This action is inappropriate because it is not accurate to say that oxygen will cause an explosion. Oxygen will fuel a fire if it comes in contact with a spark or burning object such as a cigarette, but it will not cause an explosion.**
   3. *This option is appropriate. Any room that has oxy-*

gen in use should be posted with "No Smoking" and "No Open Flame" signs for safety purposes in order to prevent fires from occurring. You are looking for an INAPPROPRIATE action.

4. *This option is appropriate. The cigarette should be extinguished immediately, and an ashtray rather than a substitute container should be used if available. You are looking for an INAPPROPRIATE action.*

9. **The nurse caring for a client who is unconscious would place the unconscious client in which position?**

1. Semi-Fowler's.
2. Trendelenburg.
3. Prone.
4. Supine.

1. *Wrong. A Semi-Fowler's position is a sitting position with the head of the bed elevated 45-60 degrees. An unconscious client cannot swallow and may therefore choke on saliva or secretions in this position. The client may also slump to one side or the other.*
2. *Wrong. A Trendelenburg position requires that the lower extremities be elevated 20 degrees above the rest of the body. This position is used for clients who are in shock.*
3. **Very good! The prone position consists of placing the client on the abdomen. This position facilitates drainage of saliva and secretions. The lateral or side-lying position may also be used provide a change in position for the unconscious client.**
4. *Wrong. The supine position involves placing the client on his back. Since the unconscious client cannot swallow, choking on saliva or secretions can occur.*

10. **A client is to receive eye drops. Which of the following nursing actions best prevents injury to the eye during administration?**

1. Apply gentle pressure over the opening to the nasolacrimal duct.
2. Hold the tip of the container above the conjunctival sac.
3. Instruct the client to look upward.
4. Deposit the drops into the conjunctival sac.

1. *Wrong. Occlusion of the nasal lacrimal ducts prevents systemic absorption, but does not protect the eye from injury.*
2. **Correct. The tip of the container can injure the client's eye and should not come in contact with the eye.**
3. *Having the client look up decreases the likelihood of a blink reflex but does not protect the eye from*

injury. This action is appropriate, but it is not the answer.

4. *Depositing the drop into the conjunctival sac helps to distribute the medication throughout the eye, but it does not protect the eye from injury. This action is appropriate, but it is not the answer.*

11. **The nurse is caring for a client who is scheduled for surgery. When the transporter arrives to take the client to the operating room, the client is sitting in a chair. To achieve the client's safe transfer onto the stretcher, the best nursing approach is to:**

1. Assist the client to get back into bed, and then move her across to the stretcher with the help of a drawsheet.
2. Have the client use the chair to step up onto the stretcher.
3. Assist the client to climb up onto the stretcher.
4. Together with the transporter, lift the client from the chair onto the stretcher, keeping a wide stance and a straight back.

1. **Very good. The client should first get back onto the bed. Then, with the bed raised to the height of the stretcher, the client should slide across to the stretcher. This is the safest option for the client and staff in preventing a fall or back injury.**
2. *This is unsafe. Different items of equipment have specific purposes and they should be used accordingly. A client could fall when climbing onto or standing on a chair, or the chair could slide out from under the client during the transfer to the stretcher. The client is at risk for a fall.*
3. *Wrong! The client could miss the edge of the stretcher and fall, which could result in an injury.*
4. *Wrong! Clients should be lifted only when necessary, to avoid a potential fall for the client and back injuries to the staff.*

12. **When caring for a client using a cane, which nursing action best provides for the client's safety?**

1. Schedule physical therapy visits to strengthen muscle mass.
2. Remind the client to place the cane on the strong side.
3. Remove the rubber tips to enhance ambulation.
4. Place the cane safely in the closet at nap and bedtime.

1. *Wrong, because this is not a nursing action! While it maybe tempting to try to strengthen the client's muscle mass, that decision is within the physician's domain and would require a physician's order.*
2. **This is correct. The cane should always be placed on the client's strong side.**

3. *No! Any ambulation aid needs to have rubber tips on the end to prevent slipping. Removing the rubber tips places the client at risk for falls.*

4. *No! If the client has to go look for the cane, the client is in danger of falling.*

13. **An elderly client is admitted with a broken right arm and contusions to the left wrist following an automobile accident. The nurse is preparing to feed the client. Which of the following nursing actions is least effective in preventing aspiration?**

1. Offer small bites of food.
2. Order pureed foods.
3. Have the client use her dentures while eating.
4. Allow enough time for the client to chew the food well before offering more.

1. *Wrong choice, this action is appropriate. Offering small bites of food helps prevent the client from choking caused by too much food in the mouth. Look for the action that is NOT appropriate.*

2. ***Good, you spotted the action that was not helpful! Pureed foods should be used for clients who are not able to chew or do not have teeth. A client who is able to chew should receive foods of normal texture.***

3. *Wrong choice, this action is appropriate. Dentures provide the mechanism for the client to chew foods. If dentures are not used, then the client is at risk for choking on unchewed foods that are too large to swallow. You are looking for the action that is NOT appropriate.*

4. *Wrong choice, this action is appropriate. Choking can occur if the client does not have time to chew food well. Attempts may be made to swallow large boluses of food, or the mouth may become too full if the nurse feeds the client at a fast pace. You are looking for the action that is NOT appropriate.*

14. **While mixing a solution of bleach and water to be used as a disinfectant spray, the nurse discovers that there is more solution than will fit in the spray bottle. Which of the following actions by the nurse is unsafe?**

1. Pour the excess solution into an empty container, label the container as to contents, and place it in the cleaning supply closet.
2. Discard the excess solution.
3. Use the excess solution for the immediate cleaning job, then discard what is left.
4. Pour the excess into another cleaning solution container that has only a small amount of an ammonia solution left in the bottom.

1. *Wrong choice, this is a correct action. All containers should be labeled with the contents and stored in the appropriate area for the contents. Cleaning*

supplies and chemicals should not be kept near supplies that are for oral consumption or other uses where a client could be injured by someone picking up the wrong bottle.

2. *Wrong choice, this is a correct action. If there are no available containers that can be safely used, then discarding the solution is the best action in order to avoid poisoning or injury by another person using the unidentified solution for the wrong purpose.*

3. *Wrong choice, this is a correct action. If the solution was prepared because of the need to clean a particular area, then the person who prepared the solution can use the excess, then discard what is left after the immediate cleaning task is completed. Any solution that is not identified has the potential for being mistakenly misused by another person.*

4. ***Great choice, you have correctly identified the unsafe action. Mixing chlorine or bleach with ammonia produces toxic fumes that can cause damage to the respiratory tract when inhaled.***

15. **During an electrical storm the lights go out for a few seconds. Some of the lights come back on, but the ventilator is not working. What is the first nursing action?**

1. Remove the client from the ventilator and ventilate with a bag and mask.
2. Quickly check the electrical outlets to determine if the ventilator is plugged into an emergency power outlet.
3. Call a code.
4. Ventilate the client with oxygen using a positive pressure bag attached to the endotracheal tube, until full power is restored.

1. *This is not correct! A client on a ventilator has an endotracheal tube in place. A mask cannot be used because a seal cannot be made.*

2. ***Good work! All emergency equipment such as ventilators should be plugged into emergency outlets in case of power failure. If the ventilator was not plugged into the appropriate outlet, then the nurse should move the plug to an emergency power outlet.***

3. *Wrong choice! It is not necessary to call a code because of equipment malfunction. A code is to be called only if the equipment cannot be readily restored and the client's condition begins to deteriorate.*

4. *Wrong. This option may be necessary if the nurse cannot get the ventilator turned back on. The nurse's first effort, however, should be to restore the functioning of the ventilator.*

16. **A client is admitted to the hospital with a compound fracture. While making the client's bed, the nurse finds a capsule of medication in the sheets. The nurse knows**

that it would be inappropriate to:

1. Administer the medication to the client.
2. Notify the physician of the missed dose.
3. Determine what medication the capsule contains.
4. Document the incident in the nurse's notes.

1. ***Excellent choice, this action might endanger the client! The nurse does not know which dose of the medication was not taken by the client. Giving the client the capsule may result in an overdose if a capsule of the same medication has recently been given.***
2. *Wrong choice! The physician should be notified to determine if the medication should be repeated.*
3. *Wrong choice! Determining what the capsule contains is necessary to determine if the client is at risk for injury if a dose was missed. Some medications are very critical for a client's well-being.*
4. *Wrong choice! All incidents that can affect the client should be charted in the nurse's notes, in order to reflect any changes that may occur as a result of the incident.*

17. **The nurse is teaching an antepartum client about the physiology of pregnancy. Which of the following statements by the client indicates to the nurse an understanding of the functions of amniotic fluid during pregnancy?**

1. "My baby receives nourishment from the amniotic fluid he drinks."
2. "My baby is able to get rid of unwanted waste by urinating the amniotic fluid he swallowed."
3. "The amniotic fluid helps to regulate my baby's body temperature."
4. "The amount of fluid around my baby doesn't really matter."

1. *Wrong. The fetus does swallow amniotic fluid, but it has no nutritive value at all.*
2. *Incorrect. It is correct that the fetus does excrete fluid, but waste is removed through fetal/maternal circulation via the placenta.*
3. ***Good choice. One of the functions of amniotic fluid is to regulate the body temperature of the fetus. The fetus has no temperature regulation while in utero.***
4. *Incorrect. The amount of amniotic fluid is important. Too much amniotic fluid (hydramnios) is associated with kidney defects; too little amniotic fluid (oligohydramnios) is associated with GI defects.*

18. **In caring for an antepartum client, the nurse knows that the onset of labor is confirmed by:**

1. Rupture of membranes.

2. Fetal engagement.
3. Progressive cervical changes.
4. Blood-tinged vaginal discharge.

1. *Wrong. Rupture of membranes usually occurs during labor, but in some clients it will occur hours, days or weeks prior to the onset of labor.*
2. *No, fetal engagement occurs two to three weeks prior to the onset of labor in a nulliparous woman. It usually occurs during labor for a multiparous woman.*
3. ***Good job! When an examiner assesses the cervix and finds changes between examinations, this confirms labor has begun.***
4. *Incorrect. Prior to the onset of labor most women pass a mucous plug that has sealed the cervix during pregnancy. This is often associated with a small amount of blood-tinged mucous. Vaginal exam with manipulation may also cause blood-tinged discharge.*

19. **Which statement made by a nursing mother would indicate to the nurse that the client has a good understanding of breast feeding?**

1. "I need to add 500 calories to my pregnancy diet to meet my own nutritional needs as well as my baby's needs."
2. "I must drink milk every day in order to assure good quality breast milk."
3. "Fluid intake is very important to adequate breast milk production."
4. "I should avoid nursing my baby more often than every four hours, or the baby will get used to it."

1. *This statement is incorrect. The antepartum client adds 300 calories to her recommended daily allowance during pregnancy. If she is breast feeding she adds an additional 200 calories following delivery, for a total of 500 calories in excess of her recommended daily allowance before pregnancy.*
2. *This statement is not completely true. There are instances in which a woman does not want to or cannot drink milk. In these circumstances, she needs to consume other foods rich in calcium to prevent dietary deficiencies, and she needs an adequate intake of other fluids.*
3. ***Correct. Inadequate intake of fluids may decrease milk volume. It is suggested that nursing women consume 8-10 eight ounce glasses of fluid daily.***
4. *This statement does not indicate a good understanding of breast feeding. In order to promote milk production, women are encouraged to nurse frequently in the first days after delivery.*

20. **An antepartum client is HIV positive, which has been confirmed by a repeat test. Which of the following will the nurse include in her antepartum/postpartum course?**

1. She will need regular blood testing to evaluate her HIV status.
2. She should abstain from sexual intercourse to reduce the risk of transmission of the virus to her partner.
3. She and her infant will need to be isolated following delivery.
4. Counseling sessions should be offered to the client.

1. *Wrong. Repeating the HIV test is of no value. Pregnancy will not change her HIV status.*
2. *Wrong. If this mother uses precautions, she can reduce the risk of transmission to her partner. After receiving complete information about the virus and its transmission, the choice of sexual abstinence is between the client and her partner.*
3. *Incorrect. As long as universal precautions are followed by the client and the health care workers, the risk of transmission is rare.*
4. ***Very true. This client not only has to deal with her own HIV positive status but also the possibility of transmitting it to her newborn infant. Counseling is an important part of her antepartum plan of care.***

21. **A client is admitted to the labor unit in early labor. Once the admission process is completed, the nurse knows that this time is best used for:**

1. Teaching baby care to the parents.
2. Quiet time for the parents together.
3. Teaching the parents the stages of labor.
4. Teaching the mother relaxation techniques.

1. *Wrong. The couple's primary concern at this time is how they will get through the labor and delivery, not infant care.*
2. *No, the parents are usually very anxious at this time, and interaction with their caregiver is reassuring to them.*
3. *No, the parents do not want to be taught the process of labor. They just want to want to know how to cope with labor to achieve a safe delivery with a healthy baby.*
4. ***Correct. When you have the luxury of client contact in early labor, the time is best used to teach or review relaxation techniques that are useful throughout labor.***

22. **You are caring for a postpartum client with cardiac disease. Which nursing intervention would be inappropriate in her plan of care?**

1. Frequent assessment of maternal vital signs.
2. Encourage increased fluid intake to promote good kidney function.
3. Gradual, progressive increase in activity.
4. Semi-Fowler's position when in bed.

1. *Wrong choice, this is an important intervention for this client. Frequent assessment of maternal vital signs is an important part of postpartum care of the client with cardiac disease. The risk of cardiac decomposition is greatest throughout the first 48 hours. You are looking for an intervention that is NOT appropriate.*
2. ***Good thinking, this intervention is incorrect! After delivery the extra fluid that accumulated gradually throughout the pregnancy returns to the blood stream for excretion. This results in increased cardiac output and blood volume. The client's intake must be carefully monitored to prevent a fluid volume overload.***
3. *Wrong choice, this intervention is appropriate for this client. The activity of client with cardiac disease is progressed gradually after delivery to prevent undue stress on the heart. You are looking for an intervention that is NOT appropriate.*
4. *Wrong choice, this intervention is appropriate for this client. The position of choice for the cardiac client is Semi-Fowler's or side lying with the head and shoulders elevated. You are looking for an intervention that is NOT appropriate.*

23. **A client calls the antepartum clinic at eight weeks gestation and tells the nurse that her nephew, whom she sees almost daily, has rubella. The client's antepartum record indicates that she is rubella negative. What information should the nurse give to the mother at this time?**

1. Reassure her that she is immune to rubella.
2. Tell her that rubella is only a concern if it is present at the time of delivery.
3. Teach her that there is no problem unless she herself actually contacts rubella.
4. Provide information regarding termination of pregnancy.

1. *Incorrect. A negative rubella titer means that the client is at risk for contacting rubella if she is exposed.*
2. *Wrong. When the client contracts rubella in the first trimester, the fetus is at high risk for congenital anomalies.*
3. ***Correct. There is no risk to the fetus unless the antepartum woman actually has rubella herself. When a rubella negative woman is exposed to the virus, she can only wait to see if she actually contracts the disease herself.***
4. *Wrong. There is no risk to her fetus unless the client herself contracts the rubella virus.*

24. **A client calls the antepartum clinic and tells the nurse that she became very dizzy while lying in bed that morning, but that the feeling went away when she turned to awaken her husband. At this time the nurse would:**

1. Instruct the client to come to clinic so that a thorough assessment of her vital signs and blood levels can be completed.
2. Instruct the client about vena caval syndrome and measures she can take to prevent it.
3. Ask the client if she has any family history of diabetes in her family, as this could be a manifestation of hyperglycemia.
4. Ask the client if she has ingested any drugs not prescribed by her physician.

1. Incorrect. Assessment of the mother is not necessary unless she has other manifestations. Try again.
2. Correct. This is the typical picture of vena caval syndrome, which responds immediately to a position change to either side.
3. Wrong. Hypoglycemia, not hyperglycemia, is associated with dizziness. Try again.
4. Wrong. This answer suggests that the dizziness could be drug induced. This is not the most likely cause of the client's problem. Try again.

25. A client reports urinary frequency at eight weeks gestation. She asks the nurse how long this will last. The correct nursing response is:

1. "It's impossible to predict, as urinary frequency differs from client to client."
2. "Urinary frequency usually lessens by the end of the first trimester."
3. "Urinary frequency usually persists throughout the pregnancy."
4. "Most clients report that urinary frequency disappears by 20 weeks gestation."

1. Incorrect. The majority of clients report that urinary frequency lessens once the uterus becomes an abdominal organ. This usually occurs by the end of the first trimester or 12 weeks.
2. Correct. The frequency usually lessens or disappears altogether by the end of the first trimester.
3. Wrong. It is a very rare client who experiences urinary frequency throughout the entire pregnancy.
4. Sorry, this is rather late in the pregnancy for the client to continue to experience urinary frequency.

26. How many vessels would the nurse expect to see in the newborn infant's umbilical cord?

1. Two arteries, one vein.
2. One artery, one vein.
3. Two veins, one artery.
4. Two arteries, two veins.

1. Correct. The vein carries oxygenated blood to the fetus, and the two arteries carry unoxygenated blood back to the placenta.

2. Wrong. The number of vessels is incorrect. An infant born with only two vessels should be assessed carefully for birth defects.
3. No, this is not correct. Try again.
4. No, this is not correct. Try again.

27. The nurse understands that the diagnosis of pregnancy is based in part on testing maternal blood or urine to determine the presence of:

1. Progesterone.
2. Estrogen.
3. Human Placental Lactogen.
4. Human Chorionic Gonadotropin.

1. Wrong. Progesterone is a hormone critical to pregnancy but is not the basis for pregnancy testing.
2. Wrong. Estrogen is critical to the survival of pregnancy but is not the basis for pregnancy diagnosis.
3. No, human placental lactogen is a hormone excreted by the placenta but it is related to maternal gestational diabetes rather than pregnancy diagnosis.
4. Correct. Human chorionic gonadotropin is excreted by the placenta and promotes the excretion of progesterone and estrogen. This hormone is the basis for pregnancy testing.

28. The first priority of the nurse caring preoperatively for a child scheduled for repair of pyloric stenosis is:

1. Prevention of infection.
2. Prevention of aspiration.
3. Provision of age appropriate activities.
4. Treatment of anorexia.

1. No, this is not the first priority. The child has no incision and this disorder does not cause immunosuppression. Think about Maslow's Hierarchy of Needs, and try again.
2. Great, you must have remembered that with pyloric stenosis there is vomiting, which may occur as long as an hour after feeding. This child is at high risk for aspiration. This question is asking you to prioritize. According to Maslow's Hierarchy of Needs, if no physiological need is identified, safety needs come first.
3. Incorrect. You haven't selected the highest need. Think about Maslow's Hierarchy of Needs, and try again.
4. No, you're not even close with this answer. The child with pyloric stenosis isn't anorexic. In fact, they are hungry, due to vomiting, in the absence of nausea. They are suffering from malnourishment. Select again.

29. Acetaminophen (Tylenol) is ordered for a nine-year-old child with a temperature of 102° F. The nurse preparing

to administer the medication to the client realizes that he looks very thin for his age. What action would the nurse take first?

1. Give him one-half the ordered dose.
2. Give the prescribed dose.
3. Measure his weight and calculate the dosage range.
4. Call the doctor and question the dosage.

1. Incorrect and illegal. It is not within the nurse's capacity to alter the dosage prescribed. Select again.

2. No! Just because it is ordered by a physician and the child has a fever, it is not necessarily correct to administer the drug. The nurse has an obligation to the client to safeguard him. Choose another answer.

3. Excellent! Perhaps he just looks thin for his age. Measuring his weight and calculating the dosage will tell the nurse if the medication is within the safe dosage range.

4. This is not necessary at this time. There is another action the nurse can take first. If necessary, the nurse should instead report to the charge nurse, who would make the decision to call the doctor. Can you identify an option that is better in terms of verifying the observation that was made?

30. At what age would the nurse expect that the anterior fontanel would be closed?

1. Three weeks.
2. Three months.
3. Eighteen months.
4. Four years.

1. Incorrect. This is too young and would not allow the brain to grow normally. Pick another answer.

2. Incorrect. Perhaps you were thinking about the posterior fontanel. Choose again.

3. Good work! A child with premature or delayed closure needs follow-up.

4. No, this is too late. The anterior fontanel should be closed well before this age. Select again.

31. When working with three-year-olds, the nurse expects to observe which speech patterns?

1. Speech that is not understood by strangers.
2. Sentences average four to five words.
3. Only direct commands are understood.
4. Practices speech by talking constantly.

1. Incorrect. This is the level of language for two-year-olds. Choose again.

2. No, years of age is approximately the same as the number of words that the child will use in a sentence. Three-year-olds would tend to use three words in a sentence. Select again.

3. No, this is below the level of three-year-olds, who should be beginning to understand concepts, such as time. Try again.

4. Yes, that's right. Ask anyone with a three-year-old! They practice speech by talking non-stop and asking many questions.

32. The mother of a four-year-old says that she is worried about her son's fine motor development. The nurse expects the child to be able to:

1. Tie shoelaces.
2. Copy a square and circle.
3. Draw a stick man with seven to nine parts.
4. Print name without errors.

1. No, this is a skill expected of five-year-olds. Pick another option.

2. Great! This is a tough question! Copying a simple shape is achieved at age four.

3. No, this would be the expectation for a five-year-old. Select again.

4. Incorrect. Preschoolers often may reverse letters or capitalize incorrectly. Select another option.

33. The nurse knows that a successful myringotomy will result in:

1. Ear drainage with less pain.
2. Bloody drainage.
3. Ear pulling and irritability.
4. Fever and purulent drainage.

1. Correct. A myringotomy is an incision into the tympanic membrane that allows drainage of serous or purulent fluid from the middle ear.

2. No, this is not an expectation. Think about the reason that a myringotomy is performed. It is done to treat otitis media. Select again.

3. No, these are manifestations of the disease process that is treated with myringotomy. Choose again.

4. Incorrect. Fever would be reportable following any surgical procedure. Select again.

34. The nurse is to explain to the parents that a barium enema is to be given to a child with intussusception. If the parents understand the diagnosis, they should be able to explain that intussusception is:

1. A piece of bowel that is telescoped like a sleeve over itself.
2. A narrow area that is very tight.
3. An interruption where bowel isn't connected.
4. An area that is bulging, ready to burst.

1. Yes, the telescoping of the bowel found in intussusception could be described this way.

2. *Wrong. This is a description of Hirschsprung's disease. Choose again.*

3. *Wrong. This describes a form of atresia. Select again.*

4. *Wrong. This describes an area of distended bowel above an area of obstruction. Try again to describe what the bowel would look like in intussusception.*

35. Genetic testing has revealed that a client is a carrier of hemophilia A, but her husband is free of the disease. The nurse determines that understanding of the disease has been achieved if the wife states:

1. "There's a 50/50 chance that each of our female children will inherit the disease."

2. "There's a 50/50 chance each male child will inherit the disease."

3. "All our male children will inherit the disease."

4. "All our female children will be carriers."

1. *Incorrect. Females do not get the disease of hemophilia A. Try again.*

2. ***Yes, correct. The same chance exists for each male child that the disease will be inherited.***

3. *Incorrect. There is not 100% inheritance with all male children. Try again.*

4. *Incorrect. There is not 100% inheritance of the carrier trait with all female children of this mother. Choose again.*

36. A newborn has a cleft palate. The nurse understands the best plan for feeding is to have the mother:

1. Come to the nursery to feed the baby.

2. Observe while the baby is fed in the nursery.

3. Go with the father to feed the baby the best they can, in private.

4. Feed her in her room while the nurse remains with her.

1. *No, this will not provide the best possible situation for feeding this infant, who may be difficult. Choose again.*

2. *No, since the nurses aren't going home with this baby, this isn't going to prepare the mother to deal with feeding when the baby is discharged. Select again.*

3. *This wouldn't be recommended. Certainly both parents should learn, but would you leave them alone to work this out?*

4. ***This is the best answer. The nurse should be making observations. This mother/baby are at risk for poor bonding, and there may be suggestions the nurse can make about feeding techniques.***

37. A child is returning from a T & A. In addition to a thermometer and BP cuff, which equipment is most impor-

tant for the nurse to gather?

1. Hot water bottle.

2. Flashlight.

3. A mouth rinse.

4. Pain medication.

1. *Incorrect. This intervention is inappropriate, since warmth will increase edema. Choose again.*

2. ***Very good! This is needed to visualize the back of the throat following surgery.***

3. *Incorrect. Until the postoperative client is fully awake and has a return of the gag reflex, this should not be given. Also, most mouthwashes have alcohol, which would be irritating to the operative site. Select again.*

4. *Incorrect. Pain medication should be delayed until initial assessments, including BP, are performed. Choose another answer.*

38. The nurse is planning to reinforce the doctor's preoperative teaching. The child is seven years old and is scheduled for repair of aganglionic megacolon (Hirschsprung's disease). The best nursing approach is to:

1. Explain the procedure to the child by pointing to the child's abdomen.

2. Discuss the procedure only with the child's parents.

3. Present an age-appropriate explanation of the procedure to the child.

4. Demonstrate the procedure to the child using a drawing or doll.

1. *No, pointing or touching the child during explanations is considered to be a threatening approach. Select again.*

2. *Incorrect. The seven-year-old is old enough to understand age appropriate information. The child will be less fearful and more cooperative if taught what to expect. Pick another option.*

3. *This is not the best choice. Retention is not the best with verbal instructions. Choose again.*

4. ***Good choice! This approach incorporates a non-threatening approach and visual props, which will increase learning.***

39. After a six-month-old has had his cleft lip repaired, in order to comfort him the nurse should:

1. Offer a pacifier.

2. Place him in the nurses' station.

3. Rock him with his favorite blanket.

4. Wrap him snugly and place him on his abdomen.

1. *No! This would put pressure on the incision line, causing edema. Select again.*

2. *This is not the recommended way to handle a child who is in need of comfort, particularly after*

this surgery and at this age. Try again.

3. **Yes, this is the best answer, since you do not want the child to cry. Crying pulls on the incision, which may affect the healing. This child should be held as much as necessary to prevent crying.**

4. *No! This will cause pressure on the incision and may allow him to rub the suture line on the bedding. Select another answer.*

40. **The most important element of nursing care for a child in sickle cell crisis is:**

1. Increased fluids.
2. Blood administration.
3. Genetic counseling.
4. Physical therapy.

1. **Correct. Adequate hydration will prevent further sickling and damage to organs. Pain control is a close second for the child in sickle cell crisis.**

2. *Wrong. Blood administration is not a priority. Recall the pathophysiology of the disease, and make another selection.*

3. *Wrong. This is never a priority of the child in a critical situation. Make another selection.*

4. *Wrong choice, this is not a top priority. PT would be helpful to maintain function of limbs and joints, but not during crisis.*

41. **The nurse is observing the chest tube drainage system of a client who had a thoracotomy yesterday. There is continuous bubbling noted in the suction control bottle. What should be the nurse's response to this observation?**

1. Encourage the client to cough and deep breathe.
2. Check the suction control outlet on the wall for air leaks.
3. Notify the charge nurse of this observation.
4. Continue to monitor the client's respiratory status.

1. *Incorrect. Although this intervention is always important in the plan of care for a client with a chest tube, it has no connection to the bubbling in the suction control bottle.*

2. *No, this action is used to detect why a suction control bottle has little or no bubbling. This was not the observation made by the nurse.*

3. *Not necessary. Continuous gentle bubbling in the suction control bottle is a desired effect.*

4. **Correct choice. Since continuous bubbling in the suction control bottle is the desired effect, the nurse will continue to monitor the client's respiratory status. Persistent bubbling in the WATER SEAL bottle requires immediate attention. Fluid in this chamber should only fluctuate as the client breathes air in and out.**

42. **In preparing a client for Buck's traction, the nurse knows that the primary purpose of Buck's traction is to:**

1. Provide temporary immobilization, support and comfort prior to definitive treatment.
2. Maintain skeletal immobilization.
3. Prevent contractures.
4. Alleviate pain.

1. **Correct. This is the primary purpose of Buck's traction.**

2. *Incorrect. Only the limb immobilized is affected by Buck's traction. Try again.*

3. *Incorrect. Range of motion exercises are utilized to prevent contractures. Try again.*

4. *Incorrect. Although Buck's traction can help to alleviate pain, this is not its primary purpose.*

43. **The nurse is caring for a client who has been fitted with a below-the-knee prosthesis. The nurse understands that the purpose of a prosthesis in clients with an amputation is to:**

1. Promote an increase in muscle mass.
2. Prevent phantom limb pain.
3. Prevent damage to the stump.
4. Provide weight bearing and assist in ambulation.

1. *This is not the purpose of a prosthesis, although a prosthesis can help to prevent excessive atrophy.*

2. *Incorrect. A prosthesis cannot prevent phantom limb pain.*

3. *This is not the purpose of a prosthesis. A prosthesis may result in damage if not worn properly.*

4. **Correct. In addition, the prosthesis also provides a cosmetic affect.**

44. **A client recently diagnosed with grand mal epilepsy following a head injury is treated with phenytoin (Dilantin) to control her seizures. Which action by the client indicates to the nurse that there has been a lack of effective client teaching?**

1. Carries a medical alert tag at all times.
2. Identifies an aura.
3. Takes medication even when seizure free.
4. Uses alcohol in moderation.

1. *Wrong choice, this action by the client is correct. The client should always have a medical alert tag identifying her condition. Look for something the client should NOT do.*

2. *Wrong choice, this action by the client is correct. The client has learned to recognize the aura that may proceed the seizure. Look for something the client should NOT do.*

3. *Wrong choice, this action by the client is correct. The client should always take the medicine on a*

consistent basis. Look for something the client should NOT do.

4. **Correct choice. Alcohol is contraindicated with phenytoin (Dilantin). Even moderate use of alcohol by the client indicates that client teaching was not successful.**

45. A client is scheduled for a gastroscopy. His wife is with him and will wait for him to return from the procedure. Which nursing measure must be included in his immediate post-gastroscopy plan of care?

1. Connect the nasogastric tube to gravity drainage.
2. Keep him flat in bed for at least two hours.
3. Have him cough and deep breathe every two hours.
4. Instruct his wife not to give him ice chips.

1. *Wrong! Following gastroscopy, the client will most likely not have a nasogastric tube in place.*
2. *Wrong! There is no rationale for the client remaining flat in bed following this procedure.*
3. *Wrong! A gastroscopy requires local anesthesia, not general anesthesia. Coughing and deep breathing will not be a priority following this procedure.*
4. **Good choice! A gastroscopy requires local anesthesia, which will paralyze the gag reflex. Until the gag reflex returns in several hours, the client should receive nothing by mouth.**

46. A client diagnosed as having diabetes mellitus has been stabilized with insulin injections daily. The nurse should include which information when planning discharge teaching for this client?

1. Increase insulin dose prior to unusual exercise.
2. Acetone in the urine indicates a need for less insulin.
3. Always keep insulin vials refrigerated.
4. Systematically rotate insulin injection sites.

1. *Wrong! Exercise enhances the action of insulin and causes increased utilization of carbohydrates. Prior to unusual exercise, the client should increase her intake of food, particularly carbohydrates. The dose of insulin should remain unchanged.*
2. *Wrong! When inadequate insulin is available, the body metabolizes fat for energy. The resulting ketones are excreted in the urine. When acetone is present in the urine, the need for insulin is increased, not decreased.*
3. *Wrong! It is recommended that insulin vials be refrigerated whenever it is convenient. However, vials may remain at room temperature if refrigeration is not available.*
4. **Yes! You are correct! Systematic rotation of injection sites will prevent hardened, painful lumps under the skin. Since insulin injections**

will be required chronically, care must be taken to maintain injection sites for future use. Rotation allows healing to occur between injections.

47. In addition to routine postoperative care, immediate plans by the nurse for a laryngectomy client will focus on the need for:

1. Adequate fluid and electrolyte balance.
2. Prevention of hemorrhage.
3. Pain control.
4. Patent airway.

1. *Wrong choice. Although this will be an important postoperative assessment, there is another option that is more critical for the client's safety. The question is asking you to focus on the special needs of a laryngectomy client.*
2. *Wrong choice, because this is an important postoperative focus for ALL clients. The question asks for specific concerns for a laryngectomy client.*
3. *Wrong choice. This is not a priority intervention for a client after neck surgery.*
4. **Excellent! A patent airway is always the immediate priority for a postoperative client, especially after neck surgery.**

48. A client is being discharged after insertion of a permanent pacemaker for complete heart block. Which instruction, if given to him by the nurse, could endanger his physical safety?

1. Wear loose fitting clothing around the area of the pacemaker.
2. Take your radial pulse for a full minute once each week.
3. You may participate in any sport that doesn't involve physical contact.
4. Avoid exposure to metal detectors at airport security check points.

1. *No, this directive is appropriate because of the reduced incidence of trauma to the pacer insertion site if the client wears loose fitting clothing.*
2. **Yes, you have identified the incorrect instruction! This information is NOT appropriate and could jeopardize the client's safety. Instead, the client should be instructed to take the radial pulse daily, usually upon arising. Any sudden slowing or increasing of the pulse rate should be reported immediately to the physician, because it may indicate pacemaker malfunction.**
3. *No, this instruction is accurate and would not endanger the client. The client may participate in physical activity, with the exception of contact sports such as football and basketball.*

4. *No, this directive is appropriate. The client will need to avoid exposure to electromagnetic fields that are produced by technologic equipment such as metal detectors, microwave ovens, and magnetic imaging (MRI) equipment.*

49. **Universal precautions requires that a nurse wear which protective equipment when performing a nasogastric tube irrigation on a client with acquired immunodeficiency syndrome (AIDS)?**

    1. Sterile gloves.
    2. Goggles and nonsterile gloves.
    3. Nonsterile gown, sterile gloves.
    4. Nonsterile gloves.

    1. *No. Universal precautions does not require the use of sterile gloves when performing a nasogastric tube irrigation, although the nurse must protect herself from contact with blood and certain body fluids. Another option is more appropriate and more cost effective!*
    2. *No, it would not be necessary for the nurse to wear goggles. These are indicated when the nurse can anticipate a splash, such as during a surgical procedure or when suctioning a tracheostomy.*
    3. *Incorrect choice. It is not necessary for the nurse to wear a gown when performing a nasogastric tube irrigation. The gown is worn when the nurse anticipates being splashed by body fluids or blood. A splash is not likely to occur with this procedure.*
    4. ***Right choice! Universal precautions requires the use of clean gloves and other protective barriers to reduce the risk of occupational exposure to blood and certain body fluids. Nonsterile gloves are indicated for this procedure.***

50. **What is the nurse's primary concern when caring for a client who has acquired immunodeficiency syndrome (AIDS)?**

    1. Prevention of infection.
    2. Relief from pain.
    3. Restoration of fluid and electrolyte balance.
    4. Provision of psychological support to client and significant others.

    1. ***Yes, absolutely! Because the client is already immunocompromised, any infection can further debilitate the client and even lead to death. Almost all AIDS clients develop at least one opportunistic infection during the course of their disease. Some never fully recover and are at increased risk for developing a second infection or malignancy.***
    2. *Wrong choice. Although the client with AIDS may experience pain from an opportunistic disease, it is*

not the primary concern for this group of clients.

3. *Incorrect choice. Not all clients with AIDS have problems with fluid and electrolyte balance; it is seen more in those AIDS clients with persistent diarrhea.*
4. *Wrong choice. This is a concern for every client with AIDS, but it is not the priority. Remember to initially consider the needs that threaten a client's physical safety.*

51. **A client was in an automobile accident. The initial assessment revealed fractures of the left femur and pelvis and a large contusion on the head. Which assessment would best help the nurse determine the client's neurological status?**

    1. Pupillary responses.
    2. Verbal responses.
    3. Limb movements.
    4. Level of consciousness.

    1. *Wrong choice. The nurse might do this assessment to determine the client's neurological status, but this is not the best answer.*
    2. *Wrong choice. The nurse might do this assessment to determine the client's neurological status, but this is not the best answer.*
    3. *Wrong choice. The nurse might do this assessment to determine the client's neurological status, but this is not the best answer.*
    4. ***You are correct! Level of consciousness includes verbal responses, limb movements and pupillary responses.***

    > **TEST-TAKING TIP:** This is the most inclusive or global response, so this is the best option.

52. **In preparing a client to be discharged, the nurse teaches him to position himself for postural drainage. To achieve success in this teaching program, which information about the client is most important?**

    1. The type of bed the client will be using at home for the procedure.
    2. The amount of time required for the client to change positions.
    3. The client's goal concerning his ability to be self-sufficient.
    4. The client's ability to move about without assistance from others.

    1. *Not the best choice! The type of bed the client will be using at home is important information, since a mechanical bed greatly facilitates the procedure. However, postural drainage can be done without a mechanical bed, using things normally found in the home such as pillows and a straight-back chair. The key word in the stem of this question is "most."*

Which of the priority setting guidelines should be applied in answering this question?

2. *Not the best choice! The amount of time required for the client to change positions is important, but it is not "most important." Look at the other options. Which of the priority setting guidelines should be applied in answering this question?*

3. ***Excellent! The client's motivation and goals are essential for success, and they are a primary concern in any teaching program. Teaching/Learning theory tells us that if the client is not motivated or goal directed, the discharge teaching program is unlikely to be effective.***

TEST-TAKING TIP: This option is also more general than any of the other options, which refer to very specific assessments. You may wish to review the test-taking strategy of looking for a global response option.

4. *Not the best choice! The client's ability to move about without assistance from others is important, but it is not the "most important" consideration. Which of the priority setting guidelines should be used in answering this question? What is the priority according to those guidelines?*

53. **A client had a myocardial infarction. The nurse visits him at home one week following his discharge. He is taking chlorothiazide (Diuril) 500 mg daily and digoxin (Lanoxin) 0.25 mg daily. The nurse should give priority to assessing the client's knowledge of:**

1. Sources of potassium.
2. Sources of sodium.
3. Activity restrictions.
4. Signs of a heart attack.

1. ***Very good! Because the client is taking both Diuril and digoxin, the nurse should focus on his knowledge related to sources of potassium. Diuril depletes potassium. If the potassium level is too low, digoxin toxicity may lead to serious cardiac arrhythmias. This is the top priority because lack of understanding may be life-threatening very quickly.***

2. *Wrong choice. The client is probably on a sodium restricted diet. Too much sodium will increase the cardiac workload. The nurse should assess the client's knowledge of sources of sodium but, based on the information provided in the case situation, this is not the top priority.*

3. *Wrong choice. The client will increase his activity gradually as he recuperates from the myocardial infarction. The nurse should assess the client's knowledge of activity restrictions but, based on the information provided in the case situation, this is not the top priority.*

4. *Wrong choice. The nurse should assess the client's knowledge of the signs of another heart attack*

but, based on the information provided in the case scenario, this is not the top priority.

54. **A client has been diagnosed with paralytic ileus. Auscultation of the client's abdomen by the nurse reveals the bowel sounds to be:**

1. Absent.
2. Decreased.
3. Hyperactive.
4. Normal.

1. ***Correct. An ileus is indicative of an immobile bowel.***
2. *Incorrect. Try again.*
3. *Incorrect. What does "paralytic" mean? Try again.*
4. *Incorrect. What does "paralytic" mean? Try again.*

55. **The physician orders a urine test. The nurse understands that specific gravity of urine is used to determine the amount of:**

1. Proteins in the urine.
2. Uric acid crystals in the urine.
3. Solutes in the urine.
4. Epithelial cells in the urine.

1. *Incorrect. Although proteins may be present in the urine, they are not measured in this test.*
2. *Incorrect. Although uric acid crystals may be present in the urine, they are not measured in this test.*
3. ***Correct. Specific gravity varies with fluid intake and the quantity of solutes dissolved in the urine. Normal value is 1.005 to 1.025.***
4. *Incorrect. Although epithelial cells may be present in the urine, they are not measured in this test.*

56. **The nurse has been assigned to care for a recently diagnosed IDDM client who is resistant to learning self-injection of insulin. The client insists that the nurse administer all the injections. What is the appropriate nursing response in dealing with the client's resistance?**

1. "You won't be able to go home unless you learn to give yourself the insulin injection."
2. "I will have to tell your doctor that you refuse to give yourself the insulin injections. I'm sure she will be angry with you."
3. "Don't worry about it. Your daughter can come over to your house every morning to give you the insulin injections."
4. "It is important that you learn to give yourself the insulin injections. What can I do to help you overcome your fear of giving the injections?"

1. *Incorrect. This is an inappropriate response as well as an untrue statement. It is also a threat to the client, which is uncalled for and unprofessional.*
2. *Incorrect. This is an inappropriate response that is*

intended to coerce the client into doing what the nurse wants. Notice that it uses the communication block of referring to an inappropriate person.

3. *Incorrect. This response refers to an inappropriate person and uses false reassurance, because the nurse cannot assume that the daughter is able to give her mother daily insulin injections. The nurse needs to help the client become knowledgeable and independent in the care of her diabetes.*

4. **Correct. The nurse shows acceptance of the client's feelings and emphasizes the importance of self-care. The nurse is responsible for assisting the client in overcoming her fear of injections, by offering support and encouragement as well as client education materials. Referral to a home health nurse may be indicated for follow-up.**

57. **At 8:45 p.m., a client tells the nurse that he is feeling short of breath and requests that the nurse assist him in changing position. In addition to repositioning the client, the nurse should give highest priority to which nursing action?**

    1. Put the client on 15 minute checks.
    2. Call the charge nurse to report the shortness of breath.
    3. Observe the rate, depth, and character of the client's respirations.
    4. Give a back rub to help the client to relax.

    1. *Wrong choice. Any client with a breathing problem must be monitored closely, because a medical emergency may develop. However, this option is an implementation action. The nurse's decision to check the client every fifteen minutes implies that the shortness of breath does not represent a medical emergency at this time. There is not enough information to support this as the correct answer.*
    2. *Wrong choice. This is an implementation action. Additional data should be collected before the charge nurse is notified. The nurse needs to complete collecting data by further monitoring the respirations.*
    3. **Congratulations! This is an assessment activity and should be done first. Before initiating 15 minute checks, calling the doctor, or giving a back rub, an assessment should be made. Following the assessment, one or more of the actions in the other options may be done, as appropriate.**

    TEST-TAKING TIP: *The nursing process calls for assessment always to come first. When prioritizing, consider whether more data is required by the nurse.*

    4. *This is an implementation action. Giving a back rub implies that the assessment has already been*

done. There is not enough information to support this as the correct answer.

58. **A client is admitted to the hospital with a head injury and is unconscious. The nurse would place this client in which position?**

    1. Supine, to promote adequate blood volume to the cerebral vessels.
    2. Side lying, to prevent aspiration of secretions into the lungs.
    3. Semi-Fowler's, to help alleviate edema of the cerebral tissues.
    4. Modified Trendelenburg, to decrease the risk of shock.

    1. *Wrong! For any unconscious client, aspiration is a potential risk. Supine position is not the best position to prevent aspiration.*
    2. **Great job! For any unconscious client, maintaining an airway is a basic physiological need with high priority, and aspiration is a potential risk. Side lying position maintains the airway and allows secretions to drain out of the mouth, rather than to be aspirated into the lungs.**
    3. *Wrong! For any unconscious client, aspiration is a potential risk. Semi-Fowler's position is not a good position to prevent aspiration. Also, an unconscious client is unable to support himself in Semi-Fowler's position.*
    4. *Wrong! Shock is not the issue in this question. The issue is unconsciousness. For any unconscious client, aspiration is a potential risk. Modified Trendelenburg position will increase the risk of aspiration.*

59. **A client will receive her first dose of heparin today for treatment of thrombophlebitis. While the client is receiving heparin, which of the following medications should the nurse have available?**

    1. Warfarin (Coumadin).
    2. Protamine sulfate.
    3. Vitamin K.
    4. Dicumarol.

    1. *Wrong! Coumadin is an oral anticoagulant frequently used for anticoagulant therapy following treatment with heparin. Availability of this drug would not be needed while the client is taking heparin. Try again!*
    2. **Good choice! Protamine sulfate is a heparin antagonist used for treatment of heparin overdose. It should be available whenever a client is receiving heparin.**
    3. *Wrong! Vitamin K neutralizes the effect of Coumadin. It should be available for clients re-*

ceiving Coumadin, but it is not needed for clients receiving heparin. Try again!

4. *Wrong! Dicumarol is an anticoagulant. Dicumarol is contraindicated for a client receiving heparin. Try again!*

60. **During cardiopulmonary resuscitation (CPR), the preferred method that the nurse should use for opening the airway is:**

1. Turning the head and opening the mouth.
2. Performing a finger sweep of the mouth.
3. Using the jaw thrust and head tilt method.
4. Tilting the head and lifting the chin.

1. *No, this is not the preferred method for opening the airway, because the tongue may still be blocking the airway.*
2. *Incorrect. This method will not change the position of the tongue, which is the most common cause of airway obstruction.*
3. *Wrong choice. Although the head tilt is part of the correct method, the jaw thrust is not as successful at bringing the tongue forward as another technique. The jaw thrust method is recommended when there is suspicion of neck injury, because it does not alter the alignment of the cervical spine.*
4. ***Yes! The head tilt/chin lift method is preferred when establishing an open airway in the initiation of CPR. This maneuver repositions the trachea and tongue so that the airway is open.***

61. **When a nurse performs cardiopulmonary resuscitation (CPR) on an adult victim, the ratio of chest compressions to lung inflations is:**

1. Five compressions to one ventilation.
2. Ten compressions to one ventilation.
3. Ten compressions to two ventilations.
4. Fifteen compressions to two ventilations.

1. *Incorrect. This is the proper ratio when there are two rescuers to perform CPR.*
2. *No, this is the proper ratio for infant CPR.*
3. *Not correct. This ratio is not indicated in any standards of CPR.*
4. ***Yes! This is the correct ratio for one-person CPR. This will provide rescue breathing at a rate of 12 per minute and chest compressions at a rate of 80 to 100 per minute, which closely approximates the normal respiratory and heart rates.***

62. **Four days after admission for a myocardial infarction, a client becomes short of breath and complains of pain in his chest. What is the nurse's priority action?**

1. Give the client a sublingual nitroglycerin tablet.
2. Report this information to the nurse in charge.
3. Assess the client's lung sounds.
4. Place the client in modified Trendelenburg position.

1. *Incorrect. The chest pain may not be related to tissue ischemia of the heart. The nitroglycerin tablet may not be indicated at this time.*
2. ***Correct action! These manifestations may be indicative of another myocardial infarction OR may be evidence of a pulmonary embolism or other disease pathology. In either case, the charge nurse should be notified immediately.***
3. *No. Assessing the client's lung sounds would not be the priority action at this time. The chest pain would take priority over the shortness of breath because of the client's admitting diagnosis.*
4. *No, this is not an appropriate action at this time. Remember that the modified Trendelenburg position (legs elevated and head flat) is indicated in conditions of shock. This position aids in the pooling of blood in the trunk of the body, allowing the blood to be accessible to the vital organs.*

63. **A client is transferred to the recovery room after a colon resection for adenocarcinoma. The client develops internal abdominal bleeding postoperatively. Which finding would be reported by the nurse as an early sign of postoperative bleeding?**

1. Tachycardia.
2. Oliguria.
3. Hyperthermia.
4. Bradypnea.

1. ***Excellent observation! Because of decreased circulating blood volume due to internal bleeding, there is decreased oxygen carrying capacity of the blood. The body attempts to relieve the hypoxia by increasing the heart rate and cardiac output along with increasing the respiratory rate.***
2. *No, this is not an initial sign of hypovolemic shock, although it is part of the clinical picture due to decreased circulating blood volume through the glomerulus. Choose again.*
3. *No, this is not an initial sign of hypovolemic shock. One of the classic signs of shock is cool, moist skin. Hyperthermia is seen in septic shock. Make another selection.*
4. *Incorrect. Initially, in shock, respirations are deep and rapid, progressing to an even more rapid and then shallow rate as the body attempts to take in more oxygen to reduce the hypoxia.*

64. **The nurse is admitting a client who is suspected of having diabetes mellitus. Which characteristics would the nurse expect to observe?**

1. Shallow, labored respirations.
2. Increased blood pressure associated with slight periorbital edema.
3. Periods of altered pulse rate.
4. Increased urinary output.

1. *This is a good distractor! It is a possibility, because it appears to be Kussmaul's breathing, characteristic of ketoacidosis, which is a complication of diabetes mellitus. Kussmaul's breathing is deep and rapid, however, not shallow and labored. Note also that the stem of the question asks for a characteristic of diabetes, not a complication. Make another selection.*
2. *This is not characteristic of diabetes. Make another selection.*
3. *Although this may be a sign of ketoacidosis, it is not characteristic of diabetes. This option is a distractor. Make another selection.*
4. ***Correct! Increased urinary output is the only characteristic of diabetes presented in these four options! Remember the "three P's" associated with the diagnosis of diabetes mellitus: polyuria, polyphagia and polydipsia. The other three options are distractors. Option 1 might appear to be Kussmaul's breathing — which is characteristic of ketoacidosis, but not of diabetes itself. Option 2 is not characteristic of diabetes. And Option 3 may be a sign of ketoacidosis, but is not characteristic of diabetes.***

65. **To monitor a client for the most common complication arising from the administration of total parenteral nutrition, the nurse should:**

1. *Weigh the client at the same time each day using the same scale.*
2. Keep accurate records of total intake and total output.
3. Determine the increase or decrease in body weight each day.
4. Take the client's temperature at least every four hours.

1. *Try again. The issue in this question is TPN. Weighing the client daily is an appropriate nursing action to assess whether the primary purpose of TPN is being met, but the stem is asking you to select a nursing action that monitors for the most common complication. Poor weight gain can be a problem, but it is not a complication. Note also that the same idea is expressed in Option 3. Similar distractors generally are wrong and can be eliminated.*
2. *Wrong choice. The idea in this option is to record intake and output. This is an appropriate nursing action, but it does not monitor for the most common complication. Try again!*
3. *Wrong choice. Weighing the client daily to assess weight and nutritional status is an appropriate nurs-*

ing action, but it is not the answer to the question. The issue is TPN, and the stem asks you to select a nursing action that monitors for the most common complication. Note that the same idea is expressed in Option 1. Similar distractors must be wrong and can be eliminated.
4. ***Yes, you are correct! Catheter-related infections are the most common complication. Taking the client's temperature at least every four hours is the nursing action that monitors for the most common complication.***

> **TEST-TAKING TIP:** Note that Options 1 and 3 are very similar to each other—so neither of them can be correct!

66. **Ileostomy and colostomy are two types of fecal diversion. In explaining the differences between an ileostomy and a colostomy, the nurse would state that the stool of the ileostomy is:**

1. More liquid.
2. Hard and brown in color.
3. Firm and formed
4. Similar in consistency to that from a colostomy.

1. ***Correct. The stool is not formed and has a more liquid consistency.***
2. *Incorrect. The stool is not hard.*
3. *Incorrect. The stool is not firm.*
4. *Incorrect. There is a difference. The stool of a colostomy has a more solid consistency.*

67. **The nurse is to insert a Levin nasogastric tube. The nurse understands that an inappropriate use of the NG tube is:**

1. Maintaining NPO status.
2. Decompression.
3. Lavage.
4. Gavage.

1. ***Correct. Maintaining NPO status is an inappropriate use of the NG tube. However, it is true that the nurse would not offer any food or liquids to the client while he/she is NPO.***
2. *No, using the NG tube to relieve abdominal distention by removing secretions and gaseous substances from the GI tract is an appropriate and common use of the NG tube.*
3. *No, irrigation of the stomach in cases of active bleeding, poisoning, or gastric dilation is an appropriate and common use of the NG tube.*
4. *No, instillation of liquid nutritional supplements of feedings for clients unable to swallow fluid is an appropriate and common use of the NG tube.*

68. **A client has been recently diagnosed with cirrhosis of the liver. Which nursing measure is inappropriate for this client?**

1. Administer supplemental vitamins to compensate for the liver's inability to store vitamins A, B complex, D, and K.
2. Administer tube feedings if the client's condition necessitates it.
3. Encourage use of sodium to correct electrolyte imbalances.
4. Begin planning discharge teaching about the impact of cirrhosis on the client's ability to tolerate common over-the-counter medications.

1. *Sorry, this measure is appropriate. The client is nutritionally compromised and requires the use of additional vitamins. You are looking for an INAPPROPRIATE measure in this question, which has a false response stem.*
2. *Sorry, this measure is appropriate. Depending on the severity of the client's condition, the physician may order tube feedings to prevent malnutrition. You are looking for an INAPPROPRIATE measure in this question, which has a false response stem.*
3. **Good work, you have identified the inappropriate action. Sodium intake is usually restricted, not encouraged, with fluid retention, which commonly occurs with cirrhosis of the liver.**
4. *Sorry, this measure is appropriate. Planning for discharge teaching begins with assessing the client's level of knowledge and readiness to learn. You are looking for an INAPPROPRIATE measure in this question, which has a false response stem.*

69. **A 22-year-old sustained a fracture of the tibia and fibula while playing football. A long leg cast has been applied, and the client is admitted to the orthopedic unit. In providing nursing care for the client, which of the following is a vital consideration?**

    1. Elevation of the leg in the cast on a pillow will minimize edema.
    2. Healing of a fractured bone requires an extended period of time.
    3. A long period of immobility may lead to atrophy of the muscle.
    4. Analgesics may be needed for pain associated with the fracture.

    1. **Excellent! When caring for a client with a newly applied cast, it is important to keep the affected extremity elevated to reduce swelling. Note that the words "leg" and "cast" appear in the stem as well as in this option.**
    2. *Wrong choice. While this is a true statement, it does not answer the question asked in the stem. The issue is a newly applied cast, and the stem asks you to select an option that is a vital consideration. Select another option.*
    3. *Wrong choice. While this is a true statement, it does not address the question asked in the stem.*

The issue is a newly applied cast, and the stem asks you to select an option that is a vital consideration. Select another option.
4. *Wrong choice. While this is a true statement, it does not address the question asked in the stem. The issue is a newly applied cast, and the stem asks you to select an option that is a vital consideration. Select another option.*

70. **In providing care to a client with COPD, what is the primary nursing consideration?**

    1. To not overtire the client.
    2. To plan adequate rest periods.
    3. To give only low flow oxygen.
    4. To allow the client to move at his own pace.

    1. *Incorrect. This option focuses on the client's need for rest. While this is important, it is not the primary nursing consideration. Note also that the idea of this option is the same as in Options 2 and 4. Similar options must be wrong and can be eliminated.*
    2. *Incorrect. This option focuses on the client's need for rest. While this is important, it is not the primary nursing consideration. Note also that the idea of this option is the same as in Options 1 and 4. Similar options must be wrong and can be eliminated.*
    3. **Yes! You are correct! Clients with COPD have a chronically elevated CO_2. The respiratory stimulus for this client is a low level of O_2. Too much oxygen may remove the hypoxic drive, leading to hypoventilation.**

    > **TEST-TAKING TIP:** Note that the idea in the three other options is the client's need for rest. Similar options must be wrong, and similar distractors can be eliminated.

    4. *Wrong! This option focuses on the client's need for rest. While this is important, it is not the primary consideration in nursing care. Note also that the idea of this option is the same as in Options 1 and 2. Similar options must be wrong and can be eliminated.*

71. **A 38-year-old is admitted to the hospital for a severe episode of gastrointestinal bleeding secondary to a peptic ulcer. He is scheduled for an upper GI series. In preparing the client for this diagnostic procedure, which explanation by the nurse is accurate?**

    1. "An upper GI series will take five or six hours to complete. Since you will be waiting much of this time, you should take something to read with you."
    2. "This is a series of x-rays in which the entire GI tract is delineated. A liquid suspension of barium sulfate taken orally is the contrast medium."

3. "You should not eat or drink anything after midnight on the evening before the test. Following the first x-rays, full liquids are allowed."
4. "A laxative is administered the day before the test. On the morning of the test, you will be given soap suds enemas are given until the returns are clear."

*1. **Good choice! An upper GI series is a series of x-rays that delineates the upper portion of the GI tract. It takes five to six hours to complete because the series of x-rays follows the progress of the contrast medium through the GI tract. The client waits during much of this time, and reading material helps to pass the time. Note that the test-taking strategy of looking for similar words would be a clue in answering this question, because the phrase "upper GI series" appears both in this option and in the stem.***

2. The absolute word "entire" makes this option wrong. An upper GI series delineates only the upper portion of the GI tract.

3. This is incorrect. The client should be NPO after midnight and should continue fasting until the test is over.

4. This is incorrect. Laxatives and enemas are contraindicated prior to an upper GI.

72. A client with atelectasis of the left lower lung is to receive intermittent positive pressure breathing (IPPB) four times a day. It would be appropriate for the nurse to instruct the client that:

1. The treatment will last 45 minutes to an hour each time.
2. The client should take short, quick breaths during the treatment to get the maximum benefit from the medication.
3. The medication used in the treatment may cause nausea, so the physician has prescribed an antiemetic to be given beforehand.
4. The client should notice an increase in productive coughing during and after the treatment. This means that the medication is working.

1. Wrong. IPPB treatments are usually administered for 15 to 20 minutes at a time. This is to prevent tiring of the client and to decrease the risk of side effects from the medications.

2. Wrong. The client is instructed to maintain a slow respiratory rate and to use diaphragmatic breathing during the IPPB treatment.

3. Wrong. The medications used in the IPPB treatment may cause nausea and vomiting if administered too soon after meals. Prevention would mean scheduling the treatments so that they do not take place around mealtime. An antiemetic would, therefore, be unnecessary.

*4. **Yes! Coughing is encouraged and indicates that the aerosol medication is liquefying the secre-***

tions. IPPB treatments may be followed by chest physiotherapy or postural drainage treatment. The end result is the effective removal of secretions that have accumulated in the lower respiratory tract.

73. A client with a chest tube drainage system is being transported to the x-ray department for a chest film. Which action by the nurse indicates proper knowledge of caring for the chest drainage system?

1. The nurse keeps the drainage system below the level of the client's chest at all times.
2. The nurse pins the excess tubing to the client's gown to prevent pulling at the entry site.
3. The nurse clamps the chest tube prior to transferring the client to the wheelchair.
4. The nurse attaches the drainage system to portable suction while the client is transferred to the x-ray department.

*1. **Yes, this technique is correct! The chest drainage system should not be raised above the level of the chest at any time. If it is raised above the chest, this may cause air and possibly drainage fluid to reenter the thoracic cavity.***

2. No, the tubing should never be pinned to the client's gown or to the bed clothes! This action could result in a puncture of the chest tubing, causing an air leak and an ineffective drainage system. Remember that the pleural cavity is an airtight compartment: the drainage system and all connections must remain sealed at all times.

3. Incorrect choice. The chest tubing should never be clamped unless the physician orders it, usually when there is evidence that the lung has re-expanded. Clamping the tubing may lead to a tension pneumothorax (collapse of the lung) because of increased pressure from gas and fluid that cannot be drained.

4. Not necessary. Even if suction is ordered (usually at 20 cm of water pressure), it is not required while the client is transferred off of the nursing unit or while ambulating. When the client is returned to bed, the suction must be reconnected. If the client must have suction at all times, a portable chest x-ray would have to be done.

74. A client has been given instructions about taking enteric-coated erythromycin (E-Mycin). Which statement by the client indicates the need for further teaching?

1. "I can take these pills with my meals."
2. "The medicine has been coated so that it dissolves in my intestine, not my stomach."
3. "It's okay to crush a tablet as long as I make sure it dissolves completely in water before swallow-

ing it."

4. "It's important that I finish the entire prescription, even if I don't feel sick anymore."

1. *No, this statement by the client is correct. Enteric-coated tablets may be taken with meals. The client understands the drug therapy. You are looking for an INCORRECT statement.*

2. *No, this statement indicates that the client understands where the medicine is absorbed. Enteric-coated means that the medication is protected from the acid media of the stomach and can thus pass safely into the duodenum, where it is absorbed. You are looking for an INCORRECT statement.*

3. **Good work, this statement by the client is incorrect. You remembered that enteric-coated tablets cannot be crushed. Another drug form that should not be crushed is the sustained release form, often identified with key suffixes attached to the drug's name: Dur (as in duration), SR (sustained release), CR (controlled release), SA (sustained action), and Contin (continuous). Trade names may also imply sustained release: spansules, extentabs, extencaps.**

4. *Wrong choice, this client understands a key principle of antibiotic therapy: take the medication for as long as prescribed, usually seven to 10 days, even if beginning to feel better. This question asks you to find a statement that indicates the client does NOT understand and requires further instruction. Try again.*

75. **Which of the following statements by a client would indicate to the nurse that the client has an accurate understanding of oral cloxacillin (Tegopen) administration?**

1. "I'll take the medicine with milk or an antacid so that my stomach won't get upset."

2. "I'll take the Tegopen with a large glass of fruit juice so that I get extra Vitamin C for wound healing."

3. "I'll take the medicine either one hour before or two hours after meals so that it will work better."

4. "I'll take the Tegopen at the same time as my blood pressure and heart pills so that I don't forget to take it."

1. *No. The client should not need milk or antacids. If abdominal cramping, diarrhea and weight loss occur, pseudomembranous colitis should be suspected. Select another option.*

2. *Incorrect. Penicillins should not be taken with acidic fruit juices or carbonated beverages, since both may facilitate decomposition of penicillins. Try another choice.*

3. **Correct! You remembered that most oral penicillins are bound to food and are poorly absorbed in acid media. They should be taken on an empty stomach to minimize bonding. NOTE: Amoxicillin is one penicillin that is well absorbed orally and maybe given with meals.**

4. *Not a wise choice. The client may take his other medications with meals or at different time intervals than suggested for antibiotics. Most antibiotics should be given at evenly-spaced intervals, usually every four to six hours, to maintain proper serum concentrations, not on a q.i.d. or b.i.d. regimen. Try again.*

76. **The nurse is caring for a client with a myocardial infarction who is taking chlorothiazide (Diuril) and digoxin (Lanoxin). Which diet is indicated?**

1. Diet low in sodium and saturated fats, high in potassium.

2. Diet low in unsaturated fats, sodium and potassium.

3. Diet high in potassium, Vitamin C and protein.

4. Diet low in sodium and saturated and unsaturated fats.

1. **Good choice! Sodium would be restricted to decrease the circulating blood volume and reduce the cardiac workload. Saturated fats would be decreased to prevent further atherosclerotic heart disease. Potassium should be increased in his diet because Diuril causes the excretion of potassium in the urine. It is vital to keep potassium within the normal limits because a low potassium level may lead to arrhythmias in a client who is taking digoxin.**

2. *Incorrect! Both saturated and unsaturated fats are restricted in a weight reduction diet. However, we have no information that this client needed to be placed on a weight reduction diet. Also, additional potassium is needed to offset potassium loss due to the medications the client is taking and to prevent resultant cardiac arrhythmias.*

3. *Incorrect. A diet high in potassium is needed because of the loss of potassium due to digoxin and Diuril. There is no reason for increased Vitamin C or protein.*

4. *Both saturated and unsaturated fats are restricted in a weight reduction diet. However, we have no information that this client needed to be placed on a weight reduction diet! Also, additional potassium is needed to offset potassium loss due to the medications the client is taking and to prevent resultant cardiac arrhythmias. Note that Option 2 also includes low unsaturated fats. Both of these options are incorrect.*

77. A client is to be medicated with narcotics for four to five days after surgery. What precautions should the nurse take?

1. Provide bed rest for the first two to three days.
2. Put the client's water and cigarettes close to her bed, within her reach.
3. Encourage the client to call for help to ambulate.
4. Suggest that the client limit the use of her medications, as addiction may result.

1. This is incorrect. This is much too long to be on bed rest. Make another selection.

2. Wrong! The client should not be smoking at all; but if allowed, someone should be with her since she is using narcotics. Try again.

3. Correct! Hypotension can occur, and she should have help with ambulating to prevent falling.

4. This is incorrect. Fewer than one percent of clients become addicted to narcotics used after surgery for pain. Choose again.

78. A client is pregnant and has iron deficiency anemia. The physician orders an injection of iron dextran (Imferon) IM. How should the nurse plan to administer the injection?

1. Use a size 23-25 gauge needle and administer in the deltoid muscle.
2. Use a size 20 or 22 gauge needle and administer deep in the thigh.
3. Select a 19-20 gauge needle and use the Z-track method to administer.
4. Select an 18 gauge needle and give deep in the buttocks.

1. Wrong. Review your needle sizes. A 23-25 gauge is very small, and would not be suitable for iron, which is thicker than this gauge allows. Remember, too, that iron must be given deep into the muscle, and a 23-25 gauge needle is short. Iron is never given in the deltoid, only the buttocks, as this is a larger muscle mass.

2. Wrong choice. Please review your needle sizes. A 20-22 gauge is too small for iron injections. Iron must be given in the buttocks—not the thigh.

3. Correct. Iron must be given in the Z-track method to prevent staining of tissue. A 19-20 gauge needle is the correct size. It should be at least two inches long.

4. Incorrect. An 18 gauge needle is not the correct size—this is too large. What method would you use? Try again.

79. The nurse observes that, in the first few days of hospitalization, an 18-month-old client sits quietly sucking

her thumb in the corner of her crib. When the nurse approaches the crib, the client shyly turns her head away from the nurse. The nurse understands that the toddler's behavior:

1. Indicates a pathological reaction to being hospitalized.
2. Indicates that the relationship between parents and child should be assessed.
3. Demonstrates an anxiety reaction to the stress of hospitalization.
4. Is an example of negative behavior and a beginning attempt at autonomy.

1. At 18 months, the client is able to identify the nurse as a stranger. Her behavior is appropriate. There is no evidence of pathology.

2. No data about the relationship between the client and her parents is provided. The conclusion that the relationship between parents and child need to be evaluated is an assumption. Do not "read into" the question! As a general rule, you should not make assumptions when answering NCLEX Exam questions.

3. Yes! You are correct! Hospitalization is stressful, regardless of the age of the hospitalized client. For an 18-month-old, separation from her parents adds to that stress. The client is demonstrating an anxiety reaction to the stress of hospitalization.

4. Erikson's development theory identifies the developmental conflict for children age one to three as autonomy versus shame and doubt. An 18-month-old may be beginning to develop autonomy. However, since the client is hospitalized, her behavior has most likely regressed to the developmental conflict of trust versus mistrust.

80. An eight-year-old client with a diagnosis of acute rheumatic fever is admitted to the hospital. Which age-appropriate activity would the nurse recommend for this client?

1. Playing computer games in the game room.
2. Visiting with several school friends.
3. Completing school assignments.
4. Listening to favorite cassette tapes.

1. Wrong! The client should be on bedrest during the acute phase of rheumatic fever. It is very important that the nurse promote rest because it decreases the cardiac workload. Make another selection.

2. No! Visiting with several school friends does not promote rest during the acute phase. It is very important that the nurse promote rest because it decreases the cardiac workload. Make another selection.

3. No! Completing school assignments does not promote rest during the acute phase. It is very important that the nurse promote rest because it decreases the cardiac workload. Make another selection.

4. **Yes! This is the best answer! The client should be on bedrest during the acute phase of rheumatic fever. It is very important that the nurse promote rest because it decreases the cardiac workload.**

81. Before she is discharged from the hospital, the client and her husband attend a client education class on the topic of depression and learn to recognize behaviors that could indicate a recurrence of depression. The nurse knows which of the following is inconsistent with signs of depression?

   1. Psychomotor retardation.
   2. Grandiosity.
   3. Self-devaluation.
   4. Insomnia.

   1. *Psychomotor retardation is a sign of depression. This option is not the answer because this question has a false response stem. Try to identify the behavior that is NOT a sign of depression.*
   2. **Correct. Grandiosity is not associated with depression. It is associated with the manic phase of bipolar depression.**
   3. *Self-devaluation is an important sign of depression. This option is not the answer because this question has a false response stem. Try to identify the behavior that is NOT a sign of depression.*
   4. *Insomnia and hypersomnia, both interrupted sleep patterns, can be signs of depression. This option is not the answer because this question has a false response stem. Try to identify the behavior that is NOT a sign of depression.*

82. A client with blastomycosis is being treated with amphotericin B (Fungizone). Which of the following statements by the client indicates to the nurse an accurate understanding of amphotericin B?

   1. "The nurse told me that the drug is destroyed by light, so I'll be getting the medicine on the 11:00 p.m. to 7:00 a.m. shift."
   2. "It sure would be nice if they used my Hickman catheter for administration of this medicine, but I guess the medicine is too irritating to the material in the catheter."
   3. "I'm glad that I'll only have to take this medicine for 10 days because of the numerous side effects."
   4. "I'll be given some Tylenol before the medicine is given to help decrease the fever that I'll probably get when the medicine is being given."

   1. *Incorrect. Although amphotericin B is light sensitive, no significant deterioration occurs within the six to eight hours required for infusion of a single*

dose. *It's not standard practice to protect the medicine from light as once was the case. The client needs further teaching, select again.*

   2. *No!! Amphotericin B should be given through a central venous access device if one is available, in order to maximize the dilution of the medicine as it enters the systemic circulation. A Hickman catheter is a central access device, and the chance of extravasation is minimal with this method of IV delivery. The client needs further teaching, select again.*
   3. *Incorrect. Amphotericin B therapy must be continued for long periods, perhaps several months, to create the possibility of a cure for disseminated fungal disease. Administering the drug on alternate days and over a six-hour period may reduce the incidence of side effects. The client needs further teaching, select again.*
   4. **Correct! The client understands this premedication protocol to help decrease the side effect of fever. The client may also be premedicated with an antiemetic, antihistamine and corticosteroids to decrease other side effects of chills, nausea/vomiting, headache and anorexia. These manifestations typically subside within the first four hours of administration.**

83. A nurse observes a client on the psychiatric unit muttering to herself and standing near a window. The client states, "The voices are telling me to jump. They say test the glass and then jump through." Which is the best nursing response to this statement?

   1. "Where are these voices coming from? Do you recognize them as belonging to anyone that you know?"
   2. "I think you are hallucinating. The only voices in this room are yours and mine."
   3. "Tell the voices that you are not going to listen to them."
   4. "You say you are hearing voices that make you feel like jumping through the window. I understand the voices are frightening to you, but I want you to know that I do not hear any voices."

   1. *This is not correct because the nurse is conveying the belief that the hallucinations are real.*
   2. *This statement is not correct because it denies the validity of the client's perceptions. Attempts to reason with the client, argue about, or challenge the perceptions will only tend to further reinforce them.*
   3. *This is not correct because the nurse is supporting the client's belief in the voices. The nurse's role is to provide a link with reality.*
   4. **Good choice! Hearing voices telling her to jump from the window is a very unsafe situation for the client who might carry out these "commands." It is important for the nurse to acknowledge the client's perceptions while also**

casting doubt on them by stating clearly that she does not share them. Additional measures may have to be taken to ensure this client's safety.

84. **A woman is crying continuously after the death of her husband. The son is distressed over his mother's crying and reports to the nurse that she has said that she wants to die. He asks the nurse to help "calm her down." The nurse's best response to the son's request is:**

    1. "All right, I'll talk with her and see if I can comfort her."
    2. "If you just sit quietly with her, I'm sure she will calm down when she gets these feelings out."
    3. "It's hard to see her so upset, but she needs to let these feelings out. We can both stay with her for a while."
    4. "This seems to bother you more than it does her."

    1. This is not the best option because the nurse is ignoring the son's feelings of distress and is not basing her response on an understanding of the grief process.
    2. This option is partially correct in that the nurse recognizes his mother has a need to express her feelings through crying. However, this response does not recognize that the son is having difficulty with his feelings and his understanding of the grief process.
    3. Correct. The nurse's response acknowledges the son's feelings while also informing him of his mother's need to express her feelings through crying. The nurse is also offering self by offering to stay with both of them.
    4. This is not an accurate response, and it is not therapeutic for the son.

85. **A women is distressed over the death of her husband. The son remarks to the nurse, "My father has been dead for six months now. I think my mother needs to get on with her life." What is the most helpful response by the nurse to the son?**

    1. "A death is usually a crisis for the whole family. How has your father's death affected you?"
    2. "I agree. How can you help her find more pleasure in her life?"
    3. "I think it would be helpful if you could give her more support."
    4. *"Perhaps she needs more time. Grieving often takes a year or more to complete."*

    1. This response does not address the son's concern, so it is not the correct option. This might be an appropriate question for the nurse after she has responded to the son's concern.

    2. This response is not appropriate, based on current information about the grief process.
    3. This response does not recognize the nature of the grief process. It also is not helpful to the son because the nurse does not explain what is meant by "support."
    4. Correct. This response communicates the correct information that acute grieving often takes one to two years to complete for the loss of a spouse or other loved one.

86. **A client with Type I insulin dependent diabetes mellitus (IDDM) usually walks two miles each day after breakfast. She is planning to participate in a Walk-a-Thon, in which she may walk as much as six miles. Which of the following responses by the nurse would be best in preparing the client for the Walk-a-Thon?**

    1. "Participating in a Walk-a-Thon is much too strenuous for you."
    2. "Ask your doctor to increase your insulin dose the day of the Walk-a-Thon."
    3. "Test your blood glucose immediately following the Walk-a-Thon."
    4. "Eat some additional carbohydrates before you begin the Walk-a-Thon."

    1. Incorrect response. Since the client walks regularly, there is no data to support the idea that a Walk-a-Thon is too strenuous for her.
    2. No! Since insulin acts more quickly when the injection is followed by vigorous exercise, an increased dose of insulin on the day of the Walk-a-Thon may cause a hypoglycemic reaction.
    3. This is not correct. Blood glucose should be monitored before meals and at bedtime.
    4. YES! Exercise causes increased utilization of carbohydrates. Prior to unusual exercise, an insulin dependent diabetic should consume an extra amount of complex carbohydrates to prevent a hypoglycemic reaction. This is the only correct response.

87. **A newly diagnosed adult diabetic is doing a return demonstration of the proper technique for insulin injection. He draws up the correct dose of insulin using the proper technique, but when he is ready to inject the needle, he hesitates and says, "I'm not sure I can do this." Which response by the nurse would be best initially?**

    1. "I'll show you again how to inject the needle."
    2. "I'll inject the needle for you this time."
    3. "You're doing fine so far. Give it a try."
    4. "Why are you so nervous? Do you need help?"

    1. Wrong choice. With this response, the nurse will inject the needle. This is not the best response, because the nurse should be encouraging the client to do the injection. Note that almost the same idea, with the same result, is expressed in Option 2. Similar distractors must be wrong and can be eliminated.

2. Good try, but with this response, the nurse will inject the needle instead of encouraging the client to do the injection. Note that almost the same idea, with the same result, is expressed in Option 1. Similar distractors must be wrong and can be eliminated.

3. **Congratulations! You are correct! With this response, the nurse encourages the client to do the procedure for himself. This response is client-centered.**

> **TEST-TAKING TIP:** Note that Options 1 and 2 are similar to each other, since in each case the nurse will inject the needle. These similar distractors must be wrong and can be eliminated.

4. Wrong response! Being nervous and unsure is an appropriate feeling for this newly diagnosed adult diabetic. However, this response by the nurse focuses on the client's nervousness and need for help, and blocks communication by making the client feel defensive. Instead, the nurse's response should enhance the client's feelings of competency. Remember, "why" responses are not therapeutic! Make another selection.

88. **Soon after being admitted to a rehabilitation unit, a chronic alcoholic says to the nurse, "I don't really need to be here. My wife and family make me drink. My wife spends all my money. My kid just had an accident with his car that will cost me a fortune in repairs." The therapeutic nursing response is:**

1. "Tell me more about how your wife is spending all your money."
2. "Could you tell me more about why your child's car accident cost you money?"
3. "It sounds like you are having a great deal of financial difficulty."
4. "Tell me more about your feelings about being here in the hospital."

1. Wrong choice! The client is a chronic alcoholic who is in denial ("I don't really need to be here"). Before the client can accept help for his problem, he must examine his feelings and acknowledge that he is an alcoholic who needs help. This option focuses on his financial difficulties rather than his feelings. Note that Options 2 and 3 also focus on financial difficulties; these similar distractors can all be eliminated.

2. Wrong choice! The client is a chronic alcoholic who is in denial ("I don't really need to be here"). Before the client can accept help for his problem,

he must examine his feelings and acknowledge that he is an alcoholic who needs help. This option focuses on his financial difficulties rather than his feelings. Note that Options 1 and 3 also focus on financial difficulties. These similar distractors can all be eliminated.

3. Wrong! The client is a chronic alcoholic who is in denial ("I don't really need to be here"). Before the client can accept help for his problem, he must examine his feelings and acknowledge that he is an alcoholic who needs help. This option focuses on his financial difficulties rather than his feelings. Note that Options 1 and 2 also focus on financial difficulties. These similar distractors can all be eliminated.

4. **You are correct! The client is a chronic alcoholic who is in denial ("I don't really need to be here"). Before the client can accept help for his problem, he must examine his feelings and acknowledge that he is an alcoholic who needs help. This option focuses on the client's feelings about being in the hospital.**

> **TEST-TAKING TIP:** Note that the other three options all focus on money and financial difficulties. Options that express the same idea can be eliminated.

89. **A 25-year-old client was admitted to the hospital with a diagnosis of diabetes mellitus. She tells the nurse that she is very concerned about being placed on a calorie-controlled diet, since she has been losing weight even though she has been eating more food. The best response by the nurse is:**

1. "You won't have to worry about weight loss once your sugar is regulated."
2. "The doctor will order enough food for you."
3. "You have been losing weight because your body is not producing insulin, which is needed to use the calories you eat. When you start receiving insulin, a calorie-controlled diet will be recommended to help maintain your weight."
4. "You probably needed to lose some weight to decrease your need for insulin."

1. Incorrect. This response may appear to address the client's concern, but the statement is not necessarily true. This response fails to explain the cause of the client's present weight loss, and it does not present a rationale for the reduced calorie diet. This response does not correctly address the client's concerns and is not therapeutic.

2. Wrong! This response focuses on an inappropriate person (the doctor) and is not therapeutic. To address the client's concerns, the nurse's response should explain the cause of the client's present weight loss and present a rationale for the reduced calorie diet.

3. *Best choice! This response briefly explains the relationship between calorie intake and insulin. It is therapeutic because it gives correct information that addresses the client's concern.*

TEST-TAKING TIP: Note that the words "calorie-controlled diet" occur in both the case scenario and this option. This is a clue that this might be the correct answer.

4. *Wrong! This response devalues the client's concerns. Furthermore, the nurse does not know that the client needed to lose weight prior to hospitalization. This response is not therapeutic. To address the client's concerns, the nurse's response should explain the cause of the client's present weight loss and present a rationale for the reduced calorie diet.*

90. **A confused, elderly client has wet herself and is standing in the hospital corridor in a puddle of urine. She looks ashamed and says to the nurse, "I want to go outside for a walk now." At this time, what is the most appropriate response by the nurse?**

1. "Before we go for a walk, perhaps we can make a list that will help you make your bathroom trips easier."
2. "Right now, let me wipe up the urine on the floor, and let's get a change of clothing for you. I am sure that this problem is upsetting for you."
3. "This has been a problem for you. Let's see if we can find a solution together."
4. "Wetting yourself is very upsetting. Yes, let's take a walk."

1. *Wrong! The issue in this question is a wet client standing in a puddle of urine. This response does not address the current problem. Also, since the client is confused, making a list is not appropriate, since she is not likely to remember to consult the list.*
2. *Good work! This response is therapeutic because it deals with the here and now by helping the client focus on her current need, which is dry clothes, and by informing the client that the nurse will first wipe up the urine off the floor. The nurse is also showing empathy. This option also indicates that the nurse is giving priority to the immediate safety issue of urine on the floor. The client, along with other clients and staff, is at risk to fall.*

STRATEGY ALERT! Note that the phrase "puddle of urine" in the question is similar to the words "urine on the floor" in this option. This is a clue that this may be the correct answer.

3. No. The client is feeling uncomfortable, and her basic needs for dry clothes and a safe environment must be met. The client is also confused, and she is feeling ashamed. Discussing possible solutions to the problem of not getting to the bathroom in time will not be helpful.
4. Wrong. In this response, the nurse is showing empathy, however, the response does not address the client's basic need at this time for dry clothes, or the nursing priority of wiping up the urine off the floor.

91. **A 78-year-old client is admitted to the hospital for an exploratory laparotomy. The client's daughter says to the nurse, "I wish I could stay with my father, but I need to go home to see how my children are doing. I really hate to leave my father alone at this time." The most helpful response by the nurse to the daughter is:**

1. "Your father needs opportunities to be independent. This will help him become self-sufficient."
2. "Your father is capable of taking care of himself. Try to allow him more independence."
3. "Stress is not good for your father at this time. Perhaps you could call your children."
4. "You are feeling concern for both your dad and your children. Let me know when you are leaving, and I'll stay with him."

1. *Wrong! This response is not focused on the client. The client in this question is the daughter, who has shared with the nurse her need to go home to see her children and her reluctance to leave her father. This response is focused on an inappropriate person.*
2. *Incorrect! This is focused on an inappropriate person and an inappropriate issue. The client in this question is the daughter, who has shared with the nurse her need to go home to see her children and her reluctance to leave her father. This response is focused on the father, not the daughter. It also uses the communication block of giving advice.*
3. *No! This response is focused on an inappropriate person. The client in this question is the daughter, and the issue is her need to go home to check on her children as well as care for her father. There is no data to indicate that the father would find it stressful if his daughter went home, or that his condition requires the daughter to remain constantly at the hospital. This response also uses the communication block of giving advice, and denies the daughter the opportunity to make her own decision and to meet her own needs.*
4. *Excellent! This option illustrates the tools of showing empathy and offering self. The client in this question is the daughter. The issue is her need to go home to check on her children. This response recognizes her feelings about both her father and her children. In offering*

to stay with the father while she is away, the nurse is offering self.

92. A 20-day-old infant is recovering from surgery for pyloric stenosis. The client's mother asked the nurse, "Now that my son has had this surgery, is it likely that pyloric stenosis will cause trouble later?" An appropriate nursing response to the mother would be:

1. "Why don't you talk to the doctor about your uncertainties regarding your son's future?"
2. "He might develop obstructive manifestations later. If so, take him immediately to an emergency room."
3. "He will not have manifestations again in childhood, but may have digestive difficulties in his adult life."
4. "Recurrence of the obstruction or repetition of the surgical procedure would be unlikely."

1. *Wrong! This is a block that places the client's concerns on hold. An answer to the client's question is within the realm of nursing.*
2. *Wrong! This response provides incorrect information. A child who has had a surgical repair of pyloric stenosis is not likely to develop obstructive manifestations later. There is no need to evoke fear in the mother by responding in this way.*
3. *The words "will not" make this an absolute statement, which is wrong. The primary manifestation of pyloric stenosis, projectile vomiting, can be caused by a variety of factors. It is incorrect for the nurse to say that the client will not have this manifestation again.*
4. ***Good choice! This option is the correct answer because the nurse is providing correct information. Following surgical repair of pyloric stenosis, recurrence of the obstruction or the surgical procedure is not expected.***

93. A chronic alcoholic has been hospitalized following a drinking binge. During a lengthy conversation with the nurse about his long history of alcoholism, the client becomes tense and uncomfortable. Which of the following is the initial response by the nurse?

1. "What did I say to make you feel so uncomfortable?"
2. "Drinking for a long time can make anyone feel uncomfortable."
3. "At what point did you begin to feel uncomfortable?"
4. "Talking about your drinking will help you to recover."

1. *Wrong! This response is an illustration of the non-therapeutic communication block of focusing on an inappropriate person. The response is focused on the nurse rather than on the client. The nurse is also accepting responsibility for the client's feel-*

ings. Try again.
2. *Wrong, try again! This response is an assumption by the nurse. The nurse should seek additional information (do an assessment) before stating the cause of the client's feelings.*
3. ***Right! This response illustrates the therapeutic communication tool of clarification. The nurse needs to gather more information about the client's feelings (do an assessment).***
4. *Try again! This response illustrates the non-therapeutic communication block of giving advice. It also does not focus on the issue, which is the client's discomfort.*

94. A 62-year-old female has been diagnosed with breast cancer. She has become quiet and thoughtful and says to the nurse, "What do you think people will say about me when I'm gone?" Which response by the nurse is the most helpful to the client?

1. "You will be remembered as a very nice person."
2. "Do you feel that people will be talking about you after your death?"
3. "At this time, a positive attitude can influence your recovery."
4. "The thought of your breast cancer must seem hopeless."

1. *Wrong! This response uses the communication block of false reassurance. We have no data to indicate that the nurse would know what others might say about the client. More importantly, however, this response is not therapeutic because it does not address the client's feelings of hopelessness.*
2. *Not the best choice because this response does not focus on the appropriate issue. The nurse's response should address the client's feelings of hopelessness.*
3. *Wrong! This response blocks communication by giving advice. The nurse's response should encourage the client to explore her feelings.*
4. ***Great choice! This response uses the tool of restatement to focus on the client's feelings of hopelessness. This response is therapeutic because it allows the client to talk about what she has been thinking since she learned of her diagnosis.***

95. A woman is admitted to the ICU on a ventilator after attempting suicide. As the husband is talking with the nurse, he begins to cry. He says, "It's all my fault. I should have been home more often to keep an eye on her." Which response to the husband by the nurse would be most helpful initially?

1. "You seem to regret not being there for your wife. How can you feel that way when you have to earn

a living?"

2. "At this time you need your privacy. I will return later, and we can talk then."

3. "This is an important issue that you need to bring up at your family therapy session."

4. "It must have been hard to be away when your wife was so sick."

1. *This response is partly correct, since it begins with the nurse showing empathy for the client. However, the second part of the nurse's response actually rejects the client's feelings and minimizes them, while appearing to show approval for his actions. This response is not therapeutic. When part of an option is a communication block, the option is incorrect.*

2. *Wrong! In this response, the nurse abandons the client when he needs to talk about his feelings, putting his feelings on hold. The client's feelings must be dealt with at this time. Remember, the client in this question is the husband.*

3. *This response puts the client's feelings on hold. The nurse's response should address the client's feelings and encourage him to express them. Remember, the client in this question is the husband.*

4. ***Good! This response shows empathy by showing that the nurse understands the husband's feelings. Note that Options 2 and 3 block communication by putting his feelings on hold.***

96. **A client is admitted to the psychiatric unit with a diagnosis of acute depression. After being hospitalized for a few weeks, the client says to the nurse, "I'm a terrible person, and I should be dead." Which response by the nurse would be appropriate initially?**

1. "That is why you are here. We are trying to help you with your bad feelings."

2. "Feeling that way must be awful. What makes you feel so terrible?"

3. "Feeling like a terrible person is part of your illness. As you get better, those feelings will lessen."

4. "You are not terrible. You are not a bad person."

1. *No! This response appears to support the client's feelings that she is a terrible person. The second part of the response also blocks therapeutic communication by focusing on inappropriate persons — the nurse and others who "are trying to help" the client. This response is not therapeutic.*

2. ***Good choice! This response shows empathy, and then seeks clarification of the client's feelings. These two communication tools combine to make a therapeutic response that allows the client to talk about her feelings.***

3. *Wrong! This response does give the client information about her illness, but the client's feelings*

must be addressed before information is given. When a client is distressed and upset, giving an explanation is inappropriate.

4. *Absolutely not! The nurse's opinion is not important! This response blocks therapeutic communication by putting the nurse in the role of an authority figure, using false reassurance, and devaluing the client's feelings. The nurse's response should encourage the client to explore her feelings with the nurse.*

97. **The nurse observes a depressed client in the day room. The client is shivering. Which response by the nurse would be most helpful to this client?**

1. "Come with me to your room, and we will get a sweater for you."

2. "Why do you sit here without a sweater when you are cold?"

3. "What color sweater do you want me to get from your room for you?"

4. "When you are in the day room, you should dress so that you are not cold."

1. ***You made the right choice! By volunteering to go with the client to get a sweater, the nurse is communicating therapeutically by offering self.***

2. *Wrong! This option uses a "Why" question. This is an example of the communication block of requesting an explanation.*

3. *In this option, the nurse is offering self by volunteering to get a sweater for the client. However, this is not the best option. It would be more therapeutic to assist the client in meeting her own need. Also, the color of the sweater is not significant, and making decisions is often difficult for depressed clients.*

4. *Wrong! In this option, the nurse is giving advice. Giving advice is not therapeutic.*

98. **After a depressed client is discharged, her husband stops attending family counseling sessions. The husband states, "I do not have time for all that talking." Which response to the husband by the nurse would be most appropriate?**

1. "Because your wife's condition is improving, you will be less involved in family therapy."

2. "You should continue attending the counseling sessions until the therapist tells you to stop."

3. "It must be difficult for you to talk about these family problems."

4. "Continuing counseling is necessary if your wife is to continue making progress."

1. *Wrong! An improvement in the client's condition does not mean that therapy can be discontinued.*

Also, this response is inappropriate because it is the therapist's role to determine the length of family therapy, not the nurse's.

2. *Wrong! This option is an example of the nurse giving advice. This is a communication block. It is unlikely that the client will return to counseling sessions as a result of this response.*

3. **Good choice! This option is an example of the nurse showing empathy. The husband's comment to the nurse states that he is having difficulty with "talking" sessions, and the nurse is showing an understanding of his feelings. The nurse is also helping the client focus on what it is about the counseling that bothers him. Helping the client explore his feelings at this time is pivotal to the family's continuing therapy and for the long-term benefit for his wife.**

4. *The husband is the client in this question, and his feelings about the family therapy are the issue. This response focuses on an inappropriate person (his wife), and an inappropriate concern (his wife's progress). This response also blocks communication by giving advice. To be therapeutic, the nurse's response must deal with the client's feelings about the family therapy.*

99. **A client was admitted to the psychiatric unit with a diagnosis of manic-depression. At 3:00 a.m., the client ran to the nurses' station, demanding to see her therapist immediately. Which response by the nurse would be best initially?**

1. "Calm down, go back to your room, and I'll try to get in touch with your therapist right away."
2. "Regulations state that I can't call the therapist in the middle of the night, except in an emergency."
3. "You must be very upset about something to want to see your therapist in the middle of the night."
4. "You are being unreasonable and I will not call your therapist at 3:00 in the morning."

1. *Wrong! It is difficult for an agitated client to follow complex directives, and this option gives several directives at one time. Also, this response is not therapeutic because it does not address the client's feelings. Finally, there is no indication that it is necessary for the nurse to call the therapist at this time. Try again!*

2. *Wrong! This option focuses on regulations, which is an inappropriate issue, and it does not address the client's feelings. This response is not therapeutic.*

3. **Good choice! This option is an example of the nurse showing empathy. This response addresses the client's feelings and offers an opportunity for the client to clarify the situation.**

4. *Wrong! The nurse is showing disapproval. This is a communication block.*

100. **A client who has a broken leg is to be discharged from the hospital after crutch training by physical therapy. His friend, who recently recovered from a similar injury, brings in a pair of crutches for him. What is the best nursing action?**

1. Since the friend knows how to use crutches, cancel the physical therapy order and allow the client to go home with his friend.
2. Inform the client that crutches are custom fitted for each client, and that he cannot use his friend's crutches.
3. Have the client try the crutches to see if they are the right size.
4. Send the crutches to physical therapy with the client for evaluation by that department.

1. *Wrong. This option is not appropriate because of the risk of falling if the crutches are used incorrectly. Before discharge, the client must be evaluated for his understanding and correct usage of crutches. Try again.*

2. *This is not true. Although crutches are sized and adjusted for proper fit for each client, crutches are not customized for each individual. The client may be able to use his friend's crutches if both men are similar in size. Read the options again and make another choice.*

3. *Wrong. Merely trying out the crutches is not sufficient. A client must receive instruction in the proper use of crutches before trying to use them, in order to avoid potential falls.*

4. **Correct! Since it may be possible for the client to use his friend's crutches, it is most appropriate to have them evaluated during crutch training by physical therapy personnel.**

NOTES

NCLEX-PN

Test 10
Pharmacology

NCLEX-PN TEST 10

1. The nurse understands that epinephrine (Epifrin) can be used for open angle glaucoma because of which of the following effects?

    1. Pupil dilatation.
    2. Pupil constriction.
    3. Reducing aqueous formation and enhancing outflow.
    4. Increasing aqueous formation.

2. In administering atropine to a client, the nurse knows that the medication is contraindicated in clients with glaucoma because of which side effect of the drug?

    1. Pupil constriction (miosis).
    2. Decreased production of aqueous humor.
    3. Pupil dilatation (mydriasis).
    4. Decreases in intraocular pressure.

3. In caring for an elderly or debilitated client on piperacillin (Pipracil), the nurse should give immediate attention to:

    1. Unusual weight loss, abdominal cramps.
    2. Blurred vision.
    3. Prolonged prothrombin time.
    4. Skin rashes.

4. Amoxicillin (Amoxil) is absorbed more effectively when the nurse administers it with:

    1. Orange juice or grapefruit juice.
    2. Milk or Amphojel.
    3. A complete meal.
    4. A full glass of water on an empty stomach.

5. Cefoperazone (Cefobid) has been prescribed to a client allergic to penicillin. To what complication should the nurse give priority?

    1. Drug resistance.
    2. Hypersensitivity reactions.
    3. Drug tolerance.
    4. Interactions with other drugs.

6. In caring for a client taking cefoperazone (Cefobid), the nurse would warn the client about significant drug interactions if taken with:

    1. Wine.
    2. Orange juice.

3. Food.
4. Maalox.

7. The nurse should teach the client that the best way to take a tablet of erythromycin (E-Mycin) that is not enteric coated is:

    1. With meals.
    2. With a full glass of water on an empty stomach.
    3. With a snack.
    4. Crushed and added to food.

8. A client is to receive cefazolin (Ancef) 500 mg IM every six hours. Which of the following nursing actions will most effectively decrease irritation at the injection site?

    1. Using the Z-track method, and injecting into the dorsogluteal site.
    2. Not massaging the site after the medication is administered, instead using gentle pressure only.
    3. Giving the medication slowly, over one minute, to allow dispersal time into the muscle.
    4. Using a 1 1/2 inch needle and injecting into the ventrogluteal site.

9. A 23-year-old client is being treated with erythromycin base (E-Mycin) 250 mg P.O. every six hours for strep throat. The nurse instructs the client to take the drug with:

    1. Milk or an antacid.
    2. Water one hour before or two hours after meals.
    3. Fruit juice.
    4. Food.

10. A client, age 63, is being treated for Legionnaires' disease with erythromycin estolate (Ilosone). Which of the following conditions, if given in his medical history, would the nurse identify as contraindicating the use of this drug?

    1. Pyelonephritis.
    2. Cirrhosis.
    3. Coronary artery disease.
    4. Emphysema.

11. A diabetic client, age 75, has ampicillin (Amcill) prescribed by his physician. Before the client leaves the clinic, the nurse should give highest priority to asking the client:

1. "What method do you use to monitor your glucose level?"
2. "Do you have any food allergies?"
3. "Do you have any difficulty swallowing capsules?"
4. "Do you have a history of liver disease?"

12. The nurse is preparing to instruct a diabetic client who is prescribed cefonicid (Monocid). The client regularly tests his urine for glucose. The most appropriate information for the nurse to give the client before taking cefonicid is:

    1. "Use a second-voided urine specimen when testing for glucose using the Clinitest method."
    2. "Have your physician adjust your insulin dosage to reflect the need for increased insulin during cephalosporin therapy."
    3. "Use an alternate method of urine testing (Clinistix or Tes-Tape) while taking Monocid."
    4. "Have the diabetic clinician teach you the use of a Glucometer to test for capillary blood sugar while taking Monocid."

13. In caring for a client who is highly allergic to penicillin, the nurse knows that which antibiotic would be safe to administer?

    1. Ampicillin (Amcill).
    2. Cefazolin (Ancef).
    3. Erythromycin ethylsuccinate (E.E.S.).
    4. Moxalactam (Moxam).

14. Which manifestations should the nurse report immediately to the charge nurse when a client is beginning a course of penicillin therapy?

    1. Indigestion, nausea.
    2. Hives, itching.
    3. Ringing in the ears, dizziness.
    4. Headaches, drowsiness.

15. A diabetic client is taking cephalexin (Keflex). The nurse understands that effective client teaching has occurred when the client knows that:

    1. A Clinitest or copper sulfate urine glucose test may yield false-positive results.
    2. The blood sugar may drop without warning.
    3. A source of sugar should always be carried.
    4. A medic alert bracelet should always be worn.

16. A six-month-old client has been prescribed erythromycin ethylsuccinate (Pediamycin) for an infection. The nurse needs to remind the client's mother that, before giving this medication, she should:

    1. Mix the medication in the client's formula.
    2. Be sure to keep the medication refrigerated and

shake it well before giving to the client.
    3. Keep the medication near the client's bed as a reminder to give it to him around the clock.
    4. Mix the medication in the client's baby food and give it at each meal.

17. It is the beginning of summer, and a 14-year-old client is taking minocycline (Minocin) for her acne. What advice should the nurse give the client?

    1. Take the medication on an empty stomach with a glass of water.
    2. Minocin makes the skin photosensitive—so shield your skin from the sun and use a sun screen.
    3. Stay inside, as this medication will react with the sun.
    4. Take this drug at night before bedtime.

18. The nurse sees a 22-year-old client in the clinic. The client has been taking a tetracycline drug for months for her acne. She is now trying to conceive a child. The nurse understands that which of the following is essential for this client to know about tetracycline therapy?

    1. Its use in pregnancy is not established.
    2. Any tetracycline can cause discoloration and mottling of fetal teeth and, therefore, cannot be used in pregnancy.
    3. The client should notify her doctor but should continue the drug as usual.
    4. This drug is dangerous and causes fetal deaths.

19. A client with a urinary tract infection is prescribed sulfisoxazole (Gantrisin). The nurse should advise the client to:

    1. Limit water intake to a quart a day.
    2. Drink plenty of juices to acidify the urine.
    3. Take extra vitamin C for healing.
    4. Drink up to three quarts of fluids a day.

20. The nurse should avoid administering sulfisoxazole (Gantrisin) to pregnant Caucasian women near term, to nursing mothers, or to infants under two months of age because of the danger of:

    1. Leukopenia.
    2. Renal damage.
    3. Kernicterus.
    4. Photosensitivity.

21. The physician prescribes minocycline (Minocin) for a 35-year-old female client with a urinary tract infection. Which question is important for the nurse to ask before starting the drug?

    1. "Are you allergic to penicillin?"
    2. "Are you currently taking an oral contraceptive?"

3. "Do you have a history of urinary tract infections?"
4. "Are you currently taking any heart medication?"

22. **A client is newly diagnosed with an upper respiratory tract infection. In caring for this client, the nurse knows that which of the following problems would contraindicate the use of norfloxacin (Noroxin) for the client's infection?**

    1. Emphysema.
    2. Epilepsy.
    3. Hiatal hernia.
    4. Cirrhosis.

23. **A 75-year-old client is being discharged on sulfisoxazole (Gantrisin) for treatment of a urinary tract infection. The nurse should emphasize which of the following to report as an early indication of possible renal impairment?**

    1. Dysuria.
    2. Weight gain.
    3. Jaundice.
    4. Oliguria.

24. **A client reports side effects she is experiencing as a result of oral clindamycin (Cleocin) therapy. The nurse should give immediate attention to:**

    1. Dysphagia.
    2. Nausea.
    3. Flatulence.
    4. Tarry stools.

25. **A client is admitted with pneumocystis carinii pneumonitis. The physician prescribes co-trimoxazole (Bactrim) and a Foley catheter is inserted to monitor urinary output. Which of the following nursing interventions would be most effective in reducing the risk of crystalluria secondary to sulfonamide therapy?**

    1. Encouraging fluid intake to 3000 cc/24 hours.
    2. Irrigating the Foley catheter with normal saline every eight hours.
    3. Monitoring specific gravity of urine every eight hours.
    4. Providing foods/fluids to maintain an acidic pH of the urine.

26. **A client has developed a urinary tract infection and sulfisoxazole (Gantrisin) 2 grams P.O., q.i.d. has been prescribed. The nurse should instruct the client to:**

    1. Take the medicine with meals or a snack.
    2. Take the medicine with a full glass of water on an empty stomach.
    3. Request a liquid form if swallowing is a problem,

since the pill cannot be crushed.
4. Use an antacid with the Gantrisin if GI upset should occur.

27. **The nurse understands that which groups of clients are most prone to the possibility of ototoxicity from tobramycin (Nebcin) therapy?**

    1. Elderly.
    2. Pregnant women.
    3. Children.
    4. Those previously sensitized to aminoglycosides.

28. **A client experiences photosensitivity while taking co-trimoxazole (Septra). The client describes photosensitivity manifestations to the nurse as:**

    1. Blurred vision.
    2. Pain in the eyes upon exposure to sunlight.
    3. Sunburn reaction with minimal sun exposure.
    4. Generalized rash and itching.

29. **A client is currently being treated with kanamycin (Kantrex). The nurse would note which condition in the client's medical history as requiring cautious use of this drug?**

    1. Hypertension.
    2. Myasthenia gravis.
    3. Diabetes mellitus.
    4. Epilepsy.

30. **A physician has prescribed sulfonamide therapy for an elderly client. Which lab work finding would the nurse identify as suggestive of a blood dyscrasia, which is a concern for this client's age group?**

    1. Hgb: 13.8.
    2. WBC: 2,000.
    3. Platelets: 200,000.
    4. RBC: 4,800,000.

31. **An elderly client is diagnosed with Klebsiella pneumonia. He is being treated with gentamicin sulfate (Garamycin). The nurse should give immediate consideration to the possibility of which side effect?**

    1. Hearing loss.
    2. Palpitations.
    3. Prolonged prothrombin time.
    4. Seizures.

32. **The nurse is caring for a client who is receiving isoniazid (INH) and who has developed peripheral neuropathy, a side effect from the use of isoniazid. The nurse knows that peripheral neuropathy is treated by administering which of the following at the same time INH is given?**

1. Vitamin C.
2. Vitamin B6 (Pyridoxine).
3. Steroids.
4. Combinations of vitamins and steroids.

33. Before beginning a client's rifampin (Rifadin) therapy, the nurse should warn him that this medication:

1. Turns urine, sweat, tears and saliva to a red-orange color.
2. Causes stools to turn black.
3. Stains teeth.
4. Causes constipation.

34. A client is scheduled for a colon resection in two days. She is started on a full liquid diet and neomycin sulfate (Neobiotic) by mouth four times a day. The nurse understands that the purpose of the administration of the neomycin sulfate before surgery is:

1. Sterilization of the bowel mucosa.
2. Reduction in bacterial content of the colon.
3. Treatment of any secondary infection that might be present prior to surgery.
4. Decreasing the rate of peristalsis during surgery.

35. The nurse understands that the purpose of treating a client in labor with naloxone (Narcan) is to:

1. Increase the effects of narcotics.
2. Depress the activity of the central nervous system (CNS) in the woman who received narcotics.
3. Block the effects of narcotics on the CNS.
4. Withdraw narcotics from the body.

36. Methylergonovine maleate (Methergine) is ordered for a client following a normal vaginal delivery. The nurse would recognize which of the following as a side effect of Methergine?

1. Marked oliguria.
2. Severe hypoglycemia.
3. Sudden hypertension.
4. Uterine rupture.

37. The doctor orders ergonovine (Ergotrate) for a client. Which condition warrants caution when the nurse is administering Ergotrate?

1. Diabetes.
2. Pre-eclampsia.
3. Uterine atony.
4. Anemia.

38. Isoxsuprine (Vasodilan) is a uterine relaxant used to treat premature labor. Which of the following findings could indicate an adverse reaction to Vasodilan and should be reported to the charge nurse?

1. Maternal apical pulse 116.
2. Fetal heart rate 164.
3. Maternal temperature 101° F.
4. Rapid decrease in blood pressure from 130/90 to 110/68.

39. A six-month-old took two ounces of expressed breast milk, provided by the mother, at 8:00 a.m., three ounces at 11:00 a.m. and two and one-half ounces at 1:00 p.m. What should the nurse record on this client's intake record for the shift?

1. 150 cc.
2. 225 cc.
3. 240 cc.
4. 375 cc.

40. The physician ordered gr 3/4. On hand are 15 mg tablets. What number of tablets should be given by the nurse?

1. Three tablets.
2. One tablet.
3. Two tablets.
4. One and one-half tablets.

41. The nurse caring for clients receiving antipsychotic medications knows that a medication often prescribed for treating the extrapyramidal side effects associated with antipsychotics is:

1. Phenelzine (Nardil).
2. Bupropion (Wellbutrin).
3. Amantadine (Symmetrel).
4. Hydroxyzine (Atarax).

42. A 19-year-old client is in crisis and is admitted for drug abuse. In caring for this client, the nurse understands that which type of medication should be prescribed only in limited amounts for this client?

1. Antipsychotics.
2. Antiparkinsonian agents.
3. Tricyclic antidepressants.
4. MAO inhibitor antidepressants.

43. The nurse is caring for a chronic alcoholic client who is experiencing alcohol withdrawal. The nurse knows which of the following medications is indicated to manage the client's alcohol withdrawal?

1. Buspirone (BuSpar).
2. Propranolol (Inderal).
3. Hydroxyzine (Atarax).
4. Chlordiazepoxide (Librium).

44. A client with COPD requests "cough medicine." The nurse's response is guided by the knowledge that the use of antitussives is only justified:

    1. If a cough is productive.
    2. In viral infections.
    3. If a cough interferes with recovery.
    4. When used in combination with expectorants.

45. The nurse is caring for a client who overdosed on codeine. The nurse knows that the effects of this overdose can be reversed by giving the client:

    1. Albuterol (Proventil).
    2. Atropine.
    3. Naloxone (Narcan).
    4. Protamine sulfate.

46. In teaching the client how to avoid unpleasant side effects when using benzonatate (Tessalon), the nurse should instruct the client to:

    1. Swallow the capsule whole.
    2. Use only for chronic coughs.
    3. Use for short periods of time to avoid addiction.
    4. Taper doses when discontinuing the medication.

47. In assessing a client with frequent allergies, the nurse would expect to find:

    1. Increased heart rate.
    2. Anorexia.
    3. Increased mucous secretion.
    4. Vertigo.

48. A 27-year-old client states that she frequently uses over-the-counter antihistamine preparations for her small child. The nurse would place priority on teaching the mother:

    1. Recommended safe dosages for children.
    2. Signs of antihistamine poisoning.
    3. The importance of keeping an antihistamine antidote on hand.
    4. The necessity of safe storage precautions.

49. When administering an antihistamine to an elderly client, the nurse would consider which of the following a priority?

    1. The elderly require increased doses of antihistamines.
    2. Paradoxical restlessness can occur in an elderly client.
    3. Sustained release preparations are contraindicated in an elderly client.
    4. Many brands of antihistamines are available in non-child-resistant containers.

50. When the nurse evaluates the client's knowledge regarding the use of antihistamines, which statement made by the client indicates a knowledge deficit?

    1. "I should be careful when driving."
    2. "Hard candy will relieve my dry mouth."
    3. "This medication may be taken with food."
    4. "If I am pregnant, I should take half the dose."

51. The nurse is teaching a client who is receiving a thiazide diuretic. The client would demonstrate understanding of his drug therapy by selecting which of the following foods?

    1. Apricots.
    2. Milk.
    3. Beef.
    4. Pork.

52. A newly diagnosed diabetic indicates a possible lack of understanding about his daily injections of insulin when he tells the nurse that:

    1. He will change injection sites.
    2. He needs to buy some alcohol.
    3. His brother also is a diabetic, and he will be able to share all of the supplies with him.
    4. His wife will be giving him the injections.

53. The nurse suspects an allergic reaction to penicillin. At this time, which of the following medications would the nurse be prepared to administer?

    1. Diphenhydramine (Benadryl).
    2. Prednisone.
    3. Ipratropium (Atrovent).
    4. Morphine sulfate.

54. A client is receiving cyclophosphamide (Cytoxan) for treatment of her leukemia. The nurse has noticed that the client vomited after each of her previous doses. To prevent vomiting, what should the nurse do?

    1. Have the charge nurse contact the physician for an antiemetic order prior to treatment.
    2. Withhold fluids prior to and during treatments.
    3. Suggest to the client that she eat before receiving her treatment.
    4. Explain that vomiting cannot be prevented and provide the client with an emesis basin during treatments.

55. A client is being treated with Cisplatin (Platinol) for his cancer. After several treatments he begins to complain of fatigue and wants to sleep all day. Which is the priority nursing action?

1. Advise the client about the dangers of immobility.
2. Check lab values of RBCs, hematocrit and hemoglobin, as he is likely to be anemic.
3. Call in the family for counseling, because the client is depressed and may become suicidal.
4. Set up an exercise plan.

56. **When instructing a client on the use of cromolyn (Intal), the nurse would include the information that Intal is most effective when:**

    1. Administered orally.
    2. Used prophylactically.
    3. Combined with an anti-inflammatory drug.
    4. Used to treat non-allergic responses.

57. **After administering acetylcysteine (Mucomyst), the nurse might enhance the effectiveness of the medication by:**

    1. Providing oxygen via Venturi mask.
    2. Positioning the client for postural drainage.
    3. Encouraging deep breathing exercises.
    4. Assisting the client with mouth care.

58. **A 62-year-old client with a history of emphysema asks the nurse about the use of chlorpheniramine maleate (Chlor-Trimeton). The nurse's response is based on the knowledge that:**

    1. Antihistamines can thicken secretions, and are only cautiously used in clients with COPD.
    2. Use of antihistamines to control respiratory secretions is preferred because of the lack of major side effects.
    3. Diphenhydramine (Benadryl) is the medication of choice for clients with COPD because it is readily available without a prescription.
    4. The sedative effect of antihistamines can compromise respiratory stimulation in clients with COPD.

59. **When discontinuing a course of prednisone for a client with recurring chronic bronchitis, the nurse should plan to taper the dose because the client may experience:**

    1. Hyperglycemia.
    2. Adrenocortical insufficiency.
    3. Severe dehydration.
    4. Delirium tremens.

60. **Before administering acetylcysteine (Mucomyst) to a confused or lethargic client, which item does the nurse needs to have readily available?**

    1. Tracheostomy set.
    2. Suction equipment.
    3. A vial of epinephrine.

    4. A secondary intravenous set.

61. **A client tells the nurse that she commonly uses commercial cough preparations containing guaifenesin (Robitussin). This statement would cause concern to the nurse if the client were also taking:**

    1. Acetaminophen.
    2. Penicillin.
    3. Phenytoin.
    4. Heparin.

62. **The nurse has completed discharge teaching on the use of metered dose inhalers for both bronchodilators and anti-inflammatory medications. Which statement made by the client indicates the need for more client teaching?**

    1. "I should wait five minutes between medications."
    2. "I will repeat the dose if I get no relief."
    3. "I should use my albuterol (Ventolin) inhaler before my beclomethasone (Beclovent) inhaler."
    4. "I will chart my response to the medications."

63. **In evaluating the effectiveness of acetylcysteine (Mucomyst), the nurse would assess for:**

    1. Respiratory rate.
    2. Presence of adventitious breath sounds.
    3. Absence of a cough.
    4. The thickness of secretions.

64. **To detect an adverse interaction between antihistamines and alcohol, the nurse would be on the alert for:**

    1. Tachycardia.
    2. Vomiting.
    3. Change in level of consciousness.
    4. Bronchoconstriction.

65. **The nurse is preparing a discharge teaching plan for the client on glucocorticoid therapy. Which information by the nurse is most appropriate?**

    1. Take medication on an empty stomach to enhance absorption.
    2. Alternate day therapy may prevent some side effects.
    3. If any sign of rash occurs, stop taking the medication immediately.
    4. Take two pills at the first sign of respiratory distress.

66. **Which common side effect would the nurse expect to find in a client receiving acetylcysteine (Mucomyst)?**

1. Sore throat.
2. Headache.
3. Nausea.
4. Drowsiness.

67. **Which of the following is an inappropriate instruction by the nurse in the teaching plan for a client using expectorants?**

    1. Be sure to increase fluid intake.
    2. Take this medication on an empty stomach.
    3. Check recommended doses and follow manufacturers' recommendations.
    4. Use deep breathing and coughing exercises.

68. **The parents of a four-year-old child with asthma ask the nurse about possible medications. The nurse understands which of the following is an inappropriate medication for a pediatric client?**

    1. Metaproterenol.
    2. Cromolyn.
    3. Isoproterenol.
    4. Aminophylline.

69. **When administering oral prednisone to a client with asthma, the nurse correctly administers the drug:**

    1. Crushed in juice, served with a straw.
    2. In a strong flavored juice to mask the taste.
    3. Accompanied by food or antacids.
    4. At least one hour before meals.

70. **In order to avoid complications of inhaled beclomethasone (Beclovent), the nurse correctly does which of the following:**

    1. Assists the client to rinse his mouth.
    2. Offers food or antacids following medication administration.
    3. Monitors the client's heart rate before and after medication administration.
    4. Cautions the client to avoid caffeine.

71. **When administering atropine, the nurse observes the client for side effects. Which side effect would cause the most concern?**

    1. Bradycardia.
    2. Urinary retention.
    3. Muscle tremors.
    4. Ventricular fibrillation.

72. **A client with chronic obstructive pulmonary disease is being discharged with an ipratropium (Atrovent) metered dose inhaler. Which of the following discharge instructions would the nurse question?**

1. Take two puffs every six hours as needed.
2. The client may have two refills.
3. Continue metaproterenol (Alupent) use.
4. Call the physician for blurred vision or headaches.

73. **In preparing a discharge plan for a client who has been on long-term prednisone therapy, the nurse must be aware that these clients are prone to:**

    1. Frequent bouts of nausea.
    2. Orthostatic hypotension.
    3. Gingival ulcerations.
    4. Bone fractures.

74. **An eight-year-old boy with asthma is placed on cromolyn (Intal) via metered dose inhaler. After client teaching, which statement by the child's parents indicates the need for more instruction?**

    1. "I will give my son a dose as soon as he starts wheezing."
    2. "My son needs to rinse out his mouth after using the inhaler."
    3. "My son should breathe in slowly while depressing the canister."
    4. "If my son has difficulty breathing in the dose, I can use a spacer."

75. **The nurse administers metaproterenol (Alupent) via a metered dose inhaler. The nurse understands the drug is effective if there is:**

    1. Clear, thin secretions.
    2. Decreased respiratory rate.
    3. Effective coughing.
    4. Absence of wheezing.

76. **The nurse administers atropine via nebulizer to a client with severe asthma. The nurse would withhold the drug and call the nurse in charge if the client exhibits:**

    1. Tachycardia.
    2. Nervousness.
    3. Visual changes.
    4. Dizziness.

77. **The nurse knows which factor is most important in planning discharge teaching for the client with obstructive pulmonary disease (COPD)?**

    1. COPD is caused by a variety of etiologies.
    2. COPD is progressive and chronic.
    3. There are a variety of medications for COPD available.
    4. Different age groups are affected by COPD.

78. When preparing a teaching plan for the client being discharged on theophylline (Theo-dur), the nurse should plan to include which information?

    1. Theophylline should be taken on an empty stomach to maximize absorption.
    2. The drug levels in the client's blood will need to be checked frequently.
    3. The client should take the last dose at bedtime so that wheezing will not occur during the night.
    4. This drug may cause drowsiness and interfere with the client's ability to operate heavy machinery.

79. In preparing a teaching plan for clients at a senior center, the nurse knows that which of the following is true of beta-agonist use in the elderly?

    1. There is an increased tendency toward incontinence.
    2. Higher drug levels are often needed.
    3. Use of multiple drugs in the elderly can lead to drug interactions.
    4. Dosage intervals are often shorter.

80. In preparing to teach a client about the use of cromolyn (Intal), the nurse is guided by the knowledge that the primary purpose of cromolyn administration in the treatment of asthma is to prevent:

    1. Bronchospasm.
    2. Infection.
    3. Anaphylaxis.
    4. Inflammation.

81. A client with status asthmaticus is admitted to the emergency room. Aminophylline is ordered. The nurse would expect the drug to be administered by which route?

    1. Subcutaneously.
    2. Intravenously.
    3. Via nebulizer.
    4. Sublingually.

82. A client is on long-term theophylline (Theo-dur) therapy. In order to decrease side effects, the nurse would caution the client to avoid:

    1. Dairy products.
    2. Caffeinated beverages.
    3. Antacids.
    4. High sodium foods.

83. A client has been taking theophylline (Theo-dur) for relief of chronic bronchitis. The nurse should be alert for which manifestations of toxicity with this drug?

1. Lethargy and slurred speech.
2. Increased urinary output.
3. Agitation and tremors.
4. Wheezing and dyspnea.

84. A client with asthma is being treated with isoproterenol (Isuprel). Which finding from the client's history would the nurse identify as requiring caution when administering this drug?

    1. Bronchospasm.
    2. Peptic ulcer disease.
    3. Angina.
    4. Raynaud's disease.

85. A client with chronic emphysema is taking theophylline (Theo-dur) at home. During the home care nurse's visit, which statement by the client demands immediate action?

    1. "I just lie awake at night, worrying about the medical bills."
    2. "I must have the flu. I was vomiting all night."
    3. "I don't have my usual appetite. Nothing tastes good to me."
    4. "I feel better if I have a big glass of milk with my pill."

86. A client is admitted to the hospital after complaining of chest pain. The client's history reveals congestive heart failure. He has been receiving digoxin (Lanoxin). The nurse understands that the purpose of giving the client digoxin is to:

    1. Increase cardiac size.
    2. Decrease cardiac output.
    3. Increase the force of cardiac contraction.
    4. Slow the pulse rate.

87. The nurse is administering digoxin (Lanoxin) to a client and notices that his breakfast is untouched. He is also complaining of nausea. The nurse checks his vitals, which are BP 118/72, P 60, R 22. The nurse understands that:

    1. The client is anxious and fearful.
    2. The client needs a change in diet.
    3. This is a normal reaction to the hospital.
    4. He may be exhibiting a drug reaction.

88. A client is receiving digoxin (Lanoxin). The nurse is alert for signs of which condition likely to contribute to digoxin toxicity?

    1. Hypokalemia.
    2. Hypocalcemia.

3.   Obesity.
4.   Hyponatremia.

89.   **An elderly client is admitted to the hospital with congestive heart failure and will be digitalized (given digoxin). Vitals on admission are BP 110/60, pulse 100, respirations 22. The nurse understands that the expected outcome of digitalization is:**

1.   Respiratory rate of 26.
2.   Heart rate greater than 100.
3.   Urine output of 50 cc per hour.
4.   Increased thirst.

90.   **In caring for a client taking digoxin (Lanoxin), the nurse would give immediate attention to which statement by the client?**

1.   "I have a headache and backache."
2.   "I feel nauseated and have no appetite."
3.   "I've gained half a pound in the last two days."
4.   "I'm having muscle cramps in my legs."

91.   **The nurse knows that there are two basic types of arrhythmias. The type that makes the heart go faster and the type that makes the heart go slower, would be identified (in that order) by the nurse as:**

1.   Bradyarrhythmias and tachyarrhythmias.
2.   Tachyarrhythmias and bradyarrhythmias.
3.   Supraventricular and ventricular.
4.   Ventricular and supraventricular.

92.   **A client is taking propranolol (Inderal) for angina. The nurse understands that Inderal relieves angina because of which action?**

1.   Increase in cardiac output.
2.   Increase in heart rate.
3.   Inhibition of vasodilatation in coronary vessels.
4.   Decrease in myocardial oxygen requirements.

93.   **A client started methyldopa (Aldomet) to lower his blood pressure. The nurse must emphasize to the client the importance of keeping appointments for which lab studies?**

1.   Renal function studies.
2.   Blood cell counts and hepatic function studies.
3.   Aldomet blood levels.
4.   Cardiac enzymes.

94.   **A client's blood pressure rises to 200/120, which is considered a hypertensive emergency. Diazoxide**

(Hyperstat) is administered. The nurse should expect the response to be noticeable in which amount of time?

1.   Within one and five minutes of administration.
2.   Within one hour of administration.
3.   After the second dose.
4.   After the first few doses.

95.   **The nurse is caring for a client who is diagnosed as hypertensive and is prescribed hydralazine (Apresoline). What statement indicates that the client understands the action of his medication?**

1.   "I will eat plenty of foods high in sodium to keep my fluid level up."
2.   "I will limit my fluid intake."
3.   "I realize that I need to get up more slowly than before."
4.   "I will always remember to take this medication on an empty stomach."

96.   **A 72-year-old with gouty arthritis is prescribed naproxen (Naprosyn). The nurse understands that the geriatric implications for this drug include:**

1.   A higher incidence of agranulocytosis and aplastic anemia.
2.   A higher incidence of perforated peptic ulcers and/or bleeding.
3.   A higher incidence of central nervous system side effects.
4.   None, as all NSAIDs are relatively safe medications for any age group.

97.   **In administering acetaminophen (Tylenol) to a client, the nurse knows that this drug is used primarily for which clinical properties?**

1.   Analgesic and antipyretic.
2.   Antirheumatic.
3.   Anticlotting.
4.   Anti-inflammatory.

98.   **A client is admitted to the emergency room with an overdose of acetaminophen (Tylenol). The nurse would give immediate consideration to which manifestations:**

1.   Slow respiratory rate.
2.   Nausea, vomiting and abdominal discomfort.
3.   Decreased urine output.
4.   Convulsions.

99. A client has been taking morphine for several weeks to relieve her cancer pain. During the last two home health visits, she has complained that her dose does not seem to be working. The nurse understands that the client has:

    1. Developed an addiction to morphine.
    2. Become confused and probably is not taking her medications properly.
    3. Developed a tolerance to the medication.
    4. Abused the medication and needs counseling about her addiction.

100. A client is being treated with pilocarpine (Pilocar) for his glaucoma. He complains of blurred vision after administration of his drops. The nurse's explanation to the client should be based upon which information?

    1. The client is not using the eye drops correctly.
    2. Pilocarpine causes the pupil to constrict, making the eye accommodate for near vision; therefore, objects far away seem blurred.
    3. When the pupil is dilated, it is more difficult to adjust vision.
    4. Pilocarpine irritates the lining of the eye and causes blurring and inflammation.

NCLEX-PN

Test 10

Pharmacology Questions with Rationales

NCLEX-PN TEST 10 WITH RATIONALES

1. The nurse understands that epinephrine (Epifrin) can be used for open angle glaucoma because of which of the following effects?

   1. Pupil dilatation.
   2. Pupil constriction.
   3. Reducing aqueous formation and enhancing outflow.
   4. Increasing aqueous formation.

   1. *Epinephrine does cause the pupil to dilate, but dilatation alone is contraindicated for glaucoma. Try again.*
   2. *Incorrect. The pupil is dilated with epinephrine, not constricted.*
   3. ***Great work! Epinephrine can be used with glaucoma because it reduces aqueous production and enhances outflow.***
   4. *Wrong, try again. If aqueous production were increased, glaucoma would get worse.*

2. In administering atropine to a client, the nurse knows that the medication is contraindicated in clients with glaucoma because of which side effect of the drug?

   1. Pupil constriction (miosis).
   2. Decreased production of aqueous humor.
   3. Pupil dilatation (mydriasis).
   4. Decreases in intraocular pressure.

   1. *Sorry, try again. Atropine causes the eye to dilate, not constrict.*
   2. *Incorrect. Atropine does not have the effect of decreasing aqueous humor.*
   3. ***Correct. Atropine causes the eye to dilate so that the ciliary body blocks the canal of Schlemm, which prevents the outflow of aqueous humor. This would be a severe reaction for a client with glaucoma.***
   4. *Incorrect. Atropine does not decrease intraocular pressure.*

3. In caring for an elderly or debilitated client on piperacillin (Pipracil), the nurse should give immediate attention to:

   1. Unusual weight loss, abdominal cramps.
   2. Blurred vision.
   3. Prolonged prothrombin time.
   4. Skin rashes.

   1. ***Very good! Elderly clients are very prone to superinfections and pseudomembranous coli-***

tis. A superinfection occurs when the normal flora are eliminated by the antibiotic, making the internal environment susceptible to undesirable bacteria, yeasts, or fungi. Weight loss, abdominal cramps, diarrhea, discolored tongue, and sore mouth are manifestations of possible pseudomembranous colitis.

   2. *Changes in the eyes are not related to penicillins. Try again.*
   3. *This is not correct. Some penicillins are metabolized up to 50% in the liver, but most excretion is via the kidney. Select another answer.*
   4. *Wrong. It is true that skin rashes should be observed for in all clients, and that elderly clients are more likely to be hypersensitive to skin rashes from penicillin. In this question, however, you are to look for a manifestation that would be particularly threatening for an elderly or debilitated client. Try again.*

4. Amoxicillin (Amoxil) is absorbed more effectively when the nurse administers it with:

   1. Orange juice or grapefruit juice.
   2. Milk or Amphojel.
   3. A complete meal.
   4. A full glass of water on an empty stomach.

   1. *This is incorrect. Citrus juices destroy oral penicillins. Make another choice.*
   2. *Antacids or milk should not be needed. If stomach upset occurs, pseudomembranous colitis should be suspected. Make another selection.*
   3. *This is incorrect. Absorption of many penicillins decreases when taken with food. Try again.*
   4. ***That's right! Oral penicillins should be given on an empty stomach because they bind to food and are poorly absorbed in the acid media of the stomach.***

5. Cefoperazone (Cefobid) has been prescribed to a client allergic to penicillin. To what complication should the nurse give priority?

   1. Drug resistance.
   2. Hypersensitivity reactions.
   3. Drug tolerance.
   4. Interactions with other drugs.

   1. *Wrong choice. Drug resistance is always possible, but it is not the highest priority. Try again.*
   2. ***You are correct! Cephalosporins are chemical modifications of penicillins. The possibility of***

a cross-reaction is five to 10 percent.

3. *This is incorrect. Drug tolerance does not develop with antibiotics. Make another choice.*

4. *Wrong choice! While this may be true in general, no other drugs are mentioned in this case scenario. Look for a complication related to penicillin itself.*

6. In caring for a client taking cefoperazone (Cefobid), the nurse would warn the client about significant drug interactions if taken with:

1. Wine.
2. Orange juice.
3. Food.
4. Maalox.

1. *Correct! When Cefobid is taken with alcohol, acetaldehyde in the blood produces an Antabuse-like reaction with gastrointestinal manifestations. Clients should avoid the use of alcohol or any over-the-counter medicines that contain alcohol when taking this medication.*

2. *This is incorrect. Fruit juices are known for their effect when combined with penicillins, not with cefoperazone. Try again.*

3. *Wrong choice. Cephalosporins may be taken with food with no ill effects.*

4. *Wrong choice. Antacids would have no untoward effect.*

7. The nurse should teach the client that the best way to take a tablet of erythromycin (E-Mycin) that is not enteric coated is:

1. With meals.
2. With a full glass of water on an empty stomach.
3. With a snack.
4. Crushed and added to food.

1. *No. If the client takes a form of erythromycin that is not enteric coated with meals, much of the drug will be lost, because erythromycin can be protein bound.*

> **TEST-TAKING TIP:** *This option uses the same idea as Option 3. When two options are this similar, neither of them can be the correct answer. When you are unsure of the answer to a test question, try to eliminate similar options.*

2. *Correct! The best way to take non-enteric coated erythromycin is with water on an empty stomach. If diarrhea or stomach complications occur, the enteric coated form may be ordered.*

3. *No. Mixing with food will bind the drug and make less available for absorption.*

> **TEST-TAKING TIP:** *This option uses the same idea as Option 1. When two options are this similar, neither of them can be the correct answer. When you are unsure of the answer to a test question, try to eliminate similar options.*

4. *Wrong choice! The medication should not be crushed. If the client has difficulty swallowing the pill, a liquid form is available. If the pill were added to food, absorption would be impaired.*

8. A client is to receive cefazolin (Ancef) 500 mg IM every six hours. Which of the following nursing actions will most effectively decrease irritation at the injection site?

1. Using the Z-track method, and injecting into the dorsogluteal site.
2. Not massaging the site after the medication is administered, instead using gentle pressure only.
3. Giving the medication slowly, over one minute, to allow dispersal time into the muscle.
4. Using a 1 1/2 inch needle and injecting into the ventrogluteal site.

1. *Excellent choice! This injection technique is specific for administration of medications known to cause pain or permanent staining of superficial tissues. The dorsogluteal site uses the gluteus medius muscle of the buttocks, a large muscle mass that is preferred in this case.*

2. *Wrong. Although use of gentle pressure without massage may help to decrease irritation, it is not the most effective technique of the choices given. Make another selection.*

3. *Wrong. This intervention may assist in more even distribution of the medication, but it does not necessarily decrease the risk of irritation. Try again.*

4. *Not the best choice. You were correct in choosing the needle length, but the VENTROGLUTEAL site, using the gluteus MINIMUS muscle, would not be the preferred site. Choose again.*

9. A 23-year-old client is being treated with erythromycin base (E-Mycin) 250 mg P.O. every six hours for strep throat. The nurse instructs the client to take the drug with:

1. Milk or an antacid.
2. Water one hour before or two hours after meals.
3. Fruit juice.
4. Food.

1. *No, erythromycin may bind with the milk or antacid and decrease the amount of drug available for absorption. Make another selection.*

2. *Good choice. Erythromycin base and stearate preparations should be given on an empty stomach.*

3. *Wrong! Fruit juice with an acid base may destroy*

the drug before it's absorbed. Try again.

4.   Incorrect. Erythromycin base would bind with the food and make less drug available for absorption. Choose another response.

10.   A client, age 63, is being treated for Legionnaires' disease with erythromycin estolate (Ilosone). Which of the following conditions, if given in his medical history, would the nurse identify as contraindicating the use of this drug?

1.   Pyelonephritis.
2.   Cirrhosis.
3.   Coronary artery disease.
4.   Emphysema.

1.   Incorrect. Ninety-five percent of the excretion of erythromycin is via the liver and bile. Only five percent is excreted in urine. There is no significant effect upon renal function. Try again.

2.   **Good work! Erythromycin estolate is contraindicated in clients with hepatic disease because the drug may be hepatotoxic. The risk of liver damage is increased if erythromycin is given concurrently with other hepatotoxic agents, e.g., estrogens, piperacillin, and sulfonamides.**

3.   No, there is no known contraindication for the use of erythromycin in clients with a history of coronary artery disease. Make another choice.

4.   No, there is no known contraindication for the use of erythromycin in clients with COPD. Erythromycin may be ordered for COPD clients who develop respiratory tract infections caused by group A beta-hemolytic streptococci or other bacteria.

11.   A diabetic client, age 75, has ampicillin (Amcill) prescribed by his physician. Before the client leaves the clinic, the nurse should give highest priority to asking the client:

1.   "What method do you use to monitor your glucose level?"
2.   "Do you have any food allergies?"
3.   "Do you have any difficulty swallowing capsules?"
4.   "Do you have a history of liver disease?"

1.   **Excellent focus! You recall that clients with diabetes who use copper sulfate urine glucose tests (Clinitest) may have false-positive results when taking ampicillin. It's important for the nurse to assess which glucose testing method (urine, blood) the client uses to determine if he/she should use an alternate method, such as Tes-Tape or Clinistix.**

2.   No, asking the client about food allergies will not help the nurse determine if there is an allergy to penicillin. Try another choice.

3.   Not the best choice. This question, although relevant to determine if the client may need a liquid suspension, does not have priority over another question that addresses the ongoing assessment of the client's health status. Try to find that option.

4.   No, hepatic function is not a major concern with most penicillins. Penicillins (except Nafcillin) are excreted mostly unchanged in urine. Nafcillin is extensively metabolized in the liver. Make another choice.

12.   The nurse is preparing to instruct a diabetic client who is prescribed cefonicid (Monocid). The client regularly tests his urine for glucose. The most appropriate information for the nurse to give the client before taking cefonicid is:

1.   "Use a second-voided urine specimen when testing for glucose using the Clinitest method."
2.   "Have your physician adjust your insulin dosage to reflect the need for increased insulin during cephalosporin therapy."
3.   "Use an alternate method of urine testing (Clinistix or Tes-Tape) while taking Monocid."
4.   "Have the diabetic clinician teach you the use of a Glucometer to test for capillary blood sugar while taking Monocid."

1.   No, this will not resolve the problem. Recall that cephalosporins and penicillins may cause false-positive reactions with copper sulfateurine glucose tests. A second-voided specimen will not alter this effect. Try another option.

2.   Wrong. There should be no need for adjusting insulin dosage while taking cephalosporins. Try again.

3.   **Excellent! Glucose enzymatic tests such as these two methods will not give false-positive results to urine testing. Using an alternate urine testing method will require minimal adjustment on the client's part compared to learning to test capillary blood glucose levels.**

4.   Not the best option. It's not necessary to have a client learn a new route/technique of glucose testing when he is already familiar with urine testing. The antibiotic therapy is not a permanent change. Make another selection.

13.   In caring for a client who is highly allergic to penicillin, the nurse knows that which antibiotic would be safe to administer?

1.   Ampicillin (Amcill).
2.   Cefazolin (Ancef).
3.   Erythromycin ethylsuccinate (E.E.S.).
4.   Moxalactam (Moxam).

1.   Incorrect. This drug belongs to the penicillin family and would be contraindicated for a client with

known hypersensitivity. **NOTE:** *The generic names of all penicillins end in "cillin." Try again.*

2. *No, recall that cefazolin belongs to the cephalosporin family and that there is a possibility of cross-sensitivity (cephalosporins are chemical modifications of the penicillin structure). Choose another option.*

3. **Good choice! You remembered that macrolides are prescribed for clients who are allergic to penicillin. One of the most important antimicrobial agents is erythromycin.**

4. *Not correct. Moxam is a member of the cephalosporin family and should not be used (or should be used with caution) for clients sensitive to penicillin since cross-sensitivity may occur. Please re-read the options and select again.*

14. **Which manifestations should the nurse report immediately to the charge nurse when a client is beginning a course of penicillin therapy?**

    1. Indigestion, nausea.
    2. Hives, itching.
    3. Ringing in the ears, dizziness.
    4. Headaches, drowsiness.

    1. *No, these manifestations, although problematic, do not constitute an immediate threat to the client's life. These two manifestations of GI distress are often experienced by clients on antibiotic therapy. Read all the options before choosing the best one!*

    2. **Excellent! The development of hives, itching, and/or wheezing are indicative of a possible hypersensitivity reaction, which could progress to anaphylactic shock. Even if a client has previously taken penicillin without problems, there is still a chance of a reaction with subsequent doses. Clients should always be instructed to report these manifestations to the physician immediately.**

    3. *No, these two manifestations are not indicative of potential adverse reactions to penicillin. Try again.*

    4. *No, these two manifestations are not indicative of adverse reactions to penicillin therapy. Choose another option.*

15. **A diabetic client is taking cephalexin (Keflex). The nurse understands that effective client teaching has occurred when the client knows that:**

    1. A Clinitest or copper sulfate urine glucose test may yield false-positive results.
    2. The blood sugar may drop without warning.
    3. A source of sugar should always be carried.
    4. A medic alert bracelet should always be worn.

    1. **Yes! Clinitest or copper sulfate urine glucose tests can give false-positive results when clients are**

taking a cephalosporin or penicillin. Clients should be instructed to substitute use of Glucometers or glucose enzymatic tests such as Clinistix to monitor their glucose level.

2. *This is not correct. Such a reaction is not caused by antibiotics. Make another selection.*

3. *Wrong choice. This statement is true for all diabetics, regardless of medications. This question, however, requires an answer that relates specifically to the effect of cephalexin on diabetics. Try again.*

4. *Wrong choice. Although all diabetics should wear a medic alert bracelet, this does not address the client's need for information about the effect of cephalexin. Try again.*

16. **A six-month-old client has been prescribed erythromycin ethylsuccinate (Pediamycin) for an infection. The nurse needs to remind the client's mother that, before giving this medication, she should:**

    1. Mix the medication in the client's formula.
    2. Be sure to keep the medication refrigerated and shake it well before giving to the client.
    3. Keep the medication near the client's bed as a reminder to give it to him around the clock.
    4. Mix the medication in the client's baby food and give it at each meal.

    1. *This action is incorrect. Mixing medications in formula is not advisable and is not good practice. If the client does not take his entire bottle, much of the medication will be wasted. This option is also not correct because we do not know if the client is bottle fed or breastfed.*

    2. **Correct. You remembered that this medication comes in a suspension that needs to be refrigerated and shaken well before administration. Good work!**

    3. *No! Keeping any medication near the baby's bed is not a safe practice! Furthermore, this drug requires special storage. Try again.*

    4. *This action is incorrect. Mixing medication in food would decrease absorption. It is also not good practice to mix medications with food.*

17. **It is the beginning of summer, and a 14-year-old client is taking minocycline (Minocin) for her acne. What advice should the nurse give the client?**

    1. Take the medication on an empty stomach with a glass of water.
    2. Minocin makes the skin photosensitive—so shield your skin from the sun and use a sun screen.
    3. Stay inside, as this medication will react with the sun.
    4. Take this drug at night before bedtime.

    1. *No, this is not necessary. While this is true of most all of the tetracyclines, Minocin was developed to*

be taken with meals.

2. **You chose the correct answer! All the tetracyclines cause photosensitivity, and Minocin is no exception. Clients should stay out of the sun or at least use a sun screen. Good answer!**

3. *Wrong! It would be inadvisable to suggest that a 14-year-old stay inside during the summer. Look for a better option.*

4. *Wrong! The drug must be taken at intervals around the clock to be effective. Please reread the options.*

18. **The nurse sees a 22-year-old client in the clinic. The client has been taking a tetracycline drug for months for her acne. She is now trying to conceive a child. The nurse understands that which of the following is essential for this client to know about tetracycline therapy?**

    1. Its use in pregnancy is not established.
    2. Any tetracycline can cause discoloration and mottling of fetal teeth and, therefore, cannot be used in pregnancy.
    3. The client should notify her doctor but should continue the drug as usual.
    4. This drug is dangerous and causes fetal deaths.

    1. *No, this is not a correct statement! It is dangerous to take a tetracycline drug during pregnancy.*
    2. **Yes! Tetracycline drugs can have a permanent effect on the teeth of a developing fetus.**
    3. *No, this statement is not totally correct. Though the client should notify her doctor, she will not be able to continue the drug as usual.*

> **TEST-TAKING TIP:** *An option that is partly correct and partly incorrect can never be the correct answer!*

    4. *No, this statement is not true. Tetracycline does not cause fetal deaths, but it is not a safe drug to take during pregnancy due to the changes it causes in developing teeth. The client will not be able to continue taking this drug during pregnancy.*

19. **A client with a urinary tract infection is prescribed sulfisoxazole (Gantrisin). The nurse should advise the client to:**

    1. Limit water intake to a quart a day.
    2. Drink plenty of juices to acidify the urine.
    3. Take extra vitamin C for healing.
    4. Drink up to three quarts of fluids a day.

    1. *No! Fluids should not be limited when a client has a UTI. Select another option.*
    2. *No! Acid urine will cause sulfonamides to precipitate, causing crystalluria, hematuria and even renal failure. Try again!*

3. *No! Vitamin C acidifies urine. Acid urine will cause sulfonamides to precipitate, causing crystalluria, hematuria and even renal failure. Make another choice.*

4. **Correct. A non-hospitalized client should drink up to three quarts of fluids per day.**

20. **The nurse should avoid administering sulfisoxazole (Gantrisin) to pregnant Caucasian women near term, to nursing mothers, or to infants under two months of age because of the danger of:**

    1. Leukopenia.
    2. Renal damage.
    3. Kernicterus.
    4. Photosensitivity.

    1. *Wrong. Changes do not occur in white blood cells of Caucasian women. Hemolytic anemia occurs mostly in blacks or Mediterranean ethnics. Try again.*
    2. *Wrong. Renal damage can occur, but it is not the main danger in pregnant women. Make another selection.*
    3. **Good work! Kernicterus can occur because bilirubin is displaced from binding sites on plasma proteins. Kernicterus can be life-threatening, so this is the priority answer.**
    4. *Photosensitivity can occur but is not a priority with pregnant women or nursing mothers.*

21. **The physician prescribes minocycline (Minocin) for a 35-year-old female client with a urinary tract infection. Which question is important for the nurse to ask before starting the drug?**

    1. "Are you allergic to penicillin?"
    2. "Are you currently taking an oral contraceptive?"
    3. "Do you have a history of urinary tract infections?"
    4. "Are you currently taking any heart medication?"

    1. *No, there is no cross-sensitivity between penicillin and tetracycline. In fact, tetracycline is often prescribed for clients who are sensitive to penicillin. Make another selection.*
    2. **Yes! Clients who take tetracycline and who are on estrogen-containing oral contraceptives may experience decreased contraceptive effectiveness and an increased risk of breakthrough bleeding. An alternative means of contraception should be used during minocycline therapy and for one week after it is discontinued.**
    3. *Sorry, this is not the best option. Although this question would be part of the routine admission interview, it does not impact on the implementation of Minocin therapy. Try again.*

4. *No, there is no significant drug interaction when Minocin is taken concurrently with any heart medication. Choose another option.*

22. **A client is newly diagnosed with an upper respiratory tract infection. In caring for this client, the nurse knows that which of the following problems would contraindicate the use of norfloxacin (Noroxin) for the client's infection?**

    1. Emphysema.
    2. Epilepsy.
    3. Hiatal hernia.
    4. Cirrhosis.

    1. *No, there is no contraindication for the use of Noroxin in clients who have COPD. Try another selection.*
    2. **Excellent! Noroxin administration may result in CNS toxicity, with manifestations such as headaches, drowsiness, hallucinations, depression, and seizures. Quinolones should not be given to clients with preexisting CNS disease because they can exacerbate the problem.**
    3. *No, there is no contraindication for the use of Noroxin in clients with GI pathology. Noroxin may cause GI distress (nausea, flatulence, constipation, and heartburn), but antacids may be taken two hours after administration if needed. Choose again.*
    4. *No, this is not a contraindication. Clients with hepatic or renal impairment may require reduced dosages, but Noroxin is not known as an hepatotoxic drug. Make another selection.*

23. **A 75-year-old client is being discharged on sulfisoxazole (Gantrisin) for treatment of a urinary tract infection. The nurse should emphasize which of the following to report as an early indication of possible renal impairment?**

    1. Dysuria.
    2. Weight gain.
    3. Jaundice.
    4. Oliguria.

    1. *Incorrect. Dysuria would be indicative of a urinary tract infection (UTI) — but this client is currently taking Gantrisin to treat a UTI. Try again.*
    2. *Sorry. Although weight gain may result secondary to renal impairment (fluid volume excess), it would not be as quickly observed by the client and is not the initial indicator of renal impairment. Choose another option that would reflect early changes in an elimination pattern.*
    3. *Incorrect. Jaundice would be indicative of liver impairment, which is another possible toxic reac-*

tion to sulfonamides. It is not an indicator of renal impairment. Select again.
4. **Correct. Oliguria (urinary output less than 500 cc/24 hours) is one of the earliest indicators of renal impairment. Gantrisin is less likely to cause formation of crystals (crystalluria) than other sulfonamides, but renal toxicity remains a major concern. A common preventative measure is good hydration (increase fluids to 3000 cc/day). If the client cannot tolerate extra fluids, sodium bicarbonate may be administered to alkalinize the urine.**

24. **A client reports side effects she is experiencing as a result of oral clindamycin (Cleocin) therapy. The nurse should give immediate attention to:**

    1. Dysphagia.
    2. Nausea.
    3. Flatulence.
    4. Tarry stools.

    1. *Wrong choice. Although dysphagia (difficulty in swallowing) is a side effect of Cleocin therapy, it is not life-threatening and would not require the nurse's immediate attention. Advise the client taking the capsule form of Cleocin to take it with a full glass of water to prevent dysphagia. Make another selection.*
    2. *Wrong choice. Nausea is a side effect of Cleocin therapy, but it is not life-threatening. Look for an option that should receive immediate attention.*
    3. *Wrong choice. Flatulence as a side effect would not receive the nurses' immediate attention. Try again.*
    4. **Yes. The most serious reaction to Cleocin therapy is colitis, ranging from a mild diarrhea to a severe, life-threatening condition called pseudo-membranous colitis. The appearance of blood or mucous in the stool may be a sign of colitis and should be reported immediately to the physician.**

25. **A client is admitted with pneumocystis carinii pneumonitis. The physician prescribes co-trimoxazole (Bactrim) and a Foley catheter is inserted to monitor urinary output. Which of the following nursing interventions would be most effective in reducing the risk of crystalluria secondary to sulfonamide therapy?**

    1. Encouraging fluid intake to 3000 cc/24 hours.
    2. Irrigating the Foley catheter with normal saline every eight hours.
    3. Monitoring specific gravity of urine every eight hours.
    4. Providing foods/fluids to maintain an acidic pH of the urine.

1. *Excellent choice! Maintenance of hydration ("natural irrigation") is the most effective intervention in preventing urinary stasis, which can lead to crystalluria. The client's output should be at least 1500 cc/day.*
2. *No! Irrigating a Foley catheter should never be a routine procedure because of the increased risk of infection (interrupting a sterile system). There is a better and safer option. Select again.*
3. *No, this will not reduce the risk of crystalluria. Monitoring specific gravity of urine will give information regarding urine osmolality and the kidneys' ability to concentrate urine. It will not reduce the risk of crystalluria because it is only an assessment tool. Choose a more effective intervention!*
4. *No! The urine pH should be alkaline, not acidic. Liquids and foods that produce acid urine should be avoided. Sulfonamides precipitate because of their low solubility in normal acidic urine, increasing the risk of crystalluria.*

26. **A client has developed a urinary tract infection and sulfisoxazole (Gantrisin) 2 grams P.O., q.i.d. has been prescribed. The nurse should instruct the client to:**

1. Take the medicine with meals or a snack.
2. Take the medicine with a full glass of water on an empty stomach.
3. Request a liquid form if swallowing is a problem, since the pill cannot be crushed.
4. Use an antacid with the Gantrisin if GI upset should occur.

1. *Incorrect. Taking Gantrisin with food will decrease the rate of absorption and decrease the effectiveness of the medication. Choose another option.*
2. *Excellent choice! You remembered that sulfonamides should be taken on an empty stomach to increase absorption. A full glass of water will increase the client's fluid intake. He should drink at least 3,000 cc/day.*
3. *Not true. Gantrisin can be crushed and swallowed with water to ensure maximal absorption. Many clients, especially the elderly, will break the tablet in half because of its large size, in order to prevent choking. Try again.*
4. *Incorrect. Gantrisin should not be taken with an antacid as it will decrease the drug's ability to be absorbed. Make another selection.*

27. **The nurse understands that which groups of clients are most prone to the possibility of ototoxicity from tobramycin (Nebcin) therapy?**

1. Elderly.
2. Pregnant women.
3. Children.
4. Those previously sensitized to aminoglycosides.

1. *You are right! Tobramycin should be used cautiously, because the elderly are especially susceptible to ototoxicity due to a decline in auditory acuity as a natural course of aging. Auditory toxicity is caused by an accumulation of aminoglycosides in the perilymph of the inner ear. An early manifestation is a high-pitched tinnitus, followed by a gradual loss of auditory acuity. Hearing loss rapidly becomes irreversible if the drug is not discontinued within a few days.*
2. *Wrong. Although most aminoglycosides should be used cautiously during pregnancy, there is no increased risk of ototoxicity for these clients. Try another option.*
3. *Wrong. Aminoglycosides can be used in children with no significant increase in risk. When drug therapy is scheduled for more than a few days, an audiogram should be taken initially and then periodically during treatment to guard against changes in auditory acuity. Choose again.*
4. *Not a good choice. Aminoglycosides would be contraindicated in clients with previous sensitization and therefore would not be ordered. This question asks specifically about ototoxicity.*

28. **A client experiences photosensitivity while taking co-trimoxazole (Septra). The client describes photosensitivity manifestations to the nurse as:**

1. Blurred vision.
2. Pain in the eyes upon exposure to sunlight.
3. Sunburn reaction with minimal sun exposure.
4. Generalized rash and itching.

1. *No, blurred vision is not a manifestation of photosensitivity. Choose another option.*
2. *No, this describes photophobia, which can be a reaction to digitalis, mydriatics, or penicillin. Try again.*
3. *Correct! Sulfonamides can cause the skin to become especially sensitive to the effects of ultraviolet rays, so the client becomes sunburned with minimal sun exposure. Other reactions can be blisters, red skin, pain or discomfort over skin surfaces.*
4. *No, this is not a description of a photosensitivity reaction. A rash and pruritus are manifestations of an allergic reaction seen in a significant proportion of clients. Select another option.*

29. **A client is currently being treated with kanamycin (Kantrex). The nurse would note which condition in the client's medical history as requiring cautious use of this drug?**

1. Hypertension.
2. Myasthenia gravis.

3.   Diabetes mellitus.
4.   Epilepsy.

1.   *No, aminoglycosides are not implicated in adverse reactions affecting the cardiovascular system. Try again.*

2.   **Correct! Neuromuscular blockade (evidenced by skeletal weakness and respiratory distress) is a major concern when aminoglycosides are given intraperitoneal or intrapleural, because of the drug's rapid access to the neuromuscular receptors of the respiratory muscles. Kanamycin should be used cautiously in clients with preexisting neuromuscular diseases such as myasthenia gravis or Parkinsonism, as they are more sensitive to this effect. To prevent or reverse this effect, the client may be treated with calcium salts or an anticholinesterase agent.**

3.   *Incorrect. Adverse reactions from aminoglycosides include ototoxicity, nephrotoxicity, hypersensitivity, superinfection and neuromuscular blockade. Review the remaining options and make another selection.*

4.   *Wrong! The only adverse reactions affecting the CNS are headache, lethargy, and neuromuscular blockade. Aminoglycosides are not contraindicated in clients with known seizure disorders. Choose another option.*

30.   A physician has prescribed sulfonamide therapy for an elderly client. Which lab work finding would the nurse identify as suggestive of a blood dyscrasia, which is a concern for this client's age group?

1.   Hgb: 13.8.
2.   WBC: 2,000.
3.   Platelets: 200,000.
4.   RBC: 4,800,000.

1.   *Incorrect. This hemoglobin is within the normal range for an adult (13.5-17.5 for men; 12-16 for women). Choose another option.*

2.   **Good! This WBC level indicates neutropenia (normal WBC count is 5-10,000) and is symptomatic of bone marrow depression. Other blood dyscrasias that can result from sulfonamide therapy in the elderly are hemolytic anemia, thrombocytopenia, agranulocytosis, and aplastic anemia.**

3.   *No, this platelet count is within normal limits (150,000-350,000) and, therefore, does not reflect a blood dyscrasia. Try again.*

4.   *No, this RBC level is within normal limits (4.2-5.4 million for men; 3.6-5.0 million for women) and, therefore, does not reflect an abnormality in the blood.*

31.   An elderly client is diagnosed with Klebsiella pneumonia. He is being treated with gentamicin sulfate (Garamycin). The nurse should give immediate consideration to the possibility of which side effect?

1.   Hearing loss.
2.   Palpitations.
3.   Prolonged prothrombin time.
4.   Seizures.

1.   **Correct! Aminoglycosides are very damaging to the inner ear, causing impairments in hearing and balance.**

2.   *No, this side effect is not reported in connection with gentamicin sulfate. Make another selection.*

3.   *Wrong. Aminoglycosides are not metabolized in the liver. They are excreted by the kidneys, so the liver would not be affected. Try again.*

4.   *Wrong. Flaccid paralysis can occur from neuromuscular blockage, but seizures are not likely. Make another selection.*

32.   The nurse is caring for a client who is receiving isoniazid (INH) and who has developed peripheral neuropathy, a side effect from the use of isoniazid. The nurse knows that peripheral neuropathy is treated by administering which of the following at the same time INH is given?

1.   Vitamin C.
2.   Vitamin B6 (Pyridoxine).
3.   Steroids.
4.   Combinations of vitamins and steroids.

1.   *No! Vitamin C does not alter neuritis. Try again.*

2.   **Good choice! Peripheral neuritis results from a deficiency in Vitamin B6, which is caused when INH forms a complex with the vitamin. Oral administration of the vitamin increases its availability and eliminates neuritis.**

3.   *Steroids are not used for peripheral neuritis. Try again.*

4.   *It is not multiple vitamins that are used to treat peripheral neuritis. Steroids are not used for peripheral neuritis. Make another selection.*

33.   Before beginning a client's rifampin (Rifadin) therapy, the nurse should warn him that this medication:

1.   Turns urine, sweat, tears and saliva to a red-orange color.
2.   Causes stools to turn black.
3.   Stains teeth.
4.   Causes constipation.

1.   **Very good! Rifampin frequently causes secretions to have a red-orange color.**

2. No, it is iron that causes stools to turn black, not rifampin. Try again.
3. No, teeth are stained from taking liquid iron preparations, not from taking rifampin. Make another selection.
4. Incorrect. Although rifampin can cause gastric complaints, constipation is not one of them. Nausea is more likely. Make another choice.

34. **A client is scheduled for a colon resection in two days. She is started on a full liquid diet and neomycin sulfate (Neobiotic) by mouth four times a day. The nurse understands that the purpose of the administration of the neomycin sulfate before surgery is:**

1. Sterilization of the bowel mucosa.
2. Reduction in bacterial content of the colon.
3. Treatment of any secondary infection that might be present prior to surgery.
4. Decreasing the rate of peristalsis during surgery.

1. No, this is not possible! Although neomycin sulfate is an antibiotic, the bowel cannot be sterilized. Try another option.
2. **Yes, very good! Antibiotics, such as kanamycin sulfate (Kantrex) and neomycin sulfate, are administered to reduce intestinal bacteria in preparation for bowel surgery. This helps to decrease the incidence of wound infections postoperatively.**
3. Not true. If the client had an infection prior to surgery, it would be treated with an appropriate antibiotic to which the organism was sensitive. Neomycin sulfate is given routinely to clients prior to bowel surgery. Make another selection.
4. Not true. Neomycin sulfate is an antibiotic and has no effect upon peristalsis. Manipulation of the bowel during surgery may produce a loss of peristalsis for 24 to 48 hours postoperatively, unrelated to the preoperative administration of neomycin sulfate. Choose again.

35. **The nurse understands that the purpose of treating a client in labor with naloxone (Narcan) is to:**

1. Increase the effects of narcotics.
2. Depress the activity of the central nervous system (CNS) in the woman who received narcotics.
3. Block the effects of narcotics on the CNS.
4. Withdraw narcotics from the body.

1. Incorrect. Narcan lessens, not accentuates, the effects of narcotics. Try again.
2. Incorrect. This is incorrect, since Narcan blocks the depressing effects of narcotics on the CNS, rather than depressing the CNS system itself. Try again.
3. **Correct. By blocking the effects of narcotics on the CNS, it prevents CNS and respiratory de-**

pression in the neonate following delivery. Try again.
4. This is incorrect. The word "withdraw" makes this answer incorrect. There is no way to remove narcotics from the body following administration. Try again.

36. **Methylergonovine maleate (Methergine) is ordered for a client following a normal vaginal delivery. The nurse would recognize which of the following as a side effect of Methergine?**

1. Marked oliguria.
2. Severe hypoglycemia.
3. Sudden hypertension.
4. Uterine rupture.

1. Try again. Methergine does not affect urinary output.
2. Try again. Methergine does not affect the blood sugar.
3. **Excellent choice! Methergine often causes a rise in blood pressure.**
4. Try again. Methergine does not cause uterine rupture following delivery.

37. **The doctor orders ergonovine (Ergotrate) for a client. Which condition warrants caution when the nurse is administering Ergotrate?**

1. Diabetes.
2. Pre-eclampsia.
3. Uterine atony.
4. Anemia.

1. Wrong. Ergotrate can be used without concern in the client with diabetes.
2. **Yes, excellent choice! Ergotrate should be used with caution in the client with pre-eclampsia because of the high risk of increased blood pressure in an already hypertensive client.**
3. Wrong. Ergotrate is used to treat uterine atony, which is relaxation of the uterus following delivery.
4. Sorry! Whether or not the client has anemia has no bearing on the administration of Ergotrate.

38. **Isoxsuprine (Vasodilan) is a uterine relaxant used to treat premature labor. Which of the following findings could indicate an adverse reaction to Vasodilan and should be reported to the charge nurse?**

1. Maternal apical pulse 116.
2. Fetal heart rate 164.
3. Maternal temperature 101° F.
4. Rapid decrease in blood pressure from 130/90 to 110/68.

1. *No! An increase in pulse rate is an expected reaction to Vasodilan, but the physician does not need to be called unless it exceeds 120 bpm.*
2. *No, try again! When the mother's pulse rate increases, the fetal heart rate increases also, but we do not need to be concerned unless it exceeds 180 bpm.*
3. *No, good try. An elevated maternal temperature is cause for concern, but it is not related to Vasodilan therapy.*
4. ***Correct! This drop in blood pressure is significant, and should be reported as it is indicative of an adverse reaction to the administration of Vasodilan.***

39. **A six-month-old took two ounces of expressed breast milk, provided by the mother, at 8:00 a.m., three ounces at 11:00 a.m. and two and one-half ounces at 1:00 p.m. What should the nurse record on this client's intake record for the shift?**

1. 150 cc.
2. 225 cc.
3. 240 cc.
4. 375 cc.

1. *No, that's not right. Check your work.*
2. ***Right, this was an easy one for you! Multiply the total ounces by 30 cc per ounce: 7.5 oz. x 30 cc/oz. = 225 cc.***
3. *No, you made an error. Try this again.*
4. *Incorrect, try this math again.*

40. **The physician ordered gr 3/4. On hand are 15 mg tablets. What number of tablets should be given by the nurse?**

1. Three tablets.
2. One tablet.
3. Two tablets.
4. One and one-half tablets.

1. ***Right! You have computed the dosage correctly. 3/4 gr x 60 mg/gr = 180 divided by 4 = 45 mg. Then 45 mg/15 mg per tablet = 3 tablets.***
2. *Not correct. Go back and rethink the question. Did you convert the grains to milligrams? Try this one again.*
3. *No, this is incorrect. Did you first convert the grains to milligrams?*
4. *Incorrect. Is your equation upside down? Try again.*

41. **The nurse caring for clients receiving antipsychotic medications knows that a medication often prescribed for treating the extrapyramidal side effects associated with antipsychotics is:**

1. Phenelzine (Nardil).
2. Bupropion (Wellbutrin).
3. Amantadine (Symmetrel).
4. Hydroxyzine (Atarax).

1. *Incorrect. Nardil is an MAO inhibitor antidepressant. Read the other options to identify the medication used to treat EPS.*
2. *Incorrect. Wellbutrin is one of the newer drugs for treating depression. Try again to select the correct option.*
3. ***Correct. Amantadine (Symmetrel) is an anti-parkinsonian drug used to treat extrapyramidal side effects. Good work!***
4. *Incorrect. Atarax is an antihistamine used to treat mild to moderate anxiety states. Look again at the options to select the one used to treat EPS.*

42. **A 19-year-old client is in crisis and is admitted for drug abuse. In caring for this client, the nurse understands that which type of medication should be prescribed only in limited amounts for this client?**

1. Antipsychotics.
2. Antiparkinsonian agents.
3. Tricyclic antidepressants.
4. MAO inhibitor antidepressants.

1. *This is not correct. Antipsychotics do not have abusive properties.*
2. ***Correct. Antiparkinsonian agents, used to treat the extrapyramidal side effects of antipsychotics, can produce a state of euphoria and therefore have the potential for abuse.***
3. *This is not correct. Antidepressants do not have properties that could lead to abuse.*
4. *This is not the correct answer. MAO inhibitors are not associated with any abuse potential.*

43. **The nurse is caring for a chronic alcoholic client who is experiencing alcohol withdrawal. The nurse knows which of the following medications is indicated to manage the client's alcohol withdrawal?**

1. Buspirone (BuSpar).
2. Propranolol (Inderal).
3. Hydroxyzine (Atarax).
4. Chlordiazepoxide (Librium).

1. *This is not the correct medication. BuSpar has no CNS depressant properties, so it cannot be used in withdrawing clients from alcohol.*
2. *This is not the correct medication. Inderal is a beta-blocker used to treat clients with anxiety. It is not used in alcohol withdrawal because it is not a CNS depressant.*
3. *This is not the correct medication. Atarax is an antihistamine that can be used as a mild sedative-*

hypnotic agent. It is not used in alcohol withdrawal because it is not a CNS depressant.

4. **Correct. Librium is a relatively long acting CNS depressant that is used to treat alcohol withdrawal. It is substituted for alcohol during the detoxification process to prevent the occurrence of delirium tremens or other complications.**

44. **A client with COPD requests "cough medicine." The nurse's response is guided by the knowledge that the use of antitussives is only justified:**

1. If a cough is productive.
2. In viral infections.
3. If a cough interferes with recovery.
4. When used in combination with expectorants.

1. *No, this is incorrect! A productive cough is generally beneficial to the client. Productive coughs clear the airway of secretions. For this reason, productive coughs are not usually suppressed, but are encouraged. Try again.*
2. *No, this is incorrect. The underlying cause of a cough should always be treated. Criteria for the use of an antitussive are based on the effect of a cough on a client, regardless of its cause. Try again.*
3. **You are on your way to becoming a great nurse! Since a productive cough is generally beneficial to a client, a cough is only suppressed when it interferes with a client's recovery. For example, an antitussive might be given at night to allow a client to rest.**
4. *No, this is incorrect. The purpose of an expectorant is to thin and mobilize secretions, which are removed from the airway through client coughing, or by suctioning. Antitussives suppress the cough and would necessitate suctioning in clients with the need for airway clearance. Do you really think this is a good idea? Try again.*

45. **The nurse is caring for a client who overdosed on codeine. The nurse knows that the effects of this overdose can be reversed by giving the client:**

1. Albuterol (Proventil).
2. Atropine.
3. Naloxone (Narcan).
4. Protamine sulfate.

1. *No, this is not correct. While albuterol may produce some of the opposite effects of codeine, it will not reverse the effects of the drug. Since codeine is a narcotic, a narcotic antagonist is necessary, not a beta agonist. Try again.*
2. *No, this is not correct. Atropine is an anticholinergic, which means it is the antidote for cholinergic poisoning. A narcotic antagonist is neces-*

sary to counter the effects of a narcotic. Try again.

3. **Yes! Codeine is a narcotic, and you have correctly identified the narcotic antagonist. Narcan will block the effects of a narcotic at the opiate receptor site. Narcan is also the antidote for morphine, which also produces respiratory depression.**
4. *No, you are way off track here. Protamine sulfate is an antidote — but for heparin, an anticoagulant. Codeine is a narcotic. Try again.*

46. **In teaching the client how to avoid unpleasant side effects when using benzonatate (Tessalon), the nurse should instruct the client to:**

1. Swallow the capsule whole.
2. Use only for chronic coughs.
3. Use for short periods of time to avoid addiction.
4. Taper doses when discontinuing the medication.

1. **Yes, very good! Benzonatate is a locally acting antitussive. If it is chewed, it may anesthetize the mouth and pharynx. The client should swallow the capsule whole.**
2. *No, this is not correct. Benzonatate is also used in diagnostic testing to suppress a cough for a short period of time. It is not indicated only for chronic coughs. Try again.*
3. *No, this option is not a true statement. Although the narcotic antitussives have a high abuse potential, benzonatate is locally acting and non-narcotic. It is not addictive. Try again.*
4. *Tapering doses when discontinuing is important for some medications, which either suppress the body's own release of chemicals, as in glucocorticoids, or which can cause rebound reactions, as in some antihypertensives. This is not the case with benzonatate.*

47. **In assessing a client with frequent allergies, the nurse would expect to find:**

1. Increased heart rate.
2. Anorexia.
3. Increased mucous secretion.
4. Vertigo.

1. *Wrong. This is not a sign of allergy. Increased heart rate is a consequence of sympathetic nervous system stimulation, which occurs, for example, with use of beta-agonist bronchodilators. It is not a sign of histamine release. Try again.*
2. *Wrong. This is not a sign of allergy. Try again.*
3. **Good! Increased mucous secretion is a common sign of histamine release. Anyone with allergies should have gotten this one correct!**
4. *Wrong. This is not a sign of allergy. Although antihistamines are used to treat vertigo, for example*

in the treatment of Meniere's disease, vertigo is not specifically a sign of histamine release. Try again.

48. **A 27-year-old client states that she frequently uses over-the-counter antihistamine preparations for her small child. The nurse would place priority on teaching the mother:**

   1. Recommended safe dosages for children.
   2. Signs of antihistamine poisoning.
   3. The importance of keeping an antihistamine antidote on hand.
   4. The necessity of safe storage precautions.

   1. This might be appropriate, but it is not the nursing priority. Some antihistamines are safe for use with children. The recommended doses vary with the medication, and are usually available on the medication package. This is not a priority intervention. Try again.

   2. This is not the nursing priority. While it is important to know the signs of antihistamine poisoning, it is more important to prevent antihistamine poisoning. Try again.

   3. Sorry; there is no antidote for antihistamine poisoning! That is why prevention is so important. Try again.

   4. Yes, this is critically important. Often commercial preparations are very attractive to small children, making it extremely dangerous to leave them within reach of children. There is no antidote for antihistamine poisoning! Prevention is the best course.

49. **When administering an antihistamine to an elderly client, the nurse would consider which of the following a priority?**

   1. The elderly require increased doses of antihistamines.
   2. Paradoxical restlessness can occur in an elderly client.
   3. Sustained release preparations are contraindicated in an elderly client.
   4. Many brands of antihistamines are available in non-child-resistant containers.

   1. This is incorrect. Usually the elderly require smaller doses of medication, because of reduced hepatic and renal function.

   2. Correct. Although the usual response to antihistamines is sedation, paradoxical restlessness and agitation can occur in children and in the elderly. Nurses need to be aware of this possibility.

   3. This is incorrect. Sustained release preparations should not be crushed or chewed, but if the client can swallow the pill or capsule whole, it would

not be contraindicated. Try again.

   4. This is important, but it is not a priority. ALL preparations can be put into non-child-resistant containers if the client desires. This is something to consider with all medications if the client will have difficulty opening a child-resistant container. However, this is not a priority. Look again!

50. **When the nurse evaluates the client's knowledge regarding the use of antihistamines, which statement made by the client indicates a knowledge deficit?**

   1. "I should be careful when driving."
   2. "Hard candy will relieve my dry mouth."
   3. "This medication may be taken with food."
   4. "If I am pregnant, I should take half the dose."

   1. Wrong choice. This statement indicates client understanding of the sedative effects of antihistamines. Clients on antihistamines should be careful when driving or operating heavy machinery. You are looking for an INCORRECT statement.

   2. Wrong choice. One of the side effects of antihistamines is a dry mouth. Hard candy will relieve the dry mouth. This statement indicates accurate knowledge. You are looking for an INCORRECT statement.

   3. Wrong choice. Use of antihistamines can cause nausea or gastric distress. If the medication is taken with food, some of these side effects may be lessened. This statement indicates good client understanding. You are looking for an INCORRECT statement.

   4. Congratulations! This is the statement that indicates a knowledge deficit. Safe use of antihistamines in pregnancy has not been proven. It is important that clients understand this, since antihistamines are found in many popular over-the-counter preparations.

51. **The nurse is teaching a client who is receiving a thiazide diuretic. The client would demonstrate understanding of his drug therapy by selecting which of the following foods?**

   1. Apricots.
   2. Milk.
   3. Beef.
   4. Pork.

   1. Good choice! Of all the foods listed, apricots have the most potassium. Since the client is receiving a thiazide diuretic, potassium needs to be replaced.

   2. Wrong! Milk is higher in sodium than in potassium. Because the client is receiving a thiazide diuretic, his potassium needs to be replaced.

   3. This choice is incorrect. Because the client is receiving a thiazide diuretic, his potassium needs to be replaced. Of the four foods listed, which is the highest in potassium?

4. This choice is incorrect. Because the client is receiving a thiazide diuretic, his potassium needs to be replaced. Of the four foods listed, which is the highest in potassium?

52. A newly diagnosed diabetic indicates a possible lack of understanding about his daily injections of insulin when he tells the nurse that:

1. He will change injection sites.
2. He needs to buy some alcohol.
3. His brother also is a diabetic, and he will be able to share all of the supplies with him.
4. His wife will be giving him the injections.

1. *Wrong choice. This statement by the client indicates good understanding of the need to rotate the sites to insure absorption and prevent complications that can result from overuse of an injection site. You are looking for an INCORRECT statement by the client.*
2. *Wrong choice. This statement indicates that the client understands that alcohol is needed for disinfection. You are looking for an INCORRECT statement by the client.*
3. **Correct choice! This statement by the client indicates that the nurse needs further clarification to be sure that the client is not planning to share needles with his brother. Needles are disposable and not to be reused by anyone!**

> **TEST-TAKING TIP:** This evaluation question has a false response stem: this statement does NOT indicate an understanding by the client of how to care for his health problem. In other words, the correct option is an incorrect statement! The NCLEX/CAT-PN exam will include a certain number of false response stems, so be sure you can recognize them.

4. *Although this should be a concern for the nurse, it does not address the issue in the question, which concerns the client's understanding of injection technique.*

53. The nurse suspects an allergic reaction to penicillin. At this time, which of the following medications would the nurse be prepared to administer?

1. Diphenhydramine (Benadryl).
2. Prednisone.
3. Ipratropium (Atrovent).
4. Morphine sulfate.

1. ***Good! Your client should be fine! The allergic response is produced by histamine release. An antihistamine is used to block the histamine response.***

2. *Your thinking may be correct, since decreasing the inflammatory reaction is sort of on the right track. However, remember that prednisone is relatively slow-acting. This crisis situation requires the most specific drug available. In this case, the client requires an antihistamine. Try another selection.*
3. *An anticholinergic would not be of use to this client. This client needs a medication that will specifically counteract the action of the histamine released in the allergic reaction. Try again.*
4. *Don't even think about it! Morphine depresses the respiratory system. Bad move for a client who is already in respiratory distress! This could be life-threatening. What is needed is a drug that will block the allergic reaction by blocking histamine receptors.*

54. A client is receiving cyclophosphamide (Cytoxan) for treatment of her leukemia. The nurse has noticed that the client vomited after each of her previous doses. To prevent vomiting, what should the nurse do?

1. Have the charge nurse contact the physician for an antiemetic order prior to treatment.
2. Withhold fluids prior to and during treatments.
3. Suggest to the client that she eat before receiving her treatment.
4. Explain that vomiting cannot be prevented and provide the client with an emesis basin during treatments.

1. ***An excellent response! The nurse may be able to prevent nausea and vomiting with an antiemetic prior to treatments.***
2. *No, try again. Fluids should not be withheld prior to or during treatments. It is important that clients stay well hydrated to prevent kidney damage.*
3. *Wrong. Eating before treatments would not solve the problem of vomiting. The client could possibly even aspirate on her vomitus.*
4. *Wrong choice! While the client may indeed need the emesis basin, the nurse may prevent vomiting by administering an antiemetic before administration of the medication.*

55. A client is being treated with Cisplatin (Platinol) for his cancer. After several treatments he begins to complain of fatigue and wants to sleep all day. Which is the priority nursing action?

1. Advise the client about the dangers of immobility.
2. Check lab values of RBCs, hematocrit and hemoglobin, as he is likely to be anemic.
3. Call in the family for counseling, because the client is depressed and may become suicidal.
4. Set up an exercise plan.

1. *Incorrect. Although there are dangers of immobility, this action would not get to the cause of the*

problem. Be sure to read all of the options before selecting the best one!

2.   **Great work! If the RBCs are low, treatment may need to be delayed until the blood counts are higher.**

3.   *Wrong choice. A family session may be needed later, but physical causes, which are more easily corrected, will be assessed first.*

> **TEST-TAKING TIP:** *Maslow's Hierarchy of Needs assigns first priority to physiological needs. Always try to identify a physiological need before responding to the client's higher level needs.*

4.   *Wrong. This will not address the cause of the problem. Physical causes must be ruled out. Reread the options and try again.*

56.   When instructing a client on the use of cromolyn (Intal), the nurse would include the information that Intal is most effective when:

1.   Administered orally.
2.   Used prophylactically.
3.   Combined with an anti-inflammatory drug.
4.   Used to treat non-allergic responses.

1.   *No, this is not a correct statement. Cromolyn is not administered orally, it is administered via an inhaler.*

2.   **Right! Cromolyn is not appropriate for acute use. It is most effective when used before the client is exposed to a trigger to an asthmatic attack, for example, before exercise, or before exposure to cold air.**

3.   *No, this is not a correct statement. Since cromolyn is not effective in an emergency, it should always be supplemented with a bronchodilator, not an anti-inflammatory drug.*

4.   *No, this is not a correct statement. Cromolyn is a mast cell inhibitor and it interrupts the allergic response. Therefore, it would be of limited use in non-allergic pulmonary disease.*

57.   After administering acetylcysteine (Mucomyst), the nurse might enhance the effectiveness of the medication by:

1.   Providing oxygen via Venturi mask.
2.   Positioning the client for postural drainage.
3.   Encouraging deep breathing exercises.
4.   Assisting the client with mouth care.

1.   *No, this will not be helpful. Providing oxygen may benefit the client, but it will not enhance the effectiveness of acetylcysteine. Remember, too, that oxygen is given cautiously in clients with COPD.*

2.   **Right! Once secretions are thinned, placing the client in position for postural drainage will facilitate the removal of secretions. A little chest percussion wouldn't hurt, either.**

3.   *No, this is inappropriate. Simply encouraging deep breathing without productive coughing will not benefit the client. In fact, it may allow the secretions to move downward and further obstruct the airway.*

4.   *This would be useful, but it is not the correct answer. Assisting the client with mouth care is a good thing to do, since acetylcysteine can cause nausea because of its foul taste. However, this intervention will relieve side effects, not enhance the effectiveness of the medication. Try again!*

58.   A 62-year-old client with a history of emphysema asks the nurse about the use of chlorpheniramine maleate (Chlor-Trimeton). The nurse's response is based on the knowledge that:

1.   Antihistamines can thicken secretions, and are only cautiously used in clients with COPD.
2.   Use of antihistamines to control respiratory secretions is preferred because of the lack of major side effects.
3.   Diphenhydramine (Benadryl) is the medication of choice for clients with COPD because it is readily available without a prescription.
4.   The sedative effect of antihistamines can compromise respiratory stimulation in clients with COPD.

1.   **Good work! COPD is characterized by bronchial constriction and thick, copious secretions. Since antihistamines can further thicken the secretions and decrease their mobilization, they are used very cautiously in clients with COPD.**

2.   *Actually, antihistamines have many side effects. There are medications better suited to controlling secretions in the client with COPD. Among them are cromolyn (Intal) and prednisone.*

3.   *If a drug is available without a prescription, that means that the client may not be carefully monitored. That may be a deficit rather than a benefit of the medication! In this case, antihistamines, in general, are not preferred for use in the client with COPD. Diphenhydramine is not an exception.*

4.   *No, this option is inaccurate. There is a difference between sedation and respiratory depression, although the two are commonly caused by the same drug. You are correct in thinking that antihistamines are not usually considered appropriate for the client with COPD. This is due to thickened secretions, however, rather than sedation.*

59.   When discontinuing a course of prednisone for a client with recurring chronic bronchitis, the nurse should plan to taper the dose because the client may experience:

1. Hyperglycemia.
2. Adrenocortical insufficiency.
3. Severe dehydration.
4. Delirium tremens.

1.   This is not an effect of discontinuing this drug. While on prednisone, the client may experience hyperglycemia. The client will not experience hyperglycemia after prednisone is discontinued. Try again.

2.   Right! Administration of glucocorticoids may depress the body's adrenocortical activity. Abrupt withdrawal of the drug can lead to a syndrome of adrenal insufficiency.

3.   This is not an effect of discontinuing this drug. Withdrawing prednisone will decrease the amount of sodium and water retained by the body, but it will not cause severe dehydration. Try again.

4.   This is not an effect of discontinuing this drug. Alcohol withdrawal leads to delirium tremens. You may want to review prednisone and the glucocorticoids. Try again.

60.   Before administering acetylcysteine (Mucomyst) to a confused or lethargic client, which item does the nurse needs to have readily available?

1. Tracheostomy set.
2. Suction equipment.
3. A vial of epinephrine.
4. A secondary intravenous set.

1.   No, try again. A tracheostomy set might be useful if laryngeal/tracheal obstruction were a danger. An example of this is following a thyroidectomy. The concern with acetylcysteine, however, is possible obstruction caused by secretions.

2.   Excellent! When administering acetylcysteine to a client with an impaired or absent cough, suction equipment must be available to prevent further obstruction from the thinned and mobile secretions.

3.   No, try again. If the major concerns were allergic reaction and anaphylaxis, then a vial of epinephrine would be of vital importance. Allergic reactions, however, are not a concern with acetylcysteine.

4.   No, try again. A secondary intravenous set is necessary when administering intravenous substances that might cause an allergic or adverse reaction. A good example of this is administration of blood products. The secondary intravenous set can quickly be connected to the client, and will provide venous access without administering any more of the original substance. Since acetylcysteine is unlikely to cause a reaction, and since it is not administered intravenously, this would not be important equipment to have on hand.

61.   A client tells the nurse that she commonly uses commercial cough preparations containing guaifenesin (Robitussin). This statement would cause concern to the nurse if the client were also taking:

1. Acetaminophen.
2. Penicillin.
3. Phenytoin.
4. Heparin.

1.   No, acetaminophen is not a concern. What you are concerned about in this question is a possible drug interaction. Guaifenesin does not interact with acetaminophen. In fact, many clients who are using an over-the-counter medication may also be using acetaminophen as well.

2.   No, penicillin is not a concern. What you are looking for in this question is the possibility of drug interactions with guaifenesin. Antibiotics do not interact with this medication.

3.   No, phenytoin is not a concern. What you should be concerned about is a possible drug interaction. Dilantin interacts with many medications, but guaifenesin is not one of them.

4.   Good work! Guaifenesin can cause increased bleeding in clients who are also taking anticoagulants.

62.   The nurse has completed discharge teaching on the use of metered dose inhalers for both bronchodilators and anti-inflammatory medications. Which statement made by the client indicates the need for more client teaching?

1. "I should wait five minutes between medications."
2. "I will repeat the dose if I get no relief."
3. "I should use my albuterol (Ventolin) inhaler before my beclomethasone (Beclovent) inhaler."
4. "I will chart my response to the medications."

1.   Sorry, this statement indicates the client has an understanding of the use of metered dose inhalers. The first medication to be used, the bronchodilator, should be allowed time to act, before administering the anti-inflammatory. This facilitates maximum absorption of the second drug. You are looking for an INCORRECT statement. Try again.

2.   Right, this client requires more teaching! If the client gets no relief from the medication, the physician should be called, or the client should seek emergency assistance. Repeating doses, especially of beta-agonists can cause cardiac arrhythmias.

3.   Sorry, the client is correct. The bronchodilator inhaler should be used first. This allows the bronchioles to dilate, for maximum absorption of the anti-inflammatory medication. You are looking for an

INCORRECT statement. Try again.

4. Sorry, this statement by the client is correct. Responses to medications should be documented by the client or the client's family. This allows the client to participate in his/her own care, as well as providing valuable data on the effectiveness of the medications and the severity of the illness. You are looking for an INCORRECT statement. Try again.

63. **In evaluating the effectiveness of acetylcysteine (Mucomyst), the nurse would assess for:**

1. Respiratory rate.
2. Presence of adventitious breath sounds.
3. Absence of a cough.
4. The thickness of secretions.

1. No, this would not indicate effectiveness. Assessing the respiratory rate is a good general assessment. However, when administering a mucolytic, the specific desired effect is thinned secretions, and that is what the nurse should evaluate.
2. No, this would not indicate effectiveness. Auscultating for adventitious breath sounds is a good general assessment. However, those breath sounds may occur with or without the use of a mucolytic. It would not be useful for specific evaluation of the therapeutic effect of acetylcysteine.
3. Sorry. If the nurse were evaluating the effectiveness of an antitussive medication, the absence of a cough would indicate therapeutic effect. This medication, however, is a mucolytic, not an antitussive.
4. **Excellent! Acetylcysteine is a mucolytic, given specifically to thin secretions. The only way to specifically evaluate its effectiveness, then, is to assess the viscosity of the secretions.**

64. **To detect an adverse interaction between antihistamines and alcohol, the nurse would be on the alert for:**

1. Tachycardia.
2. Vomiting.
3. Change in level of consciousness.
4. Bronchoconstriction.

1. Wrong choice. Antihistamines can cause tachycardia. However, the interaction between alcohol and antihistamines does not increase the effect on the cardiovascular system.
2. Wrong choice. One of the side effects of antihistamines is nausea and gastric distress. However, you are looking for the effect of a drug interaction. Alcohol would not increase the incidence of nausea or vomiting.
3. **You are correct! When the sedative effect of antihistamines is added to the depressant ef-** fect of alcohol, the client may experience central nervous system depression, which can be fatal.
4. Wrong choice. What you are looking for here is a drug interaction. Although antihistamines can lead to bronchoconstriction, their combination with alcohol will not worsen this effect.

65. **The nurse is preparing a discharge teaching plan for the client on glucocorticoid therapy. Which information by the nurse is most appropriate?**

1. Take medication on an empty stomach to enhance absorption.
2. Alternate day therapy may prevent some side effects.
3. If any sign of rash occurs, stop taking the medication immediately.
4. Take two pills at the first sign of respiratory distress.

1. No! Glucocorticoids can cause significant gastrointestinal distress and can lead to ulcer formation. Steroids should not be taken on an empty stomach.
2. **Good! Some of the side effects of long-term glucocorticoid therapy can be avoided by using alternate day therapy.**
3. No! You may be thinking of some antibiotics. A client should never stop taking a glucocorticoid abruptly. The dosage should always be tapered before being discontinued completely.
4. No! Respiratory distress requires a fast acting bronchodilator. A slower acting anti-inflammatory is therapeutic over a longer course, but does not provide relief in an acute episode.

66. **Which common side effect would the nurse expect to find in a client receiving acetylcysteine (Mucomyst)?**

1. Sore throat.
2. Headache.
3. Nausea.
4. Drowsiness.

1. Sorry, you may be thinking of cromolyn (Intal), which does cause a sore throat. Here's a hint: remember what acetylcysteine smells like?
2. Wrong. It's true that almost every medication lists headache as a common side effect, but this is one of the few medications that doesn't. Here's a hint: remember what acetylcysteine smells like?
3. **You got it! Remember, acetylcysteine smells and tastes like rotten eggs. It often causes nausea in clients. Rinsing the mouth or gargling may relieve nausea, and it is important to remember not to give a Mucomyst treatment at mealtime.**

4. *Wrong. Acetylcysteine does not cause drowsiness. Here's a hint: remember what acetylcysteine smells like?*

67.   Which of the following is an inappropriate instruction by the nurse in the teaching plan for a client using expectorants?

1. Be sure to increase fluid intake.
2. Take this medication on an empty stomach.
3. Check recommended doses and follow manufacturers' recommendations.
4. Use deep breathing and coughing exercises.

1. *No, clients should increase fluid intake to two to three liters per day in order to liquefy secretions. This is an appropriate instruction. Look for an instruction that is INAPPROPRIATE.*
2. ***Right, this would be inappropriate to include in client teaching. Most expectorants will cause some gastrointestinal distress if taken on an empty stomach.***
3. *No, this instruction is appropriate. Many clients do not realize that over-the-counter medications can have as many adverse affects as prescription medications. It is important to make clients aware of the need to comply with recommended doses. Look for an instruction that is INAPPROPRIATE.*
4. *No, this instruction is appropriate. Expectorants will be much more effective if the medication is enhanced by deep breathing and coughing exercises. If the client cannot cough, consider the use of suction equipment. Look for an instruction that is INAPPROPRIATE.*

68.   The parents of a four-year-old child with asthma ask the nurse about possible medications. The nurse understands which of the following is an inappropriate medication for a pediatric client?

1. Metaproterenol.
2. Cromolyn.
3. Isoproterenol.
4. Aminophylline.

1. *Wrong choice, metaproterenol is approved for pediatric use, particularly in pediatric asthma. You are looking for the medication that is INAPPROPRIATE.*
2. *Wrong choice, cromolyn has few side effects and is highly effective in the prophylactic treatment of pediatric asthma. You are looking for the medication that is INAPPROPRIATE.*
3. ***Yes, this drug would be inappropriate for a child. Isoproterenol is a non-selective, highly potent bronchodilator. Because of its intense side effects, it is not the drug of choice for use with children.***

4. *Wrong choice. Aminophylline is used in neonatal apnea. It is approved for use with children, and is the treatment of choice for status asthmaticus. You are looking for the medication that is INAPPROPRIATE.*

69.   When administering oral prednisone to a client with asthma, the nurse correctly administers the drug:

1. Crushed in juice, served with a straw.
2. In a strong flavored juice to mask the taste.
3. Accompanied by food or antacids.
4. At least one hour before meals.

1. *No, this is not correct. Are you thinking of oral iron preparations that may stain the teeth? Prednisone does not cause such side effects and does not need to be administered in this way. Try again.*
2. *No, oral prednisone does not have a particularly bad taste. You may be confusing it with a mucolytic, which does have a bad taste. Try again.*
3. ***Yes, good work! Since prednisone is irritating to the GI tract, it must be administered with food or antacids.***
4. *No, this is not correct! If the drug were administered one hour before meals, that would be on an empty stomach, right? Prednisone given on an empty stomach would cause severe GI distress.*

70.   In order to avoid complications of inhaled beclomethasone (Beclovent), the nurse correctly does which of the following:

1. Assists the client to rinse his mouth.
2. Offers food or antacids following medication administration.
3. Monitors the client's heart rate before and after medication administration.
4. Cautions the client to avoid caffeine.

1. ***Yes, good choice. Metered dose inhaler use of glucocorticoids can allow a fungal overgrowth in the mouth. Rinsing after their administration can lessen the likelihood of this complication.***
2. *No, this would not be helpful. This would be the correct choice if this medication were offered by mouth. Glucocorticoids administered enterally can cause gastrointestinal distress, which can be lessened by offering food with these drugs. Beclovent, however, is inhaled, and therefore has some different side effects. Try again.*
3. *No, this would not be helpful with Beclovent. If you were administering a beta-agonist or xanthine, this would be an excellent choice, as both of those medications can cause tachycardia. Beclovent, however, does not cause cardiac side effects. Try again.*

4. No, this is not specifically indicated for a client taking Beclovent. Try again.

71. **When administering atropine, the nurse observes the client for side effects. Which side effect would cause the most concern?**

    1. Bradycardia.
    2. Urinary retention.
    3. Muscle tremors.
    4. Ventricular fibrillation.

    1. No, you should know better! Atropine is a para-sympathetic blocking agent. By blocking the para-sympathetic, it allows the sympathetic impulses to predominate. Use your understanding of the autonomic nervous system, and try again.
    2. No, this would not be of urgent concern. Although it is important to assess clients for urinary retention if they are on atropine therapy, urinary retention is not immediately fatal. Read all the options carefully and try again.
    3. No, this is not the most urgent concern. Although atropine can cause muscle tremors, which are annoying to the client and can add to the client's anxiety, they do not pose a significant danger. Try again.
    4. Ventricular fibrillation is life-threatening and necessitates immediate action. This is the side effect of utmost concern.

72. **A client with chronic obstructive pulmonary disease is being discharged with an ipratropium (Atrovent) metered dose inhaler. Which of the following discharge instructions would the nurse question?**

    1. Take two puffs every six hours as needed.
    2. The client may have two refills.
    3. Continue metaproterenol (Alupent) use.
    4. Call the physician for blurred vision or headaches.

    1. Good work, this is not correct for ipratropium. Ipratropium is much more effective if used on a consistent basis. Use on a PRN or "as needed" basis is not appropriate.
    2. No, this is a valid and appropriate order. There is no reason why clients should not be allowed refills of ipratropium. Look for the option that is NOT appropriate.
    3. No, this is a valid and appropriate order. Ipratropium can be used as an adjunct to beta-agonist therapy. Concurrent use with medications such as metaproterenol is common and would not be questioned. Look for the option that is NOT appropriate.
    4. No, this is a valid and appropriate order. Headaches are a side effect of ipratropium. The physician should be aware of the presence of this side effect. In addition, since ipratropium should not be used by clients with glaucoma, visual changes

should always be reported. Look for the option that is NOT appropriate.

73. **In preparing a discharge plan for a client who has been on long-term prednisone therapy, the nurse must be aware that these clients are prone to:**

    1. Frequent bouts of nausea.
    2. Orthostatic hypotension.
    3. Gingival ulcerations.
    4. Bone fractures.

    1. Not the best choice. While prednisone can cause gastrointestinal distress, this more often comes in the form of peptic ulcers, rather than frequent nausea. Read the other options and try again.
    2. This is not correct. Prednisone causes sodium and fluid retention and hypertension, not hypotension. Try again.
    3. This is not correct. You may be thinking of phenytoin (Dilantin), which is a completely different drug altogether. Try again.
    4. Excellent! Prednisone can cause demineralization of the bones, leading to osteoporosis and fractures. Nice work!

74. **An eight-year-old boy with asthma is placed on cromolyn (Intal) via metered dose inhaler. After client teaching, which statement by the child's parents indicates the need for more instruction?**

    1. "I will give my son a dose as soon as he starts wheezing."
    2. "My son needs to rinse out his mouth after using the inhaler."
    3. "My son should breathe in slowly while depressing the canister."
    4. "If my son has difficulty breathing in the dose, I can use a spacer."

    1. Good work, you found the incorrect statement by the parents. Cromolyn has a very slow onset and is only used prophylactically. In the event of an acute attack, a bronchodilator should be used to immediately open the airways.
    2. No, this statement does not indicate the need for more instruction. Cromolyn can cause mouth and throat irritation. This is best relieved by rinsing the mouth or gargling after use. You are looking for an INCORRECT statement.
    3. No, this is the correct method for using a metered dose inhaler. The client understands use, and does not require further teaching. You are looking for an INCORRECT statement.
    4. No, this would be appropriate. A spacer allows clients with difficulty breathing in the entire dose in one inhalation to continue to receive medication in subsequent breaths. This is often useful

with children. You are looking for an INCORRECT statement.

75. **The nurse administers metaproterenol (Alupent) via a metered dose inhaler. The nurse understands the drug is effective if there is:**

1. Clear, thin secretions.
2. Decreased respiratory rate.
3. Effective coughing.
4. Absence of wheezing.

1. Wrong. Generally, respiratory secretions should be clear and easily mobilized. Metaproterenol, however, is a bronchodilator and does not affect secretions.

2. Wrong. A decreased respiratory rate, without other baseline data, is a poor indicator of respiratory function. In fact, a respiratory rate that is too slow indicates a compromised condition. It is true that the respiratory rate may decrease if labored breathing is eased; however, this is not the best indicator of open airways.

3. Wrong. The purpose of a bronchodilator is to open the airways. Effective coughing may be one of the means of achieving that goal, however, it is not a good measure of the condition of the bronchioles.

4. Very good! Wheezing occurs as air is forced through narrowed passageways. Therefore, the absence of wheezing indicates that the airways are open, and that the bronchodilator metaproterenol has been effective.

76. **The nurse administers atropine via nebulizer to a client with severe asthma. The nurse would withhold the drug and call the nurse in charge if the client exhibits:**

1. Tachycardia.
2. Nervousness.
3. Visual changes.
4. Dizziness.

1. No, tachycardia is expected with an anticholinergic. If the client does not have a history of cardiac disease and if the increased heart rate is not accompanied by chest pain or other signs of a compromised cardiac system, tachycardia is not a cause for alarm.

2. No. Anticholinergics like atropine will cause sympathetic-type side effects. One of the most common is a feeling of nervousness. While this may be unpleasant for the client, it is not a reason to withhold the medication.

3. Yes! Visual changes may indicate exacerbation of glaucoma. Atropine can increase intraocular pressure and should not be given to clients with glaucoma, as permanent vision loss can occur. Good work!

4. No. Dizziness is a common, though not life-threatening, side effect of atropine. The nurse would be wise to watch the client carefully to prevent injury, but dizziness does not warrant withholding the medication.

77. **The nurse knows which factor is most important in planning discharge teaching for the client with obstructive pulmonary disease (COPD)?**

1. COPD is caused by a variety of etiologies.
2. COPD is progressive and chronic.
3. There are a variety of medications for COPD available.
4. Different age groups are affected by COPD.

1. Although it is true that obstructive pulmonary disease is caused by a variety of etiologies, this factor is not important in discharge teaching. Etiologies are more important when teaching health prevention/promotion.

2. Right! The fact that the disease is progressive and chronic means that clients will be responsible for a large part of their care. Teaching on respiratory hygiene and medications is particularly important for those clients who will be on lifelong medication therapy.

3. Although it is true that there are a variety of medications available, this is not really important to discharge teaching. Before discharge, the client should know what specific medications he/she will be taking at home. Teaching those specific medications would be more important.

4. The nurse should know the age of the client before planning discharge teaching, but the fact that different age groups are affected has little bearing on a specific client teaching plan.

78. **When preparing a teaching plan for the client being discharged on theophylline (Theo-dur), the nurse should plan to include which information?**

1. Theophylline should be taken on an empty stomach to maximize absorption.
2. The drug levels in the client's blood will need to be checked frequently.
3. The client should take the last dose at bedtime so that wheezing will not occur during the night.
4. This drug may cause drowsiness and interfere with the client's ability to operate heavy machinery.

1. No, this is not true. Theophylline causes gastric irritation and should be taken with meals, or with a glass of milk. Taking the drug on an empty stomach increases the gastric distress.

2. Good work! There is a narrow therapeutic range with theophylline. When therapy begins, blood levels need to be checked frequently. Once sta-

bilized, these levels can be done once or twice a year.

3.   No, this is not true. Side effects of theophylline include nervousness and insomnia. Taking a bedtime dose may interfere with the client's ability to rest. It is not recommended.

4.   No, this is not true. Theophylline does not cause drowsiness. Theophylline causes excitability and nervousness.

79.   In preparing a teaching plan for clients at a senior center, the nurse knows that which of the following is true of beta-agonist use in the elderly?

1.   There is an increased tendency toward incontinence.
2.   Higher drug levels are often needed.
3.   Use of multiple drugs in the elderly can lead to drug interactions.
4.   Dosage intervals are often shorter.

1.   Although we tend to think of the elderly as often incontinent, this is not correct. In fact, use of beta-agonists increases the risk of urinary retention.

2.   No, this is not correct. Lower drug levels are often indicated because of the decreased metabolism and excretion rates in the elderly.

3.   **Yes! The elderly often use a variety of medications because of their increasing medical problems. Drug interactions are common with a variety of drugs and beta-agonists. Polypharmacy (use of multiple drugs) in the elderly is a serious medical concern.**

4.   Can you think of a reason why dosage intervals would be shorter? This isn't true! Dosage intervals tend to remain unchanged in the elderly.

80.   In preparing to teach a client about the use of cromolyn (Intal), the nurse is guided by the knowledge that the primary purpose of cromolyn administration in the treatment of asthma is to prevent:

1.   Bronchospasm.
2.   Infection.
3.   Anaphylaxis.
4.   Inflammation.

1.   No, this is not correct. Cromolyn does not directly dilate bronchioles. Instead, it prevents release of chemicals that cause constriction, edema, and inflammation. One of the few side effects of cromolyn is bronchospasm. Try again.

2.   No, cromolyn cannot prevent infection. Infection is prevented by prophylactic use of antibiotics, good respiratory hygiene, and by avoiding contact with microorganisms. Try again.

3.   No, cromolyn should not be used to correct an anaphylactic reaction, because it has an extremely slow onset and does not correct an anaphylactic

reaction. Anaphylaxis is caused by allergies and is sudden and severe. A fast acting medication, such as epinephrine, is appropriate for treatment. Try again.

4.   **Very good! While it does not have steroid-like anti-inflammatory effects, cromolyn inhibits the release of the chemicals that cause edema and inflammation.**

81.   A client with status asthmaticus is admitted to the emergency room. Aminophylline is ordered. The nurse would expect the drug to be administered by which route?

1.   Subcutaneously.
2.   Intravenously.
3.   Via nebulizer.
4.   Sublingually.

1.   No, this is not correct. Subcutaneous medications must be absorbed through the subcutaneous layer before the therapeutic effect can begin. Wouldn't you want the quickest route for someone in crisis? Can you find a more appropriate route for this medication?

2.   **Yes, the aminophylline should be administered intravenously. This answer is easy if you remember that aminophylline is most often given intravenously. If you didn't remember that, you probably chose the quickest route of administration. Either way, you were correct.**

3.   No, this is not correct. The respiratory route offers fairly rapid onset of therapeutic effect. However, in status asthmaticus, a therapeutic blood level of aminophylline is desired. That is best achieved with IV aminophylline.

4.   There are very few drugs given sublingually. Aminophylline is not one of them. Look at the options again. The client in respiratory crisis needs the fastest route possible. Which option offers the fastest route?

82.   A client is on long-term theophylline (Theo-dur) therapy. In order to decrease side effects, the nurse would caution the client to avoid:

1.   Dairy products.
2.   Caffeinated beverages.
3.   Antacids.
4.   High sodium foods.

1.   No, dairy products have no specific effect on theophylline and need not be avoided. Food, in general, may delay absorption but does not decrease or increase side effects. In fact, taking theophylline with meals is advised in order to minimize GI effects.

2.   **Yes, the client should avoid caffeinated beverages. Caffeine is in the same chemical class as theophylline. When caffeine is taken in con-**

junction with the drug, the side effects of CNS stimulation and GI upset are increased. Clients should be advised to avoid caffeine.

3. *No, antacids will delay theophylline absorption, but they have no effect on the side effects of theophylline and need not be avoided.*

4. *No, avoiding high sodium foods is not necessary for the client on theophylline. Depending on the client's health, it may be wise to avoid foods high in sodium for cardiovascular reasons. Sodium, however, does not increase or decrease the side effects of theophylline.*

83. **A client has been taking theophylline (Theo-dur) for relief of chronic bronchitis. The nurse should be alert for which manifestations of toxicity with this drug?**

1. Lethargy and slurred speech.
2. Increased urinary output.
3. Agitation and tremors.
4. Wheezing and dyspnea.

1. *No, this is not an indication of theophylline toxicity. Theophylline is a central nervous system stimulant. An increase in the blood level of theophylline will cause an increase in CNS stimulation. Lethargy and slurred speech are more indicative of CNS depression.*

2. *No, this is not an indication of theophylline toxicity. Increased urinary output is expected in theophylline therapy, because of the diuretic effect of the drug. The nurse should assess urinary output to prevent excessive fluid loss, but it is not a good indicator of toxicity.*

3. **Good work! The earliest sign of theophylline toxicity is central nervous system stimulation, often seen as agitation and tremors. Other signs include insomnia, confusion, and irritability.**

4. *No, this is not an indication of theophylline toxicity. Too low a level of theophylline will decrease the therapeutic effect and may cause wheezing and dyspnea. The nurse would be on the alert for these manifestations when assessing for an ineffective blood level.*

84. **A client with asthma is being treated with isoproterenol (Isuprel). Which finding from the client's history would the nurse identify as requiring caution when administering this drug?**

1. Bronchospasm.
2. Peptic ulcer disease.
3. Angina.
4. Raynaud's disease.

1. *No, this is not a contraindication for use of isoproterenol. This drug is primarily used to prevent or relieve bronchospasm. This is an indication for*

use, not a contraindication! Try again.

2. *No, this is not a contraindication for use of isoproterenol. Isoproterenol does not increase secretions in the GI tract and does not cause gastric irritation. It will not worsen a peptic ulcer condition. Try again.*

3. **Yes, good work! The beta-1 effects of isoproterenol will cause increased cardiac rate and force of contraction. This can cause a worsening of angina in the client with compromised cardiac circulation. Isoproterenol would be used with extreme caution in these clients.**

4. *No, this is not a contraindication for use of isoproterenol. Isoproterenol does not produce the alpha stimulation that produces vasoconstriction. In fact, isoproterenol is a vasodilator. Raynaud's disease, which is characterized by peripheral vasoconstriction and impaired circulation, is not worsened by the use of isoproterenol.*

85. **A client with chronic emphysema is taking theophylline (Theo-dur) at home. During the home care nurse's visit, which statement by the client demands immediate action?**

1. "I just lie awake at night, worrying about the medical bills."
2. "I must have the flu. I was vomiting all night."
3. "I don't have my usual appetite. Nothing tastes good to me."
4. "I feel better if I have a big glass of milk with my pill."

1. *Wrong. Insomnia is a common side effect of theophylline. While it is annoying and interferes with the client's rest, it is not life-threatening and does not call for immediate action. Try again.*

2. **Yes, very good. You have identified a sign of theophylline toxicity. The client may indeed have the flu, but one of the early signs of theophylline toxicity is vomiting. Since there is no antidote for theophylline, and since toxicity can be fatal, the nurse should immediately explore other possible signs of toxicity and request a serum theophylline level.**

3. *Wrong. A client receiving theophylline may have anorexia as a side effect of the drug. The client's nutritional status should be monitored, but loss of appetite does not pose a life-threatening situation. Try again.*

4. *Wrong. This statement indicates that the client understands how to minimize the gastric irritation caused by theophylline. There is no reason why milk cannot be taken with theophylline, and there is also no reason why the nurse should act immediately. Try again.*

86. **A client is admitted to the hospital after complaining of chest pain. The client's history reveals congestive heart**

failure. He has been receiving digoxin (Lanoxin). The nurse understands that the purpose of giving the client digoxin is to:

1. Increase cardiac size.
2. Decrease cardiac output.
3. Increase the force of cardiac contraction.
4. Slow the pulse rate.

1. *Incorrect. The client has a history of congestive heart failure. His heart is not pumping effectively, so the blood is backing up in the pulmonary system and increasing his heart size. Digoxin helps reduce (not increase) the size of the poorly working heart. Try again.*
2. *No. The client has a poorly functioning heart due to congestive heart failure. His heart is not pumping adequately. Digoxin increases (not decreases) cardiac output. Choose another.*
3. **Congratulations! Digoxin increases the strength of the heart's contractions, increases output, and slows the heart rate, which decreases the heart size, reduces edema, and increases urine output.**
4. *Incorrect choice! Digoxin slows the heart rate but its primary effect is to increase cardiac output.*

87. The nurse is administering digoxin (Lanoxin) to a client and notices that his breakfast is untouched. He is also complaining of nausea. The nurse checks his vitals, which are BP 118/72, P 60, R 22. The nurse understands that:

1. The client is anxious and fearful.
2. The client needs a change in diet.
3. This is a normal reaction to the hospital.
4. He may be exhibiting a drug reaction.

1. *There is no information that would lead to the conclusion that the client is feeling anxious. Do not "read into" the question!*

> **TEST-TAKING TIP:** *Always consider first whether there is a physiological cause for a problem, before selecting a psychological cause.*

2. *This is not the best choice! This might be true if the client were not taking digoxin.*
3. *Wrong! Nausea is not normal. The nurse needs to further assess what is causing the client's nausea.*

> **TEST-TAKING TIP:** *Always consider first whether there is a physiological cause for a problem, before selecting a psychological cause.*

4. **Good job! Digoxin toxicity includes nausea and vomiting, and bradycardia. In the assessment the nurse notes that the pulse rate is**

marginal. Bradycardia is usually defined as 60 or less. Therefore, the client may be exhibiting a drug reaction.

> **TEST-TAKING TIP:** *Always consider first whether there is a physiological cause for a problem, before selecting a psychological cause.*

88. A client is receiving digoxin (Lanoxin). The nurse is alert for signs of which condition likely to contribute to digoxin toxicity?

1. Hypokalemia.
2. Hypocalcemia.
3. Obesity.
4. Hyponatremia.

1. **Correct! Potassium inhibits the excitability of the heart; therefore, a depletion of potassium will increase excitability. Potassium loss increases the likelihood of digoxin cardiotoxicity.**
2. *Wrong. Hypocalcemia may cause bradycardia, but it does not cause digoxin toxicity.*
3. *Incorrect. Obesity does not contribute to digoxin toxicity. Try again.*
4. *Incorrect. Digoxin has no effect on hyponatremia. Choose again.*

89. An elderly client is admitted to the hospital with congestive heart failure and will be digitalized (given digoxin). Vitals on admission are BP 110/60, pulse 100, respirations 22. The nurse understands that the expected outcome of digitalization is:

1. Respiratory rate of 26.
2. Heart rate greater than 100.
3. Urine output of 50 cc per hour.
4. Increased thirst.

1. *No. Digoxin does not speed up the respiratory rate. Try again.*
2. *Sorry, try again. Digoxin does not speed up the heart rate. Choose again.*
3. **Excellent work! As the cardiac output improves, kidney perfusion will improve, and urine output will increase.**
4. *Sorry, try again. Increased thirst is not related to digitalization, but may be indicative of diabetes. Make another choice.*

90. In caring for a client taking digoxin (Lanoxin), the nurse would give immediate attention to which statement by the client?

1. "I have a headache and backache."
2. "I feel nauseated and have no appetite."

3. "I've gained half a pound in the last two days."
4. "I'm having muscle cramps in my legs."

1. *Wrong choice. Headaches and backaches are not related to use of digoxin. Make another selection.*
2. ***Excellent! Anorexia, nausea, vomiting and abdominal discomforts are early signs of digoxin toxicity.***
3. *No, a weight gain of half a pound is not significant. Diuresis is likely to occur, with some weight loss.*
4. *No, this usually indicates other electrolyte abnormalities like hypokalemia. It is not a direct manifestation of digoxin toxicity. Try again.*

91. **The nurse knows that there are two basic types of arrhythmias. The type that makes the heart go faster and the type that makes the heart go slower, would be identified (in that order) by the nurse as:**

1. Bradyarrhythmias and tachyarrhythmias.
2. Tachyarrhythmias and bradyarrhythmias.
3. Supraventricular and ventricular.
4. Ventricular and supraventricular.

1. *No. You chose the correct terminology, but in the wrong order. Remember, arrhythmias that make the heart go faster are called tachyarrhythmias, and arrhythmias that make the heart go slower are called bradyarrhythmias.*
2. ***You are right! Arrhythmias that make the heart go faster are called tachyarrhythmias, and arrhythmias that make the heart go slower are called bradyarrhythmias.***
3. *Wrong! These types of arrhythmias do not make the heart go faster and slower. These two classifications of arrhythmias refer to the area in the heart from which the arrhythmia arises: supraventricular (from above the ventricles), and ventricular (from within the ventricle).*
4. *Incorrect. In addition to the arrhythmias that make the heart go faster or slower, arrhythmias can arise from different areas in the heart as well. These areas are usually divided into ventricular (from within the ventricle) and supraventricular (from above the ventricles) arrhythmias.*

92. **A client is taking propranolol (Inderal) for angina. The nurse understands that Inderal relieves angina because of which action?**

1. Increase in cardiac output.
2. Increase in heart rate.
3. Inhibition of vasodilatation in coronary vessels.
4. Decrease in myocardial oxygen requirements.
1. *Incorrect! The effect of Inderal is to lower cardiac output, heart rate, conduction velocity, and myocardial contractility. Make another selection.*
2. *Incorrect! Inderal lowers the heart rate. Try again.*

3. *Wrong choice. Inderal does inhibits vasodilatation and arterial spasms, and can be used for vascular headaches. However, this is not the action that relieves angina. Try again.*
4. ***Excellent! Inderal lowers the heart rate and contractility, which causes the heart to use less oxygen. This effect prevents angina.***

93. **A client started methyldopa (Aldomet) to lower his blood pressure. The nurse must emphasize to the client the importance of keeping appointments for which lab studies?**

1. Renal function studies.
2. Blood cell counts and hepatic function studies.
3. Aldomet blood levels.
4. Cardiac enzymes.

1. *This is incorrect. Liver toxicity is of prime importance with this medication, not kidney function. Make another selection.*
2. ***Correct! Aldomet may cause hepatotoxicity within two to four weeks of beginning the drug. Hemolytic anemia occurs in four percent of clients.***
3. *This is incorrect. Blood levels are not drawn for Aldomet. Choose again.*
4. *This is incorrect. Cardiac enzymes are not indicated for this drug.*

94. **A client's blood pressure rises to 200/120, which is considered a hypertensive emergency. Diazoxide (Hyperstat) is administered. The nurse should expect the response to be noticeable in which amount of time?**

1. Within one and five minutes of administration.
2. Within one hour of administration.
3. After the second dose.
4. After the first few doses.

1. ***Excellent! Results occur within one minute, and peak action is within two to five minutes. The duration of the effect is from two to twelve hours.***
2. *Not true! Results occur more quickly.*
3. *This is incorrect. Results occur more quickly. Make another selection.*
4. *This is incorrect. Results occur more quickly. Make another selection.*

95. **The nurse is caring for a client who is diagnosed as hypertensive and is prescribed hydralazine (Apresoline). What statement indicates that the client understands the action of his medication?**

1. "I will eat plenty of foods high in sodium to keep my fluid level up."

2. "I will limit my fluid intake."
3. "I realize that I need to get up more slowly than before."
4. "I will always remember to take this medication on an empty stomach."

1. *Not right! Sodium intake should be reduced, as it causes water retention, which in turn raises blood pressure.*
2. *This is not correct. An adequate fluid volume is needed. As vasodilatation occurs, urine output will increase. Make another choice.*
3. ***Correct! Orthostatic hypotension occurs due to vasodilatation and lowering of the diastolic pressure.***
4. *Not correct! Taking this medication with food would minimize the first pass metabolism and enhance bio-availability.*

96. **A 72-year-old with gouty arthritis is prescribed naproxen (Naprosyn). The nurse understands that the geriatric implications for this drug include:**

1. A higher incidence of agranulocytosis and aplastic anemia.
2. A higher incidence of perforated peptic ulcers and/or bleeding.
3. A higher incidence of central nervous system side effects.
4. None, as all NSAIDs are relatively safe medications for any age group.

1. *Wrong! These effects occur with the drug phenylbutazone (Butazolidin), not with naproxen. Make another selection.*
2. ***Good choice! Ulcers and bleeding are more common because administration results in a higher proportion (up to twice than in a younger person) of unbound naproxen, which causes more side effects.***
3. *This is incorrect. It's Indomethacin (Indocin) that is responsible for causing confusion in the elderly, not naproxen. Try again.*
4. *This is incorrect! Naproxen, Indocin and other NSAIDs have many side effects. Make another selection.*

97. **In administering acetaminophen (Tylenol) to a client, the nurse knows that this drug is used primarily for which clinical properties?**

1. Analgesic and antipyretic.
2. Antirheumatic.
3. Anticlotting.
4. Anti-inflammatory.

1. ***Correct! Acetaminophen (Tylenol) has analgesic and antipyretic properties equivalent to aspirin.***

2. *This is incorrect. Tylenol does not have the clinical usefulness of an anti-inflammatory or antirheumatic. Make another selection.*
3. *Incorrect. Tylenol does not have clinical usefulness in preventing clotting. Make another choice.*
4. *Try again. Tylenol is not primarily used for anti-inflammatory effects.*

98. **A client is admitted to the emergency room with an overdose of acetaminophen (Tylenol). The nurse would give immediate consideration to which manifestations:**

1. Slow respiratory rate.
2. Nausea, vomiting and abdominal discomfort.
3. Decreased urine output.
4. Convulsions.

1. *Although acetaminophen affects the central nervous system by blocking prostaglandins, it does not depress respiration. Make another selection.*
2. ***Excellent! The principal feature of a Tylenol overdose is hepatic necrosis, which is manifested by these early manifestations.***
3. *Wrong! Hepatic failure is the major concern in Tylenol overdose, not renal failure. Try again.*
4. *Wrong choice. Coma may occur as a late manifestation but it is not one of the immediate manifestations for which the nurse observes. Try again.*

99. **A client has been taking morphine for several weeks to relieve her cancer pain. During the last two home health visits, she has complained that her dose does not seem to be working. The nurse understands that the client has:**

1. Developed an addiction to morphine.
2. Become confused and probably is not taking her medications properly.
3. Developed a tolerance to the medication.
4. Abused the medication and needs counseling about her addiction.

1. *Wrong. Addiction may occur, but with cancer pain and long-term use, the medication is still needed to relieve the pain. It would not be helpful to discuss this with the client.*
2. *Incorrect. Not enough information is given to support this answer. When answering test questions, do not "read into" the question. Make another selection.*
3. ***Excellent choice! Tolerance is an undesirable side effect of narcotic analgesics. It occurs when a larger dose is needed to produce the same response. Tolerance, however, is unpredictable and sporadic, and does not occur for every client. The information in the case scenario indicates that this client is experiencing this effect.***

4. *Not enough information is given to assume this answer. Try again.*

100. **A client is being treated with pilocarpine (Pilocar) for his glaucoma. He complains of blurred vision after administration of his drops. The nurse's explanation to the client should be based upon which information?**

1. The client is not using the eye drops correctly.
2. Pilocarpine causes the pupil to constrict, making the eye accommodate for near vision; therefore, objects far away seem blurred.
3. When the pupil is dilated, it is more difficult to adjust vision.
4. Pilocarpine irritates the lining of the eye and causes blurring and inflammation.

1. *Incorrect. This would not be the best explanation. The client needs more facts.*
2. **Correct. Pilocarpine is a miotic that makes the eye adapt to near vision.**
3. *Wrong choice. Pilocarpine does not dilate the pupil. Reread the options.*
4. *Incorrect. Blurred vision is caused by pupil changes.*

NOTES

NCLEX-PN

Alternate Test Item Formats

Section I: Overview

A. NCLEX Item Types
   1. Standard Multiple Choice Question
      a. The traditional format of NCLEX questions.
      b. Still the most commonly seen type of question on the NCLEX.
      c. Has four options, only one of which is correct ("one best option").
      d. Mastering this format is critical to your success on the NCLEX.
   2. Since April 2003, the NCLEX has included formats other than standard multiple choice questions. These items are known as Alternate Test Item Formats.
      a. Fill-in-the-Blank
      b. Drag and Drop
      c. Multiple Response
      d. Hot Spot
      e. Charts, Tables, Graphic Images
   3. The average standard question takes 60 to 70 seconds to answer.

POINTS TO REMEMBER:
You should allot a slightly longer time for alternate test items.

Section II: Fill-in-the-Blank

A. Overview
1. Definition: Fill-in-the-blank items are a type of alternate question that will be numerical. This type of question typically involves solving a math problem. Read the question carefully. If you see the question is asking for the answer in a specific unit amount, it is not necessary to put units in your answer.
2. Method of Answer: To answer these questions, you will need to type a number into the answer box on the screen.

POINTS TO REMEMBER:
1. Write equation down on your scrap paper.
2. Be certain you are solving for the correct unit value!
3. Show all of your work.
4. Bring up drop-down calculator.
5. Double-check your work.

GRAPHIC 13-1.
FILL-IN-THE-BLANK ITEM

There are 13 clients being seen in the emergency room and 5 clients in the waiting room. What is the total number of clients?

Type your answer in the box below.

| 18 |

Section III: Drag and Drop

A. Overview
  1. Definition: Drag and Drop items are the newest type of alternate test question. In this type of question, you will use every option, placing each item in the correct sequence as indicated by the prompt.
  2. Choose items for which there is only one correct sequence to maintain the client's safety at each step in the care continuum.
  3. Avoid including actions which would properly be done both prior to and after an intervention (i.e. hand washing).

The nurse is preparing to insert a Foley catheter for a client. Place the actions the nurse takes when inserting the Foley in the appropriate order. **Use all the options:**

Unordered Options

- Don sterile gloves.
- Insert the catheter into the urethra.
- Drape the client exposing only genitalia.
- Instill saline into the balloon of the catheter.
- Cleanse the meatus with bactericidal solution.

Ordered Response

Section IV: Multiple Response

A. Overview
  1. Definition: Multiple response items are a type of alternate item that require you to choose more than one answer from up to six options. Any number of the options may be correct.
  2. Method of Answer: To answer these questions, you will need to click on all the answers that apply.
  3. On the NCLEX, you will receive credit only for completely correct answers--there is no "partial credit" given for these item types.

POINTS TO REMEMBER:

> Consider each response as you would a true-false question--is that statement true about the question or false? Click on all you determine to be true.

GRAPHIC 13-3.
MULTIPLE RESPONSE ITEM

> Which of the following are types of vegetables?
>
> Select all that apply.
>
> ☑ 1. Broccoli
> ☑ 2. Cucumber
> ☐ 3. Peach
> ☐ 4. Orange
> ☐ 5. Grape

Section V: Hot Spot

A. Overview
1. Definition: Hot spot items are a type of alternate item that will be a "point and click" exercise. Hot spot items will usually require you to identify an anatomical location on a figure.
2. Method of Answer: To answer these questions, you will need to point at an area on the screen with your cursor and click on the correct spot. As you move your mouse around the screen, you will see an arrow. Once you select a spot and click, the arrow will change into a circle with an "X" in it.
3. Read the question carefully, then analyze the image.
4. The NCLEX will allow you to reclick as many times as necessary.

POINTS TO REMEMBER:

> It is very important to remember that the screen is NOT a mirror image! If you see that the question is asking for an answer on the right or left side of the body, make sure you are clicking on the correct side.

GRAPHIC 13-4.
HOT SPOT ITEM

The nurse is performing a cardiac assessment.
Identify where the nurse will place the stethoscope
to best auscultate the apical pulse.

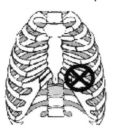

Section VI: Charts, Tables, & Graphic Images

A. Overview
1. Any of the NCLEX standard multiple choice or alternate items may also include charts, tables or other graphic images that you must analyze and understand in order to correctly answer the question.
2. It is important that you read the question carefully first, then analyze the image.

GRAPHIC 13-5.
CHARTS, TABLES, GRAPHIC IMAGES ITEM

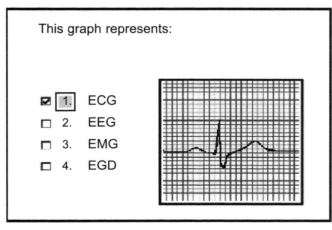

This graph represents:

☑ 1. ECG
☐ 2. EEG
☐ 3. EMG
☐ 4. EGD

CD-ROM INSTALLATION INSTRUCTIONS

MEDS Publishing Software requires 50 MB of available Hard Drive space.

To install our software, follow these steps:

1. Insert CD into CD-ROM drive.
2. Double click the "My Computer" icon.
3. Double click the icon for your CD-ROM drive.
4. Double click "Setup.exe."

NOTE:

Windows 2000 installation may receive an InstallShield dialog box "1207:Windows (R) Installer found." This occurs with use of an older version of Windows (R) Installer. Click "OK" to Continue. Click "OK" again.

3. Click the "NEXT" button to start the install and follow the on-screen instructions. A status bar displays the progress of the installation.
4. A window will appear, saying, "Install Complete."
5. Click "Finish."

To run MEDS' Software:

1. Go to Start, Programs, meds Software...
2. Locate and select the appropriate title.

You are ready to begin! Remember to visit www.medspub.com for other great NCLEX study resources, MEDS elements Nursing Student e-newsletter, and more! MEDS wishes you the best of luck in your nursing career.

NCLEX-PN

INDEX

Prepare for the NCLEX Exam with MEDS StarNurse™ Exam-A-Day Gold Online

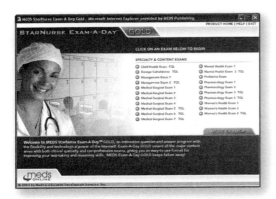
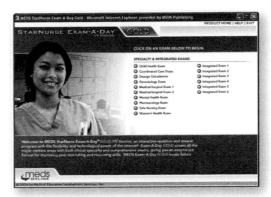

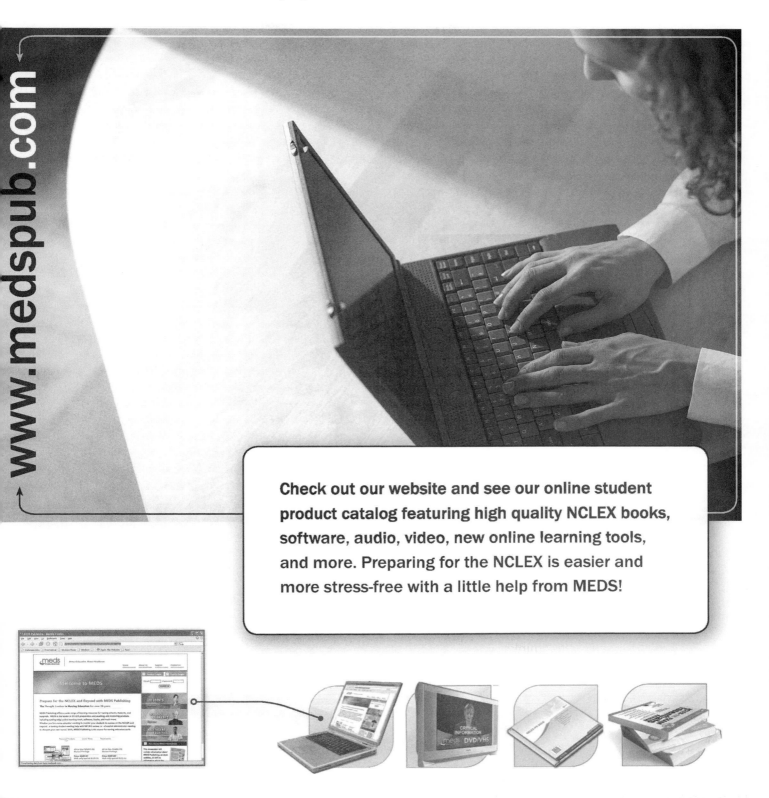

NOTES

NOTES